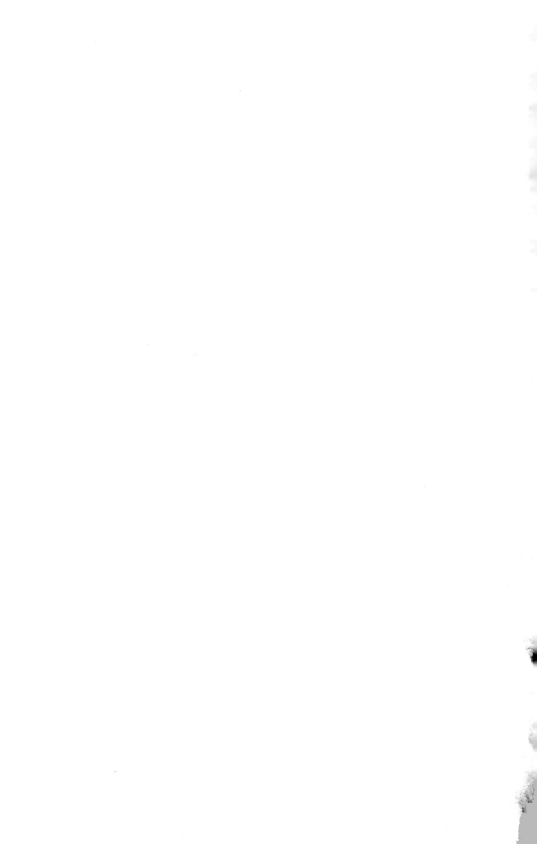

MICROCIRCULATION

MICROCIRCULATION

Volume I

Edited by

Gabor Kaley, Ph.D.

Professor and Chairman
Department of Physiology
New York Medical College
Valhalla, New York

and

Burton M. Altura, Ph.D.

Professor
Department of Physiology
State University of New York
Downstate Medical Center
Brooklyn, New York

University Park Press
Baltimore · London · Tokyo

UNIVERSITY PARK PRESS
International Publishers in Science and Medicine
Chamber of Commerce Building
Baltimore, Maryland 21202

Typeset by The Composing Room of Michigan, Inc.
Manufactured in the United States of America by Universal Lithographers,
Inc., and The Optic Bindery, Inc.

Library of Congress Cataloging in Publication Data
Main entry under title:

Microcirculation

Dedicated to B. W. Zweifach.
Includes bibliographical references and indexes.
1. Microcirculation. I. Kaley, Gabor.
II. Altura, Burton M. III. Zweifach, Benjamin Wil-
liam, 1910-   [DNLM: 1. Microcirculation. WG103
M625]
QP106.6.M5   596'.01'1   76-53805
ISBN 0-8391-0966-0 (v. 1)

CONTENTS

CONTENTS OF VOLUME II

COMPARATIVE ASPECTS OF VERTEBRATE MICROCIRCULATION

CONTENTS OF VOLUME III

CONTRIBUTORS

Emil Aschheim *Department of Physiology, New York Medical College, Valhalla, New York 10595*

Silvio Baez *Departments of Anesthesiology and Physiology, Albert Einstein College of Medicine of Yeshiva University, New York, New York 10461*

Sol Bernick *Department of Anatomy, University of Southern California School of Medicine, Los Angeles, California 90033*

John R. Casley-Smith *Department of Zoology, University of Adelaide, South Australia*

Elof Eriksson *Department of Surgery, The University of Chicago, Chicago, Illinois 60637*

Yuan-Cheng Fung *Department of Aerospace and Mechanical Engineering, University of California at San Diego, La Jolla, California 92037*

Guilio Gabbiani *Department of Pathology, University of Geneva, Faculty of Medicine, Geneva, Switzerland*

Joseph F. Gross *Department of Chemical Engineering, College of Mines, The University of Arizona, Tucson, Arizona 85724*

Zdenek Hruza *Department of Pathology, New York University School of Medicine, New York, New York 10016*

Marcos Intaglietta *Department of Aerospace and Mechanical Engineering, University of California at San Diego, La Jolla, California 92037*

Jen-shih Lee *Division of Biomedical Engineering, University of Virginia, School of Engineering and Applied Science and School of Medicine, Charlottesville, Virginia 22901*

Guido Majno *Department of Pathology, University of Massachusetts Medical School, Worcester, Massachusetts 01605*

Abel Lazzarini Robertson, Jr. *Department of Pathology, Case Western Reserve University School of Medicine, Cleveland, Ohio 44106*

Lee A. Rosen *Department of Pathology, Case Western Reserve University School of Medicine, Cleveland, Ohio 44106*

William I. Rosenblum *Division of Neuropathology, Medical College of Virginia of Virginia Commonwealth University, Richmond, Virginia 23298*

Sidney S. Sobin *Department of Physiology, University of Southern California School of Medicine, Los Angeles, California 90033*

Don D. Stromberg *Departments of Anesthesiology, Physiology, and Biophysics, University of Washington, School of Medicine, Seattle, Washington 98195*

Herta M. Tremer *Department of Physiology, University of Southern California School of Medicine, Los Angeles, California 90033*

Curtis A. Wiederhielm *Microcirculation Laboratory, Department of Physiology and Biophysics, University of Washington School of Medicine, Seattle, Washington 98195*

Joachim R. Wolff *Department of Neuroanatomy, Max-Planck-Institute for Bio-*

physical Chemistry, 34 Göttingen-Nikolausberg, Federal Republic of Germany

Harvey A. Zarem *Department of Plastic Surgery, University of California at Los Angeles, Los Angeles, California 90024*

Benjamin W. Zweifach *Department of Aerospace and Mechanical Engineering, University of California at San Diego, La Jolla, California 92037*

PREFACE

The purpose of this treatise is to present a comprehensive view of the field of microcirculation. The study of small blood vessels, which forty short years ago was the domain of morphologists only, has grown in the intervening years into a most important subject from physiologic, pharmacologic, and pathologic as well as clinical points of view. Microcirculation is currently an intensively investigated field and yet a comprehensive approach to this subject, one that would focus on its functional entities and interrelatedness to other disciplines, has not yet, to our knowledge, been attempted.

Our concept concerning individual sections of this treatise was to evaluate critically work done in the past, to describe the present state of the art, and to point out future directions that seem profitable and challenging. It is hoped that *Microcirculation* will not be merely a collection of monographs and a reference source but that it will facilitate a synthesis of all the information available and will provide new approaches to the study of small blood vessels. We also hope that the sheer size of *Microcirculation* will not discourage students, research workers, and biologists in related areas, as well as clinicians, from becoming acquainted with the field of microcirculation.

It is inevitable that some duplication of material will occur in a work of this size. It is also not possible, mostly because of limitations of the size of this treatise, to include among the authors all investigators who have contributed significantly to this research field. Nevertheless, we have been fortunate in being able to bring together so many active and outstanding workers in this field to join us in this endeavor.

There is another, equally compelling reason to put together a volume on microcirculation. It is to honor Benjamin W. Zweifach, the individual who, more than any other, has left his personal mark on this research field. It is rare in science for any one man to become as influential as he has through the years. Almost everyone who has contributed significantly to the field of microcirculation has taken a turn in Dr. Zweifach's laboratory and has been enriched by his exceptional knowledge of, and insight into, research problems. His own contributions, which span four decades and a host of scientific disciplines, encompass every important new development in the field of microcirculation and are the cornerstones of our knowledge in this area of biology. The measure of his success is also exemplified by the number and quality of his students, all of whom, including the editors of this treatise, are proud to trace their lineage to him. This book is a collaborative effort of his students and colleagues, to whom he served as mentor and for whom he continues to be a constant source of help and inspiration.

We are proud to dedicate this treatise to Benjamin W. Zweifach.

G. Kaley and B. M. Altura

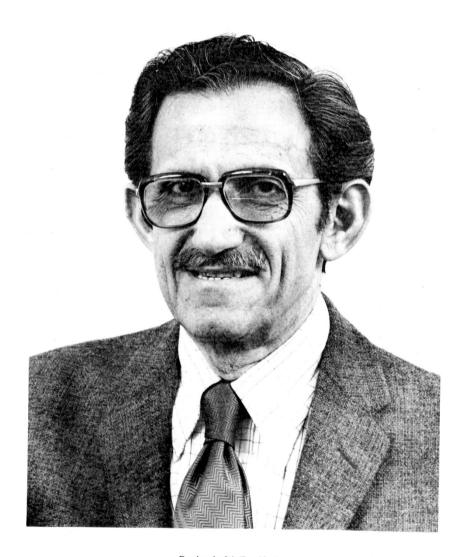

Benjamin W. Zweifach

INTRODUCTION:
Perspectives in Microcirculation

Benjamin W. Zweifach

STRUCTURE–FUNCTION RELATIONSHIPS

VASOMOTOR CONTROL OF MICROCIRCULATION
Endothelial Contractility
Intermittency
Autoregulation

CAPILLARY EXCHANGE
General Properties
Fluid Exchange

The broad outlines of the microcirculation as a separate entity were established more than half a century ago primarily on the basis of direct observational studies. Much of the information was perforce descriptive in nature. As new procedures were developed for the in vivo examination of different tissues, it was recognized that the terminal portion of the vascular tree was, in fact, an independent organic unit with intrinsic mechanisms for the local regulation of blood flow. The minute size and inaccessibility of the capillary vessels have made it difficult to utilize conventional quantitative methods to define these activities. For the most part, investigators had to be satisfied with quantitative data obtained by indirect approaches—particularly for exchange processes—using averaged values for whole organs or comparatively homogeneous tissues, such as skeletal muscle.

The substantial advances that have been made in our knowledge of the microcirculation are attested to by the very size of the present treatise. Some 25 years ago, it would have been impossible to put together so comprehensive a treatment of the small blood vessels. A combination of circumstances has made it possible to describe microcirculatory behavior in more precise quantitative terms: the application of electron microscopy, major advances in cell biology, and the development of electronic instrumentation and modern data handling procedures. These advances have, in turn, led to more rigorous theoretical and

Aided by United States Public Health Service Grant-in-Aid HL-100881.

1

physical analyses of the basic features governing tissue homeostasis. In view of the extensive coverage of microcirculatory phenomena presented in these volumes, there is little that can be added in an introductory sense, aside from a critical discussion in a historical perspective of as-yet-unresolved issues, particularly those biological characteristics that enable the microcirculation to perform as the keystone of bodily homeostasis.

Microtechniques (Intaglietta, Pawula, and Tompkins, 1970) and computer-assisted analysis of video images (Intaglietta, Tompkins, and Richardson, 1970) have made it possible to use intravital microscopy to subject individual segments of the blood capillary system to more precise analysis and to use such information to reconstruct the operational characteristics of an entire microbed. There are considerable differences in opinion as to the best approach to the problem. Some investigators (Wayland, 1973; Grafflin and Bagley, 1953) believe that the random nature and diversity of capillary patterns preclude the use of data on single vessels as a productive approach for a systematic appraisal of the capillary bed as a whole. They favor instead studies of groups of vessels representing what may be considered basic or modular subunits.

There has been a tendency to emphasize differences between species and tissues rather than similarities. Nevertheless, a meaningful discussion of the capillary bed as a discrete organic unit requires that certain common organizational and functional features be identified. The only other alternative would be to treat the myriads of vascular beds separately.

Our approach to the problem (Zweifach, 1961) has been based on the premise that all circulatory beds share certain common structural features and that these are modified by the peculiar terrain of the various parenchymal structures supplied by these vessels. Because of its two-dimensional format, the mesentery seemed to be a particularly appropriate starting point where the entire microvascular bed could be examined unencumbered by parenchymal tissue limitations.

Perhaps the most valuable asset of such two-dimensional tissue preparations is that pressure, flow, reactivity, and permeability data for single microvessels can be obtained with full knowledge of their location and structural makeup. Past attempts to handle data on single vessels have been fraught with difficulties because they were compared by setting up categories on the basis of vessel diameter alone.

In a continuously branching system, this criterion is not reliable and classification must be based on other characteristics, such as the location of the vessel in the arborizing sequence. Without a framework of this kind, it is not possible to develop models of the microcirculation that can be used to analyze blood flow through the many solid tissues of the body where intravital microscopy cannot be applied.

The term "microcirculation" would serve no useful purpose if it merely referred to the microscopically small blood vessels. The striking differences between the behavior of the large and small blood vessels cannot be explained by obvious physical features such as the lesser distensibility of the thick walled arterioles, the non-Newtonian blood flow through the narrow capillaries, or the repeated dichotomies and interdigitation of the microvasculature. Two key functions of the microcirculation require special intrinsic mechanisms: (a) the capacity to adjust blood flow in line with the changing metabolic requirements of the tissue, and (b) the local autoregulatory adjustments that serve to stabilize flow as well as pressure.

Earlier concepts depicted the capillary bed as a set of microscopic irrigation channels interposed between the arterial and venous conduits with no active participation in local regulation. In such a framework, the only important intrinsic variable was the permeability of the blood–tissue barrier. It has become obvious that the mere act of transporting a given volume of blood to the tissue was not enough to sustain tissue vitality and that a whole array of pathologic conditions are either initiated by or sustained by the failure or loss of active microcirculatory adjustments.

The literature is replete with observations on different tissues which demonstrate that the complex of minute blood vessels displays a considerable degree of local control or autonomy (Mellander and Johansson, 1968; Nicoll, 1969). Substantive data defining the mechanics of such local readjustments are not always available, although it is obvious that in some way the controls must be related to the metabolic requirements under different conditions.

We are obviously only beginning to unravel the complexities of microcirculatory behavior and, despite substantive agreement on broad principles, fundamental details remain controversial. Krogh, in his classical monograph (Krogh, 1922), presented a fairly convincing argument that under basal conditions microcirculatory flow is intermittent; this point of view has been more or less accepted by contemporary investigators. On the basis of injection studies in skeletal muscle, Krogh proposed that only a fraction of the available microvessels are perfused in so-called resting muscle and that with an active flow, the number is then increased at least four- to fivefold when higher volume flow rates are required to meet the metabolic demands of the contracting muscle. This type of local adjustment goes hand in hand with observations in other tissues that show a waxing and waning of flow in different portions of the same structure. On the other hand, in still other tissues including several skeletal muscle preparations, all of the available capillaries appear to be perfused, so that with vasomotion of the feeding arterioles the flow in all of the vessels is sped up or slowed accordingly. The question at issue is particularly germane to the discussion of blood flow in skeletal muscle or cardiac muscle where the total number of capillaries seems to be much greater than would be needed to sustain the metabolic requirements of the tissue at rest.

A direct corollary of the unresolved issue of intermittency is the mechanism responsible for the ebb and flow of the microcirculation. Structural and functional evidence (Folkow, Sonnenschein, and Wright, 1971) has led to the concept that on the proximal or precapillary side, muscular sphincters are the structural elements whose contraction and dilation modulates local blood flow. There is no question but that such sphincters are present in many tissues. In other tissues, however, the same homeostatic adjustments appear to be performed by the terminal arterioles (Eriksson and Myrhage, 1972). With the controls located more proximally in the microcirculatory system, the net effect would be an overall shifting of flow through the capillary network as a whole. Such a mechanism would preclude active adjustments within the tissue, except for minor differences due to the distribution of pressure and flow. In contrast, separate controls more distally in the precapillaries would make such adjustments independent of the resistance function of the arterioles, which are subject to continuous modulation in line with the maintenance of systemic blood pressure. Let us examine some of these questions in greater detail.

STRUCTURE–FUNCTION RELATIONSHIPS

In view of their common nutritive function in most tissues, it would seem plausible to assume that all microcirculatory beds share certain fundamental features that permit them to fulfill these basic functions. In broad operational terms, the purpose of the microcirculation is to deliver blood to the parenchymal constituents of the tissues in accord with their metabolic activity. This is accomplished by allowing a given volume of blood to perfuse the terminal network of vessels at a rate that is compatible with an adequate exchange of fluids and materials across the blood–tissue interface. Because parenchymatous organs display a range of activity, some provision must be made to vary the volume and distribution of blood accordingly. The volume flow of blood to resting as contrasted to working skeletal muscle may differ by as much as tenfold. Furthermore, local mechanisms must exist to permit pressure, flow, and resistances to be maintained in a range appropriate for steady-state conditions. Inasmuch as the kinetics of exchange differ from tissue to tissue, it is highly probable that some structural basis exists for such a selective process.

The layout for particular microvascular networks is modified by the peculiar architecture of each tissue to the extent that some investigators have concluded that there was no overall structural design and that microcirculatory networks are more or less randomly distributed (Hammersen, 1970). The strongest argument for a structural module at the capillary level of organization was originally made on the basis of studies on mesenteric tissues (Zweifach, 1957). Despite the fact that these tissues are not made up of a mass of specialized parenchymal cells that exhibit extremes in metabolic demands, they possess the functional attributes of other microcirculatory beds in large parenchymatous organs such as skeletal muscle. They exhibit an ebb and flow of microcirculation, an intrinsic capacity to redistribute blood flow, and a distinctive local autonomy.

From the structural point of view, the most prominent landmark of the terminal vascular bed is its arteriolar parent trunk. When the direct extensions of these feeding vessels penetrate into the microvascular network, they are already of capillary dimensions, but can be recognized by the high velocity of the blood stream and their scalloped appearance due to the presence of vascular smooth muscle. In some tissues, such as the mesentery, anatomic pathways can be traced from arteriole to venule, and have been referred to as preferential channels (Zweifach, 1957). In other tissues, the arteriolar stem is distinctive but its extensions do not appear to have selective pathways to the collecting venules (Eriksson and Myrhage, 1972). It is interesting to note that developmental studies (Bar and Wolff, 1973) have shown the capillary networks in major tissues such as the brain, skin, and skeletal muscle to originate as preferential channels and only secondarily to develop side branches that form the capillary network proper.

The general construction of the capillary bed using the arteriolar stem as the central framework carries with it a number of ancillary features that contribute to local regulation. The smooth muscle of the distal continuations of the terminal arterioles is progressively thinned out and within the microcirculation is found only on the extremely fine terminal arterioles ($10-12$ μ) and the immediate junctional portions of their branches. These muscular junctions, which serve as sluice gates, have been termed precapillary sphincters (Wiedeman, 1967). Beyond this, the capillary network proper consists of endothelial tubes that show no vasomotor activity. The precise point within the microcirculation where vascular smooth muscle no longer occurs varies somewhat in the different tissues.

In most tissues, the precapillary branch has a muscular investment for only a short distance (some $20-50$ μ), while in others the muscular branch may be as long as several hundred microns. These longer vessels usually distribute as many as seven to eight capillaries, which in turn dichotomize, so that in effect vasomotor adjustments of one parent vessel directly influence up to $20-30$ capillaries, whereas in most tissues the activity of a short precapillary will effect the flow in only some four to six capillaries. The disposition of smooth muscle on these delicate arterioles can be determined in intravital preparations only by the spontaneous vasomotor activity and responses of these vessels. None of the capillaries and earliest venules show physiologic evidence of smooth muscle activity (Clark and Clark, 1943).

The structural keystone to the regulatory activities of the arteriolar-precapillary functional complex is the physics of the branching complex (Zweifach, 1974). The pressure drop and resistance in a branching system are governed by the relative size of the parent and daughter vessels. Because most of the precapillary side branches are of capillary dimensions, the ratio of the branch diameter to that of the parent trunk ($40-50$ μ wide) is between 0.3 and 0.35. In addition, such branchings have a neck-like configuration so that entry conditions into the branch contribute substantially to the resulting pressure drop (Vawter, Fung, and Zweifach, 1974). Branching vessels with ratios of 0.3 and below are in the critical range where only a slight narrowing of the entry is sufficient to cut off flow completely into the offshoot.

Earlier concepts emphasized an all-or-none effect, a critical pressure below which precapillaries narrowed to shut off flow into the downstream capillaries (Nichol et al., 1951). Other recent studies indicate that the branching complex as a whole, rather than a sphincter per se, represents the important regulatory mechanism (Zweifach, 1974). The most appropriate term for this structural unit would be the arteriolar-precapillary junctional complex; most of the terminal arterioles have from five to ten such complexes. Minor changes in entry conditions (narrowing of terminal arteriole) or in size of the branch (narrowing of precapillary) can cut off capillary perfusion temporarily and lead to the intermittency observed in many tissues.

Another structural feature, which has been reported in some tissues but not in others, is the presence of anatomic "shunts" at the microvascular level (Chambers and Zweifach, 1944). Here again there has been a tendency to oversimplify and to cast aside the functional implications of the preferential flow channels because of variations in the distribution of small blood vessels to different tissues. There is, however, indirect evidence for the presence of preferential paths even in skeletal muscle (Hyman, 1971). For example, simultaneous recording of pressure in arterioles and venules that supply and drain a common area of the spinotrapezius muscle of the rat, or the mesentery of the cat, shows that a small percentage (15–20%) consistently have an AV pressure drop of as little as 10–12 cm H_2O, whereas in the majority of vessels, the pressure drop is 26–30 cm H_2O. Even in a random network of capillaries, as in the cat mesentery, not all of the capillaries have the same diameter. Several low-resistance paths are always present that allow a greater convective flow and in an operational sense can be considered as shunts. Low resistance AV paths of this kind are especially numerous in the mesentery, the omentum, the skin, and the ear microcirculation.

Other two-dimensional preparations, such as the bat wing and the hamster cheek pouch, do not show a definitive thoroughfare pattern (Webb and Nicoll, 1954). Nonetheless, the fact that even here the direct extensions of the arterioles form the backbone of the microcirculation and penetrate well into the capillary network, allows for the distribution of parallel precapillary offshoots that can confine blood flow almost entirely to the parent trunk. In skeletal muscle, the orderly parallel array of striated muscle fibrils is matched by a comparable alignment of the capillaries (Spalteholz, 1888). Thoroughfare channels are not a striking feature here, although the arrangement of the terminal arterioles in a transverse direction to the muscle fibers and their associated capillaries permits a high percentage of the flow to be restricted to a small percentage of the available channels.

Several other structural modules for the microcirculation have been described. In the cat mesentery, circumscribed areas of tissue are demarcated by pairs of interarcading arteriole-to-arteriole and venule-to-venule connections (Frasher and Wayland, 1972). The tissue within these walled-off zones is supplied by delicate arteriolar offshoots of these arcades. Although the arrangement of capillaries within this type of module is more or less random, differences in the caliber and length of the different vessels allow for a rapid shunt-like flow through paths that offer the least resistance. It is obvious that an arcading configuration by itself cannot serve as modular building blocks in three-dimensional arrays.

The term "functional shunting" has been used to describe an increase in regional blood flow that is not associated with a proportionate increase in exchange (Renkin, 1971). Various explanations have been proposed to account for this phenomenon. Such a discrepancy can arise if different groups of vessels have different permeability properties, e.g., throughfare type channels. Another possible mechanism would involve diffusional short circuiting, either between paired arterioles and venules, or between adjacent capillary networks (Crone, 1970). Finally, changes in pressure and flow may by themselves result in shifts in the permeability of the capillary barrier, either through changes in wall tension, or modification of the sieving properties of the vessel barrier.

In view of the existence of capillary vessels with substantially different permeabilities, selective shunting requires the presence of some type of regulation by means of which flow could be diverted selectively into or away from particular vessels. The observation that a reduced permeability to hydrophilic substances analogous to shunting develops at increased flow rates in skeletal muscle suggests that the restriction to diffusion through porous channels in the capillary wall may become more pronounced as blood flow is increased. It has been suggested that some form of pore plugging by plasma proteins may be responsible for such an effect (Trap-Jensen and Lassen, 1971). On the other hand, there is good evidence that "functional shunting" is present in skeletal muscle for gases (hydrogen) that presumably penetrate the vessel wall along its entire cell surface and do not require aqueous channels for their diffusion into the tissue compartment (Grunewald, 1968). Equally plausible alternatives would be either some type of redistribution of blood within the capillary network, or a change in the permeability of the vessel wall.

VASOMOTOR CONTROL OF MICROCIRCULATION

Endothelial Contractility

It is generally accepted that active vasomotor adjustments within the microcirculation of mammalian tissues occur only in those vessels with recognizable

smooth muscle in their walls. The most numerous microvessels, the true capillaries, are essentially endothelial tubes and can be considered to be non contractile in a regulatory sense. They do not respond to conventional stimuli such
as vasoactive chemicals, electrical stimulation, mechanical stimulation, or even to
substantial changes in transmural pressure (Crone, 1970). Under some situations,
endothelial cells are seen to swell (presumably by taking up water) and to bulge
into the capillary lumen sufficiently to increase the resistance to flow.

Mammalian blood capillaries behave as rigid, nondistensible tubes that
withstand static pressures of up to 200 mm Hg without a measurable increase in
diameter even at magnifications of 900X (Lamport and Baez, 1962). In perfused
preparations, the capillaries may narrow by between 15 and 20% when pressures
are dropped below 6–8 mm Hg. Under normal conditions, however, capillary
pressures do not fall below 10–12 mm Hg, the pressure prevailing in the venular
outflow vessels.

The possibility has been raised that vascular endothelium is contractile in a
limited sense, particularly in certain tissues such as the retina of the eye
(Kuwabara and Cogan, 1960). Under pathologic conditions, as in the case of
mild tissue injury, contiguous endothelial cells move apart to create pathways
through which plasma and even blood cells can penetrate. This phenomenon has
been explained as a "contraction" of the endothelial cell and attributed to the
fact that the microtubules that are attached to the sites of tight intercellular
junctions contain contractile proteins (Becker and Nachman, 1973). It should be
pointed out that identical proteins are known to be present in cell membranes in
general and in the organellae of many cells that clearly have no contractile
function. The possibility that hydration or dehydration of endothelium might
influence capillary dimensions is supported by the observation that capillaries
frequently shrink away from the basement membrane when the tissue is fixed
and processed for electron microscopy (Rhodin, 1968). The endothelial cells in
such preparations are frequently 3–4 μ thick. The consensus, based on direct
observations of the microcirculation in accessible tissues of mammals, is that the
capillaries show no measurable changes in caliber over a wide range of experimental situations, pressures, and flow rates (Nicoll, 1969).

The narrow capillaries of the mesentery in mammals are embedded in an
interstitial gel that is 40–60 μ thick, so that they behave as rigid tubes with
essentially no distensibility over the physiologic pressure range. On the other
hand, in lower forms such as the frog, the capillaries of the mesentery are much
wider, up to 20–24 μ, and have only a thin layer of connective tissue support.
Cross sections of the mesentery of the frog show the capillary endothelium to
abut against the outer mesothelial layer. These capillaries can be distended by
pressures of 60–70 mm Hg. It is thus probable that capillaries in different
regions of the body exhibit varying degrees of distensibility, as for example in
the alveoli of the lung, or in the subcutaneous tissue of the skin.

Intermittency

Perhaps the most striking impression from direct visual study of the microcirculation is the nonuniformity of red cell flow and distribution (Krogh, 1922). At the single capillary level, the erratic movement of the blood is the result of a number of different physical adjustments. Inasmuch as the capillary vessels are fairly rigid tubes, the distribution of blood in the interanastomosing network is governed in the main by shifting pressure differentials. Blood no longer behaves as a Newtonian fluid during perfusion through the capillaries. Entry dimensions into the precapillary side branches are borderline for flow. Comparatively small changes in entry conditions are sufficient to cause substantial slowing or speeding of flow. Thus, patterns are seen with forward flow for some 10–15 sec, followed by a slowed or even no flow for 20–25 sec. At another period, the duration of the on–off cycles may be reversed. The result of such discontinuities occurring simultaneously in dozens of capillaries is a nonlinear pressure–flow relationship for the network as a whole, which in turn makes it difficult to treat exchange across the capillary barrier in a simple manner.

In addition to the random variations in red cell velocity observed in the individual capillary vessels, an overall ebb and flow can also be recognized. Such vasomotion has been assumed to meet the need for redistribution of blood in line with the local needs of the tissue and is believed to reflect the spontaneous narrowing of the feeding arterioles and precapillaries (Wiedeman, 1967). Tissues maintained under exteriorized conditions for several hours show progressively less local vasomotion and remain in a partially dilated state. A similar reaction is seen during the development of reactive hyperemia induced by temporary occlusion of the arterial inflow. The increased blood flow following temporary obstruction is associated with a suppression of spontaneous vasomotion. During the period when spontaneous vasomotion is reduced or absent, the precapillary vessels show a diminishing responsiveness to vasotropic agents.

Autoregulation

Perturbations in systemic blood pressure lead to a corresponding change in blood flow which in many organs is then compensated for by local readjustments so as to restore flow to control levels. The phenomenon of autoregulation is presumed to reside in the terminal arterioles and their intermediate branches (Mellander and Johansson, 1968), which are the sites of major vascular resistance.

Intermittency involving the periodic restriction of flow to fewer capillaries has been linked to the vasomotion of the precapillary vessels. Vasomotion has also been used to describe the narrowing and dilation of feeding arterioles as well as precapillaries. Precapillary activity, however, is for the most part irregular and apparently not related to the more periodic arteriolar vasomotion. This has led to the assumption that these two key structures are controlled by different mechanisms (Folkow et al., 1971). Recent studies of pressure–flow relationships within the microvascular system (Zweifach and Lipowsky, 1975) indicate that in the arterioles proper, pressure is maintained despite changes in flow of several hundred percent. On the other hand, within the immediate precapillary vessels (20–15 μ wide), flow is maintained within a narrow range despite wide fluctuations in pressure. The sporadic fluctuations observed in the precapillary vessels thus reflect primarily the response to local environmental factors and to a lesser degree mechanically mediated myogenic adjustments. A difficulty in ascribing local autoregulatory adjustments to the larger arterioles is the lack of evidence for a retrograde or ascending feedback that would make it possible to link flow to changes in local metabolic needs.

Several possible explanations have been proposed to support the involvement of arteriolar vessels in locally mediated adjustments. The feeding arterioles and their associated venules are distributed as paired vessels separated at most by 50–100 μ. In view of the comparatively high diffusibility of gases such as O_2 and CO_2 across even vessels as large as these, a countercurrent type of exchange may occur whereby the concentration gradient of O_2 and/or CO_2 between the paired vessels would determine the state of smooth muscle tone (Granger and Shepherd, 1973). Such a mechanism implies that changes in O_2 or CO_2 tension will have a direct effect on smooth muscle tone and indirectly on their response to transmural pressure. Another possibility would be a retrograde myogenic response that begins with the dilation or constriction of the precapillary vessels and then spreads to the terminal arterioles. In effect, a myogenic mechanism here would be activated when the volume of blood diverted into the microvascular network was of sufficient magnitude to affect pressure in the more proximal arterioles.

As indicated, two types of vasomotor adjustments at the microcirculatory level are seen; one is centered about the stabilization of the pressure in the precapillary vessels. Such a mechanism was brought to light by direct measurement of pressures in arterioles and precapillary vessels (Zweifach and Richardson, 1971). Thus, in a given terminal arteriole, readjustments tend to keep the pressure between 30 and 25 mm Hg despite shifts of systemic pressure of as much as 50 mm Hg. The activity of the precapillaries that is geared to the flow distribution within the network is responsible for much of the intermittency observed in capillary blood flow.

The moment-to-moment adjustments of the small muscular vessels are believed to be mediated by a myogenic response to shifts in transmural pressure or wall tension. Myogenic activity of this kind is especially striking in the terminal arterioles which are well supplied with smooth muscle and have only sparse connective tissue. The wall-thickness-to-lumen ratio is greatest in the 20–30-μ arterioles (Baez, 1969).

On the functional level, a contributing factor to the relative autonomy of the microvascular system is the gradual increase in reactivity by virtue of which the smallest muscular vessels are the most responsive to stimulating agents, including catecholamines and polypeptides (Altura, 1971). Explanations for the heightened response characteristics of the terminal arterioles and precapillaries range from the decreased wall tension in such vessels (Gore, 1974) to the effect of environmental influences such as oxygen tension, pH, or products of cell metabolism (Haddy and Scott, 1968). The adjustments of flow at the local level within the microvascular system are thus not under the control of a specific mechanism, but reflect the interaction of multiple factors, including smooth muscle reactivity, physical makeup, the geometry of the network, myogenic responses, and the flow properties of blood (Zweifach, 1973).

CAPILLARY EXCHANGE

General Properties

Two aspects of the exchange process have been a major concern for many years. It has not been possible to identify with any degree of certainty the structural components of the blood vessel wall that determine the permeability of the barrier. There is, in addition, surprisingly little definitive data concerning local regulatory mechanisms that keep transcapillary fluid exchange in balance under widely different physiologic states. Most of our information about the barrier that separates the blood and the extravascular compartment has been obtained by modifications of three principal techniques: (1) exchange of tagged molecules of graded size from the blood, either in situ for different organs (Winne, 1965), or in perfused structures (Friedman, 1971) where conditions can be regulated more precisely, but where the physiologic conditions may be compromised; (2) dye-tagged molecules can be injected into the bloodstream and estimates are then made under the microscope of the rate of loss into the tissue from single vessels (Wiederhielm, 1966). Such methods lack some of the precision provided by exchange in whole organs, but permit a comparison of in vivo permeability data with the structural makeup of the same vessels as determined by electron microscopy. (3) Electron microscopy can be used to establish the pathways by which electron-dense materials cross the capillary barrier (Karnovsky, 1968).

The blood capillary wall acts as a selective filter for water-soluble materials. The range of this selectivity varies considerably in different tissues and, even within a given tissue, capillaries with seemingly identical structural features have substantially different permeability coefficients. Until the advent of electron microscopy, it was only possible to speculate on the physical basis for transcapillary exchange.

With this new tool it became possible to follow sequentially the passage of markers through the vessel wall. Ultrastructural evidence in general (Rhodin, 1968) has supported the intercellular pathway for movement of water-soluble materials. Electron microscopy has, however, directed attention to the possible involvement of other structures in transcapillary movement of substances. These include endothelial cytoplasmic vesicles (Simionescu, Simionescu, and Palade, 1975), fenestrae within the endothelial cell (Clementi and Palade, 1969), the basement membrane (Simionescu, Simionescu, and Palade, 1973), and tight junctional complexes between cells in capillaries with a relatively low permeability (Farquhar and Palade, 1963). Direct observational procedures have been used to follow the exchange of fluid (Majno, 1965) and even macromolecules (Witte and Hagel, 1971) in the mesentery. Perhaps the chief drawback of the direct observational approach is the difficulty of measuring diffusional exchange in a three-dimensional structure. In the past such studies have been limited to the movement of dyes, alone or in combination with plasma proteins or with synthetic macromolecules. Measurements of this kind have been made largely in the mesentery where the rate of diffusion is sufficiently slow to permit accurate recording of density (Wiederhielm, 1966). An increasing permeability has been demonstrated for macromolecules (Hauck, 1969) from the arterial to venous side of the microcirculation, but there is as yet no quantitative characterization of such differences in permeability, nor is there a plausible explanation for the physiologic significance of these gradients.

The permeability properties of the capillary barrier are usually expressed in quantitative terms as filtration coefficient, L_P or K_F, which represents the hydrodynamic conductivity of the barrier, and as a reflection coefficient (σ) to account for the relative permeability of the wall to particular molecules with respect to that for water. Such calculations permit one to characterize the perviousness of the barrier in terms of a pore equivalent of a given size (e.g., $r = 40$–50 Å for water-soluble materials), and to estimate the total number of such pores. The fact that a small amount of protein continuously permeates the capillaries and venules into the interstitium has been taken to indicate the presence of a small number of larger pores (Arturson, Groth, and Grotte, 1972).

Many observers believe that the convective flow of water-soluble substances occurs through the intercellular material in the cleft between contiguous cell borders (Chambers and Zweifach, 1947). The inability to identify "pores" by electron microscopy does not rule out the above explanation because similar channels in the interstitial gel cannot be visualized by such techniques. On the other hand, movement of water across the endothelial cell proper has not been evaluated, although compared to other pathways, such movement may be comparatively small. The presence of large numbers of endothelial cell vesicles has led microscopists to suggest that these structures represent transport pathways, not only for macromolecules or particulate matter (Simionescu et al., 1975), but for small water-soluble materials (Bassingthwaighte, 1970). Here again the difficulty of showing a positive correspondence between changes in permeability and vesicle activity raises the question as to whether a vesicle mechanism would have the selectivity and the physical capacity to handle the exchange of the large volumes of fluid and materials demonstrated in kinetic experiments of transcapillary exchange.

The fact that the diffusion of ions and small water-soluble substances is lowest where tight intercellular junctions are present in all likelihood indicates that the movement through the endothelial cell proper is comparatively small. In addition, the transcapillary diffusion rates calculated for different substances have been shown to parallel the free diffusion coefficient for these materials in water, again suggesting that their movement occurs through aqueous channels in the capillary wall. Blood capillaries with apparently identical structure and dimensions do not exhibit uniform permeabilities, some vessels being more pervious than others, even to the extent of allowing plasma proteins to leave the bloodstream. Vessels that have a higher permeability to plasma proteins also show a substantially higher hydrodynamic conductivity (L_P is 3–5 times higher). Although the continued loss of plasma proteins has been accounted for by a small number of large pores, the positive correlation between L_P levels and protein permeability has led other investigators (Michel, 1972) to suggest that the greater permeability can be explained equally well by a large number of so-called small pores.

Under abnormal conditions, as during an inflammatory reaction, the increase in permeability to proteins is associated with the spotty development of leaks or defects between contiguous cells, without affecting the permeability properties of the remainder of the vessel wall (Levick and Michel, 1973). Such defects are more numerous in the collecting venules, possibly because the accompanying vasodilation results in a proportionately greater increase in transmural pressure in these 20-μ-wide vessels than in the narrow 6–8-μ capillaries. August Krogh suggested over 50 years ago (Krogh, 1922) that an increase in transmural pressure could lead to the separation of endothelial cell borders and, thereby, to an increased permeability. It is more likely that in addition some alteration in cell-to-cell adhesion must also occur, because increases in pressure of up to 20–25 mm Hg have not resulted in any significant change in the filtration coefficient (Michel, 1972).

Fluid Exchange

For the most part, because of the minute size of the microcirculatory elements, and the difficulty of making direct measurements in solid tissues, fluid exchange has been studied in whole organs (Pappenheimer and Soto-Rivera, 1948), or in isolated masses of tissue such as skeletal muscle (Diana and Shadur, 1973) on the basis of second or third approximations of such mass transfer. Analyses of the exchange of fluid between the blood and tissue compartments must take into account not only the permeability properties of the blood vessel barrier, but those of the lymphatic capillary barrier, and the surface area available, in addition to the driving forces involved.

The Starling equation for the flux of fluid between the blood and extravascular compartments can be expressed as

$$J_V = A \times L_P(P_c - \pi_{p\ell} - (P_t - \pi_t))$$

where

J_v = rate of fluid movement μ^3/sec/cm H_2O,
A = area,
L_P = filtration coefficient,
P_c = capillary pressure,
$\pi_{p\ell}$ = plasma colloid osmotic pressure,
P_t = tissue pressure,
π_t = tissue colloid osmotic pressure.

For single vessels, fluid movement is expressed as the rate of exchange per unit of surface area per unit driving force. The basic tenets of the concept were confirmed by the work of Landis (1927) on single capillaries and that of Pappenheimer and Soto Rivera (1948) on isogravimetric preparations. However, the mechanisms by which the terminal vascular bed achieves a steady state through an interplay between hydraulic and osmotic forces are not well documented. The problem has been oversimplified without taking full cognizance of other factors such as nonuniformity, geometric considerations, the reflection coefficient of the capillary wall, tissue contribution, and lymphatic exchange.

The commonly accepted schema by which fluid exchange is balanced has filtration occurring on the arterial side of the circuit and reabsorption on the venous side, with the progressive fall in hydrostatic pressure through frictional losses leading to this straddling of the colloid osmotic pressure. What is lacking is the mechanism by which pressure, flow, and surface area are balanced to bring about equivalent filtration and absorption of fluid. Direct pressure measurements in different tissues (Zweifach and Richardson, 1971) do not support such a simple picture.

The colloid osmotic pressure of the blood in mammals ranges between 24 and 30 mm Hg (Zweifach and Intaglietta, 1971). Precapillary pressures average about 30–35 mm Hg. The net drop in hydrostatic pressure within the capillary network proper averages no more than 6–8 mm Hg so that filtration would be the primary mode of fluid exchange in the majority of vessels. During the steady-state condition, blood flow through the capillaries fluctuates with different groups of capillaries slowing almost to a standstill for periods of about 30–180 sec. It has been shown by the microneedle occlusion procedure that absorption of fluid occurs principally in those capillaries where flow has come to a standstill because of precapillary narrowing. Under such conditions the magnitude of fluid uptake is limited by the volume of plasma trapped in the static vessels. In an operational sense, absorption thus occurs, not as a continuous process in the venous capillaries, but in quanta depending upon the number of capillaries involved in the periodic waning and waxing of flow. On this basis, the steady-state fluid exchange involves a comparatively small but continuous fluid filtration into the lymphatic capillaries. This concept implies that either the net driving force is small, or that the filtration coefficient is considerably less than calculated in the past for mammalian vessels (Landis and Pappenheimer, 1963).

Estimates of fluid exchange cannot be made without taking tissue factors into account. The net force opposing transcapillary filtration (F_a) would be

$$F_a = P_t - (\pi_{p\varrho} - \pi_t)$$

where P_t is the tissue hydrostatic pressure, $\pi_{p\varrho}$ the blood colloid osmotic pressure, and π_t the tissue colloid osmotic pressure. Inasmuch as the capillary barrier is not completely impervious to plasma protein, a finite concentration of protein is built up in the interstitium of different tissues depending upon the reflection coefficient of these particular capillaries to blood proteins. As shown in the above relationship, the net filtration of fluid into the interstitium is proportional to the difference in colloid osmotic pressures in the two compartments. In turn, the difference between the rate of filtration from the blood capillaries as opposed to the removal of fluid by the terminal lymphatics determines the extent to which interstitial protein concentrations are increased or decreased. Most analyses in the literature have assumed that π_t is directly related to the volume of capillary filtrate, i.e., the interstitium is treated as a closed compartment. This approach would be valid only if the transcapillary filtration volume were many times (8–9 times) greater than the volume of lymph flow. As indicated, there is good reason to doubt the validity of this assumption (Intaglietta and Zweifach, 1974). Such a simplified explanation leaves unanswered a number of fundamental questions. The interstitium is, in fact, open ended, being drained continuously by the movement of fluid into the terminal lymphatics. There is no evidence that either the interstitial gel or the lymphatic capillary endothelium restricts the movement of plasma proteins, so that lymph fluid contains protein with the same A:G ratios as blood (Aukland, 1973). The actual volume of fluid drained by the terminal lymphatics would seem to depend on the rate of capillary filtration. During periods of increased lymph flow, the concentration of protein falls in samples collected from the large lymphatics. In view of the presumed bulk movement of interstitial fluid into the lymphatic capillaries, these findings were interpreted as indicating that the concentration of plasma proteins in the interstitial compartment had been reduced accordingly.

Here again, because of the lack of numerical information, investigators have resorted to an idealized case. There is little doubt but that the fluid in the terminal lymphatics is essentially the same as the free fluid in the interstitium. No acceptable method has been developed to measure the makeup of tissue fluids, although Aukland and Johnsen (1973) has used a cotton wick inserted through a fine catheter into the kidney parenchyma to measure tissue protein. It is likely that the lymph collected from large lymph ducts has been concentrated during its passage along the terminal lymphatic network. Our studies (Zweifach, 1972; Zweifach and Prather, 1975) indicate that the concentration mechanism would appear to be the intralymphatic pressures generated by contraction of the muscular lymphatics as the fluid is propelled centrally across a series of one-way valves. Under normal conditions, the movement of lymph fluid is slow so that the original interstitial fluid has a comparatively long transit time through these lymph capillaries, allowing the concentration process to be operative for a longer time. When vasodilation occurs and capillary filtration is enhanced, there is a speeding up of the transport of fluid through the valve-containing segments of the terminal lymphatics. During this phase, contractions of the collecting lymph channels are more moderate and P_L rises to only 4–5 cm H_2O so that there is significantly less concentration of lymph proteins as the fluid is transported centrally.

Such an analysis makes it doubtful that interstitial colloid osmotic pressure would rise and fall in proportion to capillary absorption or filtration. What is more likely is that filtration of even a slight excess of fluid into the interstitium gives rise to only a comparatively small increase in tissue pressure (P_t)—possibly only 2–4 cm H_2O; however, this is sufficient to initiate flow into the terminal lymphatics. The removal of lymph fluid is aided by stimulation of spontaneous contractions of the collecting lymphatics (Baez, 1960; Campbell and Heath, 1973), leading to a peristaltic wave of propulsion through successive valve segments.

The preceding discussion has highlighted some of the unanswered questions concerning microcirculatory behavior and organization. The broad coverage in this monograph will undoubtedly provide many of the missing links in our chain of evidence. The microcirculation as the basic building block of the cardio-vascular system represents the only access that the tissues of the body have to the bloodstream and thus bridges the gap between the cellular and molecular activities of the bodily tissues and the organism as a whole. The answer to these problems must therefore be sought at the molecular and biophysical level.

LITERATURE CITED

Altura, B. M. 1971. Chemical and humoral regulation of blood flow through the precapillary sphincter. Microvasc. Res. 3:361–384.

Arturson, G., T. Groth, and G. Grotte. 1972. The functional ultrastructure of the blood–lymph barrier. Computer analysis of data from dog heart–lymph experiments using theoretical models. Acta Physiol. Scand. 374:1–30.

Aukland, K. 1973. Autoregulation of interstitial fluid volume. Scand. J. Clin. Lab. Invest. 31:247–254.

Aukland, K., and H. M. Johnsen. 1973. Measurement of interstitial fluid colloid osmotic pressure. Acta Physiol. Scand. 87:2A.

Baez, S. 1960. Flow properties of lymph. A microcirculatory study. In A. L. Copley and G. Stainsby (eds.), Flow Properties of Blood and Other Biological Systems pp. 398–411. Pergamon Press, New York.

Baez, S. 1969. Simultaneous measurements of radii and wall-thickness of micro-vessels in the anesthetized rat. Circ. Res. 25:315–329.

Bar, T. and J. R. Wolff. 1973. On the vascularization of the rat's cerebral cortex. 7th Europ. Conf. Microcirculation, Aberdeen, 1972. Bibl. Anat. 11:515–519.

Bassingthwaighte, J. B. 1970. Blood flow and diffusion through mammalian organs. Science. 167:1347–1353.

Becker, C. G., and R. L. Nachman. 1973. Contractile proteins of endothelial cells, platlets and smooth muscle. Am. J. Pathol. 71:1−22.

Campbell, T., and T. Heath. 1973. Intrinsic contractility of lymphatics in sheep and in dogs. Quart. J. Expt. Physiol. 58:207−219.

Chambers, R., and B. W. Zweifach. 1944. Topography and function of the mesenteric circulation. Am. J. Anat. 75:173−205.

Chambers, R., and B. W. Zweifach. 1947. Intercellular cement and capillary permeability. Physiol. Rev. 27:436−463.

Clark, E. R., and E. L. Clark. 1943. Caliber changes in minute blood vessels observed in the living mammal. Am. J. Anat. 73:215−250.

Clementi, F., and G. E. Palade. 1969. Intestinal capillaries. I. Permeability to peroxidase and ferritin. J. Cell. Biol. 41:33−58.

Crone, C. 1970. Capillary permeability techniques and problems. In C. Crone and N. A. Lassen (eds.), Capillary Permeability, pp. 15−31. Academic Press, New York.

Diana, J. N., and C. A. Shadur. 1973. Effect of arterial and venous pressure on capillary pressure and volume. Am. J. Physiol. 225:637−650.

Eriksson, E., and R. Myrhage. 1972. Microvascular dimensions and blood flow in skeletal muscle. Acta Physiol. Scand. 86:211−222.

Farquhar, M. G., and G. E. Palade. 1963. Junctional complexes in various epithelia. J. Cell. Biol. 17:375−412.

Folkow, B., R. R. Sonnenschein, and D. C. Wright. 1971. Loci of neurogenic and metabolic effects on precapillary vessels of skeletal muscle. Acta Physiol. Scand. 81:459−471.

Frasher, W. G., Jr., and H. Wayland. 1972. A repeating modular organization of the microcirculation of cat mesentery. Microvasc. Res. 4: 62−76.

Friedman, J. J. 1971. Rb[86] extraction as an indicator of capillary flow. Circ. Res. 28 (Suppl. 1):15−20.

Gore, R. W. 1974. Pressures of cat mesenteric arterioles and capillaries during changes in systemic arterial pressure. Circ. Res. 34:581−591.

Grafflin, A. L., and E. H. Bagley. 1953. Studies of peripheral vascular beds. Bull. Johns Hopkins Hosp. 92:47−73.

Granger, H. J., and A. P. Shepherd, Jr. 1973. Intrinsic microvascular control of tissue oxygen delivery. Microvasc. Res. 5:49−72.

Grunewald, W. 1968. Theoretical analysis of the oxygen supply in tissue. In D. W. Lubbers, U. C. Luft, G. Thews, and E. Witzlet (eds.), Oxygen Transport in Blood and Tissue, pp. 100−114. G. Threme, Stuttgart.

Haddy, F. J., and J. B. Scott. 1968. Metabolically linked vasoactive chemicals in local regulation of blood flow. Physiol. Rev. 48:688.

Hammersen, F. 1970. The terminal vascular bed in skeletal muscle with special regard to the problem of shunts. In C. Crone and N. A. Lassen (eds.), Capillary Permeability, pp. 351−365. Academic Press, New York.

Hauck, G. 1969. Zur Frage der Existenz eines "gradient of vascular permeability":an der Endstrombahn. Arch. Kreisl. Forsch. 59:197−227.

Hyman, C. 1971. Independent control of nutritional and shunt circulation. Microvasc. Res. 3:84−94.

Intaglietta, M., R. F. Pawula, and W. R. Tompkins. 1970. Pressure measurements in the mammalian microvasculature. Microvasc. Res. 2:212−220.

Intaglietta, M., W. R. Tompkins, and D. R. Richardson. 1970. Velocity measurements in the microvasculature of the cat omentum by on-line method. Microvasc. Res. 2:462−473.

Intaglietta, M., and B. W. Zweifach. 1974. Microcirculatory basis of fluid exchange. *In* John H. Lawrence and J. G. Hamilton (ed.), Advances in Biological and Medical Physics, Vol. 15, pp. 111–159. Academic Press, New York.

Karnovsky, M. J. 1968. The ultrastructural basis of transcapillary exchanges. J. Gen. Physiol. 52:64–95.

Krogh, A. 1922. Anatomy and Physiology of Capillaries, p. 248. Yale Univ. Press, New Haven.

Kuwabara, T., and D. G. Cogan. 1960. Studies of retinal vascular patterns. I. Normal architecture. Arch. Ophthal. 64:904–930.

Lamport, H., and S. Baez. 1962. Physical properties of small arterial vessels. Physiol. Rev. 42:328–352.

Landis, E. M. 1927. Micro-injection studies of capillary permeability. II. The relation between capillary pressure and the rate at which fluid passes through the walls of single capillaries. Am. J. Physiol. 82:217–238.

Landis, E. M., and J. R. Pappenheimer. 1963. Exchange of substances through the capillary walls. *In* W. F. Hamilton and P. Dow (eds.), Handbook of Physiology: Circulation, Section 2, pp. 961–1034. American Physiology Society, Washington, D.C.

Levick, J. R., and C. C. Michel. 1973. Permeability of individually perfused frog mesenteric capillaries to T1824 and T1824 albumin as evidence for a large pore system. Quart. J. Exp. Physiol. 58:87.

Majno, G. 1965. Ultrastructure of the vascular membrane. *In* W. F. Hamilton and P. Dow (eds.), Handbook of Physiology, Section 2, Vol. III, pp. 2293–2376. American Physiology Society, Washington, D.C.

Mellander, S., and B. Johansson. 1968. Control of resistance, exchange and capacitance functions in the peripheral circulation. Pharmacol. Rev. 20:117–196.

Michel, C. C. 1972. Flows across the capillary wall. *In* D. H. Bergel (ed), Cardiovascular Fluid Dynamics, Vol. 2, pp. 241–298. Academic Press, New York.

Nichol, J. T., F. Girling, W. Jerrard, E. B. Claxton, and A. C. Burton. 1951. Fundamental instability of small blood vessels and critical closing pressures in vascular beds. Am. J. Physiol. 164:330–344.

Nicoll, P. A. 1969. Intrinsic regulation in the microcirculation based on direct pressure measurements. *In* W. L. Winters and A. N. Brest (eds.), The Microcirculation, pp. 89–101. Charles C. Thomas, Springfield, Ill.

Pappenheimer, J. R., and A. Soto-Rivera. 1948. Effective osmotic pressure of the plasma proteins and other quantities associated with the capillary circulation in the hind limbs of cats and dogs. Am. J. Physiol. 152:471–491.

Renkin, E. M. 1971. The nutritional-shunt-flow hypothesis in skeletal muscle circulation. Circ. Res. 28 (Suppl. 1):21–25.

Rhodin, J. A. G. 1968. Ultrastructure of mammalian venous capillaries, venules and small collecting veins. J. Ultrast. Res. 25:452–500.

Simionescu, N., M. Simionescu, and G. E. Palade. 1973. Permeability of muscle capillaries to exogenous myoglobin. J. Cell Biol. 57:424–452.

Simionescu, N., M. Simionescu, and G. E. Palade. 1975. Permeability of muscle capillaries to small heme-peptides. J. Cell. Biol. 64:586–607.

Spalteholz, W. 1888. Die Vertheilung der Blutgefässe in Muskel. Abdhandl. math-phys. Cl. sächs. Gesells d. Wiss. 14:509(2).

Trap-Jensen and N. A. Lassen. 1971. Restricted diffusion in skeletal muscle capillaries in man. Am. J. Physiol. 220:371–376.

Vawter, D., Y C. Fung, and B. W. Zweifach. 1974. Distribution of blood flow and pressure from a microvessel into a branch. Microvasc. Res. 8:44−52.

Wayland, H. 1973. Photosensor methods of flow measurement in the microcirculation. Microvasc. Res. 5:336−350.

Webb, R. L., and P. A. Nicoll. 1954. The bat wing as a subject for studies in homeostasis of capillary beds. Anat. Rec. 120:253−264.

Wiedeman, M. P. 1967. Architecture of the terminal vascular bed. In E. B. Reeve and A. C. Guyton (eds.), Physical Bases of circulatory Transport: Regulation and Exchange, p. 307. W. B. Saunders, Philadelphia.

Wiederhielm, C. A. 1966. Transcapillary and interstitial transport phenomena in the mesentery. Fed. Proc. 25:1789−1798.

Winne, D. 1965. Die Capillarpermeabilität hochmolekularer Substanzen. Pflüg. Arch. ges. Physiol. 283:119−136.

Witte, S., and F. Hagel. 1971. Quantitative ultraviolet microscopy. In J. Ditzel and D. H. Lewis (ed.), 6th European Conf. Microcirculation, Aalborg, 1970, pp. 86−89. S. Karger, Basel.

Zweifach, B. W. 1957. General principles governing behavior of the microcirculation. Am. J. Med. 23:684−696.

Zweifach, B. W. 1961. Functional Behavior of the Microcirculation. Charles C. Thomas, Springfield, Ill.

Zweifach, B. W., and M. Intaglietta. 1971. Measurement of blood plasma colloid osmotic pressure. II. Comparative study of different species. Microvasc. Res. 3:83−88.

Zweifach, B. W., and D. R. Richardson. 1971. Microcirculatory adjustments of pressure in the mesentery. In J. Ditzel and D. H. Lewis (eds.), 6th European Conf. on Microcirculation, pp. 248−253. S. Karger, Basel.

Zweifach, B. W. 1972. Physiology of terminal lymphatics in the mesentery. Pflüg. Arch. 336 (Suppl.):65−69.

Zweifach, B. W. 1973. Microcirculation. Ann. Rev. Physiol. 35:117−150.

Zweifach, B. W. 1974. Quantitative studies on microcirculatory structure and function. I. An analysis of pressure distribution in the terminal vascular bed in cat mesentery. Circ. Res. 34:843−857.

Zweifach, B. W., and H. H. Lipowsky. 1975. Direct measurements of the resistance to flow in microvascular networks. Biomech. Symp. 10:1−4.

Zweifach, B. W., and J. W. Prather. 1975. Micromanipulation of pressure in terminal lymphatics of rat mesentery. Am. J. Physiol. 228:1326−1335.

STRUCTURE

chapter 1

MICROVASCULAR TERMINOLOGY

Silvio Baez

Over three centuries have elapsed since Malpighi (1661) demonstrated that the "porosities in the flesh," whereby blood flows from artery to vein, were rather long, thin-walled tubes, which he termed capillaries. This first recorded observation of the microcirculation in vivo made morphologic reality of the logical necessity set forth by Harvey's first accurate description (1628) of the functioning of the heart and the concept of the blood circulation. In spite of the unrelenting study of the terminal portion of the circulatory system since Malpighi's time, the descriptions of the patterns of distribution and structure reveal persisting diversity of opinion.

In part, unnecessary semantic disagreement arises from a protracted lack of uniformity in terminology. Diversity of views on the subject also derives in some measure from generalizations. Although it is known that in most tissues and organs examined, blood flows from arteriole to collecting venules through an intervening network of endothelial capillaries, there is an increased awareness that the task performed by this segment of the circulation depends strongly on the modular patterns formed by the integrant microscopic vessels in a given tissue or organ. Progress in methodology has created a variety of tools permitting the reliable monitoring of biologic signals indicating dynamic changes in microvascular morphology, yet reliable information about dynamic morphology of the microvascular system, best obtained by vital microscopy, has been possible with sufficient detail only in superficial tissues. Hasty generalization under these circumstances might be another source of confusion or disagreement.

Information pertaining to historical development and achievement in this field of study can be found in monographs by Krogh (1929), Zweifach (1961),

---

Some of the material reported herein was supported by the United States Public Health Service, National Institutes of Health Research Grant HL-06736.

23

and Maggio (1965), and in the excellent reviews, among others, by Illig (1961) and Wiedeman (1963).

DEFINITIONS

The terminal portion of the cardiovascular system is charged with the transfer of gases and nutrients and the removal of metabolic waste products. The term microcirculation, employed by Fulton (1957) and Zweifach (1957) to describe blood flow through the small vessels of this portion of the system, is used universally. In addition to endothelial capillaries, the fine ramifications of the small arteries and veins, i.e., arterioles and postcapillary venules, are included as major components of the microcirculation.

Microvessel and *microvasculature* are terms used to describe a single vascular element or a network of microscopic vessels, respectively (without reference to the flowing blood). The term *capillary* was used to designate the endothelial tubes devoid of smooth muscle that connects the smallest arterioles to postcapillary venules. These terms are easily grasped and generally accepted.

Consensus also can be found on terms used to designate the postcapillary venous segments of the microcirculation:

Venous capillary. Capillaries formed by the confluence of two to three capillaries, diameter between 8 and 10 μ and identified as being continuous with larger postcapillary venules. The endothelium is usually thin, exhibiting occasional pericytes.

Postcapillary venule. Microvessels with a diameter of 8–30 μ formed by, and continuation of, two to four confluencing venous capillaries, with an increasing number of pericytes as the lumen increases.

Collecting venule. Microvessels of 30–50-μ diameter, with one complete layer of pericytes and a complete layer of veil cells. Occasional primitive smooth muscle appears.

Muscular venule. 50–100-μ diameter, with a thick wall of smooth muscle cells that sometime overlap to form two layers. The confluence of muscular venules forms larger, 100–300-μ diameter, *small collecting veins,* with a prominent media of continuous layers of smooth muscle cells.

However, less agreement prevails on some of the terms used in the classification of the consecutive segments of precapillary vessels. *Terminal arteriole* is a term used by Chambers and Zweifach (1944) and Zweifach and Metz (1955) to designate the final arterial ramifications (30–50-μ diameter) endowed with a continuous single layer of smooth muscle cells and scant supporting connective tissue. In addition, Nicoll and Webb (1955) noted that the branchings of the terminal arterioles continue to become nonmuscular capillary vessels. Chambers and Zweifach (1944), in their early extensive and detailed study, noticed that smaller side branches of the terminal arterioles, wherefrom arise most of the capillaries, exhibited discontinuous contractile muscle elements in the wall. These authors introduced the term metarteriole to distinguish these vessels from the continuously layered larger terminal arterioles. The distal (endothelial) portion of the metarteriole that receives confluencing capillaries, going directly to the venous side, is identified as a *preferential channel.* Finally, the term *precapillary sphincter* was used by Chambers and Zweifach (1944) to designate the muscular arrangement around the orifices of some endothelial capillaries. Webb and Nicoll (1954) proposed that the term precapillary sphincter be applied to the last smooth muscle cell along any branch of a terminal arteriole.

Introduction of the electron microscope for study of the microvasculature and microcirculation by, among others, Bennett, Luft, and Hampton (1959), Fawcett (1959), Palade (1961), and more notably by Rhodin (1967, 1968), shed considerable light on the structural arrangement and ultrastructural details of most vascular elements of the microcirculation. However, little progress has been made in establishing a universally acceptable classification. For example, Rhodin (1967), in electron microscopic examination of longitudinally sectioned micro-vessels, proposed (1) that the term *arteriole* "be used for small arteries ranging approximately between 100 μ to 50 μ," having more than one smooth muscle layer, a well-developed elastic interna, and nerve association in the outermost muscle layer; (2) *a terminal arteriole* is a vessel with a diameter of less than 50 μ that has only a single muscle layer, frequent membranous contacts between endothelium and muscle cells (myoendothelial junctions), a scant or mostly absent elastic interna, and nerves accompanying it in very close contact. Rhodin further suggested that the term *terminal arteriole* be used for two types of vessels: (1) those having "a single layer of smooth muscle cells and a diameter of 30–50 μ," and (2) those vessels "which begin to distribute capillary side branches." The study shows that the latter "include vessels with a diameter of down to 7 μ," still having a complete layer of smooth muscle cells for some distance, distally from the precapillary sphincter—a thin muscle layer with cells spaced at irregular intervals. Thus Rhodin, in his unique study, on both anatomic and morphologic grounds, identified the microvascular structure designated metarteriole by Chambers and Zweifach (1944). However, Rhodin includes the smaller musculo-endothelial vessels in the group of terminal arterioles. Rhodin also proposes the term *precapillary sphincter* as "the muscular arrangement around the orifices of the smaller branches which come off the terminal arterioles." Neither such small (18–9 μ, i.d.) terminal arterioles, discontinuously endowed with muscle cells, i.e., *metarteriole,* nor a muscular arrangement around the origin of some of the capillaries arising from the latter, i.e., *precapillary sphincter,* was found in skeletal muscle by Hammersen (1968). No doubt, a reappraisal of these differing views toward unifying designation will be in order when the functional potentiality of smooth muscle cells ubiquitously scattered toward the terminal–pre-capillary–segments of the arteriolar tree is universally realized.

Arteriovenous Anastomosis (AV Shunt)

Single vascular structures for the direct passage of blood from the arterial to the venous side of the circulation without intervening endothelial capillaries are found in superficial as well as in deep tissues and organs but are absent in others. The description based on results of studies by in vivo microscopy has been comprehensively presented and discussed by Wiedeman (1963). The older pertinent reports were reviewed by Clark (1938).

After the confirmation by in vivo microscopy of the presence of arteriovenous anastomoses in newly grown vasculature in rabbit ear chamber by Grant (1930) and Clark and Clark (1932, 1934), the search for an anastomotic vessel directly connecting artery to vein was intensified and extended to other tissues and organs amenable to study by biomicroscopy.

By using the quartz rod transillumination technique for biomicroscopy, several investigators confirmed the presence of arteriovenous anastomoses in the liver of amphibia and mammals. In frogs, mice, and rats, Wakin and Mann (1942) and Seneviratne (1950) found numerous short anastomotic vessels between the hepatic artery and the accompanying portal vein. An arteriole may also cross a lobule and on the opposite side either join a portal vein or a hepatic vein. Short direct anastomotic branches between hepatic arterioles and portal venules were also seen in guinea pigs by Knisely et al. (1947) and Bloch (1955), and confirmed in the same animal by Irwin and MacDonald (1953). The short vessel, an arterioportal anastomosis (APA), arises at irregular intervals from a larger hepatic arteriole that winds itself about the portal venule. It was described by Bloch (1955) as being well endowed with smooth muscle cells.

Passage of blood from the arterial to the venous side of the circulation via a direct anastomotic connection without passing through a capillary network has also been described in the lung of guinea pigs by Irwin, Weille, and Burrage (1955) and in stria vascularis in the same animal by Weille et al. (1954).

In the spleen of the mouse, Pappart, Whipple, and Chang (1955) describe arterioles (one in ten) making either end-to-end or end-to-side anastomoses with collecting veins. Direct anatomic shunts were seen also by direct microscopy by Bloch (1956) in the conjunctiva vasculature in humans. However, direct arteriovenous shunt vessels were absent or only occasionally seen in other important organs and tissues. Poor and Lutz (1958) found no such direct shunt vessels in the hamster cheek pouch. They were seen only occasionally in spino-trapezius muscle of the rat by Zweifach and Metz (1955), and in tenuissimus muscle by Eriksson and Myrhage (1972). Anastomotic vessels directly connecting arteries or arterioles to veins and venules were not observed by in vivo microscopy in cremaster muscle of the rat by Baez and Orkin (1967), Smaje, Zweifach, and Intaglietta (1970), Baez (1973), and Hutchins, Bond, and Green (1974). The structure was not found in cremaster muscle of the mouse by Yamaki, Baez, and Orkin (1975).

In the tissues where anatomic arteriovenous connections are seen by in vivo microscopy, most particularly in skin and liver, the structures are, by and large, short unbranched vessels 12–45 μ in diameter in the dilated state. Occasionally, the shunting vessel can be longer, tortuous, or coiled, but is always endowed with a well-developed muscle layer in over a half to two-thirds of its length, where the lumen is thinner. The lumen widens in the noncontractile endothelial portion, before it joins the collecting vein. The unbranched anatomic shunts between arterioles and venules seen in mesentery of some animal species such as the mouse, rat, rabbit, and dog are of smaller 5–7-μ diameter in the initial one-third to a half of their length and 12–18-μ diameter at the venule end during steady state of the microcirculation. In addition, the former larger arteriovenous shunts are richly innervated vessels. The smaller arteriolar-venular anastomotic structures are in less direct contact with nerve fibers. However, a characteristic shared by both types of anatomic shunts is a greater responsiveness to some stimuli (e.g., thermal, chemical, mechanical) than the parent vessel. Also, both types of shunts can exhibit vasomotion.

Vasoconstriction of anatomic cutaneous shunt vessels to cooling and dilatation to warming of the body first described by Grant (1930), Grant and Bland (1931), and Clark (1938), and substantiated, among others, by Daniel and Prichard (1956) and Prichard and Daniel (1956) has served as the basis for the concept of heat-loss regulatory function generally ascribed to these structures. Other studies, particularly by Van Dobben-Broekena and Dirksen (1960 a,b), showing a lack of correlation between temperature and diameter of the vessels in the rabbit ear, have placed some doubts as to the exclusive heat-regulating function of cutaneous arteriovenous shunts. However, numerous other observations on the responses of such vascular structures have buttressed the currently prevailing view, supported among others by Folkow (1955), that cutaneous arteriovenous shunts are specialized structures primarily engaged in the regulation of heat loss.

Preferential Thoroughfare Channel

In early studies by Zweifach (1934) and in numerous subsequent studies that relate to structure–function correlation in the terminal vascular bed, Zweifach (1937), Chambers and Zweifach (1944, 1946), and Chambers (1948) focused on the description and evaluation of the smaller metarteriole and the precapillary sphincter that are capable of local flow control or regulation. In the various tissue microvasculatures examined, including mesentery, and undersurface of the tongue of the frog, nictitating membrane, and skeletal spino-trapezius muscle, it was noted that flow can be diverted from the arteriolar to venular side of the circulation via the structural type of metarteriole that becomes a venule. Zweifach (1937) introduced the term *preferential channel* to describe the contribution of this type of microvascular structure in the microcirculatory bed.

Since they were first described, such vascular structures called preferential or thoroughfare channels, with the capability of sustaining blood flow with exclusion of dependent endothelial capillaries, have generated general interest and debate. The operational characteristics of the microcirculation as suggested by Knisely (1940) and Frasher and Wayland (1972) are that (1) flow in the exchange bed at any instant in time includes only a small fraction required for nutrition and maintenance of homeostasis of the cognate tissue, and (2) the larger fraction of flow relates to the particular function of the organ in reference to the needs of the organism.

The preferential or thoroughfare channel occurs with different frequency in the microcirculation of a variety of tissues. This vascular structure has been described in the mesentery of the guinea pig by Lee and Lee (1947), and in the human conjunctiva by Lee and Holze (1950) and Grafflin and Cordry (1953). However, Grafflin and Bagley (1953) failed to confirm the presence of a similar structure in the web and urinary bladder of the frog. Also, Lutz, Fulton, and Akers (1950), although unable to observe any preferential channels in the cheek pouch of the hamster or the retrolingual membrane of the frog, confirmed their presence in the mesentery of the latter. Stapley and Copley (1959) described the preferential channel in the labial marginal gingiva of the rat. In the mural vasculature of the ileum in the rat, Baez (1959) reported metarterioles with a preferential channel structural arrangement in external muscularis and submucosa layers with greater occurrence in the latter. Although with a lesser frequency, the structure was also observed by Baez (1973) in striated cremaster muscle of the rat and, more recently, by Yamaki et al. (1975) in the same tissue in the mouse. This vascular element was not accounted for in an early description of the microvasculature in the rabbit ear preparation by Clark and Clark (1932) and Clark (1952), and was reported absent in the terminal vasculature in the wing of the bat by Nicoll and Webb (1946).

In essence, the descriptions show that the preferential thoroughfare channel, in similarity with the direct arteriovenous anastomosis, can be present in greater or lesser number or absent in the microcirculation.

In an early consideration of structure–function correlation by Zweifach (1957), the suggestion was made that microscopic shunts may be preferentially in use when vasoconstriction of the small arterial vessels beyond the small direct shunts increases resistance to flow. Blood flow would then be diverted through these microvessel structures that seem to afford the path of least resistance. The result of more recent systematic study of pressure across the microcirculatory bed seems to lend support to such a view. An uneven blood flow distribution is customarily seen in the microcirculatory bed with a comparatively higher flow in capillaries that originate from arterioles and terminate in the nearest large venules. The micropressure measurements by Richardson and Zweifach (1970) and Zweifach (1974a,b) show high pressure (38–40 mm Hg) in the faster-flowing capillaries and much lower (18–20 mm Hg) pressure in the large-drainage venules. The observation allowed the authors to conclude that the combined effects of the shorter path length and the greater pressure difference leads to a much more rapid flow in such channels. Because of the disproportionately small surface area for exchange in such microcirculatory patterns, the term *nutritive shunting* was introduced by Zweifach (1971) and Renkin (1971) to describe the phenomenon. Metarterioles with preferential thoroughfare structural arrangements can afford such uneven patterns of blood flow distribution with high flow in situ.

Studies of the microcirculation by in vivo microscopy show that in most tissues the endothelial capillaries do not originate from the initial segments of the larger 35–50-μ-diameter terminal arterioles but rather from metarterioles, i.e., smaller 8–18-μ-diameter terminal arterioles as side branches of the latter at any point along its length. In most tissues the metarteriole, in approximately 75–80% of its length, gives off capillary side branches that form the parallel circuits of endothelial capillaries. It is only in the final 15–20% of the small arteriolar length that capillaries in series are formed. In some instances the metarteriole is devoid of muscle investment and can be traced directly into venular channels. The metarterioles in the initial portion of their length are endowed with a single layer of muscle arranged in a compact coil. Distally, as the vessel proceeds in its course the muscle cells become rare and more widely spaced until a point is reached where the muscle cells are no longer recognizable. The junctional sites of capillaries arising from the muscular segments of the metarterioles have been termed precapillary sphincters by Chambers and Zweifach (1944, 1946).

The junctional muscular precapillary sphincters are conspicuous and easily recognized in thin flat tissues such as mesentery, omentum, mesorchium, skin, and fascial tissues in general, where the exchange circuits are formed by relatively simple architectural modules. In thick tissues and organs, where higher nutritional metabolic demands must be met by a more complex organized network of capillaries, the junctional precapillary sphincters, however present, are less easily recognized. Because of their strategic location, the vasomotor activity of the last muscular outposts represents a potential determinant of flow through the dependent capillary network. The precapillary sphincter concept as originally formulated by Chambers and Zweifach (1944) envisaged local control of blood flow by chemical mediators. Because the smooth muscle in the finest ramification of the arteriolar tree is no longer covered by an outer adventitial layer of connective tissue, it is more exposed to the action of locally released mediators or metabolites, which by diffusion, can interact with the vascular smooth muscle of such structures.

The nutritional function of the microcirculation, including the orderly monitoring of fluid resources as recently discussed by Intaglietta and Zweifach (1974), is basic and universal. Lesser or greater complexity in the microvascular modules with or without additional direct shunting structures, evolved to meet particular cellular functions; this does not render invalid the basic tenets that govern microcirculatory hemodynamics.

VASOMOTION

A characteristic of blood flow through the microvascular network is the continuous fluctuation in the velocity and distribution of cellular elements, both in the same vessel and in different vessels. Careful study of the phenomenon shows that such periodic fluctuations are associated with partial narrowing and dilation of the terminal arterioles, metarterioles, or precapillary sphincters. This type of activity was termed vasomotion by Chambers and Zweifach in an early description (1944).

Vasomotion has been used by different investigators to describe either spontaneous opening and closing of microvessels, speeding and slowing of flow, or periodic fluctuation in pressure. In a generic sense, however, the term vasomotion should only be applied to describe spontaneous changes in vessel dimensions. Fluctuation in flow or velocity reflected at the level of the single capillary by the movement of the red blood cells, factors such as varying hematocrit, and cell-wall interactions by leukocytes and platelets can introduce random fluctuations of flow and mask true vasomotor patterns. However, such random modifications can be resolved by high-resolution biomicroscopy.

The spontaneous rhythmic changes in diameter may be limited to the supplying arterioles, usually resulting in changes in flow without a significant concomitant change in the number of perfusing capillaries, hence the surface area exposed to an active blood flow. Vasomotion may primarily involve the precapillary sphincter zone of the microvasculature, resulting in the redistribution of the blood within the dependent endothelial capillary circuitry. Usually, single vessels and their immediate branches are affected in the latter type of discrete vasomotor activity. The precapillary vasomotor activity tends to be irregular, and can occur either synchronously with or independent of that of the parent arterioles.

Vasomotion should not be equated with *autoregulatory reactions,* i.e., the tendency of many tissue vasculatures to maintain constancy of blood flow in the face of change in perfusion pressure. By its nature, vasomotion has a direct effect on a number of basic functions of the microcirculation: volume of blood delivered, intercapillary spacing, distribution of blood within the capillary network (hence the capillary hematocrit), hydrostatic pressure in the exchange capillary circuitry, and thereby net fluid exchange.

Vasomotion at all levels can be suppressed by factors such as anesthesia, sympathetic blocking drugs, or rising temperature, and can be significantly enhanced by stress such as hemorrhage. Venous vasomotion has been described by Wiedeman (1963) in the bat wing, and rhythmic activity was also recorded at the level of the ileo-colic vein in the rat by Baez, Laidlaw, and Orkin (1974).

However, it is rarely seen in the venous microvasculature of most other species including the rat.

LITERATURE CITED

Baez, S. 1959. Microcirculation in the intramural vessel of the small intestine in the rat. *In* S. R. M. Reynolds and B. W. Zweifach (eds.), The Microcirculation, pp. 114–129. University of Illinois Press, Urbana, Ill.

Baez, S., and L. R. Orkin. 1967. Microcirculatory reactions to chemical denervation in the anesthetized rat. 4th Conf. for Microcirculation. Bibl. Anat. 9:61–65.

Baez, S., Z. Laidlaw, and L. R. Orkin. 1974. Localization and measurement of microvascular and microcirculatory responses to venous pressure elevation in the rat. Blood Vessels 11:260–276.

Baez, S. 1973. An open cremaster muscle preparation for the study of blood vessels by in vivo microscopy. Microvasc. Res. 5:384–394.

Bennett, H. S., J. H. Luft, and J. C. Hampton. 1959. Morphologic classifications of vertebrate blood capillaries. Am. J. Physiol. 196:381–390.

Bloch, E. H. 1955. The in vivo microscopic vascular anatomy and physiology of the liver as determined with the quartz rod method of transillumination. Angiology 6:340–349.

Bloch, E. H. 1956. Microscopic observations of the circulatory blood in the bulbar conjunctiva in man in heath and disease. Ergeb. Anat. Entwicklungsgeschichte 35:1–98.

Chambers, R., and B. W. Zweifach. 1944. The topography and function of the mesenteric capillary microcirculation. Am. J. Anat. 75:173–205.

Chambers, R., and B. W. Zweifach. 1946. Functional activity of the blood capillary bed with special reference to visceral tissue. Ann. N.Y. Acad. Sci. 46:683–694.

Chambers, R. 1948. Vasomotion in the hemodynamics of the blood capillary circulation. Ann. N.Y. Acad. Sci. 49:442–549.

Clark, E. R. 1938. Arteriovenous anastomoses. Physiol. Rev. 18:229–247.

Clark, E. R. 1952. Transparent chamber techniques. *In* E. V. Cowdry (ed.), Laboratory Technique in Biology and Medicine, pp. 351–354. Williams & Wilkins, Baltimore.

Clark, E. R., and E. L. Clark. 1932. Observations on the living preformed blood vessels as seen in the transparent chamber in the rabbit's ear. Am. J. Anat. 49:441–473.

Clark, E. R., and E. L. Clark. 1934. Observations on living arterio-venous anastomoses as seen in the transparent chamber introduced into the rabbit's ear. Am. J. Anat. 54:229–286.

Daniel, P. M., and M. M. L. Prichard. 1956. Arteriovenous anastomoses in the external ear. Quant. J. Exp. Physiol. 41:107–123.

Eriksson, E., and R. Myrhage. 1972. Microvascular dimensions and blood flow in skeletal muscle. Acta Physiol. Scand. 86:211–222.

Fawcett, D. W. 1959. The fine structure of capillaries, arterioles and small arteries. *In* S. R. M. Reynolds and B. W. Zweifach (eds.), The Microcirculation, pp. 1–13. University of Illinois Press, Urbana, Ill.

Folkow, B. 1955. Nervous control of the blood vessels. Physiol. Rev. 35:629–664.

Frasher, W. G., Jr., and H. Wayland. 1972. A repeating modular organization of the microcirculation of the cat mesentery. Microvasc. Res. 4:62–76.

Fulton, G. P. 1957. Microcirculation (editorial). Angiology 8:102–104.

Grafflin, A. L., and E. H. Bagley. 1953. Studies on peripheral blood vascular beds. Bull. John Hopkins Hosp. 92:47–73.

Grafflin, A. L., and E. G. Cordry. 1953. Studies of the peripheral blood vascular beds in the bulbar conjunctiva of man. Bull. John Hopkins Hosp. 93:275–289.

Grant, R. T. 1930. Observations on direct communications between arteries and veins in the rabbit's ear. Heart 15:281–303.

Grant, R. T., and E. F. Bland. 1931. Observations on arteriovenous anastomoses in human skin and in the bird's foot with special reference to the reaction to cold. Heart 15:395–407.

Hammersen, F. 1968. The pattern of the terminal vascular bed and the ultrastructure of capillaries in skeletal muscle. In D. W. Lübbers et al. (eds.), Oxygen Transport in Blood and Tissue, pp. 184–197. Grune and Stratton, New York.

Harvey, W. 1628. Exercitatio anatomica de motu cordis et sanguinis in animalibus. W. Fitzer, Frankfurt.

Hutchins, P. M., R. F. Bond, and H. D. Green. 1974. Participation of oxygen in the local control of skeletal muscle microvasculature. Circ. Res. 34:85–93.

Illig, L. 1961. Die terminale strombahn. Springer-Verlag, Berlin. pp. 1–458.

Intaglietta, M., and B. W. Zweifach. 1974. Microcirculatory basis of fluid exchange. Advan. Biol. Med. Phys. 15:111–159.

Irwin, J. W., and J. MacDonald. 1953. Microscopic observations of the intrahepatic circulation of living guinea pig. Anat. Rec. 117:1–13.

Irwin, J. W., F. L. Weille, and W. S. Burrage. 1955. Small blood vessels during allergic reactions. Am. Otol. Rhinol. Laryngol. 64:1164–1175.

Knisely, M. H. 1940. The histopathology of peripheral vascular beds. In F. R. Moulton (ed.), Blood, Heart and Circulation, pp. 303–307. The Science Press, Lancaster, Pa.

Knisely, M. H., E. H. Bloch, T. S. Eliot, and L. Warner. 1947. Sludged blood. Science 106:431–438.

Krogh, A. 1929. The Anatomy and Physiology of Capillaries. Yale University Press, New Haven, Conn.

Lee, R. E., and N. Z. Lee. 1947. The peripheral vascular system and its reactions in scurvy. An experimental study. Am. J. Physiol. 149:469–475.

Lee, R. E., and E. A. Holze. 1950. The peripheral vascular system in the bulbar conjunctiva of young normotensive adults at rest. J. Clin. Invest. 29:146–150.

Lutz, B. R., G. P. Fulton, and R. P. Akers. 1950. The neuromotor mechanism of the small blood vessels in membranes of the frog (Rana pipiens) and the hamster (Messoericetus auratus) with reference to the normal and pathological conditions of blood flow. Exp. Med. Surg. 8:258–287.

Maggio, E. 1965. Microhemocirculation Observable Variables and Their Biologic Control. Charles C Thomas, Springfield, Ill.

Malpighi, M. 1661. De Pulmonibus Observationes Anatomicae. Bologna.

Nicoll, P. A., and R. L. Webb. 1946. Blood circulation in the subcutaneous tissue of the living bat's wing. Ann. N.Y. Acad. Sci. 46:697–709.

Nicoll, P. A., and R. L. Webb. 1955. Vascular pattern and active vasomotion as determinants of flow through minute vessels. Angiology 6:291–310.

Palade, G. E. 1961. Blood capillaries of the heart and other organs. Circulation 24:368–384.

Pappart, A. K., A. O. Whipple, and J. J. Chang. 1955. The microcirculation of the spleen of the mouth. Angiology 6:350–362.

Poor, E., and B. R. Lutz. 1958. Functional anastomotic vessels of the cheek pouch of the hamster. Anat. Rec. 132:121–126.

Prichard, M. M. L., and P. M. Daniel. 1956. Arteriovenous anastomoses in the human external ear. J. Anat. 90:309–317.

Renkin, E. M. 1971. Nutritional shunt flow hypothesis in skeletal muscle circulation. Circ. Res. 28 (Suppl. 1):21–25.

Rhodin, J. A. G. 1967. The ultrastructure of mammalian arterioles and precapillary sphincters. J. Ultrastruc. Res. 18:181–223.

Rhodin, J. A. G. 1968. Ultrastructure of mammalian venous capillaries, venules, and small veins. J. Ultrastruc. Res. 25:452–500.

Richardson, D. R., and B. W. Zweifach. 1970. Pressure relationships in the macro- and micro-circulation of the mesentery. Microvasc. Res. 2:474–488.

Seneviratne, R. D. 1950. Physiological and pathological responses in the blood vessels of the liver. Quant. J. Exp. Physiol. 35:77–110.

Smaje, L., B. W. Zweifach, and M. Intaglietta. 1970. Micropressures and capillary filtration coefficients in single vessels of the cremaster muscle in the rat. Microvasc. Res. 2:96–110.

Stapley, P. H., and A. L. Copley. 1959. Observation on the microcirculation in the gingiva of hamsters and other laboratory animals. Circ. Res. 7:243–249.

Van Dobben-Broekena, M., and M. N. J. Dirksen. 1950a. Reactions of the vessels of the rabbit's ear in response to heating the body. Acta. Physiol. Pharmacol. Neel. 1:562–583.

Van Dobben-Broekena, M., and M. N. J. Dirksen. 1950b. Influence of the sympathetic nervous system on the circulation of the rabbit's ear. Acta. Physiol. Pharmacol. Neel. 1:584–603.

Wakin, K. G., and F. C. Mann. 1942. The intrahepatic circulation of blood. Anat. Rec. 82:233–253.

Webb, R. L., and P. A. Nicoll. 1954. The bat wing as a subject for studies in homeostasis of capillary beds. Anat. Rec. 120:253–263.

Weille, F. L., S. R. Gargano, R. Pfister, D. Martinez, and J. W. Irwin. 1954. Circulation on the spiral ligament and stria vascularis of living guinea pig. A.M.A. Arch. Otolaringol. 59:731–738.

Wiedeman, M. P. 1963. Patterns of arteriovenous pathways. In W. F. Hamilton and P. Down (eds.), Handbook of Physiology, Section 2, Volume II, pp. 891–933. American Physiological Society, Wash. D.C.

Yamaki, T., S. Baez, and L. R. Orkin. Microvasculature in cremaster muscle of the mice. Proceedings of the 1st World Congress on Microcirculation, Toronto, Canada. (In press.)

Zweifach, B. W. 1934. A macromanipulative study of blood capillaries. Anat. Rec. 59:83–108.

Zweifach, B. W. 1937. The structure and reaction of the small blood vessels in amphibia. Am. J. Anat. 60:473–514.

Zweifach, B. W. 1957. General principals concerning the behavior of the microcirculation. Am. J. Med. 23:684–696.

Zweifach, B. W. 1961. Functional Behavior of the Microcirculation. Charles C Thomas, Springfield, Ill.

Zweifach, B. W. 1971. Local regulation of capillary pressure. Circ. Res. 28 (Supl. 1):129–234.

Zweifach, B. W. 1974a. Quantitative studies of the microcirculatory structure and function. I. Analysis of pressure distribution in terminal vascular bed in cat mesentery. Circ. Res. 34:843–857.

Zweifach, B. W. 1974*b*. Quantitative studies of microcirculatory structure and function. II. Direct measurement of capillary pressure in splanchnic mesentery vessels. Circ. Res. 34:858–866.

Zweifach, B. W., and D. B. Metz. (1955). Selective distribution of blood through the terminal vascular bed of mesenteric structure and skeletal muscle. Angiology 6:282–290.

appendix

Histology of Selected Microvessels

Sol Bernick

Before describing the morphology of the microcirculatory bed as viewed under the light microscope, it should be noted that variations in structure do occur based on the function of the area supplied by these vessels. (See Sobin and Tremer, 1977.) The *nutrient* microcirculatory bed exhibits relative constancy in morphology regardless of the area it maintains. On the other hand, the *operant* vessels exhibit structural modifications dependent on the specific function of the tissue supplied. The following description of the microvascular bed is limited to the morphologic characteristics as seen under the light microscope. The ultrastructure of these vessels has been described by Rhodin (1967, 1968) and is further discussed by Wolff (1977).

MICROCIRCULATORY BED

A cross section of vessels seen in a typical microcirculatory bed located in the connective tissue adjacent to skeletal muscle is seen in Figure 1.[1] An arteriole, an accompanying small vein, and a terminal arteriole and venule are seen.

ARTERIOLE

An arteriole is a small artery with up to three layers of smooth muscle. A higher magnification of the arteriole in Figure 2 shows the typical characteristics of a nutrient arteriole. The endothelial cells are flat in shape and abut against an intact internal elastic membrane that has a positive periodic acid Schiff (PAS) reaction. The fine basement membrane covering the basal surface of the endothelial cells as demonstrated in ultrastructure micrographs is not clearly demonstrated by light microscopy since it is also PAS positive and may blend with the outer coating of the elastic lamina. The muscular media are made up of up to three cell layers that are helically oriented. Although basement membrane has been demonstrated adhering to the smooth muscle cells by electron microscopy, this membrane is so thin that it is not possible to show it by light microscopy, even by PAS staining. Interspersed among the muscle cells are fine elastic fibers.

---

[1] The terminology used by Rhodin (1967, 1968) is used for the various segments of the microcirculatory bed.

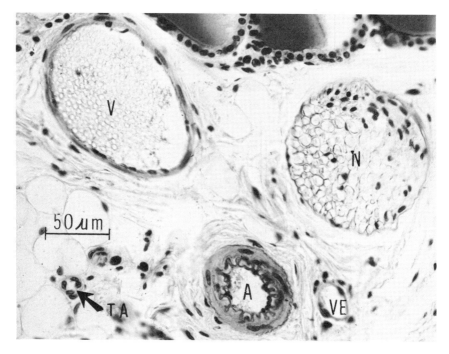

Figure 1. Epimyseal region surrounding skeletal muscle. Note arteriole, vein, terminal arteriole, and venule in the field. A, arteriole; V, small vein; VE, venule; N, nerve; TA, terminal arteriole. This and all other sections stained with PAS hematoxylin.

A definite external elastic membrane separates the media from the outer adventitia.

TERMINAL ARTERIOLE

The media consists of one single smooth muscle cell. The endothelial cell is flattened and abuts against a thin PAS positive internal elastic membrane. When the vessel diameter is less than 35 μ, the internal elastic membrane disappears and only the basement membrane separates the endothelial cell layer from the smooth muscle cell. The smooth muscle cell of the media is PAS negative (Figure 3).

CAPILLARY

The capillary morphology as seen under the light microscope is simple and, regardless of location, all capillaries are similar in appearance. However, when examined under the electron microscope, the ultrastructure shows considerable

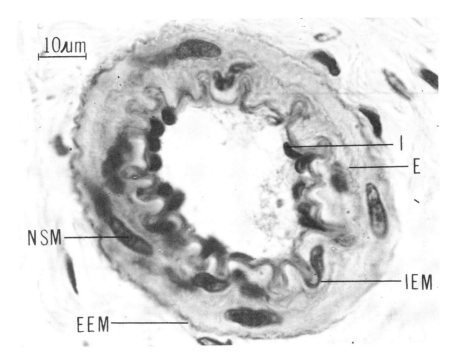

Figure 2. Higher magnification of the arteriole of Fig. 1. The internal elastic membrane is PAS positive. The media consists of smooth muscle greater than one cell layer thick. Fine elastic fibers are found in the media. I, intima; IEM, internal elastic membrane; E, fine elastic fibers; EEM, external elastic membrane; NSM, nucleus of smooth muscle cell.

variation among capillaries; that variation is not described here. The wall of the capillary in cross section consists of a single layer of flattened endothelial cells that rests on a PAS-positive basement membrane (Figure 4). As the basement membrane is PAS positive, the wall of the capillary appears red under the microscope.

COLLECTING VENULE

The venule illustrated in Figure 5 is designated as a collecting venule. The endothelium-lined vessel is surrounded only by an outer sheath of collagenous fibrils and a few fibroblasts. A smooth muscle media is absent.

SMALL VEIN (MUSCULAR VENULE)

Smooth muscle cells appear between the endothelium and the connective tissue in veins whose diameter is above 50 μ. Figure 6 illustrates such a small vein

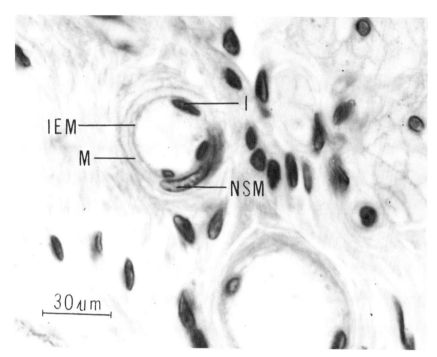

Figure 3.

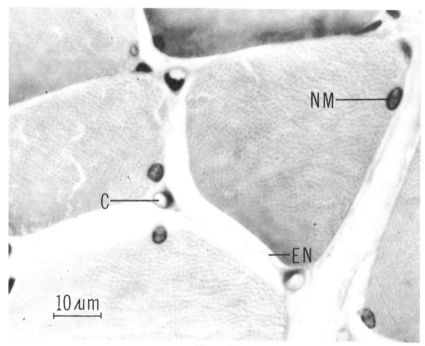

Figure 4.

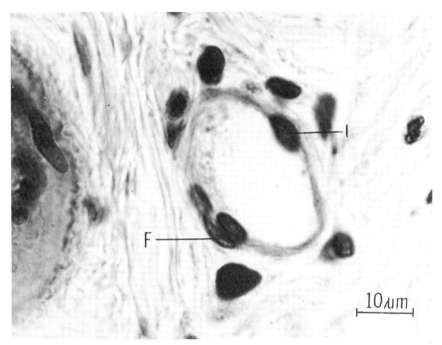

Figure 5. High-power magnification of the venule from Fig. 1. Note that the venule consists of an endothelial layer surrounded by connective tissue layer and no smooth muscle cell. F, fibroblast; I, intima.

associated with the arteriole seen in Figure 1. Between the endothelium and thin muscular media there is a fine PAS-positive internal elastic membrane. The media consists of a single smooth muscle cell layer. The tunica adventitia is made up of collagen fibers and fine elastic fibers.

VARIATIONS

As previously mentioned, the operant arterioles exhibit variants with the specific functional regions of the body. For example, the arteriolar vessels of the lungs are markedly different from the mesenteric or renal vessels of the same caliber. Unpublished studies by Sobin, Bernick, and Lindal show that typical arterioles

Figure 3. A terminal arteriole found in the connective tissue adjacent to the muscularis of the esophagus. Note the intimal endothelium, the single muslce cell layer of the media, and the fine internal elastic membrane. M, media. Other symbols as above.

Figure 4. Cross section of skeletal muscle capillaries in the endomysium. The capillary consists of an endothelial lined tube. A PAS-positive basement membrane surrounds the endothelium. The endothelial nuclei are prominent in this section. EN, endomysium; C, capillary; NM, muscle cell nucleus.

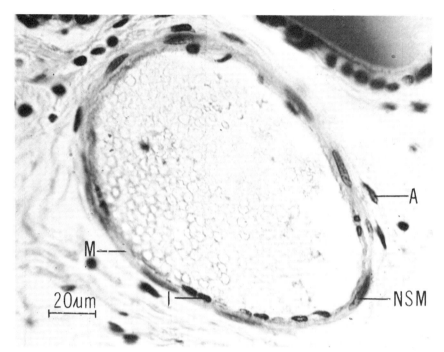

Figure 6. High-power magnification of the small vein from Fig. 1. There is a single layer of smooth muscle cell between the itima and the thick adventitia. A, adventitia. Other symbols as above.

and terminal arterioles in the kitten lung are altered in morphology beginning two days postnatally, and continue until 1 mo of age. The cytoplasm of the smooth muscle cell loses its fibrillar appearance and has a hyaline appearance; when sections are exposed to the PAS reaction, the muscle layer is intensely PAS positive. The muscle nuclei are elongated, and the chromatin is condensed in appearance. A full description of the other operant microvascular beds is beyond the scope of this presentation.

The basic reference scheme of this monograph accentuates the microvascular beds of skeletal muscle, skin, and gastrointestinal tract. The histologic morphology of the microvascular beds of these tissues seems similar.

LITERATURE CITED

Rhodin, J. A. 1967. The ultrastructure of mammalian arterioles and precapillary sphincters. J. Ultrastruct. Res. 18:181−223.

Rhodin, J. A. 1968. Ultrastructure of mammalian venous capillaries, venules, and small collecting veins. J. Ultrastruct. Res. 25:452−500.

Sobin, S. S., and H. M. Tremer. 1977. Three-dimensional organization of microvascular beds as related to function. In G. Kaley and B. M. Altura (eds.),

Microcirculation, Vol. 1, pp. 43—67. University Park Press, Baltimore (present volume).

Wolff, J. R. 1977. Ultrastructure of the terminal vascular bed as related to function. *In* G. Kaley and B. M. Alture (eds.), Microcirculation, Vol. 1, pp. 95—130. University Park Press, Baltimore (present volume).

chapter 2

THREE-DIMENSIONAL ORGANIZATION OF MICROVASCULAR BEDS AS RELATED TO FUNCTION

Sidney S. Sobin and Herta M. Tremer

The vast majority of tissues and organs of the body are solid, three-dimensional structures. Accordingly, their microcirculations are three dimensional. There are few two-dimensional structures, most of them serving a covering or lining function, for instance pleura, peritoneum, and meninges, or, as in the special case of the mesentery, serving as a protective sheet for the transit of vessels and nerves to the gut. Capillary beds of these planar structures are also two dimensional, and are not considered further here except as they specifically apply to three-dimensional microvascular beds.

The unpublished observations cited in this chapter were in part supported by Public Health Service Research Grant HE11152 and Dr. Sobin's National Institutes of Health Research Career Award No. 5 KO6 HL07064, both from the National Heart and Lung Institute. The work was carried out in the Los Angeles County Heart Association–University of Southern California Cardiovascular Research Laboratory.

43

CONCEPTUAL CONSIDERATIONS

Interior Milieu and Homeostasis

It is axiomatic that form and function of the circulatory system are interdependent, and that the anatomy clearly reflects the physiology of the part. The microcirculation is a paramount example of this. Even a cursory examination of the capillary beds of different organs such as kidney, liver, and lung shows striking differences among them, and these differences are closely related to the functional role played by the organ in its entirety. Thus organ function in broad aspect must be considered pari-passu with its microvascular anatomy. Central to the development of the microcirculation is the governing need for stabilization of the internal environment of the organism. This concept grew out of Claude Bernard's original recognition of an external and internal environment, the latter consisting of the totality of the circulating fluids of the organ system (Bernard, 1885). We have discussed this in detail elsewhere (Sobin, 1966). This circulation, in turn, can only be accomplished by the varied coordinated physiologic reactions that maintain steady or stable states in the body; this was recognized by W. B. Cannon when he coined the term *homeostasis* (Cannon, 1929).

However, Bernard's constancy of the internal environment and the homeostatic mechanisms directed toward this achievement recognized by Cannon must be viewed cautiously and critically: the constancy (for pH, O_2, CO_2, solutes, water, etc.) for most of the body covers a range and not a specific rigid level. Normal organ function proceeds within this variable range for these parameters; the exception is the central nervous system, and the significance of the central nervous system's rigid environment was clearly recognized by Barcroft when he said that for man, "the fixity of the internal environment is, in short, the condition of mental activity" (Barcroft, 1934).

Nutritional and Operant Beds

It remained for Knisely (1940) to place these concepts in their proper relationships to the role played by the microcirculation in their performance: "Thus the two different functional groups of capillary and sinusoidal systems are (1) those which merely nourish the cells around them and (2) those which not only nourish the surrounding cells but also act on the blood." We can paraphrase this classification into microvessels whose functions are (1) primarily nutritional to the tissue and (2) those whose functions are regulatory, or homeostatic or operant.[1] This classification of microscopic vessels by Knisely (1940) into groups based on the physiology of the associated tissue or organ is ultimately the basis of our recognition of three-dimensional organization in relation to function (Table 1).

---

[1] A more desirable term applied by Frasher and Wayland (1972).

Table 1. Functional classification of some microvascular beds

Nutritive	Operant
Skeletal muscle	Skin
Heart muscle	Trachea
Central nervous system	Lung
Smooth muscle	Liver
Uterus	Kidney
Bladder wall	Glands
Gut wall	Endocrine
	Exocrine

The microvascular beds of most organs and tissues clearly have both nutritional and operant components, but one or the other will usually predominate.

Multiplicity and Uniqueness of Microvascular Beds

Each organ or organ system has its own characteristic microvasculature, as individualized as are cell types or fingerprints. If the entire microvasculature of an organ is filled with an inert material (Sobin and Tremer in Volume III) and then stripped bare of its surrounding parenchyma, the revealed microvascular bed is readily recognized as a faithful representation of the organ (Figure 1). This is especially true of various operant organs (such as liver, kidney, and lung) where the tissues have been described as fitted or draped around the microvessels and where it appears that skeleton structure of the organ is determined by the microvasculature (Knisely, 1940). On the other hand, for nutritional beds, such as the central nervous system and cardiac skeletal muscle, where living cellular processes are vitally dependent on rapid and uninterrupted capillary–tissue exchange, the capillary pattern is fitted to the tissue or organ and there is more similarity among these than to microvasculatures that modify blood. However, it must not be overlooked that despite their similarities for nutritional beds, "the vessel architectural design is strictly adapted to the function of all the parts involved" (Knisely, 1940).

Microvascular Modules

A characteristic microvasculature of an organ or organ system noted above in the discussion of the multiplicity and uniqueness of microvascular beds can only be understood as a repeating organizational unit of that microvasculature. We will call this unit a microvascular module and define it as follows: It is the smallest repeating organizational unit ("building block") of a microvascular bed, which includes arterial input and venous outflow vessels and their intervening vasculature, i.e., capillaries, sinusoids, arterial-arterial, arteriolar-arteriolar, venule-venular, venous-venous, and arteriovenous vessels.

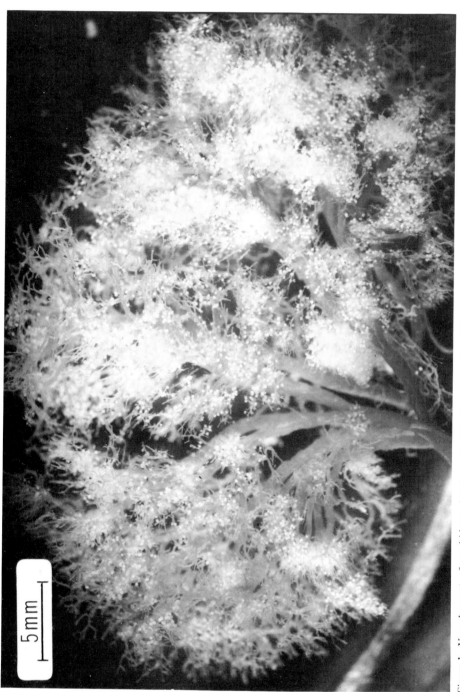

Figure 1. Vascular cast of cat kidney showing arterial and microvascular filling out to glomerular vessels; glomeruli are recognizable as small, white, glistening dots. Not all glomeruli are filled, resulting in patchy filling pattern. Vinyl corrosion preparation.

Skeletal muscle has been a prime object of physiologic study for many years, and in the past 30 or more years the microvasculature of skeletal muscle has been extensively studied by indirect ("black box") techniques for capillary filtration and other exchange properties as well as for various control or regulatory features. The description of microvascular architecture in skeletal muscle, initially described by Spalteholz in 1893, is valid; arterial and arteriolar arcades are the origin of terminal arterioles and the extensively interconnecting capillary bed (see Baez, Chapter 1 of this volume). Some years ago we noted that this is essentially the module proposed for nutritive beds; and it is also compatible with the arcuate pattern noted by Nicoll and Webb (1955) for the bat wing (Sobin, 1966).

Recently, Frasher and Wayland (1972) described a repeating modular organization (unit) for the microcirculation of cat mesentery not dissimilar in pattern to that previously noted in the bat wing. Both mesentery and bat wing are essentially planar, and Frasher and Wayland (1972) suggest that "topological elongation in the orthogonal plane of the interior of this unit may represent a common structure of the microcirculation of skeletal muscle." The reference here is to skeletal muscle with appreciable thickness. Such interrelationships between two-dimensional bed of mesentery and the three-dimensional bed of skeletal muscle should be investigated.

It may be conjectured that similar tissue structures have similar microvasculatures, i.e., connective tissue in organ capsules, organ septa, muscle fascial planes, and in subcutaneous regions may have similarly constituted microvascular beds. Likewise, the microvasculature of adipose tissue in the subcutaneous inguinal fat pads, mesentery and omentum, perirenal region and other fat depots may be similar. This possibility should be carefully investigated because, if a microvascular module can be described for various tissues, it remarkably simplifies the task of understanding microvascular control mechanisms.

Erythrocyte–Capillary Relationships

There is a vast difference in the relative importance of the erythrocyte to the organ function and blood flow in the two basic microvascular beds, nutritive and operant. Briefly, for most operant beds, the erythrocyte plays no significant role in the physiologic function of that organ. Conversely, for most nutritive beds, the erythrocyte plays a vital role in that organ function. The reasoning is as follows: Take the kidney, lung and liver as examples of operant beds. The essential physiology of these three organs is quite independent of the red cell. Neither glomerular filtration nor tubular function requires the red cell and, in fact, the kidney automatically excludes the red cell from the papilla; although the erythrocyte is essential to the transport of oxygen and carbon dioxide between the lungs and tissues, it plays no role in the process of gas exchange across the alveolar–capillary membrane; the multifaceted functions of the liver carried out by addition of substances to and removal of substances from the blood are also independent of the red cell. Basically, this is true of most operant beds, with the obvious exception of the spleen, whose function is directly involved in preferential removal of aging red cells. The capillary diameters in these beds are large relative to red cell diameter.

Skeletal and heart muscle can be taken for examples of nutritive beds. In the rat, rabbit, and cat, capillary mean diameter in the heart and gastrocnemius are 3.5, 3.8, and 3.7 μ and 4.7, 4.9, and 4.7 μ respectively; the related erythrocyte mean diameters (living cells in a wet chamber) are 6.5, 7.5, and 6.0 μ (Sobin, unpublished). In all three species, nutritive capillaries are 25–45% smaller than the erythrocytes, resulting in deformation of the red cell to allow its passage through capillaries smaller than its undeformed diameter.

The physiologic meaning of this special red cell–capillary relationship in nutritive beds is not completely clear, except that with the decreased distance between the red cell membrane and endothelium the diffusion distances are reduced, and deformation of the red cell to allow its passage through narrow capillaries increases the apposition of endothelium and red cell, and effectively increases the proximate surface areas for diffusion. The initial suggestion by Prothero and Burton (1961) that plug or bolus flow would lead to facilitated equilibration by "circus" motion of fluid between plugs has been discounted by Aroesty and Gross (1970). The type of change in red cell shape resulting from its passage through a capillary one-third smaller than its undeformed diameter is of no importance for this discussion.[2] Finally, it is conceivable that the restricted cross-sectional area of the nutritive capillaries could have unsuspected hemodynamic consequences in providing a fixed downstream resistance related to the red cell diameter. This has not been investigated.

Functional and Total Microvasculatures Compared

Because any normally operative or functionally open microvasculature may be only a part of the total bed, complete accurate quantitative data on the geometry of the total microvasculature in an organ may be essential to understanding physiologic vascular regulation and tissue exchange, as well as pharmacologic and pathologic alterations. Therefore, we distinghish between (1) total microvascular bed—the entire flow channel complex fully open—and (2) the dynamic microvascular bed or that part of the total bed which is functionally open under the specified operational event. It is modulation of the total bed by local metabolic, blood-borne, or neurally released regulatory mechanisms that selectively confines blood flow to discrete parts of that bed. The extent of that modulation and how it is accomplished are the aims of much microvascular research. As a corollary, we have noted that the need to distinguish between functionally active and total microvascular beds is important relative to techniques for their demonstration (Sobin and Rosenquist, 1973). The dynamic or

---

[2] See Chapter 12 of this volume for detailed discussion of erythrocyte deformation.

functionally open microcirculation can only be captured experimentally (or photographically) when all living processes, including blood flow, are suddenly stopped; conversely, the total microvascular bed can only be exhibited when all control or regulatory mechanisms are interrupted or abolished during life.

The methods and techniques used for demonstration and analysis of the functionally open and total microvasculatures of an organ are discussed by Sobin and Tremer in Volume III.

THREE-DIMENSIONAL
ORGANIZATION OF SPECIFIC MICROVASCULAR BEDS

Most studies of the microvasculature have been carried out in experimental animals; very few definitive studies have been done in man. The materials that follow are generally confined to various adult, nonhuman mammalian species.

Lung

The first observation of a capillary bed was made in the living frog by Malpighi in 1661, and the microvasculature of the lung has been variously and intensively studied in the intervening 300 years. Literature reviews have been written by Miller (1947), von Hayek (1960), Krahl (1964), and Nagaishi (1972). The following is based on our observations in the cat, and the results are, in general, similar to those in dogs and rabbits.

Pulmonary Arteries The pulmonary arteries closely follow the airway system and have a consistent approximate right-angle branching pattern out to and including the terminal prealveolar branches; the parent vessel usually continues in its original direction. Beyond the major lobar arteries, we have used the term *distribution* arteries, because the lobular structure of the lung is poorly differentiated in the cat as well as in the dog and rabbit (Sobin et al., 1966). The last or smallest distribution arteries are approximately 60–100 μ in diameter and show minimal tapering despite the many right-angle prealveolar branches that arise from them (Figure 2). These multiple prealveolar vessels, the precapillaries, are geometrically consistent: their diameter is 18–25 μ at the origin, and they pass into the intersecting planes of two or three alveolar walls. Frequently, they break up into the capillary network of the alveolar walls they supply within a very short distance from their origin, so that their effective length may be less than 25 μ (Figure 3). With a length–diameter ratio of 1:1 or less, these precapillary vessels function primarily as an orifice.

The arterial wall out to the last distribution artery has the general histologic characteristics of systemic arteries but with a much thinner media for vessels of comparable diameter. In vessels of 200 μ and greater diameter, there is a characteristic continuous palisading of smooth muscle nuclei. At branches of 60–100-μ diameter, there is an abrupt diminution of smooth muscle, although on occasion there may be a slight condensation of smooth muscle at the origin

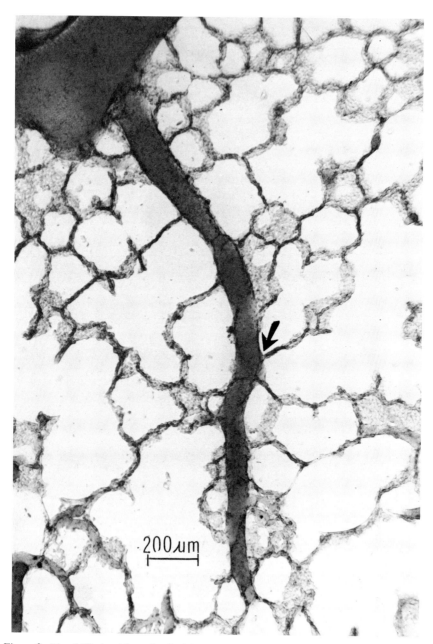

Figure 2. Blood-filled cat lung fixed with formalin instilled into trachea. Distribution artery and pre-alveolar branches. Detail at arrow shown in Figure 3. Cresyl violet stain. Section = 50 μm thick. (See text for details.)

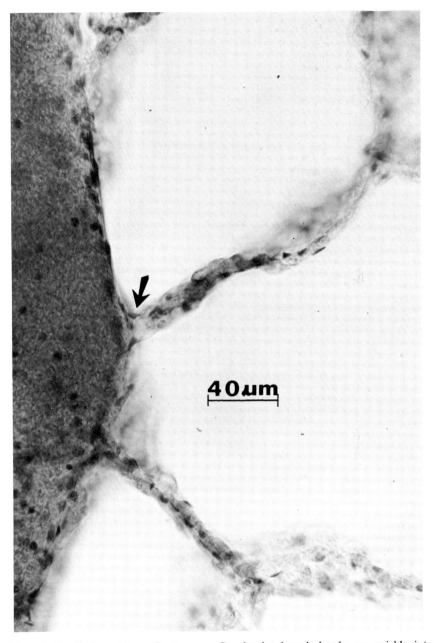

Figure 3. Detail from Figure 2 at arrow. Pre-alveolar branch breaks up quickly into interalveolar bed. Actual length of this pre-alveolar vessel is approximately same as its diameter.

of this smallest distribution artery. Smooth muscle in these latter vessels is sparse, appears to be almost randomly oriented, and gradually disappears. The internal elastic membrane also disappears, leaving an endothelial layer and external elastic layer. It is these latter vessels that most commonly have been called *pulmonary arterioles*. These have been well characterized for the human lung by Wagenvoort, Heath and Edwards (1964), and appear to be similar to the $60-100-\mu$ distribution arteries of the cat.

The short precapillary vessels that arise at regular intervals along the course of the distribution artery are devoid of smooth muscle and are essentially an endothelial conduit to the alveolar capillary bed (Figure 3). However, in the 10-day-old puppy, smooth muscle cells are found encircling the orifice of the precapillary branch at its origin from the distribution artery (Sobin and Tremer, 1966).

Alveolar Capillary Bed   For many years, the pulmonary interalveolar micro-vascular bed has been considered to be a capillary bed in which endothelium-lined tubular structures formed a vascular network (Hall, 1831; Miller, 1947). Weibel (1963) analyzed the network anatomically as a series of wedged cylinders without considering the nature of blood flow through such a model tubular system.

In 1966 we first noted that the density of capillary packing in the inter-alveolar capillary bed of the cat gave the appearance of two sheets of endothe-lium held and supported a capillary diameter apart by "stays" of septal tissue (the intercapillary connective tissue) (Sobin and Tremer, 1966). Closer examina-tion of this capillary bed led us to propose a geometric model in which the continuous space between the two endothelial layers provides the physical basis for blood to flow as a sheet (Sobin and Fung, 1967), and to advance a theory of sheet flow of blood in the interalveolar sheet or capillary bed (Fung and Sobin, 1969). The morphometric basis for sheet flow was presented simultaneously (Sobin, Tremer, and Fung, 1970).

The microvascular sheet geometry is demonstrated in Figures 4–6. Figure 4 is a low-power plan view of the cat lung, showing the relationship of alveoli to the alveolar ducts. The network pattern of capillaries is evident. The sheet detail is clearly appreciated in Figure 5, in which the vascular space is the tight continuous network of capillaries, which we have called the sheet, and the intercapillary nonvascular regions, called posts. A cross-section view of that sheet, Figure 6, demonstrates both the vascular space and post structures. An analogy can be drawn with an underground garage consisting of floor, ceiling, and supporting pillars, all of which are covered with a layer of endothelium. Thus the blood can be seen as flowing in a sheet-like layer through an essentially continuous space lined by endothelium.

Special Geometric Considerations   The three dimensions that characterize the sheet geometry are post diameter, interpost distance, and sheet thickness

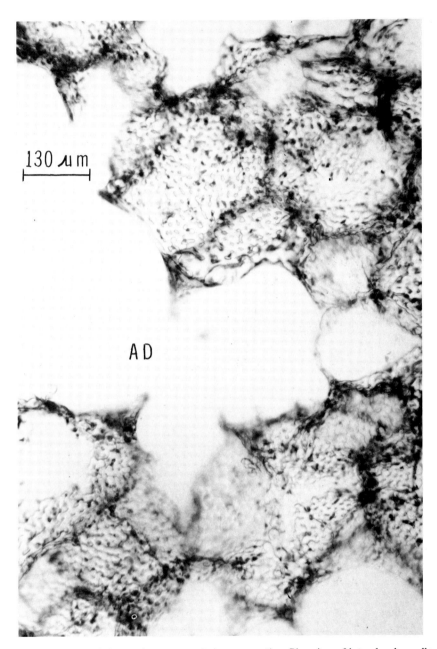

Figure 4. Cat lung. Silicone elastomer perfusion preparation. Plan view of interalveolar walls around alveolar duct (AD) showing capillary network pattern of the "sheet." Cresyl violet stain. Section = 150 μm.

54   Sobin and Tremer

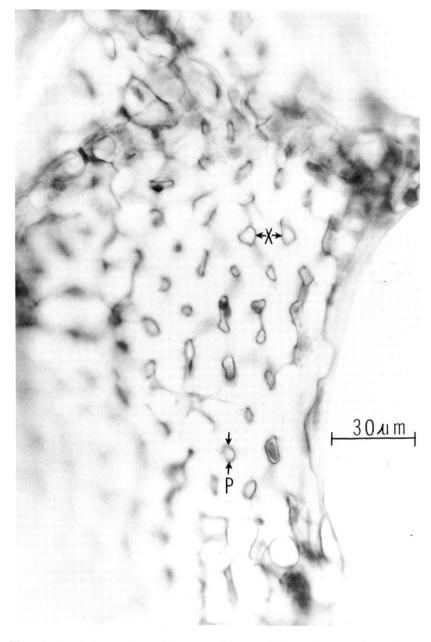

Figure 5. Detail of sheet. Post = P; Interpost distance = X. Preparation as in Figure 4.

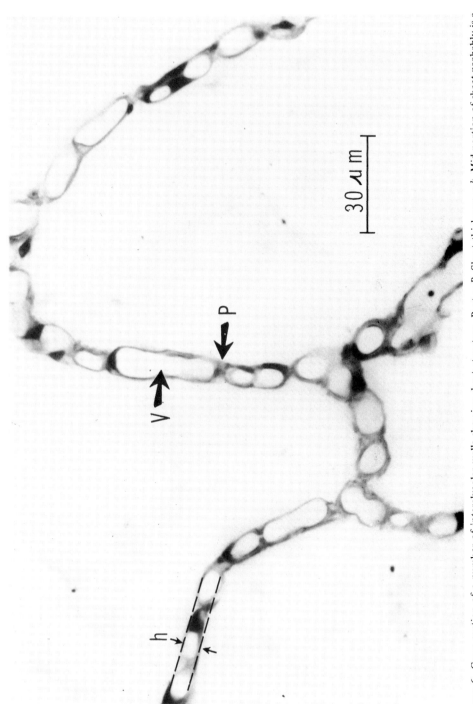

Figure 6. Cross section of a number of interalveolar walls showing sheet structure. Post = P. Sheet thickness = h. Mid-portion of sheet probably is a small venule = V. Preparation as in Figure 4.

(Figures 5 and 6). To understand how meaningful average geometric data are obtained, the methods of analysis we used are briefly given here (Sobin et al., 1970).

As a starting point, we defined for a limited segment of the interalveolar wall a vascular space–tissue ratio (VSTR) as the ratio of a vascular lumen volume to the circumscribing tissue volume. These parameters were obtained from planimetric measurements of a demarcated area of a flat or plan view of the interalveolar wall, such as in Figure 5. Various formulas were developed, based on the analysis of this plan-view field as a mosaic of hexagons of equal dimension, surrounding and including each post. From the VSTR values, the post (nonvascular) and interpost dimensions (vascular) were obtained. Sheet thickness was measured on the cross-sectioned wall (Figure 6). We found that the VSTR of 0.9035 in the cat was independent of transmural capillary pressure (Δp), that both post diameter and interpost distance were slightly sensitive to Δp, and that sheet thickness was very compliant over a broad physiologic range. (Also see Fung, Chapter 14 of this volume). At 10.3 cm H_2O transmural pressure, the geometric factors in the sheet are: sheet thickness, 6.7 μ; post diameter, 5.01 μ; and interpost distance, 9.15 μ. There is adequate space for the cat red cell (6.01-μ diameter) to pass through the capillary bed of the lung without physical restriction.

From these data it was possible to describe fully the compliant behavior of the pulmonary interalveolar microvascular sheet (Sobin et al., 1972), and further characterize its elasticity (Fung and Sobin, 1972a) and blood flow behavior (Fung and Sobin, 1972b).

Venous Drainage In contradistinction to the pulmonary arterial prealveolar vessels that supply the alveoli at their intersecting margins, the pulmonary venous drainage venule is from the "flat" free surface of the alveolus (Figure 7). Capillary segments merge and expand into a wider endothelial channel still within the interalveolar wall. As seen in Figure 6, a cross section cannot be positively identified as venule, although its central position and somewhat thicker channel suggest this vessel might be a venule. Serial section tracings would be necessary to identify this vessel with certainty, and additional morphologic data from detailed histologic and electron microscopic studies might not afford anatomic identification. As these nonmuscular venules coalesce, they become tubular and fully develop the characteristics of small venous vessels (Wagenvoort et al., 1964). Characteristically, venous channels are remote from the airway system (Miller, 1947).

Comment Although we have described as "typical" prealveolar supply and venular drainage pattern for the respiratory capillary bed, this is not constant and exclusive: variations and departures from this description are found. Therefore, our morphologic analysis of the microvasculature of the lung is still incomplete. To comprehend more fully blood flow in the lung, details of the

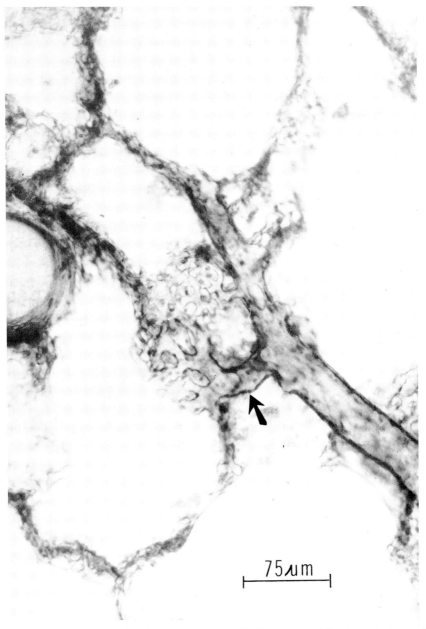

75μm

Figure 7. Pattern of venular drainage from the "flat" surface of the interalveolar wall formed by merging of capillary segments of the sheet. Venule at arrow. Preparation as in Figure 4.

exact entrance and exit conditions to the alveoli should be determined. This must include the number of vessels and their dimensions.

Examination of lung sections does not show a precapillary entrance and venule exit for each alveolus. Inflow supply and outflow drainage vessels are associated with groups of alveoli. From the sheet geometry of the interalveolar wall, it is not possible to speak of a Poiseuillean capillary length in either a physiologic or hydrodynamic sense. From the point of view of entrance to exit length, however, a path length can be defined, extending as it does over probably five or more different alveoli (Staub and Schultz, 1968). Defined entrance and exit conditions are necessary for anatomic-physiologic understanding of streamline fields in sheet-flow theory (Fung and Sobin, 1969, 1972a).

Skeletal Muscle

Proper understanding of the microvasculature of skeletal muscle is complicated by four factors: (1) muscles differ in thickness; i.e., the muscles studied most intensively are the thin membranous muscles, such as spinotrapezius and cremaster of the rat, and the tenuissimus of the cat and rabbit; (2) muscles differ in speed of contraction, slow and fast, i.e., red and white, respectively; (3) muscles differ remarkably in fiber orientation and pattern; e.g., compare gastrocnemius, gracilis, and those of the abdominal wall; (4) extrapolation between species for the same muscle group may not be justified.

The microvasculature of skeletal muscle was first described by Spalteholz (1888) for the rabbit, dog, and human newborn. Major branches of arteries run parallel to muscle fibers and are connected by interarterial loops (arcades), and the basic arcade pattern persists out to the terminal arterioles. The latter arise from the smallest arterial arcades, pass perpendicular to the muscle fibers, and ramify like a tree into capillaries that lie mainly parallel to such fibers. The venous drainage is established by capillaries uniting into venules, the latter inserted between the arterioles. Krogh (1929) adds the detail that "veins down to the smallest branches are provided with valves allowing the blood to flow in the direction of the heart only." Krogh did a careful analysis of the density of the capillary network, spatially arranged about muscle fibers, with 400 capillaries/μ^2 in the cod and 2630/μ^2 in the dog. He suggests the warm-blooded mammals would require a greater capillary density than cold-blooded species, and that small mammals, with a greater metabolic activity, would have a greater density than large mammals. Lee (1958) notes tortuous capillaries with sac-like dilatation at the arteriole-capillary branch points in rabbit "red" muscle. Red muscle contracts more slowly than white and has a greater endurance capacity.

There has been considerable controversy in recent years about the fidelity of Spalteholz's (1888) description. The many differing views given in the literature have been summarized by Stingl (1969, 1970) and the following are his own findings: In many muscles the primary and especially the secondary arcades are missing, so that "terminal" vessels are commonly found (Cohnheim, 1872). Although Stingl (1970) finds great variation in the shape and arrangement of inflow vessels in different muscles, he is not able to find a logical explanation of the variations; he notes that, although most authors were satisfied with the assumption that the variations in the small artery pattern were due to muscle shape and connective tissue partitions, he believes much information is, at present, not complete. Stingl (1969) is not able to verify the original observations of Spalteholz (1888) of anastomotic patterns of terminal arterioles, and he commonly finds terminal arterioles running parallel to muscle fibers. Stingl (1969) also notes that all precapillaries and capillaries are similar, with each arteriole ramifying tree-like into "precapillaries spreading in different directions toward the nearest muscle fibers. Consequently, one arteriole was always supplying several muscle fibers. The capillary bed looked like a network composed of longitudinally running capillaries parallel to the muscle fibers and connected by transverse capillaries." Venules begin as short tree-like trunks from fusion of capillaries, are regularly spaced between arterioles, and have a much greater number of branches than similarly placed arterioles. Less frequently, paired arterioles and venules are found. In general, the muscular venous vessels accompany arterial branches. The considerable variations among species and in different beds are noted by Stingl (1970).

Hammersen (1970), in a summary of his work, especially notes the following: Within the same muscle, most capillaries divide at a constant distance from their supplying arteriole "like a tuning-fork, into two equal limbs;" the mode of ramification of capillaries produces the observed capillary cross-anastomoses; the more rapid division of capillaries at the venous end results in an increased number of anastomoses. Hammersen (1970) especially notes that the terminal vascular bed is complicated by a difference in three-dimensional spread of arterioles and venules as well as by differences in penetration from opposite sides (Figure 8). He states that an accurate description is only possible by reconstruction based on serial sections.

There is a considerable controversy about the Chambers and Zweifach (1944) proposal of a "basic topography of a predominately nutritive type of capillary bed . . . as a central channel, of which the true capillaries are the side-branches" (Wiedeman, 1963; Hammersen, 1970). The presence or absence of thoroughfare channels is less important than the regulatory mechanisms that control flow. The discussion of the paper of Chambers and Zweifach (1946) is important in this regard:

"The evidence indicates that, irrespective of the precise structural organization of the capillary bed, the integrative feature of the capillary system, which enables it to distribute the blood circulation in accord with the needs of the tissue, resides in the activity of the muscular channels (arterioles, metarterioles, precapillaries) leading into the true capillaries."

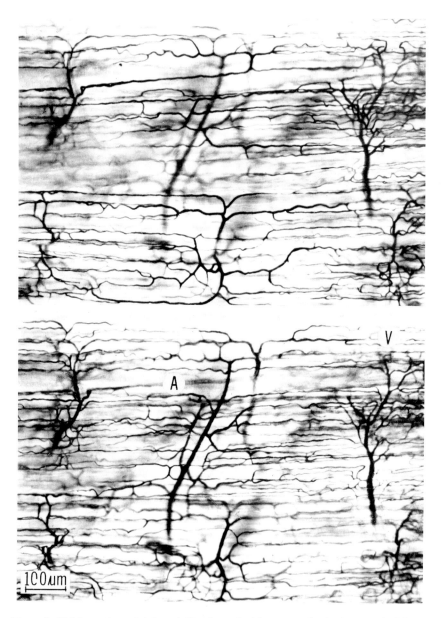

Figure 8. Thick section of injected M. plantaris (rhesus monkey) photographed in two different levels of focus to illustrate complicated three-dimensional arrangement of microvasculature. Injection preparation made with colored gelatin, subsequently cleared. (From Hammersen, 1970, by permission of the author.)

Skin

In the introduction to his book, *The Blood Vessels of the Human Skin and Their Responses* (1927), Sir Thomas Lewis says:

> "With Dr. Grant I have injected and examined many specimens of human skin, for my own satisfaction and not in the expectation of finding other than Spalteholz has found, for his skill in this field of work is unrivalled. It would not be exact to state that our personal observations have confirmed his, but truer to state that in our less perfect preparations we can see clearly the broad arrangement of vessels that he describes."

Both Spalteholz's original (1893) and subsequent (1927) publications are discussed by Lewis (1927) and include a three-dimensional block illustration (of Spalteholz) of the microvasculature of the skin and a lexicon of terms of various parts of the microvasculature used by Lewis and compared to those used by Spalteholz. Horstmann's review in 1957 included a discussion of Spalteholz's original figures. A subsequent conference publication on Montagna and Ellis (1961) presents a number of papers on microvascular anatomy of the skin in man, including its specialized appendages. Montagna (1962) briefly reviews some of the major generalizations of cutaneous vascularization in man. The review by Moreci and Farber (1962) is somewhat differently oriented and should be consulted. Reference should also be made to Hyman's (1968) critical and stimulating analysis of the cutaneous circulation.

A recent comprehensive and thoughtful publication by Ryan (1973) brings together a large volume of material on the blood vessels of the skin in an orderly manner. It covers dermal vascular embryology, wall components, precapillary sphincters, and anastomoses as well as abnormal and uncommon vascular patterns and morphology. It contains a wealth of data and literature references.

Gastrointestinal Tract

A review by Wiedeman (1963) summarizes the literature to that time and points out the major contributions of Baez (1959) in his development and utilization of special in vivo techniques for study of the gastrointestinal circulation. A prior symposium on visceral circulation (Wolstenholme, 1953) should be consulted, as should a later symposium (Jacobson, 1967) in which emphasis was placed on in vivo methods for study of the circulation. Subsequently, Guth and Rosenberg (1972) developed a technique for in vivo microscopy of the gastric microcirculation and failed to find arterial-venous anastomoses in the submucosa or superficial mucosa. Reynolds and Swan (1972) compare the canine and baboon jejunal microvasculature using the slilcone perfusion technique. In the dog villus, there are paired marginal arterial twigs and a central single drainage vein; in the baboon there are multiple parallel capillary channels that rise to midvillus level, and form an anastomotic plexus that converges at the top to a central drainage vein. A significance of these studies of Reynolds and Swan (1972) is the finding that the two species are so different, illustrating again the danger of extrapolating from one species to others.

Other Organs

Attention should be called to very recent definitive studies on the microvasculature of the heart and liver. Bassingthwaighte, Yipintsoi, and Harvey (1974) investigated the left ventricular myocardial microvasculature because of the need to obtain precise geometric data about the myocardial capillaries, so that accurate values could be used in their models describing the exchange of tracers in the heart. Details of capillary inflow and outflow vessel patterns and their densities, geometric (unbranched) and functional capillary lengths, and capillary density within muscle groups are given. It is possible to estimate the minimal capillary surface area as 500 cm^2/g of myocardium. Figure 9 illustrates the type of preparation used.

In a resumé and extension of his prior work, Rappaport (1973) presents a different appraisal of the microcirculatory hepatic unit. He abandons the hexagonal lobule for one that has microvascular unity with the terminal portal venule and sinusoid branching off from it forming a glomus (Figure 10).

COMMENTS

The purpose of an accurate and specific description of the geometry of the microvascular bed is to understand better the control features of that bed under conditions of varying physiologic and pathophysiologic activity. We have traced Bernard's concept of stability of internal environment to Cannon's ideas of homeostasis, and related both ultimately to the classification of organs on the basis of microcirculatory function: nutritional and operant beds. Yet these ideas are not that new. Marshall Hall (1831) said it quite clearly:

> "The number and distribution of the minute and capillary vessels, is accurately proportioned and adapted to the object of the circulation. When the structure of the part is simple, and the object of the circulation is its nutrition merely, the vessels are few in number; when the part is more complicated, or other objects besides its nutrition are to be fulfilled, the number, character, and mode of distribution of the vessels, are appropriately modified."

The features of microvascular control, whether by neural, circulating, or locally produced vasoactive agents, are executed against the background of the organ's total available microvasculature. The consequent establishment of dynamic flow channels that make up the active microcirculation at rest or activity, or even in disease states, can occur only as a result of modulation of the whole bed. The multiplicity of tissue and organ function is generally associated with multiplicity of microvascular beds, within the overall classification of nutritional and operant beds. The geometric features of the microcirculation

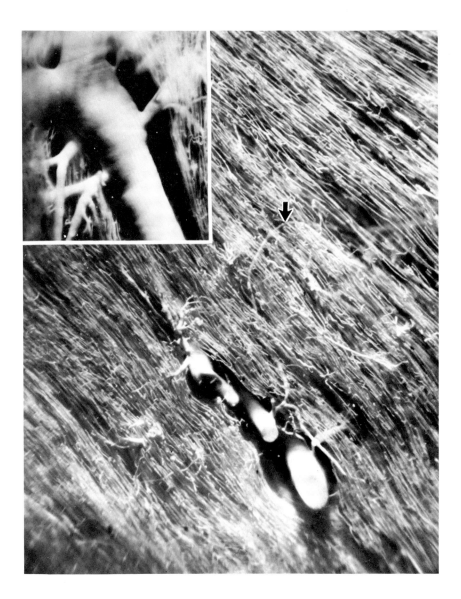

Figure 9. Subepicardial vasculature. Section parallel to epicardium, 1 mm deep. Scale divisions 10 and 100 μm. A 60-μm arteriole, accompanied by two venules, gives rise to three 10-μm arterioles, two short and one long (at arrow). The insert (same scale) shows a 160-μm vein giving rise to small venules and branching rapidly into the parallel capillaries. (From Bassingthwaighte et al., 1974. Reprinted by permission of the author and Academic Press, Inc.)

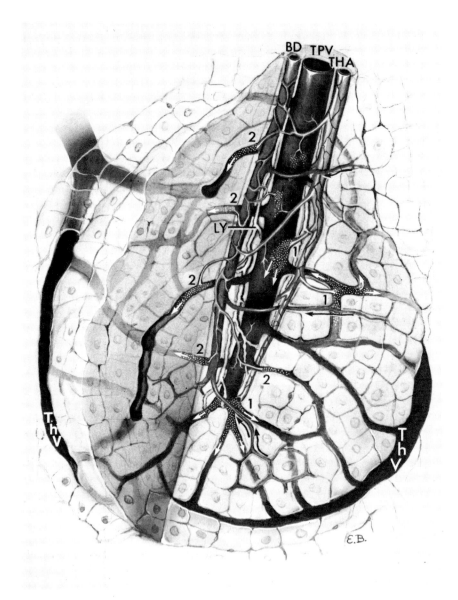

Figure 10. Microcirculatory hepatic unit. The unit consists of: (a) the terminal portal venule (TPV) with the sinusoids branching off it and forming a glomus; and (b) the hepatic arteriole (THA), lacing with its branches a plexus around the terminal bile ductule (BD). The arterioles empty either directly (1) or via the peribiliary plexus (2) into the TPV and sinusoids. The sinusoids run along the outside of cell plates and cords, inside which are the capillaries of the hepatic secretory and excretory system. The glomus of sinusoids is drained by at least two terminal hepatic venules (ThV); Ly = lymphatics. (From Rappaport, 1973. Reprinted by permission of the author and Academic Press, Inc.)

may similarly be important in the regulation of blood flow, especially as this relates to capillary–erythrocyte relationships, capillary hematocrit, etc. A defined three-dimensional microvascular geometry is essential to the understanding of these control mechanisms.

ACKNOWLEDGMENTS

We gratefully acknowledge the able technical assistance of Mrs. Roberta Lindal and Mr. Daniel J. Netto.

LITERATURE CITED

Aroesty, J., and J. F. Gross. 1970. Convection and diffusion in the microcirculation. Microvasc. Res. 2:247–267.

Baez, S. 1959. Microcirculation in the intramural vessels of the small intestine in the rat. In S. R. M. Reynolds and B. W. Zweifach (eds.), The Microcirculation, pp. 114–128. The University of Illinois Press, Urbana, Ill.

Barcroft, J. 1934. Features in the Architecture of Physiological Function. Cambridge University Press, London. p. 86.

Bassingthwaighte, J. B., T. Yipintsoi, and R. B. Harvey. 1974. Microvasculature of the dog left ventricular myocardium. Microvasc. Res. 7:229–249.

Bernard, C. 1885. Lecons sur les Phenomenes de la Vie Communs aux Animaux et aux Vegetaux. 2nd Ed., 2 vols. J.-B. Baillere et fils, Paris. Vol. 2, pp. 113–114. Cited by L. E. Bayliss, Principles of General Physiology, Vol. 2. 5th Ed. Longmans, Green and Co., London, 1960. pp. 721–722.

Cannon, W. B. 1929. Organization for physiological homeostasis. Physiol. Rev. 9:399–431.

Chambers, R., and B. W. Zweifach. 1944. Topography and function of the mesenteric capillary circulation. Am. J. Anat. 75:173–205.

Chambers, R., and B. W. Zweifach. 1946. Functional activity of the blood capillary bed, with special reference to visceral tissue. Ann. N. Y. Acad. Sci. 46 (art. 8):683–695.

Cohnheim, J. 1872. Untersuchungen über die embolischen Prozesse. Hirschwald, Berlin. Quoted from J. Stingl. 1969. Arrangement of the vascular bed in skeletal muscles of the rabbit. Folia Morphol. 17:257–264.

Frasher, W. G., and H. Wayland. 1972. A repeating modular organization of the microcirculation of cat mesentery. Microvasc. Res. 4:62–76.

Fung, Y. C., and S. S. Sobin. 1969. Theory of sheet flow in lung alveoli. J. Appl. Physiol. 26:472–488.

Fung, Y. C. B., and S. S. Sobin. 1972a. Elasticity of the pulmonary alveolar sheet. Circ. Res. 30:451–469.

Fung, Y. C. B., and S. S. Sobin. 1972b. Pulmonary alveolar blood flow. Circ. Res. 30:470–490.

Guth, P. H., and A. Rosenberg. 1972. In vivo microscopy of the gastric microcirculation. Am. J. Digest. Dis. 17:391–398.

Hall, M. 1831. A Critical and Experimental Essay on the Circulation of the Blood. R. B. Seeley and W. Burnside, London. p. 22.

Hammersen, F. 1970. The terminal vascular bed in skeletal muscle with special regard to the problem of shunts. In C. Crone and N. A. Lassen (eds.), Capillary Permeability, pp. 351–365. Academic Press, New York.

von Hayek, H. 1960. The Human Lung. Translated by V. E. Krahl. Hafner Publishing, New York.

Horstmann, E. 1957. Blutgefässe der Haut. *In* V. Mollendorff (ed.), Handbuch der Mikroskopischen Anatomie des Menschen. Vol. 3 (Part 3, Chapt. 8), pp. 198–207. Springer, Berlin.

Hyman, C. 1968. Cutaneous circulation: A clouded window. *In* D. Shepro and G. P. Fulton (eds.), Microcirculation as Related to Shock, pp. 69–78. Academic Press, New York.

Jacobson, E. D. (ed.). 1967. Symposium on the Gastrointestinal Circulation. Gastroenterology 52:327–471.

Knisely, M. H. 1940. The histophysiology of peripheral vascular beds. *In* F. R. Moulton (ed.), Blood, Heart and Circulation, pp. 303–307. Publ. No. 13, American Association for the Advancement of Science, Science Press, Lancaster, Pa.

Krahl, Vernon E. 1964. Anatomy of the mammalian lung. *In* W. O. Fenn and H. Rahn (eds.), Handbook of Physiology, Sec. 3, Respiration, Vol. 1, pp. 213–284. American Physiology Society, Washington, D.C.

Krogh, A. 1929. The Anatomy and Physiology of Capillaries. 2nd Ed. Yale University Press, New Haven.

Lee, J. C. 1958. Vascular patterns in the red and white muscles of the rabbit. Anat. Rec. 132:597–611.

Lewis, Thomas. 1927. Blood Vessels of the Human Skin and Their Responses. Shaw and Sons, London.

Malpighi, Marcello. 1661. De Pulmonibus. Translated by James Young. 1929. Proc. Roy. Soc. Med. 23:1–14.

Miller, W. S. 1947. The Lung. 2nd Ed. Charles C Thomas, Springfield, Ill.

Montagna, W., and R. A. Ellis. 1961. Advances in Biology of Skin. Vol. II: Blood Vessels and Circulation. Pergamon Press, New York.

Montagna, W. 1962. The Structure and Function of Skin. 2nd Ed. Academic Press, New York.

Moreci, A. P., and E. M. Farber. 1962. Cutaneous circulation: Anatomy. *In* D. I. Abramson (ed.), Blood Vessels and Lymphatics, pp. 489–494. Academic Press, New York.

Nagaishi, Chuzo. 1972. Functional Anatomy and Histology of the Lung. University Park Press, Baltimore.

Nicoll, P. A., and R. L. Webb. 1955. Vascular patterns and active vasomotion as determiners of flow through minute vessels. Angiology 6:291–310.

Prothero, J., and A. C. Burton. 1961. The physics of blood flow in capillaries: I. The nature of the motion. Biophys. J. 1:565–579.

Rappaport, A. M. 1973. The microcirculatory hepatic unit. Microvasc. Res. 6:212–228.

Reynolds, D. G., and K. G. Swan. 1972. Intestinal microvascular architecture in endotoxic shock. Gastroenterology 63:601–610.

Ryan, T. J. 1973. Structure, pattern and shape of blood vessels of the skin. *In* A. Jarrett (ed.), The physiology and pathophysiology of the skin, Vol. 2, pp. 577–805. Academic Press, London.

Sobin, S. S., M. Intaglietta, W. G. Frasher, and H. M. Tremer. 1966. The geometry of the pulmonary microcirculation. Angiology 17:24–30.

Sobin, S. S., and H. M. Tremer. 1966. Functional geometry of the microcirculation. Fed. Proc. 25:1744–1752.

Sobin, S. S. 1966. The architecture and function of the microvasculature. *In* Y.

C. Fung (ed.), Biomechanics (Symposium), pp. 132—150. American Society of Mechanical Engineering, New York.

Sobin, S. S., and Y. C. Fung. 1967. A sheet-flow concept of the pulmonary alveolar microcirculation. The Physiologist 10:308 (abstr.).

Sobin, S. S., H. M. Tremer, and Y. C. Fung. 1970. The morphometric basis of the sheet-flow concept of the pulmonary alveolar microcirculation in the cat. Circ. Res. 26:397—414.

Sobin, S. S., Y. C. Fung, H. M. Tremer, and T. H. Rosenquist. 1972. Elasticity of the pulmonary alveolar microvascular sheet in the cat. Circ. Res. 30:440—450.

Sobin, S. S., and T. H. Rosenquist. 1973. Determinations of dimensions and geometry in fixed specimens. Microvasc. Res. 5:271—284.

Spalteholz, W. 1888. Die Vertheilung der Blutgefässe im Muskel. Abhandl. math.-phys. Cl. sächs. Gesellsch. Wissench. 14:507—535. Quoted from J. Stingl. 1969. Arrangement of the vascular bed in the skeletal muscles of the rabbit. Folia Morph. 17:257—264.

Spalteholz, W. 1893. Die Vertheilung der Blutgefässe in der Haut. Archiv. f. Anat. u. Physiol. (Anat. Abth.), 1—54. Cited by T. Lewis. 1927. Blood Vessels of the Human Skin and Their Responses. Shaw and Sons, London.

Spalteholz, W. 1927. Blutgefässe der Haut. Hand. d. Haut u. Geschlechtskr. Bd, i. Th. i, p. 379—433. Cited by T. Lewis. 1927. Blood Vessels of the Human Skin and Their Responses. Shaw and Sons, London.

Staub, N. C., and E. L. Schultz. 1968. Pulmonary capillary length in dog, cat and rabbit. Respir. Physiol. 5:371—378.

Stingl, J. 1969. Arrangement of the vascular bed in the skeletal muscles of the rabbit. Folia Morph. 17 (No. 3):257—264.

Stingl, J. 1970. Zur Frage der Gefässversorgung der Skelettmuskulatur. Acta Anat. 76:488—504.

Wagenvoort, C. A., D. Heath, and J. E. Edwards. 1964. The Pathology of the Pulmonary Vasculature. Charles C Thomas, Springfield, Ill.

Weibel, E. R. 1963. Morphometry of the Human Lung. Academic Press, New York.

Wiedeman, M. P. 1963. Patterns of the arteriovenous pathways. In W. F. Hamilton (ed.), Handbook of Physiology: Section 2, Circulation, Vol. 2, pp. 891—933. American Physiological Society, Washington, D. C.

Wolstenholme, G. E. W. (ed.). 1953. Visceral Circulation. Ciba Foundation Symposium. Little, Brown, Boston.

chapter 3

SKELETAL MUSCLE AND GASTROINTESTINAL MICROVASCULAR MORPHOLOGY

Silvio Baez

MICROCIRCULATION IN SKELETAL MUSCLE

MICROCIRCULATION IN GASTROINTESTINAL VASCULATURES
Introduction

GASTRIC MICROCIRCULATION IN VITRO

GASTRIC WALL MICROCIRCULATION IN VIVO
Arteriovenous Anastomoses in the Gastric Wall

INTESTINAL MICROCIRCULATION

INTESTINAL MICROCIRCULATORY PATTERNS
Mural Supplying Vessels
Muscular Coat
Mucosal Microvasculature
Arteriovenous Anastomosis

COMMENTS

MICROCIRCULATION IN SKELETAL MUSCLE

Since the early careful description of the vascular arrangement in skeletal muscle by Spalteholz (1888), great strides have been made, not only in obtaining further important details about the distribution and architectural organization of the microvasculature in this tissue, but also toward meeting Professor Krogh's plea (1929) for securing a firm knowledge about "quantitative anatomy of muscle capillaries in different animals and in different muscles from each animal."

Some of the material reported herein was supported by United States Public Health Service,
National Institutes of Health Research Grant HL-06736.

69

The description of the distribution of the microvasculature in contrast-injected specimens of skeletal muscle by Spalteholz has served as a basis for pioneering intravital studies by Heilemann (1902) and by Krogh (1919). Krogh described the vascular arrangement in skeletal muscle as freely branching arteries with numerous anastomoses between them, forming a primary network. Small arteries are given off from the former; these interanastomose to form a secondary cubical network of great regularity. From the latter network arise arterioles, at regular intervals of about 1 mm, which finally divide into a large number of capillaries. The capillaries run in parallel to the muscle fiber, interconnecting between each other to form a long narrow mesh about the fibers. They then unite into venules and form the system of veins, which reproduces and follows that of the arteries. Krogh added that all veins down to the smallest branches are provided with valves and gave a remarkably accurate estimation of, for example, capillary density, surface area, and intercapillary distance, in skeletal muscle of the frog, dog, and horse. Algire (1954) and Algire and Merwin (1955) saw, in the paniculus carnosus of the transparent skin flap preparation in the back of the rat, arterial branches from the subcutaneous layers supplying the striated muscle fibers. Arterioles arise from these arteries to subdivide into capillaries that, cross connecting among each other at regular intervals, run parallel to the muscle fiber. After 0.3–1.0 mm from the origin, these join the capillaries to form collecting venules. These authors saw in paniculus carnosus arterial anastomoses and also a number of arteriovenous anastomoses. Active vasomotion was present, with intermittent capillary blood flow in the unanesthetized rat. A similar vascular pattern has been depicted by Wiedeman (1963) for skeletal muscle of the bat's wing. The terminal vasculature of the spino-trapezius muscle of the rat was observed microscopically by Zweifach and Metz (1955), who noted the large blood vessels distributed along the connective tissue cleavage planes of the muscle bundles. These vessels anastomose with comparable vessels to form a series of arterial and venous arcades. Metarterioles arise from the central portion of the interarterial arcades. They either break up into a series of capillaries or continue as preferential channels, i.e., receiving capillaries in the distal portion to become collecting venules. The endothelial capillary proper arises from metarterioles and lies directly on the surface of the muscle, running parallel along its length at a distance of 40–50 μ. In most preparations of spino-trapezius muscle, occasional direct connection between arterial and venous vessels was seen. Zweifach and Metz (1955), in careful observation of the muscle microcirculation at rest, noted spontaneous active vasomotion in the arteriolar vessels. Under conditions of drastic circulatory stress, i.e., hemorrhage, single capillaries or groups of capillaries were seen to be cut off from active circulation. The metarterioles of the thoroughfare type frequently showed an active flow of blood during periods of complete capillary ischemia, thus constituting pathways for the continuous return of arterial blood to the venous system.

The introduction of the open cremaster muscle preparation for study of the tissue vasculature in the rat has permitted a proper transillumination for observation at high magnifications (Baez and Orkin, 1967; Baez, 1968; Smaje, Zweifach, and Intaglietta, 1970). Grant (1964, 1966) gave a fine anatomic description of the major structural components of the cremaster muscle of the rat and its vascular supply and innervation. In most instances, the cremaster muscle is supplied by a single paired artery and vein (approximately 110—130- and 150—190-μm diameters), respectively, which derive from branches of external spermatic vessels. The vessels enter the cremaster of the dorsal aspect between two layers of the muscle. Occasionally the main artery divides into two or three (100—110 μ) vessels immediately on reaching the muscle. The main vessels run longitudinally toward the hind end of the muscle, giving off side branches (75—90 μ) as seen in Figure 1. The arterial side branches (8—10 in number) run

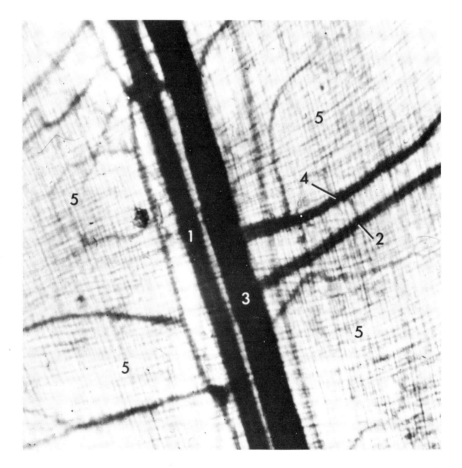

Figure 1. Microphotograph of cremaster muscle vasculature in vivo, showing the main cremasteric artery (1) and vein (3) with the corresponding arterial (2) and venous branches emerging at right angle. Also seen are venules (4) and capillaries (5). (Original magnification ×12.)

radially from the parent vessel and, after giving off numerous arterioles, anastomose with similar vessels at the anterior thinner aspect of the intact muscle sack, 1.2–1.4 cm from origin. The arteries and veins are seen as paired structures up to the third or fourth division, after which they run separately. An extensive anastomotic network is found in both the arterial and venous circuit and extends to the fourth or fifth order of branches from the main vessels. The arterioles, which run between the two muscle layers with no apparent relationship to the direction of the fibers, give off metarterioles to supply capillaries to both muscle layers. Some of the arterioles, which do not form anastomoses with similar vessels, are end-arterioles, as they in turn terminate, breaking up into numerous endothelial capillaries. The metarterioles, i.e., thoroughfare channels, for the most part, break up into 8–10 capillaries, and occasionally begin to receive capillaries in their course, thus becoming postcapillary venules. Except for these occasional thoroughfare channels, no arteriovenous anastomoses or short connections between arterial and venous pathways are seen in cremaster muscle of the rat, according to Baez (1969, 1973) and Smaje et al. (1970). In some instances, usually in the proximity of the main arteries, the capillaries are seen to arise from a short vascular structure (10–12 μ i.d., and 24–35 μ in length; lower left in Figure 2) to supply the thicker center portion of the muscle structure. In general, the endothelial capillaries arising along the length of metarterioles or as terminal ramifications of these, or terminal arterioles, run parallel to and between the muscle fibers, exhibiting multiple cross connections between adjacent capillaries in the same plane with a capillary network of planes of the muscle fibers in depth. In the two-layered cremaster muscle, three "decks" of capillary networks are seen—internal, middle, and external—with numerous, short interconnecting capillaries in depth as well, which occur at about 180–210-μ intervals. Each muscle fiber appears to be surrounded by successive modules of oblong capillary meshes. in consonance with descriptions of Wiedeman (1963), Clark and Le Gross (1952), and Wells (1960). Measurements by Smaje et al. (1970) give values of 615±194 μ for capillary length, from its origin to its termination in the primary venule, and for cross connection in the same plane occurring at 210±85 μ intervals (mean and S.D.). Smaje et al. found the internal diameter of capillaries of the arteriolar end to be 5.5±1.1 μ, and 6.1±1.4 μ at the venular end. The distance for open capillaries at rest was 34±2 μ in a portion of the tissue with fibers measuring 22.5±1.6 μ in diameter. Values for capillary density of 1,300 mm^2 and capillary surface area of 2.44 m^2/cm^3 were also calculated. In the anterior thinner portion of the cremaster muscle, a more random appearance of the capillary network is seen, as shown in Figure 3.

More recently, introduction of the tenuissimus muscle preparation by Brånemark and Eriksson (1971), permitting easy transillumination for biomicroscopy, has allowed studies by Eriksson and Myrhage (1972), Eriksson and Lisander (1972), and Ericson, Eriksson and Johansson (1973), in which further quantita-

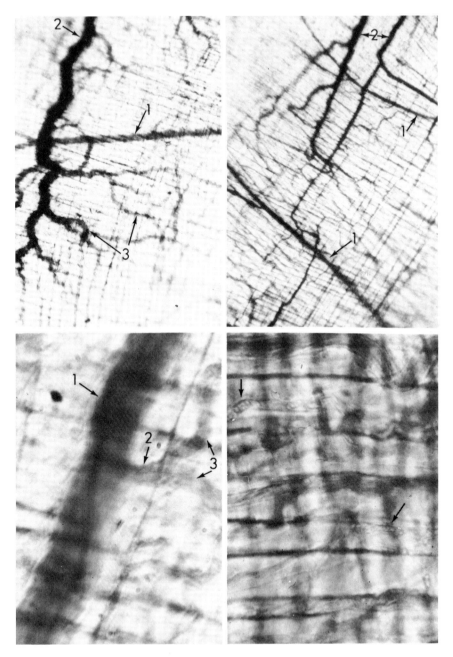

Figure 2. Microphotograph of the microvasculature in the open cremaster muscle preparation. It shows (*lower left*) a metarteriole (1) a short (18 μ length) muscle precapillary vessel (2) and the origin of two dependent capillaries (3). (Original magnification ×750.)

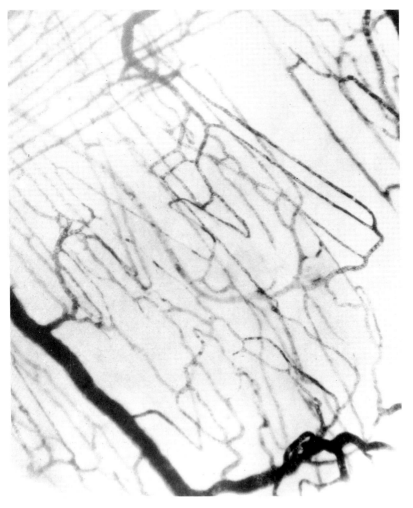

Figure 3. Photograph of India ink-injected microvasculature of cremaster muscle in the rat. It shows the random appearance of the capillaries in the lower portion with fewer muscle fibers, and capillaries oriented in parallel in the upper portion of the cremaster preparation. (Original magnification ×19.)

tive data concerning anatomic distribution, structure, and functional morphology of the microvasculature in skeletal muscle are presented. The thin tenuissimus muscle in the cat was seen to be supplied by a centrally located artery (about 70-μ diameter) and a vein (about 90-μ diameter), running together longitudinally in the tissue proper. From the central artery and vein, transverse arterioles and venules arise, forming "end-arterioles" and "end-venules" (25–50-μ internal diameter). No anastomoses between branches of similar size in the arborization of the transverse vessels are seen and an arteriovenous anastomosis was observed only occasionally ("in about 1 out of 20") in tenuissimus muscle preparations. The average endothelial capillary measures 1015 μ in length, with cross connections at every 200-μ interval. The average diameters of the capillaries were 4.7, 5.3, and 5.9 μ, at the beginning, in the middle, and at the end, respectively. In addition to the combined approach by light and electron microscopic methods for the study of the distribution and structure of the microvasculature in tenuissimus muscle, Ericson et al. (1973), by cytochemical techniques, determined the different types of fibers in the muscle and were able to quantitate the number of capillaries in close contact with each type of fiber. The values were 3.5 for A-fibers, 3.6 for B-fibers, and 3.8 for C-fibers, in the classification of skeletal muscle fibers by the presence of ATP-ase activity (Henneman and Olson, 1965). The number of capillaries per muscle fiber was counted at 0.95, and the morphological capillary surface area was calculated to be approximately 0.9 $m^2/100$ cm^3 of muscle tissue. Neither by vital microscopy nor in electron microscopic studies were Eriksson and Lisander (1972) or Ericson et al. (1973) able to observe "any arrangement of smooth muscle attributable to the morphologically defined concept of precapillary sphincter" in the tenuissimus muscle of the cat or the rabbit.

MICROCIRCULATION IN GASTROINTESTINAL VASCULATURES

Introduction

Descriptions of the vascular arrangement within the gastric and intestinal walls have been based on dissections, histology, and microangiographic investigations in fixed and dye-injected materials. There is general agreement concerning the anatomy and distribution of the major supplying arteries and draining veins. Regarding the vascular patterns of the small blood vessels in the gastric and intestinal walls, however, an uncertainty prevails. Because certain inherent factors, such as thickness of tissue, create technical problems for the ready application of currently available methodology for study by in vivo microscopy, information concerning the functional anatomy of gastric and intestinal microcirculation is scant and incomplete. In addition, the anatomic location of the viscera, in close contact with the intermittently moving diaphragm in the upper abdomen, makes in vivo examination cumbersome. Clearance studies have provided evidence of alteration in the distribution of microcirculatory blood flow, yet anatomic correlates implementing the hemodynamic and microcirculatory alterations seen under various physiologic, pharmacologic, and pathophysiologic conditions remain uncertain. As aptly noted by Wiedeman (1963), in organs such as the hollow viscera, with vast networks of freely interconnecting system of arcading arterioles and venules, it is extremely difficult to establish the path of blood flow without observing it in vivo.

GASTRIC MICROCIRCULATION IN VITRO

A considerable body of knowledge has evolved, since the early descriptions, notably by Arnold (1847) and Mall (1887), concerning the vascular topography of the gastric wall. In extensive and painstaking dissections of injected and fixed material, the branching of supplying arteries at the lesser and greater curvatures and the number and manner of formation of arterial anastomoses in different areas of the organ have been described. Disse (1904) defined and measured the distributing vessels of the submucosa and mucosal layers and concluded that the mucosal arteries are *end-arteries.* Similar conclusions were reached by Reeves (1920), Jatrou (1920), and Hoffman and Nather (1921).

In general, these descriptions agree that the arteries supplying the gastric wall arise from the lesser and greater curvatures and, unbranched, perforate the muscular layer, ramify, and form a rich submucosal arterial plexus. Mucosal arteries arise from this plexus and, anastomosing at either side the muscularis mucosa, finally divide into slender arterioles that perforate the mucosal membrane. A rich capillary network arises from these mucosal arterioles to enclose and supply glandular crypts in a honeycomb-like structure.

GASTRIC WALL MICROCIRCULATION IN VIVO

In contrast to the numerous descriptions of gastric vasculature and circulation derived from in vitro methods of study, similar reports based on in vivo observation are scant.

In a brief communication, Piasecki (1969) has described a method of transillumination for in vivo microscopy of gastric and mural microcirculation in the dog. However, it was not until a method for study in the rat was developed and applied by Rosenberg and Guth (1970) that a systematic examination of the gastric microcirculation was rendered possible in this organ by in vivo microscopy. By observing first the vasculature in the simple exteriorized stomach and then in an everted pouch of the organ in the anesthetized rat, these authors were able not only to confirm the source and distribution of the major supplying arteries and veins but also to witness the pattern of blood flow through the various tissue layers of the gastric wall. In a report of this study—the only report yet found—Guth and Rosenberg (1972) have given detailed descriptions of their observation in the living anesthetized animals. Therefore, the following discussion is based mainly on the description by these authors.

In their in vivo microscopic study, Guth and Rosenberg (1972) confirmed previous observations by Schnitzlein (1957) and Lambert (1965), namely, that the macroscopic branches of the celiac axis to the stomach of the rat are similar to those in man. In the gastric wall proper, Guth and Rosenberg found that the nutrient vessels to the muscular coat (averaging $20-35\ \mu$ in diameter) arise from the arterial branches as they pierce the muscle, before entering the submucosa. These vessels divide into smaller branches that curve in the muscle layer in a direction transverse to the long axis of the stomach. Two sets of capillaries are distinguished in the muscle coat, one deep and the other superficial, both running parallel to one another at $40-80\ \mu$ intervals. Capillaries communicate freely with those on the same plane as well as with those on different planes. The arteriole was rarely seen to continue its course to become a venule, thus forming a thoroughfare channel. Rather, it usually terminates by dividing into capillaries. The capillary network converges into venules that accompany the arterioles. These venules in turn drain into the venous plexus in the submucosa. The primary arterial branches, after giving off branches to the muscle coat, subdivide into smaller branches in outer portions of the submucosa. These vessels anastomose with each other and form the primary submucosa arterial arcades ($34-58\ \mu$ in diameter). Branches of these arterial arcades ($21-41\ \mu$ in diameter) in turn anastomose to form a secondary arcade. Smaller mucosal arterioles ($14-15\ \mu$ in diameter) arise from these arcades and pierce muscularis mucosa, and divide into two to four branches in the deep portion of the mucosa to form the rich network of mucosal capillaries. Guth and Rosenberg (1972) noted that the primary and secondary arcades, on the anterior wall and greater curvature of the stomach, form an extensive, continuous, interconnecting network. This network is much less extensive near the lesser curvature of the organ, where the main mucosal arteries give off branches to the mucosa directly with relatively few arterio-arterial anastomoses.

By careful removal of the external mucularis and direct exposure of the submucous vascular plexus, the authors were able to observe consecutive segments of interconnecting arterial branches and the direction and coloration of the blood flow (Figure 4). They gave special attention to vascular structures that might provide evidence for arteriovenous shunts, i.e., structures directly shunting blood from artery to vein, thus bypassing the intervening capillaries. No such shunts were seen. Guth and Rosenberg (1972) noted that an occasional submucous arterial branch disappeared behind a vein at a point of interception in its course through the submucosa, thus giving the impression of a direct anastomotic vascular connection. However, on careful tracing of the blood flow, and of the flow of injected contrast material, such vascular arrangements invariably proved to be merely sites of changes in the direction of the arterial vessel in its course toward the mucosa. The pattern of blood flow in the meshwork of the

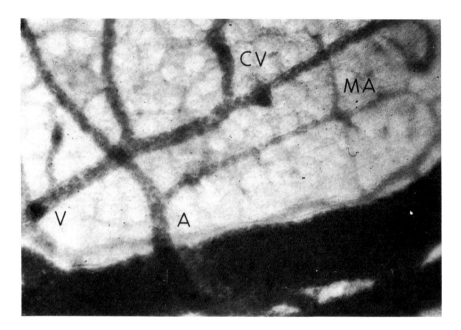

Figure 4. Photomicrograph of the submucosal preparation. The characteristic submucosal arterial (A) and venous (V) plexi are seen. The venous network can be distinguished by the larger diameter of its vessels and the presence of collecting veins (CV), seen in cross section, which drain into the venous anastomotic network. An arterial arcade gives rise to a mucosal arteriole (MA), which divides and enters the capillary network. The honeycomb-like appearance of the mucosal capillary bed is barely visible. (Original magnification ×100.) Reprinted by permission of Dr. Paul H. Guth.

interconnecting submucous arterial plexus of the stomach was found, in general, to be similar to that which was previously described by Baez (1959a) in the submucosal plexus of the small intestine of the rat, i.e., a continuous unidirectional blood flow toward the periphery through the main supplying arteries and an intermittent change in the direction of the flow in the consecutive interconnecting arterial arcades. A given arterial arcade may be first supplied with blood exclusively by one of the main arteries and then by the other main artery. The rat stomach preparation for observation of the submucosal vasculature, in combination with an everted pouch in situ, allowed Guth and Rosenberg (1972) to follow the distribution of the small blood vessels in the mucosa and to observe the flow of blood and of injected contrast material through them. Mucosal arteries were seen to arise from secondary submucosal arcades and enter the mucosa. Each mucosal artery divides into three to four smaller branches, which in turn break up into three to six capillaries in the mucosa. The pattern of blood flow could be followed from the mucosal arteries into the capillary at the base of the mucosa. Observation of the everted mucosa confirms the well-known honeycomb appearance of capillary distribution about the opening of the gastric glands (Figure 5) and the blood flow can be traced from the capillaries into collecting veins (21−24-μ diameter) in the mucosa. Because the authors were unable to find either arteriovenous anastomoses or arterial branches extending from the base to the surface of the mucosa, they questioned the presence of arteriovenous shunts in the gastric microcirculation of the rat.

Arteriovenous Anastomoses in the Gastric Wall

In a monograph by Clara (1937) and in reports by Watzka (1936), Shumacker (1938), and de Busscher (1948), two main types of arteriovenous pathways are described. One consists of a complex interlacing, knot-like arrangement of blood vessels, exhibiting an epithelioid type of cell in tunica media, a "glomus." The other, although of a sinus form, exists as a more direct channel and is endowed with typical well-developed smooth muscle cells in the wall. Barclay and Bentley (1949), noticing in the mucous membrane of human stomach the absence of radiopaque material injected immediately upon removal by surgery, proposed that in the gastric wall there were arteriovenous anastomoses. They suggest that the injected material flowed from arteries to veins through direct shunts located

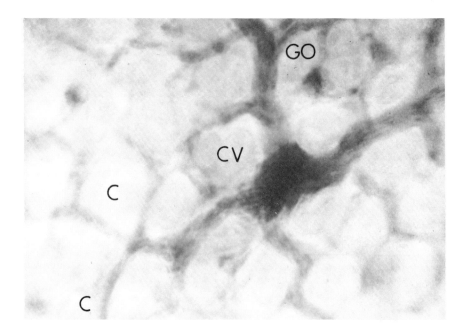

Figure 5. Photomicrograph of the mucosal preparation. Honeycomb-like appearance of the capillaries (C) surrounding the glands and ultimately draining into collecting veins (CV) is clearly observed. The orifices (GO) of the glands in the center of surrounding capillaries can be seen in some areas. (Original magnification ×200.) Reprinted by permission of Dr. Paul H. Guth.

in the submucosal plexus. Barlow, Bentley, and Walden (1951), in histologic and microradiographic studies, were unable to find any evidence of the glomus form of arteriovenous anastomoses in submucosa as described by de Busscher (1948). However, they found that arteriovenous anastomoses of the "direct sinus" type were abundantly present. Barlow (1952), using the techniques of double injections of dye and radiopaque materials, found arteriovenous anastomoses to be usually a branch of mucosal artery, but occasionally to arise from a limb of the submucosal plexus. The anastomosis consisted of an arterial end (variable in length), a short narrow junction area, and a short, wide venous channel, and terminated by either joining a distal mucosal vein or doubling back on itself, anastomosing with a tributary of its accompanying vein. He added that the anastomoses are usually found arising from each mucosal artery and are equally distributed in different parts of the stomach.

Walder (1952), accepting the presence of arteriovenous anastomoses in the submucous layer of the human stomach, carried out investigations to determine their size and responses to stimuli, both physical and pharmacologic. The results of the injection of drugs, nerve stimulation, and varying perfusion pressures were inconclusive. However, the emergence in the gastroepiploic vein of glass microspheres (140 μ in size), when injected in the gastroepiploic artery, seemed to be a confirmation of patent arteriovenous shunts, described by Barlow (1952). On the basis of these findings, as well as the results of other studies by Prinzmetal et al. (1948), which show a constancy in the proportion of large (140 μ) to small (40 μ) glass spheres passing from arterial to venous blood under different hemodynamic conditions, Barlow et al. have proposed that the arteriovenous structure in the stomach must be functionally characterized by an all-or-none type of dynamic activity, i.e., the anastomotic vessels do not maintain an intermediary position of lumen. This would be a unique type of functional morphology of the stomach arteriovenous shunt vessels, which is at variance with dynamic activity of other blood flow controlling segments of the microvasculature. It is well established that the arteriole, metarteriole, and precapillary sphincter all exhibit a measurable gradient of constriction and dilatation, brought about by physical chemical stimuli (Baez, 1961, 1968, 1969,; Altura 1971, 1972).

In spite of the various reports attesting to the existence of abundant arteriovenous shunts in the gastric wall, no general agreement has been reached regarding their precise location and distribution in mucosa and submucosa. Consequently, their significance in the regulation of the mucosal blood flow has continued to be questioned. In histologic studies in the rat, Schnitzlein (1957) described arteriolar vessels penetrating the muscularis mucosa to anastomose with venous channels, but failed to disclose their existence in submucosa. Nylander and Olerud (1961), with a microangiographic study in vagotomized rats, also failed to disclose arteriovenous shunts in submucosa. However, they described mucosal arterioles running upward within a network of interlocking capillaries and forming arteriovenous anastomoses near the mucosal surface. In a more recent study, the presence of arteriovenous anastomotic channels, similar to those noted by Barlow et al. (1951), although smaller (10–40 μ), were described in the submucosa of the rat stomach by Hase and Moss (1973). In their fixed preparations, injected with colloidal carbon and different colored silicone rubber, the presence of arteriovenous shunts was said usually to occur at a site where arteries and veins jointly penetrated the muscle coat. They claimed that in microdissection and histology of tissue of the fixed preparations, the yellow (arteriole) and red (venous) rubber mixed. The submucosal shunting vessels seemed to be more distended in the ischemic areas of the stomach preparations in the stressed animals. Although no quantitative data were given regarding the frequency of distribution of such arteriovenous channels, the authors pointed out some of the morphologic characteristics of the mucosa capillary meshwork in the antrum and corpus of the rat stomach. In the antral region the capillaries were shorter, straighter, and coarser than in the corpus.

The significance of anatomic arteriovenous shunts in the regulation of gastric mucosal blood flow has also been questioned on the basis of physiologic studies in the dog. Quantitative analysis of venous blood-microsphere content, after the injection of spheres into the celiac axis, allowed Delaney and Grim (1964) to conclude that no more than 1 or 2% of the blood flow passed through arteriovenous shunts. Also, Bell (1967) obtained evidence, using a dye dilution technique, that indicated the presence of functioning arteriovenous shunts but only to a limited degree. There is thus a need for further studies by multiple approaches to define the regulation of blood flow in the microcirculation of this organ.

INTESTINAL MICROCIRCULATION

As with descriptions of the patterns of the arteriovenous pathway in the stomach, available information concerning the microcirculation of the small intestine is derived, by and large, from the observation of injected and fixed preparations. A comprehensive review of early pertinent literature dealing with such preparations can be found in Noer's (1943) extensive and detailed report of studies of the vascular patterns in jejunum and ileum. In specimens prepared by liquid latex injection, Noer compared the vascular architecture and distribution in the mesentery and intestinal wall of over a dozen different animals and man. Except for some variation in the number of mesenteric arterial arcades, the basic architecture was found to be similar in all animals studied and in man. Branches of the intestinal arteries form mesenteric arcades. These in turn give rise to vasa recta, which, on reaching the intestinal wall, form the main arterial mural trunks. In general, in the animals studied, and in man, Noer noted that the mural trunks, after sending branches to the opposite side give, in their course, lateral arterial branches (three to four in number), which then form anastomotic arcades with similar branches from neighboring vasa recta. The main vasa recta continues to the antimesentery border of the viscera. Noer described three types of anastomoses between the terminal portions of the main arterial trunks in the antimesentery area: (1) direct interdigitation between mural trunks of the opposite sides, (2) a plexiform arrangement, and (3) short arcuate mural anastomoses. The veins were found to follow the same general pattern of distribution.

Reports on the search for an experimental animal that might exhibit a vascular architecture and distribution similar to man became available some 10 years later. Using basically the same latex injection technique on intestinal specimens of rabbit, dog, opossum, and man, Jacobson and Noer (1952) were able further to describe their observation of intestinal mucosal microvasculature. In essence, they found that (1) "the capillary network is derived from both the artery of the villus and the submucous plexus," (2) "the axial vessel is venous in nature," and (3) "arterial supply and venous drainage exist throughout the villus from tip to base." Jacobson and Noer also noted that the microvasculature of the villi in the rabbit ileum bears considerable resemblance to that of man.

In the monkey, Reynolds, Brim, and Sheehy (1967) found that the villus capillaries are derived from the capillary plexus surrounding the crypts of Lieberkühn, and not from a central villus arteriole. However, they noted that "the rat and rabbit mucosa prepared by the same technique reveal arterial and venous channels extending the length of the villi" and thus closely resemble the classical description. Reynolds et al. noted that the villus capillary bed forms a network of interconnected vessels in the upper half of the villus. The lower half of the bed is composed of vessels that essentially run parallel to each other and appear to be continuous with a plexus of capillary channels ramifying between the bases of the villi. The resulting subvillus plexus surrounds the luminal openings of the crypts of Lieberkühn, giving the characteristic honeycomb appearance. Small arterial branches bifurcate to form capillary arteriolar twigs that are distributed to the undersurface of the mucosal cryptic layer. Venous channels are also in communication with the cryptic plexus, but do not terminate at this level. Instead, the terminal branches penetrate the cryptic layer of the mucosa and a single centrally located vein enters the base of each villus, extending to the apex. In essence, the distinguishing feature of the microvascular architecture in the *Macaca mulatta* monkey consists in the arterial supply, which is distributed to the undersurface of the mucosa. The terminal arteriolar twigs run continuously into the capillary plexus surrounding the crypts of Lieberkühn. The capillary nets of the villi are derived from the cryptic plexus via a series of parallel capillary channels that extend from the lumenal surface of the cryptic plexus to approximately midlevel of the villi where they break up into a mesh of capillaries. These vessels converge near the apex of each villus into a single axially located villus vein. The central vein passes into the cryptic layer of the mucosa, where it joins other venous channel leading to the submucosal venous return system. In addition, an alternative venous return was found in the form of a second set of venous channels that arise from the cryptic capillary plexus and extend to the venous channels leading to the submucosa.

INTESTINAL MICROCIRCULATORY PATTERNS

In spite of both a thinner wall structure, amenable to transillumination for microscopy, and a relative accessibility and mobility for exposure of the small intestines, reports on systematic study by in vivo microscopy of the mural microcirculation of this segment of the viscera are remarkably few. Although some information regarding quantitation of pressure gradients in selected segments of intestinal vasculature has recently become available in the work of Bohlen and Gore (1974), descriptions of the architecture and distribution are, by and large, fragmentary. They are usually incidental to observation of the responses of submucous and mucosal capillary, to neurogenic stimuli, as by Bohlen et al. (1971), or to drugs and biogenic substances, as noted by Hambleton (1914), King and Arnold (1922), Kokas and Ludany (1934), and Wells and Johnson (1934), among others. A method for intravital examination of intestinal microcirculation introduced by Baez (1959a), which used colloidal carbon injection for further corroborative observation of the mucosal microcirculatory pattern of the observed isolated segment of intestine, has yielded the following description in the living rat.

Mural Supplying Vessels

From the last mesenteric arterial arcade, two types of vasa recta arise (at 4–6-mm intervals) to supply the intestinal wall. The main vasa recta (60–80 μ, o.d.) and the small vasa recta (30–40 μ, o.d.) both pierce the muscularis in the mesentery border of the organ at regular intervals of 4–6 mm (Figure 6). Both types of vasa recta, previously described in various mammals and man by Eisenberg (1924), Noer (1943), and Jacobson and Noer (1952), among others, are seen equally to distribute in anterior and posterior aspects of the viscera. The main arteries, after variable lengths as a single trunk in the submucosa, divide into two or three branches. Each arterial branch in turn breaks up into four to six smaller (30–40 μ, o.d.) branches, and reaching the antimesenteric border, anastomose with similar branches of the opposite side. In their course, the main arteries give off three to five secondary arteries at various degrees of angularity, which inosculate end to end with similar arterial branches originating from neighboring vasa recta (2 in Figure 7) and form the main system of mural arterial arcades in the submucosa. The small vasa recta interspaced between the large ones soon divide into four to six branches in the lower third of the mesentery border of the organ. The branches terminate by anastomosing with secondary branches of neighboring vasa recta. The meshwork of interconnected arterial vessels gives off secondary and tertiary arterial loops in the submucosa.

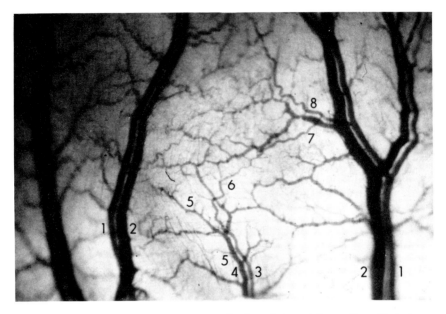

Figure 6. Photomicrograph from mesentery border of the rat ileum (from Kodachrome transparency). (1) Main incoming arteries with (2) accompanying veins (large vasa recta). Small vasa recta, artery (3), and vein (4). Mucosal arteries (5) originating from main trunk (6). End portion of small vasa recta inosculates with a secondary submucous arterial loop (7), which in turn arises from a main arterial arcade (8) in the submucosa. (Original magnification ×7.)

Muscular Coat

Vessels nourishing the muscular coat usually arise from the secondary arcade, less frequently from the proximal end of mucosal arteries. The majority of these vessels (10–14 μ, o.d.) are metarterioles that turn outward and, reaching the plane of cleavage between the circular and longitudinal muscle fibers, run in this plane in a general direction transverse to the long axis of the organ. Upon reaching the intermuscular septum, the arteriole gives off two sets of endothelial capillary vessels at regular intervals: (1) those destined to supply the circular muscle bundles remain in the same plane as the parent vessels; (2) those supplying longitudinal bundles twist further outward, running between and distributing to muscularis and serosa. These small blood vessels (Figure 8)–some equipped with precapillary sphincters, others without–run parallel to one another at 40–60-μ intervals along the cleavage between muscle fibers. They communicate freely with each other by lateral branches arising in the same plane every 200–250 μ in their course and also with similar capillary vessels of the adjacent layer of the muscle. The main arteriole or metarteriole, after variable lengths of 0.5–1 mm, may divide into two or, without further branching, may arch inward on itself to become a small venule on reaching the submucosa. The

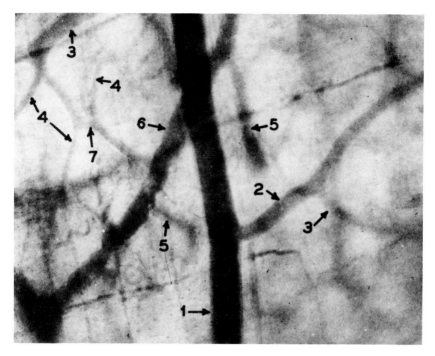

Figure 7. Photomicrograph from anterior wall of ileum (from Kodachrome transparency). (1) Main submucous anastomotic artery. (2) Secondary arterial loop, giving off (3) a mucosal artery. In the left upper corner (3), a terminal segment of a mucosal artery breaks up into branches (4) to neighboring villi. (5) Emerging mucosal venules join submucous venules (6). A final interarterial anastomosis can be seen (7) deep in submucosa. (Original magnification ×275.)

venule draining the muscular coat, enlarged by other venules formed by neighboring capillaries, finds its way to a submucous vein draining the mucosa. This type of vessel, which arose singly in the submucosa and returned to the submucosa as a small venule (22–26 μ) after giving out its capillary network in muscularis externa, constitutes a distinctly organized terminal vascular structural unit.

Microscopic observation of the pattern of blood flow in the living animal—i.e., the direction and distribution of the flowing blood, its coloration, and the lesser or greater apparent proportion of plasma to cell population, as well as the microvascular responses to various stimuli—permitted a reliable basis for determining the structural microvascular components and their respective interconnections. The network of capillaries in the muscular coat is composed of muscular and nonmuscular elements. The muscular components are the centrally located metarterioles with their precapillary sphincters (when present) at the origin of dependent capillaries. The metarteriole and the sphincters, in addition to exhibiting vasomotor activity ("vasomotion"), constitute the most reactive

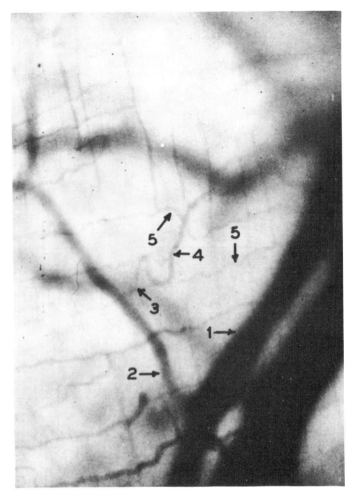

Figure 8. Photomicrograph from anterior wall of ileum (from Kodachrome transparency). (1) Main arterial and venous limbs of submucous plexus. (2) Main anastomosing arterial branch. (3) Mucosal artery which disappears from focus after giving off an arteriole (4) to muscular layer. (5) Metarterioles supplying capillaries for oppositely oriented muscle bundles. (Original magnification ×92.)

vascular elements thus far observed in the entire intestinal vasculature. The endothelial capillaries (4.5–6.2 μ, i.d.) may run in their course 700–950 μ in length before joining a neighboring capillary vessel. Thus the capillaries in muscularis externa, similarly to capillaries in striated muscle, as described by Zweifach and Metz (1955), Baez and Orkin (1967), Smaje et al. (1970), and Eriksson and Myrhage (1972), constitute some of the longest endothelial microvessels in the body.

The vasculature of the muscular layer may vary in that the supplying vessel is a rather long arteriole (24–28 μ, i.d.), which, on reaching the muscularis, gives off two to three metarterioles. The main trunk either terminates by breaking up into three to four endothelial capillaries or turns inward to become a draining venule, a thoroughfare channel. Another variation can be seen in the venous drainage toward the mesentery border of the small intestines. Small venules, formed either by the confluence of four to six capillaries in the muscle coat, or the thoroughfare channel convey blood directly to the vein accompanying the small vasa recta, thus avoiding the submucous venous plexus.

Mucosal Microvasculature

Arteries that supply the mucosal layer may arise from the first, second, or third arterial loops or arcades. Those originating from the first loop usually give off a branch to the external muscularis as described above (3 in Figure 8). The main trunk and arteries arising from secondary loops continue toward the muscularis mucosa, giving off in their course one or two short arterioles (14–18 μ). These immediately break up into three to six capillaries, which after a semicircular turn, reunite as a venule (18–22 μ), to join a submucous vein. This capillary arrangement in submucosa surrounds an area of tissue from 40 to 60 μ in diameter and seems to correspond to vascular formations described as "rete" by Mall (1887), which in the living animal appear to surround nerve cell aggregates and/or lymphatic channels. These capillaries communicate freely with each other and with similar neighboring endothelial capillary formations in the submucosa. Deeper in the submucosa all mucosal arteries, after sending a short anastomotic branch to a neighboring mucosal artery, give off one or two arteriolar vessels (at nearly right angles) before penetrating the villus. The lateral branches break up into six to eight endothelial capillaries, which again arrange themselves in a semicircular fashion, surrounding a larger 80–100-μ area of tissue. These capillary arrangements are regularly distributed throughout the deep mucosa and seem to correspond to glandular tissues forming the crypts of Lieberkühn. Venules (18–24 μ, o.d.) draining these, and capillaries from similar neighboring formations, join a venule draining two or three villi (Figure 9). The terminal portion of the mucosal artery, reduced in size (12–18 μ, o.d.), penetrates the villi as a single- or double-branched vessel.

Direct vital microscopy from serosa to mucosa of the cleared, distended loop of intestine has allowed observation of the mucosal arteries from origin to penetrations at the base of the villi (Figure 10). Using this approach, Baez (1959b) reported that the emerging villus venule was also readily seen and photographed in the living animal. In studies by Baez (unpublished), eversion of the loop of intestine permitted extension of mucosal microvasculature examination in vivo. Further verification was made with the aid of colloid carbon injection and formalin fixation of the same loop under observation. In the

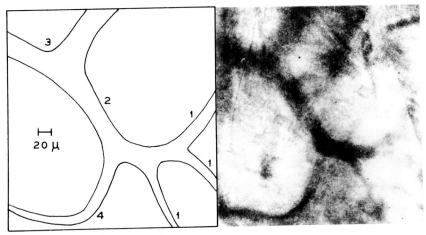

1 VILLI   VENULES
2 MUCOSAL VENULE
3 SUBMUCOUS VEIN
4 ARTERIAL CAPILLARY

Figure 9. Photomicrograph and projection drawing of base of villi (from Kodachrome transparency). (1) Converging venules from neighboring villi. (2) Mucosal venule on its way to join a submucosal venule (3). A vessel of capillary dimensions (4) which injects arterial blood into mucosal venule. (Original magnification ×275.)

everted segment of ileum, before carbon injection, a mucosal arteriole (14–18 μ) is seen penetrating the villi. It ascends towards the apex as a single trunk giving off numerous capillary side branches. Upon reaching the apex of the villus, the arteriole either divides into two or breaks up into 8–10 capillaries. On occasion (in one out of ten villi), the arteriole bifurcates into two slightly smaller branches immediately on penetration of the villus. The vessels ascending in parallel toward the apex distribute capillary side branches in a similar pattern. In both instances the capillaries in the ascending and descending portion of the villus interconnect freely with each other, resulting in the classical meshwork module of the intestinal villi (Figure 11). The capillaries given off at the apex of the villi proper soon receive other capillaries and, joining together with them, form a distinct draining venule (20–24 μ, o.d.) about one-third from the apex. The venule joins a submucous vein at the exit from the villus. A variation of mucosal microvascular pattern is found in villi surrounding Payer's patch. Here, three to four sinuous arterioles ascend to the villus from the base. In addition, numerous endothelial capillaries from neighboring Lieberkühn crypts contribute to the capillary module of the villi (Figure 12).

Arteriovenous Anastomosis

As with the gastric microvasculature, in spite of the assertion by Barlow (1952) that, "in an organ of phasic function in nature, arteriovenous anastomoses are to

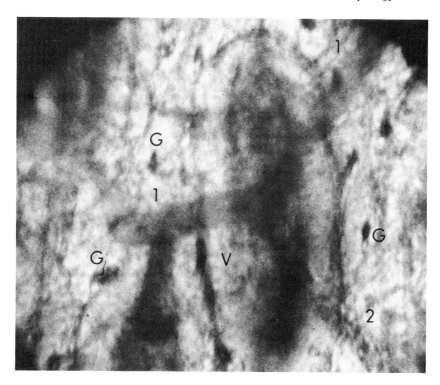

Figure 10. Photomicrograph of mucosal layer in intact loop of ileum of the rat. It shows a mucosal artery (1) penetrating a villus. A venule (2) showing glandular blood flow, emerges from villus (V). The orifices of glands (G) in the center of surrounding capillaries can be seen in some. From Kodachrome cinemicrophotography in the noninjected ileum. (Original magnification ×210.)

be expected," or postulation that the "escape" of the vasculature in the alimentary canal, either from sympathetic nerve stimulation, as suggested by Folkow et al. (1964), or from infusion of norepinephrine, as noted by Dresel, Folkow, and Wallentin (1966), is due to the opening of submucosal arterio-venous shunts, no such direct anastomosis has been observed. In no instance, upon careful search in separate zones of jejunum and ileum, has a direct short cut of blood from artery to vein been found. The only sites where blood of bright arterial coloration has been seen to divert into a vein were (1) in the mesentery border, through the throughfare channels leading from some of the muscular arterioles to the vein accompanying small vasa recta and (2) at the base of the villi, as shown in Figure 9. The latter small vessels (18–20 μ, o.d.), which on occasion receive the vein draining the villus, are not actually true arterio-venous anastomoses, for in their course they also give off a few branches to neighboring structures in the submucosa and deep mucosa. Although the vascu-lar formations do not occur at every villus, they seem to correspond in location

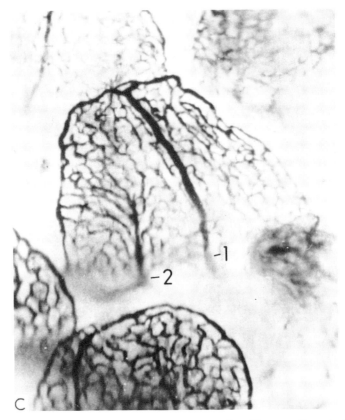

Figure 11. Photograph of India ink-injected ileum preparation. The ascending arteriole (1) after giving numerous capillaries breaks up in fountain-like arrangement upon reaching villous' apex. A single venule (2) formed at about one-third from the apex of the villus drains blood toward submucosal vein. (Original magnification × 120.)

to those described by Spanner (1932) and Muratori (1941) as arteriovenous anastomoses.

COMMENTS

The architectural module of the microcirculatory bed in the outer smooth muscle coat of the alimentary canal, functionally a motor structure for peristaltic activity, shows great similarity to microvascular modules in the several skeletal muscles studied. In essence, both motor structures exhibit endothelial capillaries in parallel, cross connected at regular intervals, forming networks in oblong meshes built around centrally located small terminal arterioles. Some of the arterioles show preferential channel arrangement, but no direct arteriovenous shunting structures. In the functionally absorptive-secretory mucosal layer of the

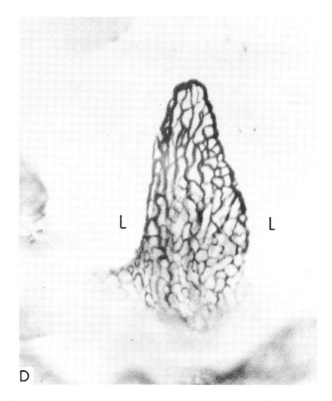

Figure 12. Photograph of India ink-injected ileum preparation. Three tortuous arterioles ascending in parallel break up into capillary network supplying the single villus bordering a lymph node (L). (Original magnification × 120.)

alimentary canal requiring a more extensive exchange surface area, the capillaries interconnect more frequently.

A particularly vexing question is the absence or infrequent occurrence of direct microscopic arteriovenous shunts in the alimentary canal. The descriptions of the pattern of distribution and structure of gastric and intestinal microcirculation, derived from study by in vivo microscopy, are as yet much too brief to clarify the problem. Precise knowledge of the nutritional requirements and metabolic priorities of these tissues will permit one to define how the microscopic structure and arteriovenous shunts of the vasculatures subserve their physiologic function.

Quantification of the dynamics of capillary blood flow in skeletal muscle, gastric and intestinal microcirculations of different mammalian species by direct in vivo microscopic techniques should help to resolve many of the uncertainties concerning the distribution and regulation of blood flow in these regions of the circulation.

LITERATURE CITED

Algire, G. H. 1954. The transparent chamber technique for observation of the peripheral circulation, as studied in mice. *In* G. E. W. Wolstenholme and I. S. Freement (eds.), Peripheral Circulation in Man, pp. 58–67. J & A Churchhill, London.

Algire, G. H., and R. Merwin. 1955. Vascular pattern in tissues and graft within transparent chambers in mice. Angiology 6:311–318.

Altura, B. M. 1971. Chemical and humoral regulation of blood flow through the precapillary sphincter. Microvasc. Res. 3:361–384.

Altura, B. M. 1972. Can metarteriolar vessels occlude their lumens in response to vasoactive substances? Proc. Soc. Exp. Biol. Med. 140:1270–1274.

Arnold 1847. Handbuch der Atatomica des Menschen II. Bd. Abt. Freiburg.

Baez, S. 1959*a*. Microcirculation in the intramural vessels of the small intestine of the rat. *In* S. R. M. Reynolds and B. W. Zweifach (eds.), The Microcirculation. Proceedings of the 5th Conference on Microcirculation Physiology and Pathology, pp. 114–129. University of Illinois Press, Urbana, Ill.

Baez, S. 1959*b*. Microcirculation in the small intestine of the rat (motion picture). *In* E. P. Fowler, Jr., and B. W. Zweifach (eds.), Intravascular phenomena: Proceedings of the 7th Microcirculation Conference, pp. 66–67. University of Illinois Press, Urbana.

Baez, S. 1961. Response characteristics of perfused microvessels to pressure and vasoactive stimuli. Angiology 12:452–461.

Baez, S. 1968. Vascular smooth muscle quantitation of cell thickness in the wall of arterioles in the living animal in situ. Science 159:536–538.

Baez, S. 1969. Simultaneous measurements of radii and wall thickness of microvessels in the anesthetized rat. Circ. Res. 25:315–329.

Baez, S. 1973. An open cremaster muscle preparation for the study of blood vessels by in vivo microscopy. Microvasc. Res. 5:384–394.

Baez, S., and L. R. Orkin. 1967. Microcirculatory reactions to chemical denervation in the anesthetized rat. 4th Conference for Microcirculation. Bibl. Anat. 9:61–65.

Barclay, A. E., and F. H. Bentley. 1949. The vascularization of the human stomach. Br. J. Radiol. 22:62–69.

Barlow, T. E. 1952. Vascular patterns in the alimentary canal. *In* G. E. W. Wolstenholme (ed.), Visceral Circulation, Ciba Foundation Symposium, pp. 21–36. J & A Churchill, London.

Barlow, T. F., F. H. Bentley, and D. N. Walder. 1951. Arteries, veins and arteriovenous anastomoses in the human stomach. Surg. Gyn. Obst. 93:657–671.

Bell, P. R. F. 1967. Gastric arteriovenous shunts. An investigation using dye dilution technique. Scand. J. Gastroenterol. 2:59–67.

Bohlen, H. G., P. Hutchins, C. Rapela, and H. D. Green. 1971. The effects of carotid occlusion on villi vessels of the small intestine. Fed. Proc. 30:716 (Abstr.).

Bolhen, H. G., and R. W. Gore. 1974. Microvascular pressure in innervated intestinal muscle. Fed. Proc. 3:393 (Abstr.).

Brånemark, P. I., and E. Eriksson. 1971. Method for studying qualitative and quantitative changes of blood flow in skeletal muscle. Acta Physiol. Scand. 84:284–288.

Clara, M. 1937. Die arteriovenosen anastomosen. J. A. Barth, Leipzig.

Clark, W., and E. LeGross. 1952. The Tissue of the Body. Oxford University Press, New York. pp. 144–145.

de Busscher, G. 1948. Les anastomoses arterioveineuses de l'estomac. Acta Neerl. Morph. 6:1–19.

Delaney, J. P., and D. Grim. 1964. Canine gastric blood flow and its distribution. Am. J. Physiol. 207:1195–1202.

Disse, E. 1904. Uber die blutgefässe der menschlichen magenschleimhaut besonders über arterien derselben. Arch. Mikr. Anat. 63:512–531.

Dresel, P., B. Folkow, and I. Wallentin. 1966. Rubidium 86 clearance during neurogenic redistribution of intestinal blood flow. Acta. Physiol. Scand. 67:173–184.

Eisenberg, H. B. 1924. Intestinal arteries. Anat. Rec. 28:227–242.

Ericson, L. E., E. Eriksson, and B. Johansson. 1973. Morphological aspects of the microvessels in cat skeletal muscle. In H. Harders (ed.), Advances in Microcirculation, pp. 62–79. S. Karger, Hamburg.

Eriksson, E., and B. Lisander. 1972. Changes in precapillary resistance in skeletal muscle vessels studied by intravital microscopy. Acta Physiol. Scand. 84:295–305.

Eriksson, E., and R. Myrhage. 1972. Microvascular dimensions and blood flow in skeletal muscle. Acta Physiol. Scand. 86:211–222.

Folkow, B., D. H. Lewis, O. Lundgren, L. Mellander, and I. Wallentin. 1964. The effect of graded vasoconstrictor fiber stimulation on the intestinal resistance and capacitance vessels. Acta Physiol. Scand. 61:445–457.

Grant, R. T. 1964. Direct observation of skeletal muscle blood vessels (rat cremaster). J. Physiol. 172:123–137.

Grant, R. T. 1966. The effect of denervation on skeletal muscle blood vessels (rat cremaster). J. Anat. 100:305–316.

Guth, P. H., and A. Rosenberg. 1972. In vivo microscopy of the gastric microcirculation. J. Digest. Dis. 17:391–398.

Hambleton, B. T. 1914. Note upon the movement of intestinal villi. Am. J. Physiol. 34:446–447.

Hase, T., and B. J. Moss. 1973. Microvascular changes of gastric mucosa in the development of stress ulcer in the rat. Gastroenterology 65:224–234.

Heileman, H. 1902. Das Verhalten der Muskelgefässe während der Kontraktion. Arch. Anat. Physiol. 45–53.

Henneman, E., and C. B. Olson. 1965. Relations between structure and functions in the design of skeletal muscle. J. Neurophysiol. 28:598.

Hoffman, L., and K. Nather. 1921. Zur Anatomie der Magenarterien, Eine chirurgische Behandlung. Arch. F. Klin. Chir. 115:650–671.

Jacobson, L. R., and R. J. Noer. 1952. The vascular pattern of the intestinal villi in various laboratory animals and man. Anat. Rec. 114:85–101.

Jatrou, S. 1920. Uber die arterielle Versorgung des Magens und ihre Beziehung zum Uicus ventriculi. Deutsche Z. Chir. 159:196–223.

King, C. E. Ed., and L. Arnold. 1922. The activities of the intestinal mucosal motor mechanism. Am. J. Physiol. 59:97–121.

Kokás, E., and G. Ludány. 1934. Nouvelles recherches sur la regulation hormonale des mouvements de villocites. Compt. Rend. Soc. Biol. 117:972–973.

Krogh, A. 1919. The number and distribution of capillaries in muscles with calculations of the oxygen pressure head necessary for supplying the tissue. J. Physiol. (London) 52:409–415.

Krogh, A. 1929. The Anatomy and Physiology of Capillaries. Yale University Press, New Haven.

Lambert, R. 1965. Surgery of the Digestive System in the Rat. Charles C. Thomas, Springfield, Ill.

Mall, F. P. 1887. Die Blut und Lymph Wege im Dünndarm. des Hundes. Abh. d. Math.-Phys. 14:153−200.

Muratori, G. 1941. Constributo alla vascolavizzazione sanguigna del linfo-noduli intestinali dell'uomo. Att. 1st Veneto 2:479.

Noer, R. J. 1943. The blood vessels of the jejunum and ileum: A comparative study of man and certain laboratory animals. Am. J. Anat. 73:293−334.

Nylander, G., and S. Olerud. 1961. The vascular pattern of the gastric mucosa of the rat following vagotomy. Surg. Gyn. Obst. 12:475−480.

Piasecki, C. 1969. In vivo transillumination of the submucous plexus of vessels in the dog's stomach. J. Physiol. 201:69 (Abstr.).

Prinzmetal, M., E. M. Ornitz, Jr., B. Simkin, and H. C. Bergman. 1948. Arteriovenous anastomoses in the liver, spleen and lungs. Am. J. Physiol. 152:48−52.

Reeves, T. B. 1920. A study of the arteries supplying the stomach and duodenum and their relation to ulcer. Surg. Gyn. Obst. 30:374−385.

Reynolds, D. G., J. Brim, and T. Sheehy. 1967. The vascular architecture of the small intestinal mucosa of the monkey (Macaca mulatta). Anat. Rec. 159:211−218.

Rosenberg, A., and P. H. Guth. 1970. A method for the in vivo study of the gastric microcirculation. Microvasc. Res. 2:111−112.

Schnitzlein, H. N. 1957. Regulation of blood flow through the stomach of the rat. Anat. Rec. 127:735−754.

Schumaker, S. 1938. Über die Bedeutung der Arteriovenosen Anastomosen und der Epitheloiden Muskelzellen. Z. mikr. Anat. Forsch. 43:107−130.

Smaje, L., B. W. Zweifach, and M. Intaglietta. 1970. Micropressures and capillary filtration coefficients in single vessels of the cremaster muscle in the rat. Microvasc. Res. 2:96−110.

Spalteholz, W. 1888. Die Vertheilung der Blutgefasse im Muskel. Abhandl. d. K.S. Ges. d. Wiss 24:507−532.

Spanner, R. 1932. Neue Befunde uber die Blutwege der Darmwand und ihre functionel. Bedetung. Morph. 69:394−454.

Walder, D. 1952. Arteriovenous anastomoses in the human stomach. Clin. Sci. 11:59−71.

Watzka, M. 1936. Über Gefässpieren und arteriovenosen Anastomosen. Z. mikr. Anat. Forsch. 39:30−54.

Wells, E. W. 1960. The microanatomy of muscle. In G. H. Bourne (ed.), Structure and Function of Muscle, Vol. 1, pp. 21−61. Academic Press, New York.

Wells, H. S., and R. G. Johnson. 1934. The intestinal villi and their circulation in relation to absorption and secretion of fluid. Am. J. Physiol. 109:387−402.

Wiedeman, M. P. 1963. Patterns of arteriovenous pathways. In W. F. Hamilton and P. Dow (eds.), Handbook of Physiology, Section 2, Volume II, pp. 891−933. American Physiology Society, Washington, D.C.

Zweifach, B. W., and D. B. Metz. 1955. Selective distribution of blood through the terminal vascular bed of mesenteric structure and skeletal muscle. Angiology 6:282−290.

chapter 4

ULTRASTRUCTURE OF THE TERMINAL VASCULAR BED AS RELATED TO FUNCTION

Joachim R. Wolff

Various sections of the terminal vascular bed are distinguished by vital microscopists and physiologists, such as arterioles, terminal arterioles, metarterioles, arterial and venous sides of capillaries, sinusoids, terminal or postcapillary, collecting, and muscular venules, and other kinds of small arterial and venous vessels (Majno, Palade, and Schoefl, 1961; Fernando and Movat, 1964a, 1964b; Movat and Fernando, 1964; Rhodin, 1967, 1968; Hammersen, 1968). However, it is difficult to describe their ultrastructure separately, not only because the definitions vary somewhat from one organ and one author to another, but also because their functional and structural characteristics show gradual transitions, i.e. no clear boundaries exist. Consequently, this chapter is confined to "terminal arterioles," "capillaries," and "venules." Their structural aspects and functional properties are treated together. Nevertheless, a short survey of the structural differences between these three types of vessels is presented.

ARTERIOLES

As already mentioned, there are no distinct boundaries between small arteries, arterioles, terminal arterioles, and—as far as they exist—metarterioles. Along this sequence the endothelial cells become gradually more flattened, while the number of interendothelial contacts per vascular cross section decreases; i.e., the endothelial cells change from a lancet-like shape with long axis parallel to that of the vessel to a more disk-like shape. The size and shape of endothelial cells depend, however, very much on the degree of contraction at which the vessel has been preserved in the fixed tissue. This may also be the reason for the varying numbers of endothelial vesicles that have been observed, especially when the tissue was fixed by immersion (Moore and Ruska, 1957; Fawcett, 1959; Stingl, 1971). One of the characteristic features of the smallest arterial vessels, often including the arterial side of capillaries, are the numerous basal protrusions of the endothelium. Breaking through the basal lamina and, if present, through the discontinuous internal elastic membrane, they adhere or even make close contacts with the smooth muscle cells. These myoendothelial contacts have also been found to be numerous at capillary sphincters and also in venules (Fernando and Movat, 1964b; Rhodin, 1967, 1968). The functional significance of these myoendothelial contacts is unknown. Some authors assume that they may be related to transport phenomena (Mohamed, Waterhouse, and Friederici, 1973). By transmitting messages from the blood (Romanul and Bannister, 1962), they may also induce contractions of the smooth muscle (Rhodin, 1968). In the vessel wall, contractility does not seem to be restricted to smooth muscle cells. At least some endothelia might be contractile, too (see below). Therefore, a similar mechanism might exist in both the close contacts between pericytes, smooth muscle cells, and contractile fibrocytes in the intestinal villi (Güldner, Wolff, and Keyserlingk, 1972), and in the myoendothelial contacts of arterioles. One could think of a synchronizing effect on the contraction of smooth muscle and endothelium. Endothelia of arterioles, as of other terminal vessels, usually contain small filaments (60–90 Å ϕ) that accumulate near the cell surfaces and are supplemented by thicker filaments and microtubules (see below and Figures 2 and 6; Fernando and Movat, 1964a; Cecio, 1967). Even cross-striated fibrils have been described in normal arterioles of the myometrium (Röhlich and Oláh, 1967), and in cerebral arteries and arterioles during hypertension (Giacomelli, Wiener, and Spiro, 1970). Although contractile proteins have been found in endothelia (Becher and Murphy, 1969), the subcellular mechanisms of the contraction of the vascular smooth muscle and endothelial cells as well as their interaction are still to be elucidated (Phelps and Luft, 1969; Heumann, 1971). Future studies have to ascertain the exact conditions for endothelial contraction, besides induction by histamine and other vasoactive drugs (Majno, Shea, and Leventhal, 1969), the normal effects of endothelial contraction aside from the formation of endothelial gaps under pathologic conditions, and also the influence of sol-gel transformations, and the consequent changes in viscosity and motility of cytoplasmic vesicles, etc. The reason for the differing amounts of glycogen in the smooth muscle cells of arteries and veins, of different age and species (Luciano and Jünger, 1968), is also unknown. A rich innervation seems to be a rather common feature of arterioles and precapillary sphincters (Han and Avery, 1963; Moffat, 1967; Mohamed et al., 1973; Cervos-Navarro and Matakas, 1974), but great variations exist between arterioles of different organs and tissues. In some the elastic membranes are lacking, while the adventitia is well developed (Hibbs, Burch, and Phillips, 1958). In other arterioles the layer of muscle cells is incomplete (Moore and Ruska, 1957). These vessels might be called metarterioles, but in most publications information about the relative position of the vessel within the terminal vascular bed, i.e., topographically controlled preparations, is lacking.

Localized areas of small arteries and arterioles, especially regions of branching, seem to be highly permeable even to large tracer molecules (Suwa, 1962; Westergaard and Brightman, 1973). It is unknown whether these regions correspond to the localized areas of high alkaline phosphatase activity in the endothelium of small arteries and arterioles (Romanul and Bannister, 1962). However, we found that ferritin, lanthanum, and alcian blue permeate into the muscular layer of arterioles, when the tracers were applied 10–20 min after the beginning of perfusion fixation. Therefore, vesiculation does not seem to be the only means of transport, as suggested by Westergaard and Brightman (1973). An open extracellular communication must exist between the vessel lumen and the media, which allows for transendothelial passage of big molecules. Further investigations of this phenomenon are necessary to decide whether it results from open intercellular clefts, transendothelial channels (see "venules"), or some other unknown structure.

CAPILLARIES

Because of their great structural variability, it is impossible to define in generally applicable terms the capillary position in relation to other parts of the terminal vascular bed and the structure of the capillary wall.

Many, but not all, capillaries are arranged in series between arterioles and venular vessels, for instance, the unbranched capillary loops in dermal papillae. Other microvessels with a capillary-like structure connect the series elements to each other or to venules. Being arranged in parallel to the former type of capillaries, the latter form more or less extended networks. Especially in organs with a high metabolic rate, the network capillaries or "true capillaries" (Majno, 1965) outnumber the series elements. Network capillaries develop late during ontogenesis, and probably contain "seamless" endothelia, because the sprout tips fuse with the wall of rather mature vessels (Wolff, Moritz, and Güldner, 1972; Wolff and Bär, 1972; Güldner and Wolff, 1973). However, in the portal system of the infundibulohypophyseal region of the CNS and of the liver (Rappaport, 1973), the capillaries are situated between venous vessels, and in the rete mirabile of the kidney the glomerular capillaries are interposed between an afferent and efferent arteriole, the latter feeding the medullary capillaries (Moffat, 1967). In all these cases, the arrangement of a capillary within the terminal vascular bed influences intracapillary pressure and pressure gradient and therefore the rate and direction of blood flow, as well as the filtration rate (Lipowsky and Zweifach, 1974; Intaglietta and De Plomb, 1973).

Moreover, the well-known structural variations of the capillary wall (Table 1) (Bennett, Luft, and Hampton, 1959; Simon, 1965; Majno, 1965) cannot be simply correlated with any of the above-mentioned variations in arrangement. The endothelium of the series elements may be continuous, fenestrated (e.g., dermal papillary capillaries; Parakkal, 1966; McLeod, 1970; Takada and Hattori, 1972) and may even become discontinuous after the application of histamine (dermal capillaries; Hammersen, 1972a). The same is true for the network capillaries, and also for capillaries in connective tissue. Fenestrated capillaries occur in muscle fascia (Karrer and Cox, 1960; Rhodin, 1962; Hammersen, 1966), in the vasa vasorum (Shimamoto et al., 1970) as well as near various types of parenchymal cells (see Table 1). These comparisons show that our knowledge is far from the level at which structure, arrangement, and function of capillaries can be correlated in general terms. However, some cellular and subcellular structures of the capillary wall have been detected, which may be correlated with functional properties of capillaries (Majno, 1965; Karnovsky, 1968; Casley-Smith, 1970; Hammersen, 1972b).

The morphologic equivalent of the capillary "membrane" (Landis and Pappenheimer, 1963) consists of several layers, which may vary independently in thickness and structure: (1) the endothelium, (2) the pericytes, (3) the basal lamina, and (4) the pericapillary tissue space. The latter, consisting of very diverse structures like connective tissue, labyrinths of intercellular clefts, or parenchymal cells, cannot be considered to be strictly a part of the capillary wall. However, terminal vessels and even capillaries in this connective tissue are often surrounded by structures that remind one of the adventitia of larger vessels. Furthermore, the lack of an extracellular pericapillary space coincides with a restricted permeability of the vascular wall (e.g., CNS, renal glomerulus, blood—air boundary in lung).

ENDOTHELIUM

Many excellent reviews on the ultrastructure of capillary endothelia exist in several languages (e.g., Simon, 1965; Majno, 1965; Florey, 1966; Karnovsky,

1968, 1970; Santolaya and Bertini, 1970; Hammersen, 1972*b*). The present chapter is confined to those structures which at present can be related to functional aspects of either the endothelium or the microvasculature. The distribution of capillaries with continuous, fenestrated, or discontinuous endothelia in various tissues and organs is summarized in Table 1. (See also Chapters 5 and 19 in this volume.)

The most characteristic constituents of *continuous endothelia* (Figures 2 and 9b, and 10a, below) are the varying numbers of micro-pinocytotic vesicles. In fixed material, (Figure 2), but also in freeze fractures (Figure 1b), and in scanning electron microscopy of freeze-substituted material, a high percentage of these vesicles (30%; Bruns and Palade, 1968*a*, 1968*b*) seems connected to the luminal surface of the endothelium. Another large fraction (about 40%) is fused with the basal surface, and only less than one-third seems to be suspended in the cytoplasm. The actual number of free cytoplasmic vesicles depends on the overall thickness of the endothelial layer. However, some apparently free vesicles in the cytoplasm can be filled by tracers after the endothelium has already been fixed by aldehydes, i.e., after vesicle movements have stopped (Figure 11c, below; see also Karnovsky, 1970). This may be explained by the fact that some vesicles in favorable sections can be seen to be connected to others, which may eventually communicate with the surface membrane (arrow, Figures 2a–2c). This view is supported by the distribution of "washed-out" vesicles after perfusion fixation with initially high pressure (for rats, 220 cm H_2O for 1–3 min, followed by 130 cm H_2O for 30 min). In most capillaries with a continuous endothelium, the empty vesicles are confined to the upper half of the endothelium, while the vesicles in the basal part contain a fuzzy material that resembles plasma protein and fills all vesicles after immersion fixation or in nonperfused capillaries (Figures 2b and 2c). Many authors agree that in thinner parts of continuous endothelia–especially on the venous side–by simultaneous fusion of vesicles with both sides small transendothelial channels may develop (Wolff, 1966; Bruns and Palade, 1968*a*, 1968*b*; Mohamed, Waterhouse, and Friederici, 1973). Also, fenestrations or open pores may be formed by this mechanism (Karrer and Cox, 1960; Elfvin, 1965; Wolff and Merker, 1966; Casley-Smith, 1970; see also Figures 3b, 13, below and the insets of Figure 4).

Because these results could not be confirmed by Karnovsky (1968), one might look for conditions that may vary the number of vesicles and induce or suppress vesicle fusion. No unequivocal answer can be deduced from the literature. High numbers of endothelial vesicles have been described in the endothelium below the sphincters of capillaries (Rhodin, 1967), in the capillaries of heart (subendocardial > subepicardial; Anversa, Giacomelli, and Wiener, 1973) skeletal and tongue muscles (Fernando and Movat, 1964*b*; Karnovsky, 1970; Hammersen, 1972*b*), as well as in the thick parts of the lung capillaries (Weibel and Knight, 1964). One of the conditions that seem to be common to all of these capillaries is that their endothelium is exposed to temporary compression,

Table 1. Ultrastructure of the capillary wall in various tissues (for literature see Simon, 1965)

Tissue	Endothelium (E)[a]	Basal lamina (BL)[a]	Pericytes (PC)[a]	Subendothelial Space (SES)[a]
Connective tissue				
Subcutis fat tissue				
Normal mesentery				
Normal subserosa and mucosa of the intestine	c	c	d	3+
Subepidermal plexus				
Perimuscular fascia				
Vasa vasorum	c + f	c	d	3+
Dermal papillae				
Hair follicle				
Synovial membranes				
Dental pulp	c − f	c	d	2+
Mucosa of				
Urinary bladder				
Gall bladder				
Uterus				
Vagina	c − f	c	d	1+
Exocrine glands				
Prostate				
Sweat glands				
Lacrymal glands				
Sabaceous glands				
Salivary glands	c − f	c	d	1+
Pancreas				
Stomach				

All endocrine glands	f	o–c		1+
Intestinal villi	f		d	1+
Kidney				
Glomerulus	f	c	o–d	o^b
Tubules	f	c	o	o^b–1+
Medulla	c + f	c	d	2+
CNS blood–brain barrier	c	c	d	o^b
Choroid plexus				
Area postrema, etc.	f	c	d	1–2+
Hypothalamo-hypophyseal system				
Muscle (endomysial: skeletal, heart, smooth)	c	c	d	1–2+
Lung	c	c	d	o^b–3+
Sinusoids of				
Liver, spleen and				
Bone marrow	d	d	d^c	o^b–3+

[a] c, continuous; f, fenestrated; d, discontinuous; o, lacking.
[b] Where the subendothelial space is lacking, the endothelial basal lamina fuses with the neighbouring epithelial one, "thick BL."
[c] The RES-cells (Kupffer and reticulum cells).

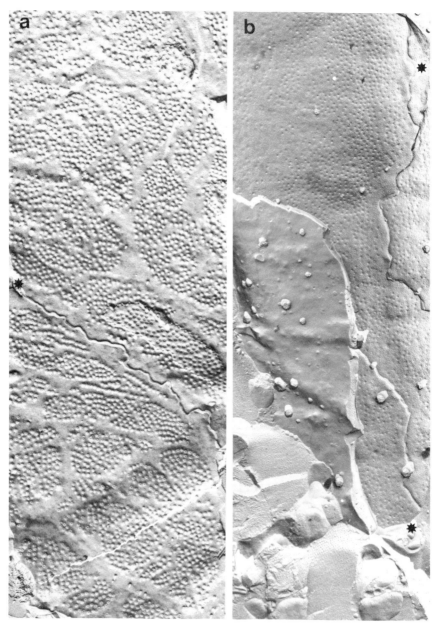

Figure 1. Freeze fractures of a fenestrated peritubular capillary of the kidney (a) and of a heart capillary (b) with continuous endothelium. (a) Note the nonfenestrated cytoplasmic strands or streaks, which surround fields of fenestrae and the intercellular contacts. (b) Note that the invaginated vesicles are distributed more evenly than the fenestrae, but are also lacking around the contact belts. About × 10,000. Reprinted with permission of Dr. St. Peter, Heidelberg.

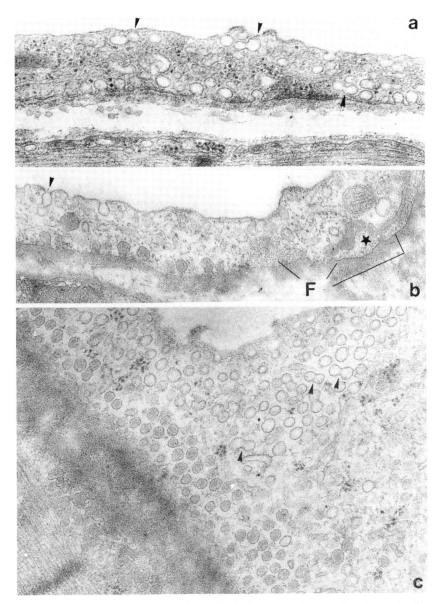

Figure 2. After perfusion fixation with initially high pressure (220 cm H_2O for 5 min, then 130 cm) in some portions of the capillaries the vesicles appear empty on both sides of the endothelium. In these cases also the subendothelial space and some vesicles at the surface of the neighbouring muscle fibers appear empty (a). Usually, however, the vesicles in the basal part of the endothelium and in the muscle fibers as well as the interstitial space are filled with an opaque material similar to precipitated plasma proteins. Only the vesicles at or near the luminal surface are electron lucent (b). This can also be seen in a tangential section through a capillary (c). Note fused vesicles (arrows). F, thin filaments forming bundles or marginal layers near the base of endothelial cells. × 52,000.

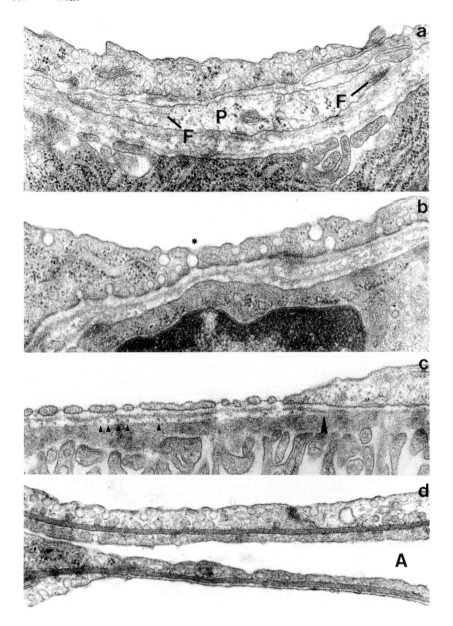

Figure 3. (a) In most organs and tissues the basal laminae (BL) of the capillary wall (endothelial, pericytic) are separated from the BL of the parenchymal cells as in the pancreas of rat. P, pericyte containing thin filaments (F), which aggregate at the plasma membrane of their processes. (b) The BL of the "endoepithelial" capillaries of the urinary bladder may fuse locally with that of the epithelium without becoming thicker at the point of fusion. Note the transendothelial channel (asterisk) originating from a vesicle that is fused with both surfaces. (c) The thin BL of renal peritubular capillaries is mostly separated from

or a variable external pressure. On the other hand, the number of vesicles and vesicle fusions increases and even fenestrations are formed when the level of steroid hormones is increased, especially estrogens (Wolff and Merker, 1966; Friederici, 1967; Haim, 1968; Kessel and Panje, 1968) or when the tissue is cooled (Basbaum, 1973), inflamed (see Hammersen, 1972a) or influenced by $N_6 O_2$-dibutyrylcyclic AMP (Joó, 1972). The latter group of experiments show that chemical and/or physical stimuli can also induce the formation of new vesicles, although ultimately this process may be mediated by rather few basic mechanisms. The number of vesicles has been found to be small in normal brain capillaries (see Karnovsky, 1968, 1970; Brightman and Reese, 1969; Joó, 1971), and in the flattened areas near fenestrations and in nonfenestrated capillaries, suggesting that the vesicles are utilized during the process of flattening and enlargement of the endothelial surfaces (Wolff, 1966, 1967). Some parts of the alveolar capillaries are extremely flattened, neither containing fenestrations nor vesicles (Figure 3D; Weibel and Knight, 1964). These facts suggest that vesicles constitute a membrane reserve by which the endothelium can easily increase its surface (Figure 13A, below). Quantitative calculations on vesicle density have been reviewed by Karnovsky (1968), Wolff (1966, 1971), and Casley-Smith and Clark (1972). Because about 125 vesicles have the surface of 1 μ^2, and because in many continuous endothelia more than 250 vesicles exist below 1 μ^2 of endothelial surface, capillaries could dilate by this mechanism and up to double the surface area of both lumen and basement. By a peculiar arrangement of the fusing cytoplasmic vesicles, microvilli are formed at the apical surfaces of several cell types (Herman, 1960; Wolff, 1966; and Figure 13B, below). At the luminal surface of endothelia, microvilli develop under various experimental pathologic conditions (see Andres, 1963; Hammersen, 1972a). However, in "normal" capillaries variable numbers of microvilli may also occur (see, for instance, for the heart, Kisch, 1957; and for the skin, Mohamed et al., 1973). In our material, microvilli were more numerous in the arterial sides of capillaries in the tongue and urinary bladder. Microvilli, microfolds, and irregular surface variations occur in early stages of vasculogenesis (Schoefl, 1963; Aminova, 1967; Aloisi and Schiaffino, 1971), as in tumors (Stehbens and Ludatscher, 1968). Unusually high numbers of microvilli, however, have only been described in vessels of the testis and in the ganglion Gasseri of the rat (Gabbiani and Majno, 1969) as well as in the conus papillaris of reptiles (Nguyen and Anh, 1970; Dieterich and Dieterich, 1974). Usually long and regularly arranged microfolds were found in the capillary endothelium of the pecten oculi of birds (Semba, 1962; Dieterich et al., 1973). The functional significance of these specialized endothelial "brush

---

the thicker epithelial BL by a narrow cleft containing thin collagen fibrils which can nevertheless fuse locally (arrow). (d) At the blood–air boundary of the lung, the BLs of the alveolar epithelium (A) and of the capillaries are fused. The endothelium of alveolar capillaries varies in thickness. The thick parts are rich in vesicles, while the very thin parts (0.02 μ) do not contain vesicles. × 40,000.

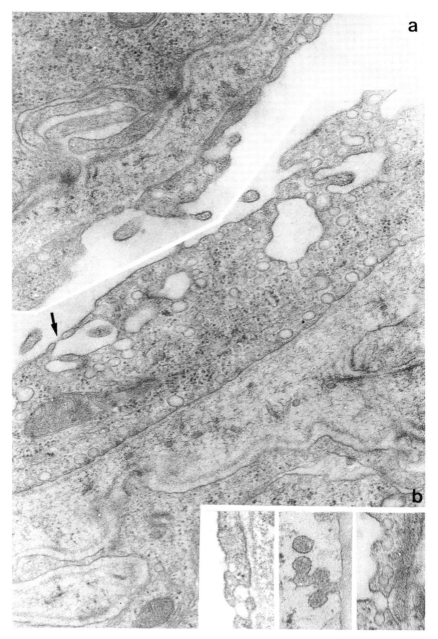

Figure 4. Subepithelial capillaries from the urinary bladder. (a) Fixed in a filled state: note the relatively smooth and small interdigitations of the epithelium, the narrow subepithelial space and the flattened, partly fenestrated endothelium. (b) Fixed in an empty state: note the wavy epithelial base, the wide subendothelial space, and the thick and irregularly formed endothelium containing numerous vacuoles fusing with vesicles and fenestrations (arrow). × 50,000. *Insets:* Various confluents of vesicles in venous sides of capillaries partly forming transendothelial channels. × 52,000.

borders" or lamellar structures, respectively, is unknown. They do not only cover the luminal, but also the basal surface of the endothelium (Figure 5). Because the endothelial contacts are sealed by tight junctions (Dieterich, personal communication), enzyme-mediated transport, as in other brush borders, may be occuring in this special type of capillary (Greenberger, 1969).

Lacerta agilis

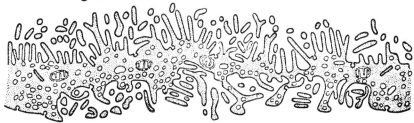

Platysaurus intermedius

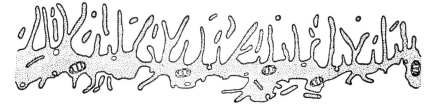

Iguana iguana

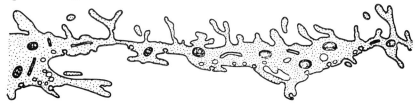

Anguis fragilis

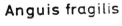
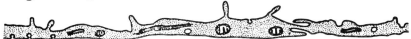

Figure 5. Comparison of the structure of the capillary endothelia in the conus papillaris of various reptiles. Note the more or less extensively developed microvilli at the luminal as well as at the basal surface. Reprinted with permission of Dr. C.E. Dieterich and Dr. H.J. Dieterich, and VEB Gustav Fischer Verlag, Publisher.

Fenestrated Endothelium

Fenestrated endothelium (Figures 1a, 3c, 4, 6a, 7, and 9a and 13c, below) shows a gradual transition toward a continuous endothelium containing single or a few isolated fenestrations (see above). In typical fenestrated endothelia, however, the fenestrations or pores cover about one-third of the total surface. They are not uniformly distributed, but are densely packed in fields of extremely flattened endothelium. The porous fields are surrounded and separated by branching strands of thicker cytoplasm that connect to the perikaryon and the more voluminous border areas between endothelia (Figure 1a). This arrangement of cytoplasmic strands resembles the venation of a leaf. This similarity may not only be formal but also functional, because the strands contain microtubules and filaments (Figure 6a), suggesting that the cytoplasm may flow and circulate in these venations (Wolff and Merker, 1966; Friederici, 1968).

Fenestrated endothelia may cover the whole length of a capillary, as in the glomerulus and peritubular capillaries of the kidney (Farquhar, 1964), in the choroidal plexus, in the sinusoidal capillaries of many endocrine glands, in the intestinal villi, and in other areas (see Table 1; Majno, 1965). In other tissues, however, only the venous ends of the capillaries contain fenestrae, while either the arterial side shows a continuous endothelium, or the density of fenestrae increases towards the venous end (Casley-Smith, 1971; Dorn, 1961; Mohamed et al., 1973). Fenestrae are not static structures. They can proliferate, e.g., in inflamed tissue (see Hammersen, 1972a), or under the influence of sexual hormones (Wolff and Merker, 1966; Mohamed et al., 1973) and unknown factors that can seemingly be produced by epithelial cells (Horstmann, 1966; Campbell et al., 1972). However, because the localization of the fenestrated parts of capillaries may vary or even change polarity in relation to the epithelial surface, other physiologic factors must also be able to induce the production of fenestrae (compare Figures 7a and 7b). The mechanism of forming new fenestrae has often been discussed (see Elfvin, 1965; Maul, 1971). They can close under various conditions in various organs (Fletscher, 1964; Wolff and Merker, 1966). A rather dramatic change can, for instance, be observed in the urinary bladder, depending on whether it has been fixed in the empty or maximally filled state (Figures 4a and 4b). The "endoepithelial" capillaries, which represent arc-shaped capillaries enclosed in folds of the epithelial basement, can be passively transformed by the surrounding epithelium. About 5 min after the relaxation of the bladder wall, most of these flattened, partly fenestrated capillaries are transformed into vessels with a highly irregularly shaped endothelium. Many vesicles are formed in the endothelial cells and seem to fuse, forming vacuoles (Figure 6).

The fenestrae, although mostly closed by a diaphragm (Maul, 1971), are permeable not only to high amounts of fluid and solutes, but also to molecules as large as ferritin (Clementi and Palade, 1969a). However, larger particles do not

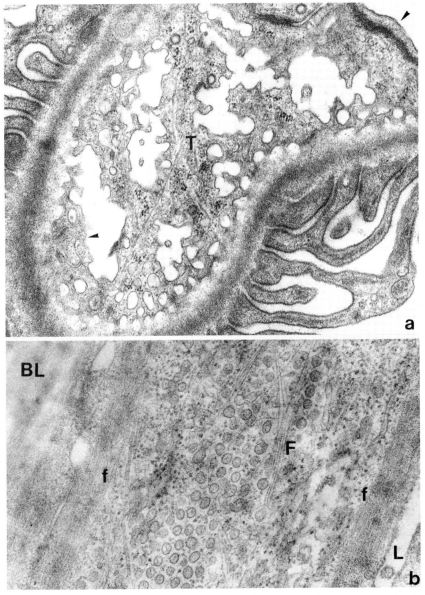

Figure 6. (a) A tangential section through a renal glomerular capillary demonstrates the cytoplasmic strands containing microtubules (T) and separating fenestrated fields. The strands always include the intercellular contact zones (arrows). Compare Figure 1. X 39,000. (b) A tangential section through the continuous endothelium of a muscle capillary reveals numerous thin filaments (f) that are aggregated near the plasma membranes, and small groups of thicker filaments (F) running through the inner part of the cytoplasm. BL, basal lamina; L, lumen. X 52,000.

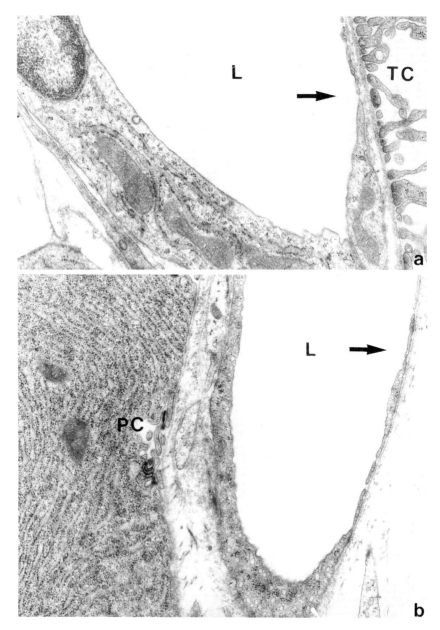

Figure 7. (a) The fenestrated parts of capillary endothelia (arrows) often face the neighboring parenchymal cells (TC) as in the case of a peritubular capillary of kidney of rat. (b) However, exceptions exist as in the exocrine pancreas of rat, where sometimes all capillaries direct their fenestrated portions to the interstitial space and not to the parenchymal cells (PC). L, vessel lumen. × 25,000.

penetrate the fenestrae (see Karnovsky, 1968; Hammersen, 1972b). This high protein permeability may be especially important when venous capillaries are fenestrated, since it may influence the reabsorbtive capacity of the blood vessels (Deen, Robertson, and Brenner, 1974; Wiederhielm, 1968).

Discontinuous Endothelia

Discontinuous endothelia represent the typical lining of the sinusoids or sinuses of liver, spleen, and bone marrow. However, similar intracellular holes and intercellular gaps have been observed in the adrenal medulla (Fletscher, 1964), and there are many similarities between the endothelia of the sinusoids of liver, spleen, bone marrow, and lymph nodes on one side and other RES cells on the other (Mori, 1967; Carr, 1972; Amreek Singh, 1974).

Because this peculiar type of "capillary" has been well described and the literature collected (Majno, 1965; Karnovsky, 1968, 1970, Wolff, 1971), we refer only to some properties derived from an analysis of the sinusoids of the spleen (Figure 8). The endothelia are fusiform cells that are oriented along the axis of the vessel (Figure 8c). They are laterally connected by simple apposition of their plasma membranes, or by primitive adhesion plaques. Each endothelial cell contains numerous cytoplasmic filaments and microtubules that traverse as bundles the basal part of the cell in various directions, and insert in localized dense structures at the basal plasma membranes. Since basal lamina material adheres to the external aspect of these attachment zones, they sometimes look like hemidesmosomes (Figures 8a and 8b). (For discussion of the contractility of endothelia, see the section on arterioles.) The cytoplasm is filled by many membrane-bound smooth and coated vesicles and vacuoles, lysosomes, dense bodies, Golgi lamellae, etc.; however, since the cells are rather thick, only a few transendothelial channels have been observed. Erythrocytes and other cells penetrate the sinusoidal wall via open intercellular clefts (Figure 8c), which otherwise are mostly closed. The discontinuous, as well as the other forms of endothelia, cannot be considered as static. Their shape, internal structure, and arrangement must rather be considered as an effect of continual complicated interactions of many cellular and extracellular, local, and humoral factors. Thus the discontinuous endothelium can even be transformed into a typical continuous one under appropriate conditions, for example, in pathologic states such as "capillarization of hepatic sinusoids" (Schaffner and Foper, 1963).

BASAL LAMINA

Quite a number of investigations have been undertaken to understand more about the structure, chemical constitution, and variability under normal and pathologic conditions of the basal lamina (Cotran and Majno, 1964; Hempel and Geyer, 1967; Misra and Berman, 1969; Fung and Kalant, 1972; Hruza, Chapter 7 of this volume). It has been demonstrated that the basal lamina is produced and

112   Wolff

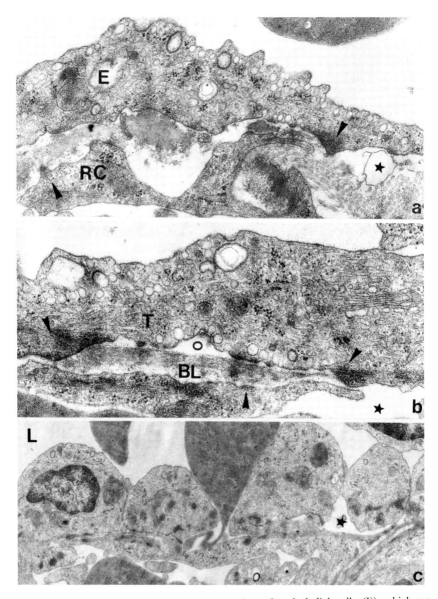

Figure 8. The wall of the splenic sinusoids consists of endothelial cells (E), which are oriented parallel to their long axis (a and b, longitudinal; c, cross section). Locally elastic elements and networks support the endothelium. (a) and (b), basal lamina material is irregularly distributed along the wall, but obviously attached locally to the plasma membranes of endothelia and reticulum cells (RC), where intracellular filaments aggregate, forming hemidesmosome-like structures (arrows). Between these attachment zones the basal lamina material is separated from the cells (O) or is lacking (*). Note numerous microtubules (T), vacuoles, and vesicles in the endothelium. (c) An erythrocyte is interposed between two endothelial cells probably leaving the sinusoid. (a), × 31,000; (b), × 3,900; (c), × 14,000.

organized locally by the adhering cells (Majno, 1965; Joó, 1969; Bär and Wolff, 1972), but disintegrates when it is separated from them by the action of vasoactive drugs or by degeneration (Cotran and Majno, 1964). However, if the regeneration of endothelia occurs in a reasonable time after degeneration, the old basal lamina is used as a microskeleton or scaffold for a regular spatial reconstruction of the vessel, and its further disintegration is halted, although the new basal lamina is forming inside the old one. By this mechanism a multi-lamellar basal lamina may be formed under many different pathologic conditions (Pease, 1960; Pardo, Perez-Stable, and Alzamora, 1972; Vracko and Benditt, 1972). In many pathologic cases the basal lamina is, however, not multilamellar, but regularly or irregularly thickened (Figure 10a, below; Cohen, Weiss, and Calkins, 1960; Churg et al., 1966; Pardo et al., 1966; Hinglais, Grunfeld, and Bois, 1972). A simple thickening is also reported in old animals and men (Bloom, Hartmann, and Jernier, 1959; Krebs and David, 1962). In spite of its high structural stability (Blinzinger, Matsushima, and Anzil, 1969), it represents an elastic sheet, which becomes thinner as the vessel is dilated (Sosula et al., 1972). However, there are significant variations in the thickness of the basal lamina between different organs and species (see Table 2 and Figure 3; Jörgensen and Bentzon, 1968). Although vasoactive substances usually do not affect the structure of the basal lamina directly (Gabbiani, Badonnel, and Majno, 1970), the concentration of Mg^{++} and Ca^{++} seems to have a significant influence (Clementi and Palade, 1969b; Mönninghoff, Themann, and Westphal, 1972), and fragile capillaries show a defective basal lamina (Han and Avery, 1963; Majno, 1965). The basal lamina functions as a sieve for particles, but only the passage of very large molecules (ferritin, Majno and Palade, 1961; Farquhar, 1964; Cotran, Suter, and Majno, 1967; Clementi and Palade, 1969a) is restricted. Recently, another function of the basal lamina has been discussed, namely, whether protein, and possibly also other molecules, may be adsorbed or even stored in it (Wendt, 1973). This would agree with the fact that the basal lamina of the glomerular capillaries becomes thicker in proteinuria (Ruckley et al., 1966). Its variable antigenic properties and the storage of amyloid in or near the basal lamina, as well as cholinesterase molecules that occur in the extracellular space of the brain, would fit into such a concept (Cohen and Calkins, 1960; Johnson and Pierce, 1970; Flummerfelt, Lewis, and Gwyn, 1973). However, much has to be done to confirm such a concept of the basal lamina as a device for regulating the microenvironment of the adhering cells.

PERICYTES

We exclude this type of cell from an extensive description. Aside from their contractile function as a precursor of smooth muscle cells (see above), there is little information about their possible role within the general functional scheme of the vascular wall. On the venous side of the capillaries, a gradual transformation of pericytes into smooth muscle cells takes place, the latter obtaining their

Table 2. Thickness of basal lamina in different organs and animal species[a] (nm)

Organ	Man	Dog Total	Dog Up to 5 yr	Rabbit, Rat	Mouse
Kidney					
glomerulus[b]	100–200[c]			100–220	
	225–323–480	250±31	>300	284±50[d]	125±21
Peritubular					
capillary				35–40	
CNS					
Cortex				40–100	
Retina		148±23	>150		
In connective tissue				25–35	
(pia mater,					
area postrema,					
neurohypophysis)					
Lung					
Blood–air					
barrier				70–100	
in alveolar-					
septum				20–35	
Muscle		76±5	70–100	20–35	
Skin				25–50	
Fat		66±10	≤150	25–50	
Connective tissue				25–35	
Endocrine glands				0–25–70[e]	

[a]The values were collected from several publications, which are not mentioned here, but which can be found in the index list of references or taken from review articles.

[b]Measured with the two laminae rarae.

[c]Children.

[d]Older than 3 yr.

[e]0 means the functional states, under which the basal lamina electron microscopically becomes insignificant or disappears (e.g., in the thyroid gland). The outer boundary as well as the width of the lamina rara is often difficult to measure.

typical structure in the muscular venules (Rhodin, 1968; Stingl, 1971) (Figure 10b). On the arterial side, however, smooth muscle cells vanish suddenly. This is most obvious at precapillary sphincters, where the muscle layer terminates with a single muscular ring (Figure 9a). This difference between the arterial and venous sides may simply be caused by the different pressure gradients. Phago-

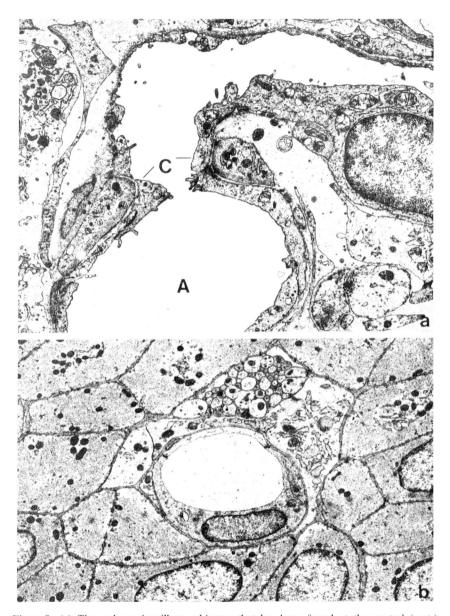

Figure 9. (a) The only pericapillary sphincter that has been found at the central (met-) arteriole (A) of an intestinal villus being reconstructed from serial thin and thick sections. × 15,000. (b) Capillaries within the smooth muscle layers of the intestine are typically tightly surrounded by muscle cells, fibrocytes, and nerves. No pericapillary space can be recognized. × 15,000.

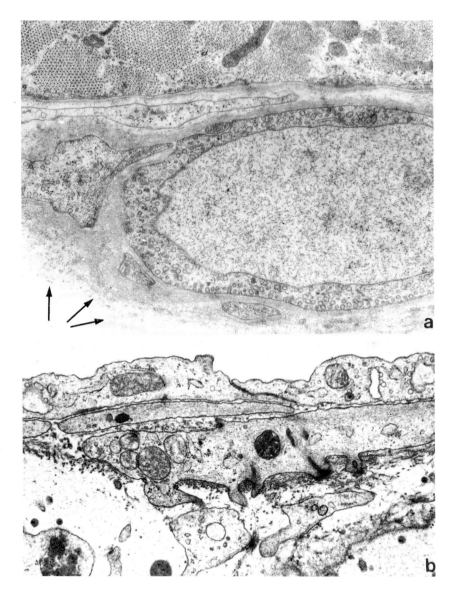

Figure 10. (a) Muscle capillary from a patient with a long-lasting hypertension (about 20 yr). The basal lamina is thickened and not clearly delimited towards the interstitial space (arrows). × 31,000. (b) Venule at the base of an intestinal villus. The smooth muscle cells from protrusions that break through the basal lamina and make contacts with the contractile fibrocytes. Note peculiar vacuoles in the endothelium.

cytosis has been discussed in earlier reviews (Majno, 1965; Hammersen, 1972a, 1972b), but to our knowledge no better evidence has been presented during the last years to confirm this function in pericytes within basal laminae. Other RES cells, for instance, the Kupffer cells in the liver and the endothelia and reticulum cells of spleen, bone marrow, and lymph nodes, are of course heavily involved in the phagocytotic activity of these organs (see Hershey in Volume III).

VENULES

At the venous side of the terminal vascular bed, ultrastructural boundaries are especially fluid between the various subsections that have been structurally distinguished, i.e., venous capillaries, postcapillary venules, collecting venules, muscular venules, and small collecting veins (see Rhodin, 1968). Most authors distinguish venules by their larger diameter. Comparing the postcapillary vessels of different organs, indeed their diameter always increases towards the venous side, but the absolute size varies strongly from one organ to another. Moreover, the diameter of venular vessels depends much more on the internal pressure during perfusion fixation than that of arterioles. Thus the diameter can only be used as a diagnostic feature if techniques allowing visual control of the vascular arrangement are applied (see Rhodin, 1968; Stingl, 1971; Ericsson and Ericsson, 1973). A better criterion is probably that, in contrast to venous capillaries, venules are more or less completely covered by pericytes that gradually change into smooth muscle cells (Rhodin, 1968; Stingl, 1971).

Some authors agree that there are more endothelio-pericytic contacts (for discussion see the section on arterioles) in venules than in capillaries, that the interendothelial contacts become more complicated by increasing interdigitation, that lysosomes appear, and that myoendothelial contacts are more numerous (Movat and Fernando, 1964; Rhodin, 1968; Claesson, Jørgensen, and Røpke, 1971; Hammersen, 1972b). One or more fenestrae have been described in the venular endothelium (Rhodin, 1968; Takada and Hattori, 1972; Mohamed et al., 1973).

One of the most characteristic properties of venules is their relatively high permeability for large molecules (permeability gradient; Intaglietta and De Plomb, 1973; Hauck, 1971) and their high sensitivity to histamine and other vasoactive drugs (Majno, Palade, and Schoefl, 1961; Cotran and Majno, 1964; Hammersen, 1972a). Until now, no morphologic correlate has been detected. However, in most publications about postcapillary venules there are pictures that show locally accumulating and partly fusing vesicles. These vesicles and vacuoles show a characteristic variability of diameters, the largest being 2000–3000 Å thick. The smallest are common micropinocytotic vesicles (400–800 Å ϕ) [compare for instance Figures 11a and 11b of the present paper with Figure 4 of Movat and Fernando (1964), Figure 36 of Rhodin (1968), and Figures 2 and 3 of Mohamed et al. (1973)]. A three-dimensional reconstruction

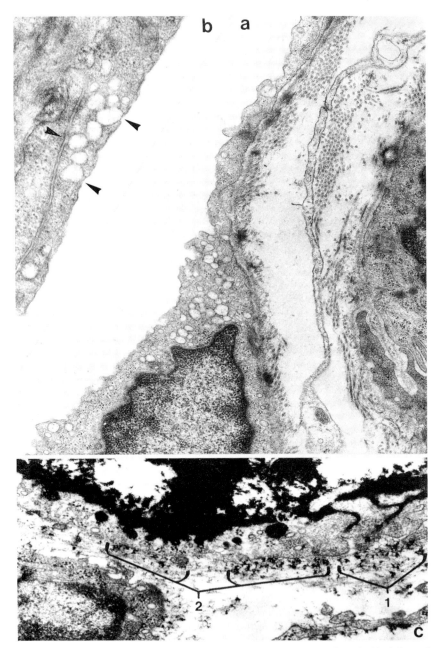

Figure 11. Local aggregates of large vesicles in a venous part of a capillary (ϕ 10 μ) from the urinary bladder (a) and in a venule in skeletal muscle (b). Note that the aggregated vesicles are partly fused with each other, forming complicated branched chains or channels and with the surface membranes (arrow heads). (c) Lanthanum infused 15 min after the beginning of the perfusion fixation entered only some of the small, but all large vesicles, penetrated the interendothelial contacts, and accumulated in the subendothelial space of the terminal venule (ϕ 18 μ) below the intercellular contact zone (1) and vesicle aggregates (2). (a), $\times$ 22,000; (b) and (c), $\times$ 43,000.

of the endothelial wall of a muscle venule reveals the following. (1) The aggregates of vesicles and vacuoles show a peculiar distribution within the venular wall. They accumulate near the intercellular adhesion belts, are often situated around the cell nuclei, and form fine strands, which connect the various aggregates to each other and cause a net-like arrangement within the endothelial cells (Figure 12). (2) Within many of the aggregates, complicated branched channels exist that consist of fused vesicles and vacuoles, often separated by a diaphragm. These channels can connect the luminal and the basal surface of the endothelium with one to several openings per channel on each side (Figure 11a), but can also be closed on one or the other side. After initially high-pressure perfusion, the channels always appear "washed out." Under these conditions the aggregated and communicating vesicles can easily be detected even when the luminal opening is not included in the section. The application of ferritin, lanthanum, and alcian blue 10–20 min after the beginning of the perfusion fixation does not inhibit the permeation of the tracers through the intercellular clefts (Karnovsky, 1968). However, the vesicles and vacuoles are also filled, and local accumulations of the tracer can be observed at corresponding sites of the endothelial basement (Figure 11b). Because the three-dimensional shape of most of the channels is too complicated to include in one section, and because the openings on both or even on one side of the cell, are likewise too complicated to include in one section, it is difficult to demonstrate directly the continuity of such channels. However, this has been confirmed by consecutive sections. To our knowledge, only Sulzmann (1965) and Riedel, Fromme, and Tallen (1966) have mentioned that they observed channels penetrating the endothelial cells of venules in the dental pulp.

The question is, what makes these channels so difficult to detect? Several factors may be responsible: Many of the relevant electron microscopic studies have used material that had been fixed by immersion. From our biopsy material, and the above-mentioned pictures of other authors, we know that under these conditions many of the vesicles and vacuoles contain a fuzzy material, probably plasma proteins. This may have caused their misinterpretation as lysosomes, dense bodies, etc., or their contents may have so resembled the surrounding cytoplasm that they have been overlooked. On the other hand, similar channels and aggregates have been called "increased vesiculation" (Alksne, 1959), "intercellular gaps," etc., because they were observed after vascular injury, on inflammation, after the application of vasoactive drugs, and in different types of edema (see Cotran et al., 1967; Hammersen, 1972a; Shea, Caulfield, and Burke, 1973). However, even in normal, untreated control animals, small particles permeate to some extent through the venous part of the terminal vascular bed (Majno and Palade, 1961), and there is only a gradual transition between the structure of the normal and injured venule (Hammersen, 1972a). Therefore, it is possible that these vesicular aggregates have been seen by several authors, but have not been accepted as "normal." This at least would explain why an excellent observer like Rhodin (1968) demonstrates vesicular aggregates with typical morphology and

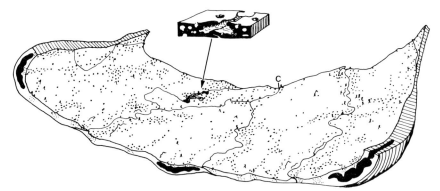

Figure 12. The distribution of large vesicles (black points), sometimes forming complicated transendothelial channels in a venule from skeletal muscle. C, interendothelial contacts; *inset*, magnified portion of a complicated part of an intercellular junction.

distribution in his summarizing diagram, but does not mention them in the text. Another possibility is that these structures are confined to venules only in some organs and that they are lacking in the others. Nevertheless, we have observed transendothelial channels and vesicular aggregates in venules of different muscles, urinary bladder, exocrine pancreas, skin, and tongue. The material was taken from several rats that did not show any indication of general or local infection or of any kind of injury or immunologic response. We therefore propose to look for these transendothelial channels in future studies of the various parts of terminal vascular bed of various organs. The distribution and size of these complicated transendothelial channels in venules, together with the more simple channels and fenestrae in the flattened venous parts of capillaries, suggest that they may be the morphologic equivalent of the so-called "fenestellae" (Hauck, 1971) that cause the increased and localized "spotty" high permeability on the venous side of the terminal vascular bed.

CONCLUDING REMARKS

History

The history of attempts to correlate vascular ultrastructure and function begins with ultrastructural research itself, i.e., in 1953 when endothelial vesicles or caveolae (Palade) and pores or fenestrae (Monroe) were discovered. This first period is characterized by the search for organotypic vascular structures. This led to several attempts to classify the ultrastructure of capillaries (Bennett et al., 1959; Simon, 1965; Majno, 1965). During the second period, investigators tried to define a more general correlation between the typical functions of microvessels (permeability to small and large molecules and fluid, fragility, and cellular emigration) and structural characteristics of the vascular wall (intercellular clefts, vesiculation, transcellular holes and gaps, as well as fenestrations of the endo-thelium, etc.). Since then evidence has accumulated for a rather high variability of all parts of the terminal vascular bed even under normal conditions. This aspect is stressed in the present chapter more than the former approaches, which have been excellently reviewed before. However, many important original papers have not been cited explicitly, but can be found in the references that have been cited.

Arrangement and Ultrastructure of Microvessels

It is concluded from the evidence presented that there is a tendency towards increasing diameter, decreasing thickness of the endothelial wall, and an in-creasing number of fenestrae and/or transendothelial channels, toward the venous end of capillaries. However, because of great variations in different organs, no general correlation can be made between the ultrastructure of a random section through a vessel and its position within the terminal vascular bed.

Permeability and Structure

From the evidence available at present, one can conclude that there is no general morphologic correlate of *filtration* through the vascular wall. It takes place through continuous endothelia at the arterial side of many capillaries, and probably also through their intercellular clefts. In organs with very high filtra-tion rates (glomerulus, choroid plexus, etc.) fenestrated endothelia are found. Hitherto, there has been no total agreement about the sites of *passage of large molecules* through the vascular wall. After an excellent series of tracer experiments, it is, however, accepted that, when and where large molecules are prevented from leaving blood vessels, e.g., the blood–brain barrier, the intercel-lular clefts must be sealed by tight junctions, and the vesiculation must be insignificant. This holds not only for capillaries, but also for arterial and venous vessels. The differences between the various authors consist mainly of their divergent views with respect to the relative importance of either intercellular clefts or vesiculation as the main pathway of large molecules. A possible morphologic equivalent of the gradient of protein permeability increasing toward the continuous endothelia of venules is presented. Aggregates of vesicles of various size increase at the venous end of capillaries and in venules. Their partial fusion causes the formation of complicated transendothelial channels, which are difficult to detect as transendothelial communications because of their complicated three-dimensional shape and branching. They may supplement single fenestrations and straight channels, which are known to occur on the venous side of capillaries. All these structures may be the morphologic equiva-lent of the "fenestellae."

Fenestrations seem to be permeable to rather big molecules, although they appear to be mostly closed by diaphragms. Enzyme-mediated or other kinds of transendothelial transport can only be effected in capillaries with tight barriers for large molecules (see above). Special transport functions are ascribed to capillaries containing endothelia with extremely numerous microvilli (brush border on one or both surfaces of the endothelium). The resistance of micro-vessels against bleeding (fragility) seems to presume that the vessel wall is continuous (endothelium and basal lamina). However, active emigration of cells can occur without any visible destruction of the wall structure. The cells seem to cause local and temporary disintegration of intercellular contacts and basal lamina. The basal lamina being produced by the adhering cells slowly disintegrates, after the latter have degenerated. However, if regeneration occurs early, the basal lamina seems to act as a microskeleton or scaffold.

Membrane Dynamics

Vesiculation has mainly been discussed with respect to its possible effect on the net shift of molecules from blood to pericapillary spaces and vice versa; i.e., vesiculation has been considered as a vehicle of the transport of vesicular contents (see Shea and Bossert, 1973). This is certainly an important aspect, but may not be the only or the most important effect of intrusion, pinching off, Brownian movement, and fusion of vesicles in endothelial cells. Another, perhaps even more important, aspect of vesiculation is that it changes locally or generally the size of endothelial surfaces; i.e., the vesicles represent a mobile membrane reserve for sudden dilations or elongations of the capillary, for the formation of fenestrations, for intracellular and intercellular gaps and holes, and for transcellular channels as well as for microvilli and folds of the endothelium (see Figures 13 and 14). In spite of the great difficulties involved, investigations are needed of the ultrastructure of capillaries that have been fixed under visual

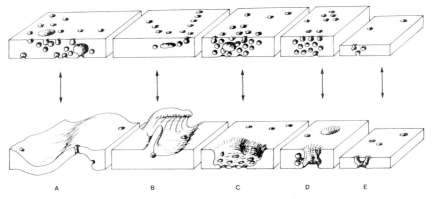

Figure 13. Schematic representation of various possible effects of the fusion of vesicles with the endothelial plasma membranes or vice versa. (A) flattening, (B) formation of folds and microvilli, (C) formation of localized fenestrated fields, (D) formation of transendothelial holes and—in a similar way—of intercellular gaps (e.g., histamine effect), (E) formation of transendothelial channels, see also (A).

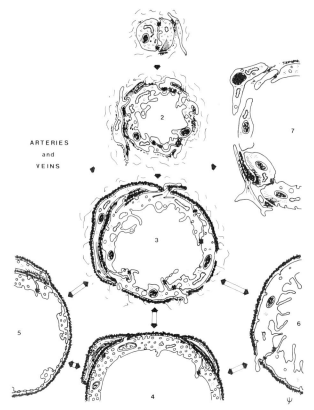

ARTERIES
and
VEINS

Figure 14. Diagram summarizes various developmental stages from sprouts (1) to immature capillaries that may occur in inflammation and granulation tissue and tumors (3). From this precursor all types of vessels and capillaries are formed, those with continuous (4), fenestrated (5), microvillous (6), and discontinuous endothelia, so-called sinus or sinusoids (7). The possibility of transformations from one type to another is indicated by arrows.

control of the diameter and of the internal pressures. Much experimental work is also necessary using substances other than the typical vasoactive substances, such as hormones, ions, etc., to learn more about the local interaction of the tissue and capillary wall. Perhaps by this type of experiment we can learn more about the reasons for the variable tendency of vesicles to fuse with certain endothelial surfaces (AV gradient, fenestrae in many flat endothelia, but not in the alveolar capillaries of the lung; see Figure 3) as well as about the reasons for variable interdigitations along the endothelial boundaries.

LITERATURE CITED

Alksne, J. F. 1959. The passage of colloidal particles across the dermal capillary wall under the influence of histamine. Quart. J. Exp. Physiol. 44:51–66.

Aloisi, M., and S. Schiaffino. 1971. Growth of elementary blood vessels in diffusion chambers. II. Electron microscopy of capillary morphogenesis. Virchows Archiv Abt. B—Zellpathologie 8:328.

Amreek Singh. 1974. Subplasmalemmal microfilaments in Kupffer cells. J. Ultrastruct. Res. 48:67—69.

Aminova, G. G. 1967. Changes in the endothelium of blood capillaries and vessels of the diaphragm during the process of development in the rabbit (Russian). Arkh. Anat. Gistol. Embriol. 53/12:99—101.

Andres, K. H. 1963. Elektronenmikroskopische Untersuchungen über Strukturveränderungen an Blutgefäßen und am Endoneurium in Spinalganglien von Ratten nach Bestrahlung mit 185 MeV-Protonen. Z. Zellforsch. 61:23—51.

Anh, J. 1970. Le cône papillaire des reptiles II. Ultrastructure chez l'oplure, Oplurus cyclurus (Iguanides). Z. Mikrosk Anat. Forsch. 82:17—28.

Anversa, P., F. Giacomelli, and J. Wiener. 1973. Regional variation in capillary permeability of ventricular myocardium. Microvasc. Res. 6:273—285.

Bär, Th., and J. R. Wolff. 1972. The formation of capillary basement membranes during internal vascularization of the rat's cerebral cortex. Z. Zellforsch. 133:231—248.

Basbaum, C. B. 1973. Induced hypothermia in peripheral nerve: Electron microscopic and electrophysiological observations. J. Neurocytol. 2:171—187.

Becher, C. G., and G. E. Murphy. 1969. Demonstration of contractile protein in endothelium and cells of the heart valves, and endocardium, intima, arteriosclerotic plaques and Aschoff bodies of rheumatic heart disease. Am. J. Pathol. 55:1—29.

Bennett, H. S., J. H. Luft, and J. C. Hampton. 1959. Morphological classification of vertebrate blood capillaries. Am. J. Physiol. 196:381—390.

Blinzinger, K., A. Matsushima, and A. P. Anzil. 1969. High structural stability of vascular and glial basement membranes in areas of total brain tissue necrosis. Experientia 25:976.

Bloom, P. M., J. F. Hartmann, and R. L. Jernier. 1959. An electron microscopic evaluation of the width of normal glomerular basement membrane in man at various ages. Anat. Rec. 133:251.

Brightman, M. W., and T. S. Reese. 1969. Junctions between intimately apposed cell membranes in the vertebrate brain. J. Cell Biol. 40:648—677.

Bruns, R. R., and G. E. Palade. 1968a. Studies on blood capillaries. I. General organizations of muscle capillaries. J. Cell Biol. 37:244—276.

Bruns, R. R., and G. E. Palade. 1968b. Studies on blood capillaries. II. Transport of ferritin molecules across the wall of muscle capillaries. J. Cell Biol. 37:277—299.

Campbell, G. R., and Y. Uehara. 1972. Formation of fenestrated capillaries in mammalian vas deferens and ureter transplants. Z. Zellforsch. Mikrosk. Anat. 134:167—173.

Carr, I. 1972. The fine structure of microfibrils and microtubules in macrophages and other lymphoreticular cells in relation to cytoplasmic movement. J. Anat. 112:383—391.

Casley-Smith, J. R. 1970. The functioning of endothelial fenestrae on the arterial and venous limbs of capillaries, as indicated by differing directions of passage of proteins. Experientia 26:852—853.

Casley-Smith, J. R. 1971. Endothelial fenestrae in intestinal villi: Differences between the arterial and venous end of the capillaries. Microvasc. Res. 3:49—68.

Casley-Smith, J. R., and H. I. Clark. 1972. The dimensions and numbers of small vesicles in blood capillary endothelium in the hind legs of dogs, and their relation to vascular permeability. J. Microsc. 96:263−267.

Cecio, A. 1967. Ultrastructural features of cytofilaments within mammalian endothelial cells. Z. Zellforsch. 83:40−48.

Cervos-Navarro, J., and F. Matakas. 1974. Electron microscopic evidence for innervation of intracerebral arterioles in the cat. Neurology 24:282−286.

Churg, J., V. A. Discala, M. Salomon, and E. Grishman. 1966. Renal structure in hypothyroidism. *In* R. Uyeda (ed.), Sixth International Congress on Electron Microscopy, Kyoto, Vol. II, p. 665.

Claesson, M. H., O. Jørgensen, and C. Røpke. 1971. Light and electron microscopic studies of the paracortical post-capillary high endothelial venules. Z. Zellforsch. Mikroskop. Anat. 119:195−208.

Clementi, F., and G. E. Palade. 1969a. Intestinal capillaries. I. Permeability to peroxydase and ferritin. J. Cell Biol. 41:33−52.

Clementi, F., and G. E. Palade. 1969b. Intestinal capillaries. II. Structural effects of EDTA and histamin. J. Cell Biol. 42:706−714.

Cohen, A. S., and E. Calkins. 1960. A study of the fine structure of the kidney in casein-induced amyloidosis in rabbits. J. Exp. Med. 112:479−490.

Cohen, A. S., L. Weiss, and E. Calkins. 1960. Electronmicroscopic observations of the spleen during the induction of experimental amyloidosis in the rabbit. Am. J. Pathol. 37:413−431.

Cotran, R. S., and G. Majno. 1964. A light and electronmicroscopic analysis of vascular injury. Ann. N.Y. Acad. Sci. 116:750−764.

Cotran, R. S., E. R. Suter, and G. Majno. 1967. The use of colloidal carbon as a tracer for vascular injury. A review. Vasc. Dis. (N.Y.) 4:107−127.

Deen, W. M., C. R. Robertson, and B. M. Brenner. 1974. Concentration polarization in an ultrafiltering capillary. Biophys. J. 14:412−431.

Dieterich, C. E., H. J. Dieterich, M. A. Spycher, and M. Pfautsch. 1973. Fine structural observations of the pecten oculi capillaries of the chicken. Z. Zellforsch. 146:473−489.

Dieterich, C. E., and H. J. Dieterich. 1974. Vergleichend-elektronen-mikroskopische Untersuchungen am Kapillarendothel des conus papillaris von Echsen (Sauria). 69. Vers. Anat. Ges. Anat. Anz.

Dorn, E. 1961. Über den Feinbau der Schwimmblase von Anguilla vulgaris L. Licht- und elektronenmikroskopische Untersuchungen. Z. Zellforsch. 55:849−912.

Elfvin, L. G. 1965. The ultrastructure of the capillary fenestrae in the adrenal medulla of the rat. J. Ultrastruct. Res. 12:687−704.

Ericsson, L., and E. Ericsson. 1973. Morphological aspects of intravascular and extravascular phenomena in cat skeletal muscle at low flow states. Advan. Microcirc. 5:72−79.

Farquhar, M. G. 1964. Glomerular permeability investigated by electron microscopy. *In* M. D. Siperstein, A. H. Colwell, and K. Meyer (eds.), Conference on small blood vessel involvement in diabetes mellitus, pp. 31−38. American Institute of Biological Sciences, Washington, D.C.

Fawcett, D. W. 1959. The fine structure of capillaries, arterioles and small arteries. *In* S. R. M. Reynolds and B. W. Zweifach (eds.), The Microcirculation, pp. 1−27. University of Illinois Press, Urbana.

Fernando, N. V. P., and H. Z. Movat. 1964a. The fine structure of the terminal vascular bed. II. The smallest arterial vessels; terminal arterioles and metarterioles. Exp. Mol. Pathol. 3:1−9.

Fernando, N. V. P., and H. Z. Movat. 1964b. The fine structure of the terminal vascular bed. III. The capillaries. Exp. Mol. Pathol. 3:87.

Fletscher, J. R. 1964. Light and electron microscopic studies of the effect of reserpine on the adrenal medulla of the guinea pig. Exp. Cell Res. 36:579–591.

Florey, Lord W. 1966. The endothelial cell. Br. Med. J. 2/2512:487–490.

Flumerfelt, B. A., P. R. Lewis, and D. G. Gwyn. 1973. Cholinesterase activity of capillaries in the rat brain. A light and electron microscopic study. Histochem. J. 5:67–79.

Friederici, H. H. R. 1967. The early response of uterine capillaries to estrogen stimulation. An electron microscopic study. Lab. Invest. 17:322–333.

Friederici, H. H. 1968. The three dimensional ultrastructure of fenestrated capillaries. J. Ultrastruct. Res. 23:444–456.

Fung, K. K., and N. Kalant. 1972. Phospholipid of the rat glomerular basement membrane in experimental nephrosis. Biochem. J. 129:733–743.

Gabbiani, G., M. C. Badonnel, and G. Majno. 1970. Intra-arterial injections of histamine, serotonin or bradykinin: A topographic study of vascular leakage. Proc. Soc. Exp. Biol. Med. 135:447–452.

Gabbiani, G., and G. Majno. 1969. Endothelial microvilli in the vessels of the rat Gasserian ganglion and testis. Z. Zellforsch. 97:111–117.

Giacomelli, F., J. Wiener, and D. Spiro. 1970. Cross-straited arrays of filaments in endothelium. J. Cell Biol. 45:188–192.

Greenberger, N. J. 1969. The intestinal brush border as a digestive and absorptive surface. Am. J. Med. Sci. 258:144–149.

Güldner, F.-H., J. R. Wolff, and D. Graf Keyserlingk. 1972. Fibroblasts as a part of the contractile system in duodenal villi of rat. Z. Zellforsch. 135:349–360.

Güldner, F.-H., and J. R. Wolff. 1973. Seamless endothelia as indicators of capillaries developed from sprouts. Bibl. Anat. 12:120–123.

Haim, G. 1968. Elektronenmikroskopische Untersuchungen der Hyperplasia gingivae gravidarum. Dtsch. Zahn-, Mund- u. Kieferheilk. 50:121–136.

Hammersen, F. 1966. Poren- und Fensterendothelien der Kapillaren in der Skelettmuskulatur der Ratte. Z. Zellforsch. 69:296–310.

Hammersen, F. 1968. The pattern of terminal vascular bed and the ultrastructure of capillaries in skeletal muscle. In D. W. Lübbers (ed.), Oxygen Transport in Blood and Tissue, pp. 184–197. G. Thieme, Stuttgart.

Hammersen, F. 1972a. The fine structure of different types of experimental edema for testing the effect of vasoactive drugs demonstrated with a flavonoid. Angiologica 9:326–354.

Hammersen, F. 1972b. Ultrastructure and functions of capillaries and lymphatics. Pflügers Arch., Suppl. 43–63.

Han, S. S., and J. K. Avery. 1963. The ultrastructure of capillaries and arterioles of the hamster dental pulp. Anat. Rec. 145:549–572.

Hauck, G. 1971. Organisation und Funktion der terminalen Strombahn. In I. Bauereisen (ed.), Physiologie des Kreislaufs I, pp. 100–144. Springer, New York.

Hempel, E., and G. Geyer. 1967. Experimentelle Untersuchungen an der glomerularen Basalmembran in der Niere der Maus. Anat. Anz. 120:84–90.

Herman, L. 1960. An EM study of the salamander thyroid during hormonal stimulation. J. Biophys. Biochem. Cytol. 7:143–150.

Heumann, H.-G. 1971. Mechanism of smooth muscle contraction. An electron microscopic study of the mouse large intestine. Cytobiologie 3:259.

Hibbs, R. G., G. F. Burch, and J. H. Phillips. 1958. The fine structure of the small blood vessels of normal human dermis and subcutis. Am. Heart J. 56/5:662–670.

Hinglais, N., J.-P. Grünfeld, and E. Bois. 1972. Characteristic ultrastructural lesion of the glomerular basement membrane in progressive hereditary nephritis (Alport's syndrome). Lab. Invest. 27:473–488.

Horstmann, E. 1966. Über das Endothel der Zottenkapillaren im Dünndarm des Meerschweinchens und des Menschen. Z. Zellforsch. 72:364–369.

Intaglietta, M., and E. P. De Plomb. 1973. Fluid exchange in tunnel and tube capillaries. Microvasc. Res. 6:153–168.

Jörgensen, F., and M. W. Bentzon. 1968. The ultrastructure of the normal human glomerulus. Thickness of glomerular basement membrane. Lab. Invest. 13:42.

Johnson, L. D., and G. B. Pierce. 1970. Changes in antigenicity of basement membrane during wound healing. Devel. Biol. 23:534–549.

Joó, F. 1969. Changes in the molecular organization of the basement membrane after inhibition of adenosine triphosphatase activity in the rat brain capillaries. Cytobios 1:289.

Joó, F. 1972. Effect of N_6O_2-dibutyryl-cyclic-3'-5'-adenosine monophosphate during enhanced permeability of the blood-brain barrier. Br. J. Exp. Pathol. 52:646–649.

Joó, F. 1972. Effect of N_6O_2-dibutyryl-cyclic-3'-5'-adenosine monophosphate on the pinocytosis of brain capillaries of mice. Experientia 28:1470–1471.

Karnovsky, M. J. 1968. The ultrastructural basis of transcapillary exchanges. J. Gen. Physiol. 52 (Suppl.):64s–95s.

Karnovsky, M. J. 1970. Morphology of capillaries with special reference to muscle capillaries. In C. Crone and N. A. Lassen (eds.), Capillary Permeability. The Transfer of Molecules and Ions Between Capillary Blood and Tissues. Proceedings of the Alfred Benzon Symposium II. Copenhagen, 1969. Academic Press, New York.

Karrer, H. E., and J. Cox. 1960. The striated musculature of blood vessels. II. Cell interconnections and cell surface. J. Biophys. Biochem. Cytol. 8:135–150.

Kessel, R. G., and W. R. Panje. 1968. Organization and activity in pre- and postovulatory follicle of necturus maculosus. J. Cell Biol. 39:1–34.

Kisch, B. 1957. Electronmicroscopy of the capillary wall. II. Filiform processes of the endothelium. Exp. Med. Surg. 15:89.

Krebs, W., and H. David. 1962. Beitrag zu elektronenmikroskopischen und funktionellen Altersveränderungen der Kapillaren. Dtsch. Gesundh. wesen 17/43:1845–1849.

Landis, E. M., and J. R. Pappenheimer. 1963. Exchange of substances through the capillary wall. In W. F. Hamilton and P. Dow (eds.), Handbook of physiology, Section 2: Circulation, Vol. II, p. 961–1034. American Physiological Society, Washington, D.C.

Lipowsky, H. H., and B. W. Zweifach. 1974. Network analysis of microcirculation of cat mesentery. Microvasc. Res. 7:73–83.

Luciano, L., and E. Jünger. 1968. Glykogen in glatten Muskelzellen der Gefäßwand von Säugetieren. Elektronenmikroskopische und spektrophotometrische Untersuchungen. Histochemie (Berl.) 15:219–228.

Majno, G., and G. E. Palade. 1961. Studies on inflammation. I. The effect of histamine and serotonin on vascular permeability: An electronmicroscopic study. J. Biophys. Biochem. Cytol. 11:571–606.

Majno, G., G. E. Palade, and G. I. Schoefl. 1961. Studies on inflammation. II.

The site of action of histamine and serotonin along the vascular tree: A topographic study. J. Biophys. Biochem. Cytol. 11:607–626.

Majno, G. 1965. Ultrastructure of the vascular membrane. *In* W. F. Hamilton and P. Dow (eds.), Handbook of Physiology, Section 2: Circulation, Vol. III, pp. 2293–2375. American Physiology Society, Washington, D.C.

Majno, G., S. M. Shea, and M. Leventhal. 1969. Endothelial contraction induced by histamine type mediators. J. Cell Biol. 42:647–672.

McLeod, W. A. 1970. Observations of fenestrated capillaries in the human scalp. J. Invest. Derm. 55:354–357.

Maul, G. G. 1971. Structure and formation of pores in fenestrated capillaries. J. Ultrastruct. Res. 36:768.

Misra, R. P., and L. B. Berman. 1969. Glomerular basement membrane: Insights from molecular models. Am. J. Med. 47:337–339.

Mönninghoff, W., H. Themann, and U. Westphal. 1972. Elektronenmikroskopische Untersuchungen über den Einfluß von Magnesium- und Calcium-Chelaten auf die Capillarpermeabilität im Herzmuskel der Maus. Res. Exp. Med. 157:123.

Moffat, D. B. 1968. The fine structure of the blood vessels of the renal medulla with particular reference to the control of the medullary circulation. J. Ultrastruct. Res. 19:532–545.

Mohamed, A. H., J. P. Waterhouse, and H. H. R. Friederici. 1973. The fine structure of gingival terminal vascular bed. Microvasc. Res. 6:137–152.

Monroe, B. C. 1953. Electronmicroscopy of the thyroid. Anat. Rec. 116:345–361.

Moore, D. H., and H. Ruska. 1957. The fine structure of capillaries and small arteries. J. Biophys. Biochem. Cytol. 3:457–462.

Mori, M. 1967. An electron microscope study on the sinus endothelial cells of lymph node with reference to their relation to the reticuloendothelial system. Sapporo Med. J. 30/2–3:65–84.

Movat, H. Z., and Fernando, N. V. P. 1964. The fine structure of the terminal vascular bed. IV. The venules and their perivascular cells (pericytes, adventitia cells). Exp. Mol. Pathol. 3:98–114.

Palade, G. E. 1953. Fine structure of blood capillaries. J. Appl. Physiol. 24:1424.

Parakkal, P. F. 1966. The fine structure of the dermal papilla of the guinea pig hair follicle. J. Ultrastruct. Res. 14:133–142.

Pardo, V., E. R. Fisher, E. Perez-Stable, and G. P. Rodnan. 1966. Ultrastrukturelle Untersuchungen bei Hypertension. II. Nierengefäßveranderungen bei progressiver systematisierter Sklerose. Lab. Invest. 15:1434–1441.

Pardo, V., E. Perez-Stable, D. B. Alzamora, and W. Cleveland. 1972. Incidence and significance of muscle capillary basal lamina thickness in juvenile diabetes. Am. J. Pathol. 68:67–81.

Pease, D. C. 1960. The basement membrane: substratum of histological order and complexity. 4. Internat. Kongr. Elektronenmikroskopie 1958, Bd. II, S. 139. Springer, Berlin.

Phelps, C., and J. H. Luft. 1969. Electron microscopical study of relaxation and constriction in frog arterioles. Am. J. Anat. 125:399–428.

Rappaport, A. M. 1973. The microcirculatory hepatic unit. Microvasc. Res. 6:212–228.

Rhodin, J. A. G. 1962. Fine structure of vascular walls in mammals. Physiol. Rev. 42, Suppl. 5:II, 48.

Rhodin, J. A. G. 1967. The ultrastructure of mammalian arterioles and pre-capillary sphincters. J. Ultrastruct. Res. 18:181–223.

Rhodin, J. A. G. 1968. Ultrastructure of mammalian venous capillaries, venules and small collecting veins. J. Ultrastruct. Res. 25:452–500.

Riedel, H., H. G. Fromme, and B. Tallen. 1966. Elektronenmikroskopische Untersuchungen zur Frage der Kapillarmorphologie in der menschlichen Zahnpulpa. Arch. oral. Biol. 11:1049–1055.

Röhlich, P., and J. Oláh. 1967. Cross-striated fibrils in the endothelium of the rat myometral arterioles. J. Ultrastruct. Res. 18:667–676.

Romanul, F. C., and R. G. Bannister. 1962. Localized areas of high alkaline phosphatase activity in the terminal arterial tree. J. Cell Biol. 15:73–84.

Ruckley, V. A., M. K. McDonald, P. R. MacLean, and J. S. Robson. 1966. Glomerular ultrastructure and function in orthostatic proteinuria. Nephron (Basel) 3:153–166.

Santolaya, R. C., and F. Bertini. 1970. Fine structure of endothelial cells of vertebrates. Distribution of dense granules. Z. Anat. Entwicklungs-Gesch. 131:148–155.

Schaffner, F., and H. Popper. 1963. Capillarization of hepatic sinusoids in man. Gastroenterology 44:239.

Schoefl, G. I. 1963. Studies on inflammation. III. Growing capillaries: their structure and permeability. Virch. Arch. 337:97.

Semba, T. 1962. The fine structure of the pecten studied with the EM. I. chick pecten. Kyushu J. Med. Sci. 13:24.

Shea, S. M., and W. H. Bossert. 1973. Vesicular transport across endothelium: A generalized diffusion model. Microvasc. Res. 6:305–315.

Shea, S. M., J. B. Caulfield, and J. F. Burke. 1973. Microvascular ultrastructure in thermal injury: A reconsideration of the role of mediators. Microvasc. Res. 5:87–96.

Shimamoto, T., T. Sunaga, and Y. Yamashita. 1970. Progress in the study of atherosclerosis by the appearance of scanning electron microscopy—new structure: Form and pathological physiology of vascular endothelial folds and intracellular bridge. Jap. J. Clin. Med. 28:1529–1543.

Simon, G. 1965. Ultrastructure des capillaires, Kap. II. Angiologica 2:370–434.

Sosula, L., P. Beaumont, F. C. Hollows, and K. M. Jonson. 1972. Dilatation and endothelial proliferation of retinal capillaries in streptozotocin-diabetic rats: Quantitative electron microscopy. Invest. Ophthalmol. 11:926–935.

Stehbens, W. E., and R. M. Ludatscher. 1968. Fine structure of senile angiomas of human skin. Angiology 19:581–592.

Stingl, J. 1971. Zur Ultrastruktur des terminalen Gefäßbettes der Skelettmuskulatur. Acta Anat. 80:255–272.

Sulzmann, R. 1965. Elektronenoptischer Nachweis von kristallinen Einschlüssen in gefensterten Venulenendothelien der menschlichen Eckzahnpulpa. Dtsche. Zahnärztl. Z. 20:973–975.

Suwa, K. 1962. The use of alcian blue 8GS for vital stain, and the mode and routes of the entrance of basic dye into tunica media across the endothelium of elastic arteries in rabbits with the light and electronmicroscopes. Acta Med. Okayama 16, Suppl.:39–52.

Takada, M., and S. Hattori. 1972. Presence of fenestrated capillaries in the skin. Anat. Rec. 173:213–220.

Vracko, R., and E. P. Benditt. 1972. Basal lamina: The scaffold for orderly cell replacement. Observations on regeneration of injured skeletal muscle fibers and capillaries. J. Cell Biol. 55:406–419.

5

Weibel, E. R., and B. W. Knight. 1964. A morphometric study of the thickness of the pulmonary air-blood barrier. J. Cell Biol. 21:367.

Wendt, L. 1974. Krankheiten verminderter Kapillarmembran-Permeabilität. Verl. E. E. Koch, Frankfurt 1973. 2. Aufl.

Westergaard, E., and M. W. Brightman. 1973. Transport of proteins across normal cerebral arterioles. J. Comp. Neurol. 152:17−45.

Wiederhielm, C. A. 1968. Dynamics of transcapillary fluid exchange. J. Cell Biol. 52:295−615.

Wolff, J. 1966. Elektronenmikroskopische Untersuchungen über die Vesikulation im Kapillarendothel. Lokalisation, Variation und Fusion der Vesikel. Z. Zellforsch. 73:143−164.

Wolff, J., and H. J. Merker. 1966. Ultrastruktur und Bildung von Poren im Endothel von porösen und geschlossenen Kapillaren. Z. Zellforsch. 73:174−191.

Wolff, J. 1967. On the meaning of vesiculation in capillary endothelium. Angiologica 4:64−68.

Wolff, J. 1971. Ultrastruktur der Capillaren. In I. Bauereisen (ed.), Physiologie des Kreislaufs, pp. 67−98. Springer, Berlin.

Wolff, J. R., and T. Bär. 1972. "Seamless" endothelia in brain capillaries during development of the rat's cerebral cortex. Brain Res. 41:17−24.

Wolff, J. R., A. Moritz, and F.-H. Güldner. 1972. "Seamless" endothelia within fenestrated capillaries of duodenal villi (rat). Angiologica 9:11−14.

BIOLOGY OF
ENDOTHELIUM AND
CONNECTIVE
TISSUE

chapter 5

FINE STRUCTURE
OF ENDOTHELIUM

Guilio Gabbiani and Guido Majno

ENDOTHELIAL STRUCTURES IN RELATION
TO PERMEABILITY
Endothelial Junctions
Fenestrations and Discontinuities
Cytoplasmic Vesicles
Cytoplasmic Filaments
Basement Membrane

INTERACTION WITH FORMED BLOOD ELEMENTS

CONCLUDING REMARKS

The endothelium is a very extensive, thin cellular layer representing the ultimate barrier between the blood and the tissues. The largest part of its surface belongs to the microcirculatory system (Figure 1): it is at this level that most of the exchanges between blood and tissues occur. (See Chapter 8–10 in this volume.)

Physiologic studies have shown that the capillary wall can be considered to be a semipermeable membrane and that the process of transcapillary exchange is, to some extent, passive in nature, dependent on diffusion, filtration, and hydrostatic and osmotic pressures (Pappenheimer, 1953; Mayerson et al., 1960; Landis and Pappenheimer, 1963; Yudilevich and Alvarez, 1967). Thus it would seem that the vascular barrier behaves as if it were a semipermeable membrane penetrated by water-filled channels or pores, through which water and small, lipid-insoluble molecules pass: such pores seem to occupy a very small fraction of the capillary surface.

Pappenheimer's concept of a pore system stimulated the interest of many investigators. On the basis of physiologic techniques, the existence of a system of small pores (40–50 Å radius) and larger pores (120–350 Å radius) has been postulated (Grotte, 1956; Mayerson et al., 1960). The smaller pores allow the passage of water and small lipid-insoluble molecules, and the larger pores (fewer

This work was supported in part by the Fonds National Suisse pour la Recherche Scientifique (Grants No. 3.356.70, 3.460.70 and 3.0330.73) and by the Zyma S.A. Nyon, Switzerland.

133

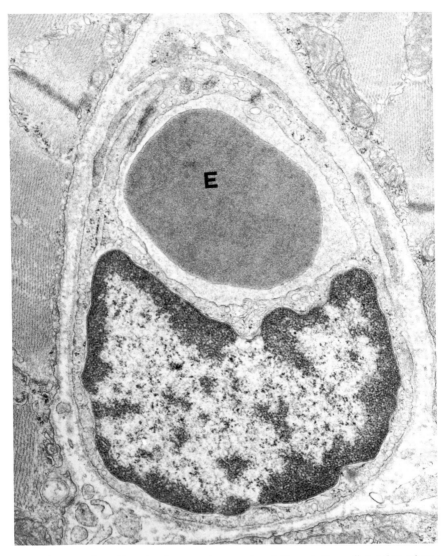

Figure 1. Normal capillary in the masseter muscle of the rat. Its wall consists of two endothelial cells: one has a large nucleus surrounded by a thin layer of cytoplasm containing rough endoplasmic reticulum and many vesicles. Some vesicles face the lumen, others open toward the continuous basement membrane. The endothelial junctions show condensations of the type macula occludens. × 21,300. E, erythrocyte.

in number) are capable of allowing the passage of molecules of varying molecular weight including large proteins or particulate matter.

Subsequent ultrastructural studies (Jennings, Marchesi, and Florey, 1962; Karnovsky, 1967; Revel and Karnovsky, 1967), using tracer particles with a radius from 25 to 250 Å, have suggested that in continuous capillaries the small pore system is represented by endothelial junctions (more or less focal tight junctions), and the large pore system by the intracytoplasmic vesicular system first described by Palade (1953). This classification of pores, however, has been called into question because recent tracer studies do not seem to provide firm evidence that the interendothelial junctions are the only site of the small pore system (Williams and Wissig, 1975). More specialized gap junctions have been described between endothelial cells of the rat aorta (Hüttner, Boutet, and More, 1973) and related to a possible electrical coupling between endothelium and smooth muscle.

These correlations, however, do not apply to all vessels in all regions of the body; e.g., (1) in the brain, the endothelial junctions form *zonulae occludentes*, which probably represent the morphologic equivalent of the blood—brain barrier (Reese and Karnovsky, 1967); and (2) the fenestrated or discontinuous endothelia (e.g., those of endocrine glands or the liver sinusoids), for obvious reasons, are more permeable than continuous capillaries (Karnovsky, 1968).

Physiologic studies of territories irrigated mostly by continuous capillaries have shown that molecular exchanges can take place differently both quantitatively and qualitatively in various organs (Majno, 1965). Moreover, it is accepted by physiologists and morphologists that permeability is generally greater in the venular part of the microcirculation rather than in the more proximal small vessels (Majno, 1965; Wiederhielm, 1968; Hauck and Schröer, 1969). Therefore, even in continuous capillaries, the overall concept that the vascular wall acts as a semipermeable membrane implies the interaction of different factors acting at various levels. In special situations and especially in pathologic conditions, these factors may cause important changes in the blood—tissue exchanges in a given territory.

ENDOTHELIAL STRUCTURES IN RELATION TO PERMEABILITY

Some of the differences in permeability between certain areas of the microcirculatory system are related to obvious anatomic variations in the endothelial cells. In some situations, however, such differences are not immediately apparent. They may become so when the microcirculatory system is subjected to a certain degree of stress or damage. We briefly review the endothelial structures that may participate in the various processes bringing about molecular exchanges, and then discuss their respective roles in altering the permeability of blood vessels. (For further discussions see Chapters 4 and 7 in this volume.)

Endothelial Junctions

By electron microscopy, apposing cell membranes in a continuous capillary appear very close, with an intervening gap of 100—200 Å (Majno, 1965). At certain points, these membranes and the adjacent cytoplasm appear darker (Figure 1). The intercellular clefts are also sealed by tight junctions or *maculae occludentes*, which are formed by the close apposition or fusion of the external leaflets of the plasmalemma to give a "quintuple-layered junction," i.e. three dark lines separated by two clear ones (Muir and Peters, 1962; Farquhar and Palade, 1963) completely obliterating the intercellular space. This phenomenon can be demonstrated between cells of many types, including vascular endo-thelium (Karrer, 1960; Farquhar and Palade, 1965; McNutt and Weinstein, 1973). In certain areas of the microcirculatory system (e.g., in the brain) it has been proposed that these junctions form an uninterrupted seal, i.e., *zonulae occludentes,* preventing the passage of molecules with a radius of 25 Å (Reese and Karnovsky, 1967).

Although there are no detailed studies on the extent of maculae and zonulae occludentes in different vessels, it seems reasonable to expect that the quantita-tive distribution of these structures may participate in the determination of the degree of permeability of blood vessels in a given vascular bed, under normal conditions.

Fenestrations and Discontinuities

Fenestrated capillaries (Majno, 1965; see Chapters 4 and 19 in this volume) are generally similar to continuous capillaries in that they have a continuous base-ment membrane and a sheet of closely apposed endothelial cells. However, they also differ in two main respects. The endothelial cells are thinner, with few organelles and pinocytotic vesicles, and contain rounded fenestrae 200–1,000 Å in diameter, usually closed by a diaphragm about 40 Å in thickness (Rhodin, 1962; Luft, 1965). This type of vessel has been described in three groups of organs: (1) endocrine glands, (2) structures engaged in the production or absorp-tion of fluids (e.g., renal glomerulus, choroid plexus, intestinal villus), and (3) retia mirabilia (e.g., renal medulla, fish swim bladder).

A peculiar feature of fenestrated capillaries is that occasionally a cell that lies outside the vessel protrudes through the endothelium into the lumen. This is seen in the renal glomerulus (Yamada, 1955), where the protrusion of mesangial cells is relatively common, and in the hypophysis and in the adrenal gland (Majno, 1965). Because these protruding cells are often phagocytic, their parti-cipation in blood–tissue exchanges becomes evident.

Discontinuities between endothelial cells are present in those vessels com-monly called sinusoids. In addition to possessing intercellular gaps, sinusoids lack a continuous basement membrane. This type of vessel is common in organs whose primary functions are to add or to extract from the blood whole cells as well as large molecules and extraneous particles, e.g., liver, spleen, and bone marrow. In the liver sinusoids "sieve plates" have been described at the level of endothelial fenestrations, after fixation of the organ by glutaraldehyde perfu-sion. These would not allow the passage of molecules larger than 1,000 Å and may have important implications in the interpretation of the filtering function of liver sinusoids (Wisse, 1969).

The phagocytic activity in the sinusoids is almost exclusively confined to specialized cells lining the vascular wall, such as the Kupffer cells in the liver. In contrast to endothelial cells, these show a characteristic pattern of endogenous peroxidase activity in the endoplasmic reticulum and perinuclear cisternae (Widmann, Cotran, and Fahimi, 1972). Thus it appears that endothelial cells and mononuclear phagocytes in the liver sinusoids are two distinct cellular entities rather than two variants of the same cell type.

Cytoplasmic Vesicles

A system of spherical vesicles is present in several cell types but is more prominent in the endothelium (Palade, 1953; Majno, 1965) (Figure 1). The vesicles are very uniform in diameter (600–700 Å) and so numerous as to occupy about one-third of the cell volume in the capillaries of rat myocardium (Palade, 1961). In cross section, the majority appear to lie just below the cell membrane along the blood and tissue fronts of the cell. Some vesicles lie free in the cytoplasm, others are in contact with the plasma membrane at the surface of the cell, and others actually open through this membrane (either toward the vascular lumen or towards the basement membrane). Palade (1953), in the first description of endothelial vesicles, suggested that these images could represent different stages of molecular transport through the cytoplasm. In the light of recent studies, the original suggestion that these vesicles represent the large pore system of endothelium would have to be modified. Simionescu, Simionescu, and Palade (1975) have demonstrated that probe molecules of the size of 20 Å cross the endothelium primarily via intercytoplasmic vesicles that quite likely form patent channels across the cells in muscle capillaries.

Cytoplasmic Filaments

Intracytoplasmic filaments, like vesicles, are present not only in endothelial cells (Majno, 1965; Rhodin, 1967; Majno, Shea, and Leventhal, 1969). If we exclude muscular tissues, they are found in a large variety of cell types (Wessels et al., 1971) and have been implicated in such phenomena as contractility, movement (Goldman, 1971; Gabbiani et al., 1972), and secretion (Orci, Gabbay, and Malaisse, 1972). Extensive studies on the distribution of intracytoplasmic filaments in the endothelial cells of different parts of the vascular tree are not available at present. In our experience they are less prominent in the rat aortic endothelium [here a very important system of microfilaments develops during hypertension (Gabbiani and Rona, 1974)] but very numerous in arterioles (Giacomelli, Wiener, and Spiro, 1970), including coronary arterioles (Figures 2 and 3) (Yohoro and Burnstock, 1973) and in small vessels of granulation tissue.

These filaments usually have a diameter of 40–80 Å (Figure 3) and occasionally of 100–120 Å; these diameters are similar to those of actin and myosin, respectively (Goldman, 1971). They are located more often at the cell periphery,

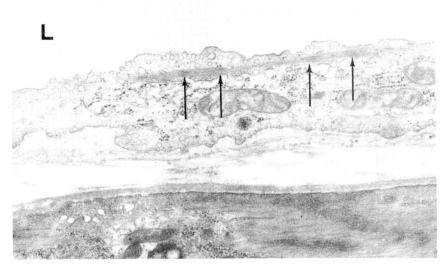

Figure 2. Wall of a coronary arteriole in the rat. The endothelial cell contains a bundle of microfilaments similar to those present in the underlying smooth muscle. Note dark bands in the filamentous bundle (arrows). There are few microtubules. × 20,800. L, lumen. Reproduced by permission of Dr. I. Joris.

toward the cell junctions or the basement membrane. When facing the cell membrane they may show zones of condensation forming hemidesmosome-like complexes (Stehbens, 1966). In view of the increased interest in the contractile ability of nonmuscular cells (Majno et al., 1969; Wessels et al., 1971; Gabbiani et al., 1972), further studies are needed to understand better the role of endothelial filaments.

Basement Membrane

The existence of a fine connective tissue sheath around small vessels (Figure 1) was established a long time ago. This sheath has been shown to be argyrophylic (Plenk, 1927) and to stain red with the PAS reaction (Gersh and Catchpole, 1949). Thus it was thought that the vascular basement membrane was composed mostly of polysaccharides. However, the finding that collagenase could almost completely hydrolyse the basement membrane (Speidel and Lazarow, 1963) indicated that the major component of basement membrane was collagen. Lately it has been shown that collagen is one of the most powerful inducers of platelet aggregation (Marcus and Zucker, 1965). Hence it seemed easy to understand why endothelial lesions that allowed free contact between basement membrane and blood elements could induce thrombus formation. There is evidence that well-formed collagen (with the typical periodicity of 640 Å) is inserted into or is closely associated with the basement membrane of small vessels (Majno, 1965). More recently, it has been proposed that basement membrane is composed not

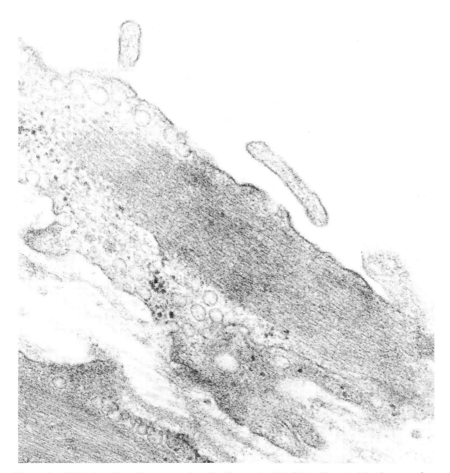

Figure 3. Thick bundle of intracytoplasmic filaments (40–80 Å diameter) in the cytoplasm of an endothelial cell from a rat coronary arteriole. × 51,100. Reproduced by permission of Dr. I. Joris.

only of collagen but mostly of microfibrils (Baumgartner, Stemerman, and Spaet, 1971) similar to those demonstrated by Ross and Bornstein (1969) in connective tissue. The modality of interaction between basement membrane and platelets seems to be different from the modality of interaction between collagen and platelets (Baumgartner et al., 1971), thus supporting the concept that basement membrane is not only composed of this protein.

The origin of basement membrane in small and large vessels (as well as in other structures such as epithelia) has been the subject of much discussion. It seems certain that endothelial cells (as well as pericytes, smooth muscle, and epithelia) actively participate in the building of the basement membrane either by synthesizing the principal constituents or by producing substances capable of organizing the surrounding connective tissue into forming a basement membrane (Majno, 1965). Where there is chronic endothelial damage, several layers of basement membrane surrounding the small vessels can be frequently observed with the electron microscope (Vracko and Benditt, 1972). This probably results from a rapid turnover of endothelial cells, which produce their own basement membrane.

INTERACTION WITH FORMED BLOOD ELEMENTS

Blood−tissue exchanges in normal and pathologic conditions are influenced by the presence and activity of various blood elements and by the interactions between these structures and the endothelium. In certain conditions the endothelium may become detached from the vascular wall and enter the circulation. This takes place when there is local or systemic vascular damage (e.g., local trauma, endotoxin administration) (Gaynor, Bouvier, and Spaet, 1968; McGrath and Stewart, 1969). This phenomenon, the consequences of which are not yet well clarified, deserves further study, particularly in view of the recent findings indicating that endothelium and platelets have similar morphologic and functional characteristics (Johnson, 1971; Booyse et al., 1973; Rafelson, Hoveke, and Booyse, 1973). On the other hand, different blood elements may influence endothelium in different ways. It has been shown in large vessels that platelet adhesion to the basement membrane after endothelial damage depends largely upon the presence of whole blood, and not simply of plasma (Baumgartner et al., 1971); these features probably apply to small vessels. Whether the factor that is lacking in plasma is Hellen's factor "R" of erythrocytes (later identified as ADP) is not yet clear (Baumgartner et al., 1971).

Adhesion of red cells to endothelium and diapedesis of red cells through the endothelial wall are well-known phenomena in inflammation, although their mechanism is not yet understood (Grant, 1965; Majno, 1965). Damage to endothelium seems, however, to be a prerequisite for red cell diapedesis. Florey (1962) has described visible roughening of the endothelium in the form of "spikes" around which red cells modify their shape because of the force of the blood stream; whether this is only a special example of erythrocyte sticking is not clear. White cell sticking and diapedesis are two of the most important phenomena in inflammation. Suffice it to mention here that in most cases the passage of leukocytes through the vascular wall takes place at the level of intercellular junctions in the venular part of microcirculatory bed (Grant, 1965; Majno, 1965). Platelets also may stick to the vascular wall (after endothelial damage) and thus initiate the process of aggregation and thrombus formation (Grant, 1965).

An interesting function of platelets is their endothelium-supporting action (Johnson, 1971). It is well established that in thrombocytopenic men or animals the vascular wall of small vessels is more fragile than normal. This results in a prolonged bleeding time and in frequent extravasation of erythrocytes into the interstitial space. The transfusion of platelets into thrombocytopenic animals greatly diminishes these phenomena. Although the mechanism of protection of the vascular wall by platelets is not fully explained, it has been proposed that platelets are incorporated into endothelial cells, thus providing some "support" for the cytoplasm (Johnson, 1971). This is an attractive hypothesis that would explain some recent findings, namely the presence of a similar contractile apparatus in platelets and endothelial cells, and the contraction of both platelets and cultivated endothelial cells when treated with thrombin (Booyse et al., 1973; Rafelson et al., 1973). (For further discussion see Chapter 6 in this volume.)

CONCLUDING REMARKS

In the last few years several new observations have greatly enhanced the knowledge of the structure and function of small vessel endothelium. Although the morphologic equivalents of small and large pores have not as yet been categorically identified as endothelial junctions and pinocytotic vesicles, the equivalent of certain blood–tissue barriers were localized at the level of the endothelial junctions. It is presently well accepted that under pathologic conditions there is a great change in the permeability of endothelial junctions, particularly in venules. However, nothing is known of the possibility that fine changes of such structures modify small vessel permeability and participate in physiologic exchanges.

The presence of new cytoplasmic organelles such as microfilaments was described in many types of vessels. However, the exact functional role of these structures is not yet known. It is also not known with certainty how endothelial cells develop. Many observations favor the possibility that the endothelium is produced locally. However, an hematogenous origin cannot be excluded. Further studies on these lines would prove important in the understanding of the turnover of such cells under normal and pathologic conditions. The possibility that platelets provide some support for the endothelial cytoplasm may stimulate further studies on the interaction between platelets, endothelial cells, and basement membrane in such major pathologic processes as inflammation and thrombus formation. It appears probable that the basement membrane is produced by endothelial cells or that the presence of endothelial cells is necessary for basement membrane formation. Little is known of the role of this structure during exchange processes, particularly in such situations as senility or increased endothelial turnover when several layers of basement membrane surround a single small vessel. Further studies on the structure and function of aging endothelium may furnish new data for the explanation of the permeability changes in old persons. (For further discussion see Chapter 7 in this volume.)

ACKNOLWEDGMENTS

We wish to acknowledge the help of: Drs. S. Mathewson and M-C. Badonnel in the writing of the manuscript; the technical help of Miss M-C. Clottu, Mrs. A. Fiaux, and A. de Almeida; and the photographic work of Messrs. J-C. Rümbeli and E. Denkinger. We are grateful to Dr. I. Joris for contributing the electron micrographs of Figures 2 and 3.

LITERATURE CITED

Baumgartner, H. R., M. B. Stemerman, and Th. H. Spaet. 1971. Adhesion of blood platelets to subendothelial surface: distinct from adhesion to collagen. Experientia 27:283–285.

Booyse, F. M., D. Shepro, M. Rosenthal, and R. I. McDonald. 1973. Properties of cultured aorta endothelial cells. Microvasc. Res. 6:244 (Abstr.).

Farquhar, M. G., and G. E. Palade. 1963. Junctional complexes in various endothelia. J. Cell Biol. 17:375–412.

Farquhar, M. G., and G. E. Palade. 1965. Cell junctions in amphibian skin. J. Cell Biol. 26:263–291.

Florey, H. W. 1962. Inflammation. In H. Florey (ed.), General Pathology, pp. 21–97. Lloyd-Luke, London.

Gabbiani, G., B. J. Hirschel, G. B. Ryan, P. R. Statkov, and G. Majno. 1972. Granulation tissue as a contractile organ. A study of structure and function. J. Exp. Med. 135:719–734.

Gabbiani, G., and G. Rona. 1974. Cytoplasmic Contractile Apparatus in Aortic Endothelial Cells of Hypertensive Rats. Lab. Invest. 32(2):227–234.

Gaynor, E., C. A. Bouvier, and T. H. Spaet. 1968. Circulating endothelial cells in endotoxin treated rabbit. Clin. Res. 16:535 (Abstr.).

Gersh, I., and H. R. Catchpole. 1949. The organization of ground substances and basement membrane and its significance in tissue injury, disease and growth. Am. J. Anat. 85:457–522.

Giacomelli, F., J. Wiener, and D. Spiro. 1970. Cross-striated arrays of filaments in endothelium. J. Cell Biol. 45:188–192.

Goldman, R. D. 1971. The role of three cytoplasmic fibers in BHK-21 cell motility. J. Cell Biol. 51:763–771.

Grant, L. 1965. The sticking and emigration of white blood cells in inflammation. In B. W. Zweifach, L. Grant, and R. T. McCluskey (eds.), The Inflammatory Process, pp. 197–244. Academic Press, New York.

Grotte, G. 1956. Passage of dextran molecules across the blood-lymph barrier. Acta. Chir. Scand. 211 (Suppl.):1–84.

Hauck, G., and H. Schröer. 1969. Vitalmikroskopische Untersuchungen zur Lokalisation der Eiweisspermeabilität an der Endstrombahn von Warmblütern. Pfluegers Arch. 312:32–44.

Hüttner, I., M. Boutet, and R. More. 1973. Gap junctions in arterial endothelium. J. Cell Biol. 57:247–252.

Jennings, M. A., V. T. Marchesi, and H. Florey. 1962. The transport of particles across the walls of small blood vessels. Proc. Roy. Soc. B 156:14–19.

Johnson, S. A. 1971. Endothelial supporting function of platelets. In S. A. Johnson (ed.), The Circulating Platelet, pp. 283–299. Academic Press, New York.

Karnovsky, M. J. 1967. The ultrastructural basis of capillary permeability studied with peroxidase as a tracer. J. Cell Biol. 35:213–236.
Karnovsky, M. J. 1968. The ultrastructural basis of transcapillary exchanges. J. Gen. Physiol. 52 (Suppl.):64–95.
Karrer, H. E. 1960. Cell interconnections in normal human cervical epithelium. J. Biophys. Biochem. Cytol. 7:181–183.
Landis, E. M., and J. R. Pappenheimer. 1963. Exchange of substances through the capillary walls. In Hamilton, W. F. and P. Dow (eds.), Handbook of Physiology, Section 2, Part II, pp. 961–1034. American Physiological Society, Washington, D.C.
Luft, J. H. 1965. The ultrastructural basis of capillary permeability. In B. W. Zweifach (ed.), The Inflammatory Process, pp. 121–159. Academic Press, New York.
McGrath, J. M., and G. J. Stewart. 1969. The effects of endotoxin on vascular endothelium. J. Exp. Med. 129:833–848.
McNutt, N. S., and R. S. Weinstein. 1973. Membrane ultrastructure at mammalian intercellular junctions. Progr. Biophys. Mol. Biol. 26:45–101.
Majno, G. 1965. Ultrastructure of the vascular membrane. In W. F. Hamilton and P. Dow (eds.), Handbook of Physiology, Section 2, Volume II, pp. 2293–2375. American Physiological Society, Washington, D.C.
Majno, G., S. M. Shea, and M. Leventhal. 1969. Endothelial contraction induced by histamine-type mediators. An electron microscopic study. J. Cell Biol. 42:647–672.
Marcus, A., and M. B. Zucker. 1965. The physiology of blood platelets. Grune and Stratton, New York. p. 162.
Mayerson, H. S., C. G. Wolfram, H. H. Shirley, and K. Wasserman. 1960. Regional differences in capillary permeability. Am. J. Physiol. 198:155–160.
Muir, A. R., and A. Peters. 1962. Quintuple layered membrane junctions at terminal bars between endothelial cells. J. Cell Biol. 12:443–448.
Orci, L., K. H. Gabbay, and W. J. Malaisse. 1972. Pancreatic beta-cell web: Its possible role in insulin secretion. Science 175:1128–1130.
Palade, G. E. 1953. Fine structure of blood capillaries. J. Appl. Phys. 24:1424.
Palade, G. E. 1961. Blood capillaries of the heart and other organs. Circulation. 24:368–384.
Pappenheimer, J. R. 1953. Passage of molecules through capillary walls. Physiol. Rev. 33:387–423.
Plenk, H. 1927. Über argyrophile fasern (gitter fasern) und ihre bildungszellen. Ergeb. Anat. Entwicklüngsgeschichte 27:302–412.
Rafelson, N. E., T. P. Hoveke, and F. M. Booyse. 1973. The molecular biology of platelet and platelet-endothelial interactions. Microvasc. Res. 6:245 (Abstr.).
Reese, T. S., and M. J. Karnovsky. 1967. Fine structure localization of a blood-brain barrier to exogenous peroxidase. J. Cell Biol. 34:207–217.
Revel, J. P., and M. J. Karnovsky. 1967. Hexagonal array of subunits in intercellular junctions of the mouse heart and liver. J. Cell Biol. 33:C7–C12.
Rhodin, J. A. G. 1962. The diaphragm of capillary endothelial fenestrations. J. Ultrastruct. Res. 6:171–185.
Rhodin, J. A. G. 1967. The ultrastructure of mammalian arterioles and precapillary sphincters. J. Ultrastruct. Res. 18:181–223.
Ross, R., and P. Bornstein. 1969. The elastic fiber. I. The separation and partial characterization of its macro-molecular components. J. Cell Biol. 40:366–381.

Simionescu, N., M. Simionescu, and G. E. Palade. 1975. Permeability of muscle capillaries to small heme-peptides. J. Cell Biol. 64:586−607.

Speidel, E., and A. Lazarow. 1963. Chemical composition of glomerular basement membrane material in diabetes. Diabetes 12:355.

Stehbens, W. E. 1966. The basal attachment of endothelial cells. J. Ultrastruc. Res. 15:389−399.

Vracko, R., and E. P. Benditt. 1972. Basal lamina: The scaffold for orderly cell replacement. Observations on regeneration of injured skeletal muscle fibers and capillaries. J. Cell Biol. 55:406−419.

Wessels, N. K., B. S. Spooner, J. F. Ash, M. O. Bradley, M. A. Luduena, E. L. A. Taylor, J. T. Wrenn, and K. M. Yamada. 1971. Microfilaments in cellular and development processes. Science (Washington) 171:135−143.

Widmann, J. J., R. S. Cotran, and H. D. Fahimi. 1972. Mononuclear phagocytes (Kupffer cells) and endothelial cells. Identification of two functional cell types in rat liver sinusoids by endogenous peroxidase activity. J. Cell Biol. 52:159−170.

Wiederhielm, C. A. 1968. Dynamics of transcapillary fluid exchange. J. Gen. Physiol. 52 (1, Pt. 2):29S.

Williams, M. C., and S. L. Wissig. 1975. The permeability of muscle capillaries to horseradish peroxidase. J. Cell Biol. 66:531−555.

Wisse, E. 1969. An electron microscopic study of the fenestrated endothelial lining of rat liver sinusoids. J. Ultrastruc. Res. 31:125−150.

Yamada, E. 1955. The fine structure of the renal glomerulus of the mouse. J. Biophys. Biochem. Cytol. 1:551−556.

Yohoro, T., and G. Burnstock. 1973. Filament bundles and contractility of endothelial cells in coronary arteries. Z. Zellforsch. 138:85−95.

Yudilevich, D. L., and O. A. Alvarez. 1967. Water, sodium, and thiourea transcapillary diffusion in the dog heart. Am. J. Physiol. 213:308−314.

chapter 6

THE ARTERIAL ENDOTHELIUM: Characteristics and Function of the Endothelial Lining of Large Arteries

Abel Lazzarini Robertson, Jr., and Lee A. Rosen

COMPARATIVE EMBRYOLOGY AND MORPHOLOGY OF
ARTERIAL ENDOTHELIUM

FUNCTIONAL ASPECTS OF ARTERIAL ENDOTHELIUM
AND ITS METABOLISM
Biochemistry
Cell Multiplication
Respiration
Endothelial Permeability
Hemodynamics

INTERACTION OF CIRCULATING BLOOD ELEMENTS
WITH ARTERIAL ENDOTHELIUM

MORPHOLOGY AND FUNCTION OF ARTERIAL
ENDOTHELIUM IN VITRO

DIFFERENCES BETWEEN ARTERIAL AND OTHER
VASCULAR ENDOTHELIA

FUTURE DEVELOPMENTS

It is our main purpose to review and emphasize the unique morphologic and functional characteristics of the endothelial lining of large and medium size arteries. Much of this recently acquired cytochemical, pharmacologic, and ultrastructural data is currently under intensive investigation in a number of laboratories around the world. What follows is a summary of available results as well as promising research trends.

COMPARATIVE EMBRYOLOGY
AND MORPHOLOGY OF ATERIAL ENDOTHELIUM

In adult man, the normal endothelial lining of large arteries constitutes a single and essentially continuous cell monolayer measuring 0.5–1.2 μ in thickness.

Silver nitrate *en face* staining methods have shown that arterial endothelium is arranged in a characteristic "mosaic" configuration, with occasional multi-nucleated or even giant cells. Endothelial cells, typically elongated in the direction of the vascular axis, are claimed to have fewer intracellular organelles (from mitochondria to endoplasmic reticulum) than most cells. This is not the case, however, with arterial endothelial cells. The presence of fewer organelles may simply represent different stages of the cell cycle; it may not indicate lower metabolic activity at all.

One specific organelle, first described in endothelial cells of small arteries in rats and man by Weibel and Palade (1964), is approximately 3 μ long and 0.1 μ thick, containing small tubules embedded in a dense matrix. While the nature and significance of this cytoplasmic element, known as "Weibel-Palade bodies," is still unclear, it provides a useful ultrastructural marker for arterial endothelial cells.

A significant aspect of endothelial morphology is the junctional configuration between individual cells. The degree of complexity of the intercellular junctions is related to the function of this layer in the regulation of intimal permeability, which is discussed at length in a succeeding portion of this chapter.

In the female Wistar Firth/Mai rat, Schwartz and Benditt (1972) described four types of cell junctions. The least complex and least common forms included the single end-to-end and simple overlap type junctions, while the most common was the "mortice" junction characterized by the interposition of a tongue of one cell into a corresponding invagination of an adjoining endothelial cell. The final type was described as a more complex folded relationship between the two cells involved and was thought by the authors to be almost as common as the "mortice" type. This latter junction type was also described by Robertson and Khairallah (1973) as the most common kind of endothelial junction found in the thoracic aorta of the adult Sprague-Dawley rat.

In hiw review of endothelial embryology, Altschul (1954) discussed the many contradictions and discrepancies that appear in the literature regarding vascular ontogenic origin and concluded that the question was in no way settled. In the 20 years that have elapsed since his review and the present date, little new information has come forth. It has been suggested that blood vessels have their phylogenic origin in the lacunary system of primitive animals. Many authors agree that, ontogenically, the endothelium and the vessel wall is of mesodermal–mesenchymal origin. Blood vessels first appear in the yolk sac of mammals as clusters and cords, forming the vitelline blood vessels and bearing the name of blood islets. Peripheral cells then flatten out, forming the first endothelial layer, while the cells in the center form blood elements (Gilchrist, 1968). Other vessels are known to form in the same manner: angioblasts form cell clones in situ and hollow out to form the endothelial lining. Endothelial differentiation ceases with either development of the aorta (Evans, 1912) or establishment of the circulation (Benninghoff, 1930). Further growth or replacement results from expansion of preformed endothelium.

FUNCTIONAL ASPECTS
OF ARTERIAL ENDOTHELIUM AND ITS METABOLISM

Biochemistry

The limited availability of "pure" arterial endothelial samples for direct quantitative analysis has seriously handicapped collection of meaningful biochemical data. Qualitative histochemistry and quantitative radioisotopic techniques have produced some interesting results, however, particularly in relation to pathologic conditions. A comprehensive monograph by Kirk (1969) reviewed current knowledge on vascular enzymology. Relatively few detailed data were provided on the enzymic activity of the various components of the vascular wall, and reference to specific endothelial enzymes was not made.

Hadjiisky, Scebat, and Renais (1970) reported on their histochemical findings with various enzymes of the adult pheasant (*coturnix coturnix*) aorta, including reductases, dehydrogenases, and ATPase, and concluded that endothelial enzymes have only partial activity in comparison to those of medial smooth muscle cells. In the rabbit, catechol-*o*-methyl transferase has shown greater activity in smooth muscle cells than in endothelium of the aorta, while monoamine oxidase activity was similar in both cell types (Verity, Su, and Bevan, 1972). By contrast, a 15-fold greater histidine decarboxylase activity was found by Hollis and Rosen (1972) in isolated bovine aortic endothelium compared to that of its adjacent media. A recent report indicates that angiotensin-converting enzyme is localized in arterial endothelium and also in endothelial cells of other types of blood vessels of a number of organs in the rabbit, including lung, liver, pancreas, kidney, and spleen (Caldwell et al., 1976). Rabbit and human small arteries showed variations in alkaline phosphatase activity seemingly related to vessel location and diameter (Romanul and Bannister, 1962). In the rat aorta, cytochrome oxidase and DPNH dehydrogenase activities in the endothelial layer have been reported to be only about 20% of that found in liver cells in the same species (Pearl and Cascarano, 1963). Using electron microscopy, it was shown that neutral phosphatase activity of the rabbit aortic endothelial cells is located primarily in cell membrane invaginations at the intercellular junctions and in neighboring pinocytotic vesicles (Hoff and Graf, 1966).

Studies on the biochemistry of lipid metabolism of arterial endothelium have been limited by the methodological difficulties in extrapolating data from homogenates of whole arteries or intimal-medial samples that presuppose a uniformity in cell behavior not verified by in vitro studies. Nevertheless, knowledge of endothelial lipid metabolism is essential for an understanding of the initial stages of vascular pathology such as atherogenesis. Such problems disallow inclusion of many interesting studies on arterial lipid metabolism (Whereat, 1967; Stein and Stein, 1973) in this section on arterial endothelium. Until more sensitive methods of detection or improved techniques of endothelial cell isolation are presented, lipid studies must be based on difficult qualitative conjectures and ultrastructural comparisons. In rabbits, esterified and free cholesterol concentrations in plasma and endothelium demonstrate a greater ratio of free cholesterol in the intimal tissue (Böndjers and Björkerud, 1973), suggesting that hydrolytic activity of the cholesterol esters is a primary step in lipid uptake (Jensen, 1969). Analysis of electron density of lipid droplets further suggests metabolic transformation of lipids (Hoff and Gottlob, 1969).

An important aspect of endothelial function involves the clearing of fibrin from the circulation. Todd (1972) recently reviewed information available on fibrinolysis in relation to the high activity of plasminogen activators in the human endothelial lining, and proposed that this activity is of considerable physiologic import with regard to the regulation of blood clotting and blood flow. Endothelial fibrinolytic activity appears to be site- and species-related. Todd (1959) reported on absence of fibrinolytic activity in most large human arteries, yet arteries and arterioles in specialized tissues such as retina, myocardium, pulmonary arteries, and kidney (Todd, 1958) possess high activity. Warren (1964) demonstrated this function in endothelial cells of the aortas of a number of animals and described an inverse relationship between fibrinolytic activity and the diameter of the vessel. Fujinami and Gore (1967) found that fibrinolytic activity of the aorta increased progressively as one moved away from the heart, and Kwaan and Astrup (1967) reported the presence of numerous confluent zones of fibrinolytic activity in the intima of human arteries covering atherosclerotic plaques.

Fibrinolysis facilitates blood flow by clearing fibrin from the circulation. Anoxia and mechanical damage have been reported to be important stimuli for the appearance in endothelium of plasminogen activators in humans (Todd, 1972). Gader, Clarkson, and Cash (1973) have proposed adrenergic, beta-receptor mediation of fibrinolysis, while Biggs, MacFarlane, and Pilling (1947) found earlier that exercise induces increased fibrinolytic activity in healthy patients. These latter effects could also be mediated by the release of plasminogen activators from endothelium. On the other hand, Pugatch et al. (1970) extracted and isolated both fibrinolytic activators and inhibitors from human endothelium.

Direct endothelial involvement in the clotting mechanism has been suggested, but this is also open to question. O'Brien (1959) scraped cells from the luminal surface of human aortas and showed that, using these cells, blood clotted at a faster rate than with platelet suspensions. He also reported partial inactivation of heparin. Al'Fonsov and Kuznik (1968) demonstrated that human aortic endothelial extracts induce blood coagulation. They proposed that this activity is discharged with endothelial injury, while under normal conditions endothelial cells release substances that inhibit clotting. Differential centrifugation of human aortic intima revealed strong antithrombin activity in the 105,000 G fraction, and procoagulant activity in the microsomal and mitochondrial fractions (Tsubohawa, 1970). Intimal extracts of arterial endothelium from children possessed the strongest antithrombin activity, while sclerotic intimas have a procoagulative activity proportional to the severity of involvement (Tsubohawa, 1970), in contrast to the findings of Kwaan and Astrup (1967) mentioned above. No activity was found in any fraction of other vascular layers. Antihemophilic factor (AHF, factor VIII) has been localized in the cytoplasm of vascular endothelium of human arteries, including the aorta (Hoyer, de los Santos, and Hoyer, 1973) by immunofluorescent techniques suggesting endothelial synthesis. Activity is reported to increase under stressful stimuli (Green, 1970; Bennett and Ratnoff, 1972; Prentice, Forbes, and Smith, 1972).

Cell Multiplication

Owing to wear and tear, endothelial replacement under physiologic conditions occurs throughout life. A number of investigators, including Wright (1972), have shown that mitotic activity in endothelium of mammalian aorta is very low. The estimated life span of an endothelial cell in the guinea pig aorta is approximately 100–180 days, but is considerably shorter in areas prone to injury. These studies using labeled thymidine allowed the reevaluation of Altschul's thesis (1954) and the earlier findings of Efskind (1941) that suggested that both mitotic and amitotic cell divisions were infrequent. Stchelkounoff (1936) proposed that arterial endothelial replacement may occur by growth of undifferentiated subendothelial cells, an hypothesis that has been strengthened by similar findings in rabbits (Ts'ao, 1968).

Interesting patterns of endothelial cell division were reported in autoradiographic studies by Wright (1972), who found significant differences in ^{3}H thymidine incorporation in the normal guinea pig aorta, with mitotic activity decreasing proportionately with greater distance from the heart. Gaynor (1971) reported higher endothelial mitotic activity in the normal renal and pulmonary arteries than in the aorta of the rabbit. However, aortic endothelium showed proportionately higher mitotic response than other vessels following endotoxin-induced injury. Seventy-two hours of cholesterol feeding was found adequate to cause a two- to threefold increase in endothelial uptake of ^{3}H thymidine in swine abdominal aorta (Florentin et al., 1969). In addition, primates exhibit localized thymidine incorporation in the aorta, especially in areas prone to injury or with preexisting atherosclerotic plaques (Murata, 1967).

Respiration

Investigation of endothelial respiration could add significantly to the study of vascular physiology as a possible indicator of tissue metabolic activity. Literature concerning the endothelium, however, is scanty. As indicated earlier in this section, most studies extrapolate results from data obtained using whole artery or intima-media preparations and neglect the fact that the predominant cell type is smooth muscle and not endothelium.

Whereat (1967) has pointed out that an interesting feature of arterial tissue is the lack of a Pasteur effect. Recently Scott, Morrison, and Kroms (1970) speculated that such a lack of respiratory control may be an artifact due to the common practice of cooling tissues preceding respiratory measurement. Data on direct measurement of endothelial oxygen consumption is very limited. Robertson (1968) reported a control value of 0.094 μl O_2/hr/10^7 cells measured manometrically, for cultured human aortic and coronary "intimacytes" (cells with many ultrastructural and cytochemical characteristics of vascular smooth muscle cells). Rosen and Hollis (1973) reported a value of 0.20 μl O_2/hr/mg protein measured polarographically, for freshly isolated rabbit thoracic aortic endothelium. These two studies are not exactly compatible, because methods and species were different. Further investigation is urgently needed fully to elucidate the various parameters of endothelial metabolism, including respiration.

Endothelial Permeability

Structurally, the inner portion of the normal aorta of all species is avascular; the vasa vasorum, when present, seldom penetrate beyond the outer third of the medial layer. Considering the diffusion capacity of various molecules, nutrients must then reach the intima and inner media by crossing the endothelial barrier. Endothelial permeability of large arteries appears to be selective; nonstimulated normal endothelium usually allows passage of small macromolecules (Schwartz and Benditt, 1972) and limited passage of cholesterol (Böndjers and Björkerud, 1973). The major portion of lipids found in the arterial wall is not synthesized in situ, but is developed from plasma (Day, Wahlquist, and Campbell, 1970; Dayton and Hashimoto, 1970; Somer and Schwartz, 1971).

Aortic intimal permeability varies according to species and location, and reportedly decreased with age in the rabbit (Friedman and Byers, 1963) and pig (Klynstra and Bottcher, 1970). Permeability to protein is focal, being confined primarily to the sinuses of Valsalva, ostea of branches, and curved regions (Packham et al., 1967; Jørgensen et al., 1972; Somer, Evans, and Schwartz, 1972) in the pig, rabbit, and human. Comparative studies have demonstrated a similar focal permeability to cholesterol in porcine aortas (Somer and Schwartz, 1971). In addition to focal areas, long streaks along the rabbit (Packham et al., 1967) and pig (Packham et al., 1967; Klynstra and Bottcher, 1970; Somer et al., 1972) aortas are permeable to Evans blue and trypan blue dyes. In the pig (Packham et al., 1967) and in the dog (Duncan, Buck, and Lynch, 1963), the thoracic aorta is more permeable to protein than the abdominal aorta. The canine aorta demonstrates a gradient of labeled cholesterol deposition along its length (Duncan and Buck, 1960). It is also of interest that Pries and Klynstra (1971) found that focal areas in normal porcine aortas demonstrated excess accumulation of cholesterol esters with a decrease in total lipid and phospholipid content.

The mechanism of permeability is generally described using the concept of a two-pore system as proposed by Chambers and Zweifach (1947). There is agreement among investigators concerning the importance of vesicular transport of material through endothelial cells in the aorta; passage of molecules between cells, however, is still presently in dispute. Cellular clefts forming total or partial occlusions of 40 Å (Stein and Stein, 1972) have been demonstrated by electron microscopy. Passing of horseradish peroxidas (250 Å) by vesicular transport has been shown in the rat (Schwartz and Benditt, 1972; Florey and Sheppard, 1970; Hüttner, Boutet, and More, 1973) and mouse (Stein and Stein, 1972), and ferritin (about 110 Å) has been demonstrated in vesicles in the rat (Hüttner et al., 1973). Conversely, only horseradish peroxidase has been reported intercellularly (Florey and Sheppard, 1970; Hüttner, More, and Rona, 1970). Under nonstimulated conditions, when high concentrations of the marker were injected, intercellular peroxidase activity was demonstrated (Stein and Stein, 1972). Schwartz and Benditt (1972) proposed that the presence of peroxidase in interendothelial spaces in the Wistar/Firth Mai rat may in fact result from vesicular transport (see Chapters 4 and 5 in this volume for further discussion.)

On the other hand, some investigators contend that the absence of markers in endothelial junctions may represent methodological differences rather than variation in endothelial behavior. In more recent studies, Giacomelli and Wiener (1974) reported regional differences in permeability of the rat thoracic aorta to horseradish peroxidase. The endothelial junctions were shown to contain a considerable amount of marker. The authors further reported that the results are transient. These findings are in agreement with the report by Robertson and Khairallah (1973), who found that increased endothelial permeability in rat thoracic aortas, lasting 60 sec or less, was induced by subpressor doses of various vasoactive amines or peptides. These authors reported that interendothelial gaps opened in response to amines, but the number of opened gaps and degree of permeability to lipoprotein or albumin decreased rapidly during the initial 60 sec. In addition, Robertson and Khairallah (1973) demonstrated the presence of tracers in endothelial junctions, with only minimal amounts of tracer in cellular vesicles, suggesting intercellular passage. It has been proposed that this passage is a result of endothelial cell contraction, based on the estimation of nuclear membrane pinching (Majno, Shea, and Leventhal, 1969). The term "trap door" has been proposed (Robertson and Khairallah, 1973) to describe these transient permeability increases due to endothelial contraction.

Table 1 illustrates the results obtained with tissues fixed in vivo with a mild buffered aldehyde fixative. Tritiated lipoprotein fractions, injected by cardiac puncture (Robertson, 1965), were taken up to varying degree in the

Table 1. Incorporation of tritiated lipoprotein fractions by rat aortic intima[a] after endothelial stimulation with angiotensin II[b]

% Radioactivity from plasma		(A) Simultaneous injection with Angio II	(B) Injected 60 sec after Angio II	(C) Injected 480 sec after Angio II
VLDL		7.8	5.4	—
	$\overline{S}$	1.24	1.82	—
LDL		16.2	8.4	0.4
	$\overline{S}$	4.64	1.49	—
HDL		4.8	0.4	—
	$\overline{S}$	1.47	0.12	—

[a]Intima and inner medial layers.

[b]Left intraventricular injection of 0.1 ng angiotensin II in 0.2 ml Ringer's solution in a 200-g Sprague-Dawley rat.

subendothelial and inner medial layers in response to 0.1 ng of angiotensin II. When the lipoprotein fractions were injected simultaneously with angiotensin II, a higher percentage of uptake occurred for all fractions than when the lipoprotein was injected 60 or 480 sec after the octapeptide. Furthermore, low-density lipoproteins (LDL) showed the highest radioactivity in the arterial wall. Whether this difference relates to higher uptake or retention of the lipoprotein is under investigation.

Table 2 summarizes aortic endothelial permeability to ^{125}I albumin in the same animal model. The method used for administration of the vasoactive agents at varied concentrations and the labeled albumin was similar to the above lipoprotein study. It was determined by autoradiography that the degree of permeability was dose related. Angiotensin II induced the greatest permeability

Table 2. Changes in arterial endothelial permeability to ^{125}I albumin induced by circulating vasoactive agents

	Total injec. ($\times 10^{-9}$ g)[a]	Av. time (sec.)	Subendothelial[b] space
Norepinephrine	100–200	42	++[c]
Serotonin	10–200	54	+++
Prostaglandin E_1	10–20	51	++
Angiotensin II	0.1–10	42	++++
Control Ringer's sol.	2 ml	280	—

[a]In 1 ml Ringer's solution injected in left ventricle of a 200-g Sprague-Dawley rat.

[b]Intima and inner media

[c]+ = 25%; ++ = 50%; +++ = 75%; ++++ = 100% labeled cells, by autoradiography.

to the marker at the lowest concentration in the shortest time, followed by prostaglandin E_1, serotonin, and norepinephrine.

Endothelial vesicular transport is a complex mechanism. Stein and Stein (1972) reported that mouse aortic endothelia transport horseradish peroxidase and bovine milk lactoperoxidase via different forms of vesicles. In addition, Still and Prosser (1964) showed that, following injection of thorium and cholesterol in rabbits, these markers could be localized to mitochondria and pinocytotic vesicles of aortic endothelial cells. The endothelium represents a structural semipermeable barrier to molecular transport across the aortic wall, and in particular against the excess influx of cholesterol and other lipids. Loss of endothelial integrity could constitute an important pathologic aspect of lipid accumulation.

Hemodynamics

The effect of changes in dynamics on endothelium is a highly complex and controversial question. It has been hypothesized that the reaction of the vessel wall to hemodynamic alterations is a causative factor in focal changes in permeability (Jørgensen et al., 1972; Somer et al., 1972). In this context, it is noteworthy that similar flow patterns in certain locations could explain long streaks of permeable areas in the rabbit and pig thoracic aorta (Packham et al., 1967; Klynstra and Bottcher, 1970; Somer et al., 1972).

The development of mathematical (Kuchar and Ostrach, 1971) and structural (Robbins and Bentor, 1967) model systems has been complicated by the unique complexity of the vascular wall (McDonald, 1960). Other major contributing factors include the dynamic flow characteristics of blood (Merill, 1969) and the rheologic alterations induced by the presence of blood cells at high concentrations (Goldsmith, 1970). Each of these problems has been reviewed recently and is included only as complementary information. Focal permeability alterations, discussed in the preceding section, have also been explained on the basis of hemodynamic stress (Jørgensen et al., 1972; Björkerud and Böndjers, 1972). The arterial endothelial response to normal blood flow has been studied by *en face* preparations. The nuclear alignment (Flaherty et al., 1972) and mitotic activity (Wright, 1972) of endothelial cells have been related to the direction of blood flow. Variations in nuclear alignment were found in endothelial cells at sites of curvature of the aorta in dogs and guinea pigs. Surgical alteration of the endothelial cell alignment at right angles with blood flow produced realignment of endothelial cells to the original pattern within 10 days (Flaherty et al., 1972).

While a number of hypotheses have been put forth to explain the mechanism of blood flow-induced injury to endothelium, causative factors are still in dispute. Following a unique series of experiments, Fry (1968) proposed that endothelia are injured if the shearing stress (frictional forces) at the endothclial interface exceeds an "acute yield stress" resulting in an increase in protein accumulation. Aortic plugs and electromagnetic flowmeter probes in canine aortas permit quantitation of increases in shearing stress with proportional morphologic correlation of sequential endothelial changes, beginning with Evans blue staining, followed by cell swelling, yielding, dissolution, and erosion. Similar results have been reported using extraaortic tapered vanes and clamps (Fry, 1969). Mathematical and fluid models confirm the shear stress distribution developed by plug insertion (Ray and Davids, 1970), while heated-film techniques and electromagnetic flowmeters demonstrate eddy turbulence in the canine aortic arch (Ling et al., 1968). Calculations based on the above measurements demonstrate that shear stresses reached peaks of 80–160 dynes/cm^2, values below the acute yield stress of 378 dynes/cm^2 proposed by Fry (1969). Blood flow in the descending aorta was laminar with low shear stress values.

Scharfstein, Gutstein, and Lewis (1963) put forth the hypothesis that a boundary layer is established as a protective buffer against transient turbulent shearing stress normally present in the flow core under conditions of stable flow. Such a model has been described and confirmed mathematically, taking into account the various parameters of wall elasticity, fluid viscosity, and pulsatile flow. As flow rate and, therefore, Reynolds number and turbulence increase, the velocity profile flattens, resulting in an increased viscous shearing stress at the fluid–vessel interface. The viscous shearing stress, being proportional to fluid viscosity and velocity gradient, is more injurious than and separate from the stresses of the turbulent flow core. Local flow disturbances, such as stenoses and/or alterations in vessel configuration, including curvatures and bifurcations, also alter the velocity profile resulting in increased shear stress (Scharfstein et al., 1963). Even minute disruption of the endothelial surface causes microscopic alterations and injury leading to the progressive development of a plaque (Stemerman, 1973).

Confirming evidence has come from studies using heated filament probes and anemometer circuitry (Gutstein, Farrell, and Armellini, 1973). Probes inserted in various positions in the porcine trifurcation area demonstrated highly disturbed blood flow patterns in the area of the ilio-aortic angle when compared to straight areas of the abdominal aorta and iliac artery. Light and electron microscopy confirmed the relationship between endothelial integrity, edema, and the shearing stress exposure discussed previously.

In addition to shearing stress, the effects of pressure and tensile stresses are also important to endothelial permeability. Carew and Patel (1973) recently reported that circumferential tensile stress rather than fluid friction induces endothelial permeability to Evans blue dye in canine coronary arteries. Aars and Solberg (1971) showed that turbulence did not influence the localization or degree of lipid deposition in partially constricted or normal aortas of cholesterol fed rabbits.

Rosen, Hollis, and Sharma (1974) described a model flow chamber that permits one to subject bovine endothelium grown in vitro to quantitative shearing stress. With this technique the endothelial enzymatic formation of histamine increased relative to control cultures in two stages, in response to low, physiologic shearing stresses. Despite in vitro conditions, the results suggest a possible correlation between shearing stress and endothelial injury and contraction. An additional investigation in which rabbit aortas were perfused in situ and subjected to low shearing stress in vitro helped to confirm the above proposal. Histidine decarboxylase activity of the aortic wall increased proportionately with shearing stress, and the results demonstrated that half of the enzyme activity was related to the endothelial lining (Hollis and Ferrone, 1974).

INTERACTION OF CIRCULATING
BLOOD ELEMENTS WITH ARTERIAL ENDOTHELIUM

Under both normal and experimental conditions, some relation seems to exist between injury, endothelial permeability, and blood cell deposition. Normal aortas have shown leukocyte and platelet deposition in endothelial areas permeable to Evans blue dye in pig, rabbit, and man. In contrast, erythrocyte deposition has only been found in human aortas (Jørgenson, Haerem, and Moe, 1973). Experimentally, mechanical injury results in similar leukocyte and platelet deposition in areas of permeability or denudation (Ashford and Freiman, 1968; Björkerud and Böndjers, 1971; Stemerman, 1973) and infusion of amines produces platelet aggregation (Robertson and Khairallah, 1973) and leukocyte deposition (Shimamoto, 1963).

Since blood platelets have been the subject of intensive investigation, the reader is referred to any one of many excellent books and monographs available concerning platelet biochemistry, morphology, and pathology (for recent reviews see Mason, Read, and Shermer, 1974; and White, 1974). ADP is the principle factor in platelet aggregation (Mustard, 1967), but a variety of tissue components such as collagen, microfibrils, and elastin (Baumgartner and Haudenschild, 1972), or blood-borne substances such as thrombin, antigen–antibody complexes and some hormones (Mustard, 1967), are known to induce aggregation of platelets either directly or by stimulation of ADP release. These substances vary in their affinity to endothelium and their platelet aggregating activity (Baumgartner and Haudenschield, 1972); species variations are also reported (Niewiarowski and Thomas, 1970). The endothelium normally provides a physiologic, nonthrombogenic surface to the blood. Any disruption of the cell surface or integrity of the endothelial layer may result in platelet aggregation. Recently, Jørgensen et al. (1973) reported platelets in contact with structurally seemingly normal endothelium in the mouse aorta. Ashford and Freiman (1968), however, found by electron microscopy that the apparently intact endothelial surfaces contain minute lesions that only become obvious when fibrinolysis is inhibited. While more data are needed, it is obvious that circulating blood elements play a vital role in the function and preservation of arterial endothelium.

MORPHOLOGY AND FUNCTION
OF ARTERIAL ENDOTHELIUM IN VITRO

The increasing interest in the physiology and pathology of arterial endothelium has required development of new approaches for its investigation. Endothelial culture techniques have been available for many years. Lewis (1921) described the morphology of endothelium and smooth muscle cells, finding the two readily distinguishable. Altschul (1954) reviewed much of the work on cultured endothelium; the reading of the experimental results indicates discrepancies regarding morphology, identification, differentiation, and culturability.

Since Altschul's monograph (1954), improvement of culture methods has permitted isolation of meaningful quantities of cells without severe contamination with other cell types (Lazzarini-Robertson, 1959). Identification techniques have also improved, permitting standardization by biochemical (Robertson, 1965; Iwanaga et al., 1969), morphologic (Robertson, 1968; Iwanaga et al., 1969; Jaffe et al., 1973; Rosen et al., 1974) and immunofluorescent procedures (Jaffe et al., 1973). Endothelial culture permits biochemical determinations when homogeneous populations are available by cloning. Robertson (1965) utilized cell cloning to identify two distinct cell types of intimacytes in the human and animal arterial wall that maintain morphologic and biochemical characteristics for several generations. Other investigators have contributed additional information on the physiology of endothelial cells in culture. Cultured rabbit aortic endothelia have been reported to synthesize and secrete sulfated mucopolysaccharides. Comparative studies led Buonassisi (1973) to propose that the cells synthesize heparin and secrete two forms of proteoglycans. Bovine aortic endothelium grown in vitro demonstrates histidine decarboxylase activity only half as often as normal endothelium; subjection of endothelium in vitro to low shearing stresses restores enzyme levels to normal (Rosen et al., 1974). The presence of factor VIII has been demonstrated in human endothelium in vitro (Jaffe et al., 1973). This factor cannot be detected in the media, however, suggesting either a lack of secretion or immediate degradation.

Some functional aspects of endothelium have been substantiated by the activity of cultured cells. Lewis (1921) reported the presence of contractile elements in cultured endothelium and observed a fibrillation in the cytoplasm similar to that seen in smooth muscle cells. While Lewis (1921) considered such a structure a response to fixation, Levi (1923) suggested that it was an indication of cellular contraction. Ptokhov (1963) reported phagocytic properties of endothelium removed from various portions of the vascular system of the rabbit, including the abdominal aorta. In vitro, intracellular incorporation was particularly intense when melanin and muscle fragments were added; in addition, changes in cellular morphology indicated the presence of injury. Such activity is not just a phenomenon seen in cell culture, because phagocytosis and pinocytosis have also been observed in arterial endothelium in vivo, particularly under conditions of reticuloendothelial system overload.

An interesting application of cultured cells may be in the implantation of prostheses in vascular surgery. Prosthesis material is in most cases thrombogenic, owing either to surface unevenness or to chemical attraction of formed elements. With experimental implantation of prostheses in canine (O'Neal et al., 1964; Sun and Shidone, 1971) and porcine (O'Neal et al., 1964) aortas, a cellular covering of the luminal surface, thought by some to be endothelium, is in evidence. There is disagreement as to whether the mechanism involved is migration (Sun and Shidone, 1971) or differentiation of blood-borne cells (O'Neal et al., 1964). There is also some doubt as to whether the cellular covering is actually endothelium (Robertson, 1965). Current studies in several laboratories have proposed the use of cell culture techniques to coat the luminal surface of prostheses prior to implantation. The clinical need of providing a living, nonthrombogenic surface is of importance but has not yet been proved feasible.

DIFFERENCES BETWEEN
ARTERIAL AND OTHER VASCULAR ENDOTHELIA

The endothelium forms a tight, continuous layer throughout the vascular system, but regional differences in endothelial morphology, metabolism, and function are becoming evident. These differences may explain well-known variations in susceptibility of the vascular system to pathologic conditions. Both capillary and arterial endothelium contain relatively large numbers of vesicles, endoplasmic reticulum and mitochondria. Functionally, both cell types exhibit responses to pharmacologic agents that resemble contraction, but the focal changes that follow are varied, particularly in relation to the resulting permeability changes. Cerebral capillaries are part of what is referred to as the blood–brain barrier. They appear to be virtually seamless (Wolff and Bär, 1972; also see Chapter 4 in this volume) and are relatively impermeable. Other capillaries, however, demonstrate varying degrees of permeability to small and large particles depending on the size of the interendothelial gaps.

Metabolically, enzymic dissimilarities include a uniform, high alkaline phosphatase activity in capillaries as opposed to regional variations found along the arterial system (Romanul and Bannister, 1962). Neutral phosphatase is localized predominantly in pinocytotic vesicles along the cell surface of capillaries, while the enzyme activity of arterial cells is localized on the surface of invaginations at intercellular spaces and in neighboring pinocytotic vesicles (Hoff and Graf, 1966). Capillary endothelial cells do not show the same response to β-glycerophosphate and phenylphoshate found in the arterial intima. Comparative evaluation of arterial and venous endothelium indicates some similarities in cellular organelle content and structure, but differences are reported in mitochondrial content between calf mammary artery and vein (Huyoff and Hackensellner, 1965). Recently, cultured human umbilical vein endothelial cells have been shown to secrete a prostaglandin E-like substance. This secretion is inhibited by indomethacin and substantially stimulated by angiotensin II (Gimbrone and Alexander, 1975). These same cells in culture exhibit both a renin-like activity and an angiotensin I converting enzyme activity (Hial et al., 1976). The above findings, while not as yet extended to arterial endothelium, nevertheless indicate that vasoactive mediators are generated in endothelium and thus may participate in the local regulation of clotting, vascular permeability, and vascular tone.

Injury studies have shown that venous endothelia respond amitotically at first, with subsequent mitosis caused by crushing (Sinapius, 1966) and chemical injury (Sinapius and Rittmeyer, 1966). The authors calculated that reendothelialization of the denuded areas originated from preexisting surrounding cells at an average rate of 0.5–1.0 mm daily. Stchelkounoff (1936) proposed that surface cell replacement in veins, rather than replacement with cells from the subendothelial layer as has been proposed in arteries, may explain differences between venous and arterial pathology. Venous endothelia exhibit a higher level of fibrinolytic activity than arteries in many animal species (Warren, 1964; Fujinami and Gore, 1967) and are the principal source of this activity in the human vasculature (Todd, 1972). Only specialized arteries exhibit activity similar to that of veins. Venous endothelial cells have also been shown immunologically to possess antihemophilic factor activity, both in vivo (Hoyer et al., 1973) and in vitro (Jaffe et al., 1973).

Table 3 illustrates the functional differences between arterial and venous permeability in vivo. Arteries exhibit a greater permeability to most markers; only the higher-molecular-weight markers show decreased passage presumably as a result of their inability to penetrate temporarily distended interendothelial junctions (Robertson and Khairallah, 1973). Elastic and large muscular arteries demonstrate similarities in permeability, but wide variations exist between vena cava and umbilical veins, the former exhibiting a relatively low uptake of markers. The predominance of pinocytosis in venous endothelium may explain the increased uptake of markers by umbilical veins. Stimulation of endothelium maintained in vitro induces uptake of LDL similar to the in vivo condition in both arteries and veins as shown in Table 4. Of interest is the fact that venous endothelia respond with greater activity to hypoxia while arterial cells exhibit greater uptake of ^{3}H thymidine. As indicated above, umbilical cells possess greater pinocytotic activity. The above differences in functional response and metabolism between venous and arterial endothelium may present an interesting tool for future investigation of vascular pathophysiology.

Table 3. Functional differences between stimulated[a] "arterial" and "venous" endothelium in vivo

	Markers					
Arterial	Fe	HRP	LDL[b]	VLDL[b]	HDL[b]	Chylo[b]
Elastic arteries	+++	+++	++++	+++	+	+
L. muscular arteries[c]	++	+++	++++	+++	+	+

Permeability > Pinocytosis

Venous						
Vena cava	+	++	++	++	++	+
Umbilical vein (F)	++	++++	+	+++	++++	++++

Pinocytosis > Permeability

[a]Angiotensin II, 0.1 ng/ml; prostaglandin E_1, 10 ng/ml; serotonin, 10 ng/ml.
[b]^{3}H Labeled.
[c]Exceptions: renal, pulmonary, cerebral.

FUTURE DEVELOPMENTS

The preceding overview of arterial endothelial metabolism and function can hopefully provide the reader with a summary of current knowledge of the physiology of this seemingly forgotten key component of the vascular wall. Undoubtedly, more questions have been raised than specific answers provided. It is our hope that further application of both in vitro and in vivo techniques for endothelial study will be forthcoming, ranging from mass cultivation and quantitative biochemistry to immunologic and morphologic identification of regional peculiarities and functional characteristics of specialized endothelium. The

Table 4. Functional differences between stimulated[a] "arterial" and "venous" endothelium in vitro (cell or organ culture)

Arterial	Hypoxia	^{3}H Thy	Pinocytosis	^{3}H LDL[b]
Elastic arteries	+	+++	+	++++
L. muscular arteries[c]	++	+++	+	++++
Venous				
Vena cava	+++	+	+++	+
Umbilical vein (F)	++++	+	++++	+

[a]Angiotensin II, 0.1 ng/ml; prostaglandin E, 10 ng/ml; serotonin, 10 ng/ml.
[b]Intracellular uptake.
[c]Exceptions: renal, pulmonary.

acquisition of new data will undoubtedly provide further insight into the true physiologic function of endothelium.

LITERATURE CITED

Aars, H., and L. A. Solberg. 1971. Effects of turbulence on the development of aortic atherosclerosis. Atherosclerosis 13:283–287.

Al'Fonsov, V. V., and B. I. Kuznik. 1968. Study of tissue factors of blood clotting in endothelial cells of the aorta (human). Lab. Delo. 8:480–481.

Altschul, R. 1954. Endothelium. MacMillan and Co., New York.

Ashford, T. P., and D. G. Freiman. 1968. Platelet aggregation at sites of minimal endothelial injury. Am. J. Pathol. 53:599–607.

Baumgartner, H. R., and C. Haudenschild. 1972. Adhesion of platelets to subendothelium. Ann. N.Y. Acad. Sci. 201:22–36.

Bennett, B., and O. D. Ratnoff. 1972. Changes in antihemophilic factor (AHF, factor VIII) procoagulant activity and AHF-like antigen in normal pregnancy and following exercise and pneumonencephalography. J. Lab. Clin. Med. 80:256–263.

Benninghoff, A. 1930. Blutgefässe und Herz. In W. von Mollendorf (ed.), Handbuch der mikroskopischen Anatomie des Menschen, Vol. 6, Part 1. J. Springer, Berlin.

Biggs, R., R. G. Macfarlane, and J. Pilling. 1947. Observations on fibrinolysis; experimental activity produced by exercise or adrenaline. Lancet 1:402–405.

Björkerud, S., and G. Böndjers. 1971. Arterial repair and atherosclerosis after mechanical injury 1. Permeability and light microscopic characteristics of endothelium in nonatherosclerotic and athersclorotic lesions. Atherosclerosis 13:355–363.

Björkerud, S., and G. Böndjers. 1972. Endothelial integrity and viability in the aorta of the normal rabbit and rat as evaluated with dye exclusion tests and interference contrast microscopy. Atherosclerosis 15:285–300.

Böndjers, G., and S. Björkerud. 1973. Cholesterol accumulation and content in regions with defined endothelial integrity in the normal rabbit aorta. Atherosclerosis 17:78–83.

Buonassisi, V. 1973. Sulfated mucopolysaccharide synthesis and secretion in endothelial cell culture. Exp. Cell Res. 76:363–368.

Caldwell, P. R. B., B. C. Seegal, K. C. Hsu, M. Das, and R. L. Soffer. 1976. Angiotensin-converting enzyme: Vascular endothelial localization. Science 191:1050–1051.

Carew, T. E., and D. J. Patel. 1973. Effect of tensile and shear stress on intimal permeability of the left coronary artery in dogs. Artherosclerosis 18:179–189.

Chambers, R., and B. W. Zweifach. 1947. Intercellular cement and capillary permeability. Physiol. Rev. 27:436–463.

Day, A. J., M. L. Wahlqvist, and D. J. Campbell. 1970. Differential uptake of cholesterol and of different cholesterol esters by atherosclerotic intima in vivo and in vitro. Atherosclerosis 11:301–320.

Dayton, S., and S. Hashimoto. 1970. Recent advances in molecular pathology: A review—cholesterol flux and metabolism in arterial tissue and in atheromata. Exp. Mol. Pathol. 13:253–268.

Duncan, L. E., and K. Buck. 1960. Quantitative analysis of the development of experimental atherosclerosis in the dog. Circ. Res. 8:1023–1027.

Duncan, L. E., K. Buck, and A. Lynch. 1963. Lipoprotein movement through Canine aortic wall. Science 142:972–973.

Efskind, L. 1941. Die Regenerationsverhaltnisse in Intimaepithel nach Gefäss-Satur. Acta Chir. Scand. 84:283–309.

Evans, H. M. 1912. The development of the vascular system. In F. Keibel and F. Mall (eds.), Manual of Human Embryology, Vol. 2. Lippincott, Philadelphia.

Flaherty, J. T., J. E. Pierce, L. J. Ferrans, D. J. Patel, W. K. Tucker, and D. L. Fry. 1972. Endothelial nuclear patterns in the canine arterial tree with particular reference to hemodynamic events. Circ. Res. 30:23–33.

Florentin, R. A., S. C. Ham, K. T. Lee, and W. A. Thomas. 1969. Increased ^{3}H-thymidine incorporation into endothelial cells of swine fed cholesterol for three days. Exp. Mol. Pathol. 10:250–255.

Florey, H. W., and B. L. Sheppard. 1970. The permeability of arterial endothelium to horseradish peroxidase. Proc. Roy. Soc. London (Biol.) 174:435–443.

Friedman, M., and S. C. Byers. 1963. Endothelial permeability in atherosclerosis. Arch. Pathol. 76:99–105.

Fry, D. 1968. Acute vascular endothelial changes associated with increased blood velocity. Circ. Res. 22:165–197.

Fry, D. 1969. Certain chemorheologic considerations regarding the blood vascular interface with particular reference to coronary artery disease. Circulation 39–40 (Suppl. 4):38–57.

Fujinami, T., and I. Gore. 1967. Fibrinolytic activity of the endothelium (of the aorta and inferior vena cava). Jap. Circ. J. 31:267–273.

Gader, A. M. A., A. R. Clarkson, and J. D. Cash. 1973. The plasminogen activator and coagulation factor VIII responses to adrenaline, noradrenaline, isoprenaline and salbutanol in man. Thromb. Res. 2:9–16.

Gaynor, E. 1971. Increased mitotic activity in rabbit endothelium after endotoxin: An autoradiographic study. Lab. Invest. 24:318–320.

Giacomelli, F., and J. Wiener. 1974. Regional variation in the permeability of rat thoracic aorta. Am. J. Pathol. 75:513–28.

Gilchrist, F. G. 1968. A Survey of Embryology. McGraw-Hill, New York.

Gimbrone, M. A., Jr., and R. W. Alexander. 1975. Angiotensin II stimulation of prostaglandin production in cultured human vascular endothelium. Science 189:219–220.

Goldsmith, H. L. 1970. Motion of particles in a flowing system. Thromb. Diath. Haemorrh. Suppl. 40:91–110.

Green, D. 1970. Factor VIII (anti-hemophilic factor). J. Chronic Dis. 23:213–225.

Gutstein, W. H., G. A. Farrell, and C. Armellini. 1973. Blood flow disturbances and endothelial cell injury in preatherosclerotic swine. Lab. Invest. 29:134–149.

Hadjiisky, P., L. Scebat, Y. Renais. 1970. Aspects histochini ques et histoenzymatiques de l'aovte de coturnix coturnix (caille) (phasianides). Atherosclerosis 12:265–277.

Hial, V., M. A. Gimbrone, Jr., G. Wilcox, and J. J. Pisano. 1976. Human vascular endothelium contains angiotensin I converting enzyme and renin-like activity. Fed. Proc. 35:705 (Abstr.).

Hoff, H. F., and R. Gottlob. 1969. An electron microscope study of fat uptake by endothelial cells by doubly-ligated carotid artery segments. Experientia 24:1018.

Hoff, H. F., and J. Graf. 1966. An electron microscope study of phosphatase activity in the endothelial cell of rabbit aorta. J. Histochem. Cytochem. 14:719–729.

Hollis, T. M., and R. Ferrone. 1974. Effects of shearing stress on aortic histamine synthesis. Exp. Mol. Pathol. 20:1–10.

Hollis, T. M., and L. A. Rosen. 1972. Histidine decarboxylase activity of bovine aortic endothelium and intima-media. Proc. Soc. Exp. Biol. Med. 141: 978–981.

Hoyer, L. W., R. P. de los Santos, and J. R. Hoyer. 1973. Antihemophilic factor antigen: localization in endothelial cells by immunofluorescent microscopy. J. Clin. Invest. 52:2737–2744.

Hüttner, I., B. Boutet, and R. H. More. 1973. Studies on protein passage through arterial endothelium I. Structural correlates of permeability in rat arterial endothelium. Lab. Invest. 28:672–677.

Hüttner, I., R. H. More, and G. Rona. 1970. Fine structural evidence of specific mechanism for increased endothelial permeability in experimental hypertension. Am. J. Pathol. 61:395–404.

Huyoff, H., and H. A. Hackensellner. 1965. On the number of mitochondria in the vascular endothelial cells in various locations. Naturwissenschaften 52:163–164.

Iwanaga, Y., A. Tanimura, H. Kitsukawa, J. Tanigawa, M. Aikara, T. Kawashima, A. Maw, and T. Nakashima. 1969. The role of endothelial cells in the pathogenesis of atherosclerosis. Acta Pathol. Jap. 19:161–178.

Jaffe, E. A., R. L. Nachman, C. G. Becker, and C. R. Minick. 1973. Culture of human endothelial cells derived from umbilical veins: Identification by morphologic and immunologic criteria. J. Clin. Invest. 52:2745–2756.

Jensen, J. 1969. A further study of the kinetics of cholesterol uptake at the endothelial cell surface of the rabbit aorta in vitro. Biochem. Biophys. Acta 173:71–77.

Jørgensen, L., J. W. Haerem, and N. Moe. 1973. Platelet thrombosis and nontraumatic intimal injury in mouse aorta. Thromb. Diathes. Haemorrh. 29:470–489.

Jørgensen, L., M. A. Packham, H. C. Rowsell, and J. F. Mustard. 1972. Deposition of formed elements of blood on the intima and signs of intimal injury in the aorta of rabbit, pig and man. Lab. Invest. 27:341–350.

Kirk, J. E. 1969. Enzymes of the Arterial Wall. Academic Press, New York.

Klynstra, F. B., and C. J. F. Bottcher. 1970. Permeability patterns in pig aorta. Artherosclerosis 11:451–462.

Kuchar, N. R., and S. Ostrach. 1971. Unsteady entrance flows in elastic tubes with application to the vascular system Amer. Inst. Aeronaut. Astronaut. J. 9:1520–1526.

Kwaan, H. C., and T. Astrup. 1967. Fibrinolytic activity in human atherosclerotic coronary arteries. Circ. Res. 21:799–803.

Lazzarini-Robertson, A. 1959. Studies on the effects of lipid emulsion on arterial intimal cells in tissue culture in relation to atherosclerosis. Thesis, Cornell Graduate Medical School, Cornell University.

Levi, G. 1923. Struttura e proprieta degli endoteli vascolari. Richerche su culture in vitro. Gio. Biol. Med. Sperimentale 1:233–237.

Lewis, W. H. 1921. Smooth muscle and endothelium in tissue culture. Anat. Rec. 21:72.

Ling, S. C., H. B. Atabek, D. L. Fry, D. J. Patel, and J. S. Janicki. 1968.

Application of heated-film velocity and shear probes to hemodynamic studies. Circ. Res. 23:789−801.

Majno, G., S. M. Shea, and M. Leventhal. 1969. Endothelial contraction induced by histamine-type mediator. J. Cell Biol. 42:647−672.

Mason, R. G., M. S. Read, and R. W. Shermer. 1974. Comparison of certain functions of human platelets separated from blood by various means, Am. J. Pathol. 76:323−332.

McDonald, D. A. 1960. Blood flow in arteries. Williams and Wilkins, Baltimore. 328 p.

Merrill, E. W. 1969. Rheology of human blood; in vitro observations and theoretical considerations. In S. Sherry, K. M. Brinkhous, E. Genton, and J. M. Stengle (eds.), Thrombosis, pp. 477−495. National Academy of Science, Washington, D.C.

Murata, K. 1967. Tritiated thymidine incorporation into aortic cells in vivo. Cell regeneration in spontaneous atherosclerosis in monkeys. Experientia 23:732−733.

Mustard, J. F. 1967. Recent advances in molecular pathology: A review−platelet aggregation, vascular injury and atherosclerosis. Exp. Mol. Pathol. 7:366−377.

Niewiarowski, S., and D. P. Thomas. 1970. Platelet release reaction: The effects on the vessel wall. Thromb. Diathes. Haemorrh. Suppl. 40:199−210.

O'Brien, J. R. 1959. Some properties of endothelial cells. Nature 184:1580−1581.

O'Neal, R. M., G. L. Jordon, E. R. Rabin, M. E. DeBakey, and B. Halpert. 1964. Cells grown on isolated intravascular dacron hub: An electron Microscope study. Exp. Mol. Pathol. 3:403−412.

Packham, M. A., H. C. Rowsell, L. Jørgensen, and J. F. Mustard. 1967. Localized protein accumulation in the wall of the aorta. Exp. Mol. Pathol. 7:214−232.

Pearl, W., and J. Cascarano. 1963. Cytochrome oxidase and DPNH dehydrogenase activity in endothelium, vascular smooth muscle and mesothelium of the rat. Fed. Proc. 22:180 (Abstr.).

Prentice, C. R. M., C. D. Forbes, and S. M. Smith. 1972. Rise in factor VIII after exercise and adrenaline infusion, measured by immunological and biological techniques. Throm. Res. 1:493−506.

Pries, C., and F. B. Klynstra. 1971. Aortic permeability, lipids, and atherosclerosis. Lancet 1:750−751.

Ptokhov, M. P. 1963. Phagocytic properties of endothelium in cultures. Arkh. Anat. Gistol. Embriol. 45:75−83.

Pugatch, E. M. J., E. A. Foster, D. E. MacFarlane, and J. C. F. Poole. 1970. The extraction and separation of activators and inhibitors of fibrinolysis from bovine endothelium and mesothelium. Br. J. Haematol. 18:669−681.

Ray, G., and N. Davids. 1970. Shear stress analysis of blood-endothelial surface in inlet section of artery with plugging. J. Biomech. 3:99−110.

Robbins, S. L., and I. Bentor. 1967. The kinetics of viscous flow in a model vessel. Lab. Invest. 16:864−874.

Robertson, A. L. 1965. Intracellular incorporation of plasma lipoproteins by arterial intima in relation to early stages of intravascular thrombosis. In P. M. Sawyer (ed.), Biophysical Mechanisms in Vascular Homeostasis and Intravascular Thrombosis, pp. 267−274. Appleton-Century-Crofts, New York.

Robertson, A. L. 1968. Oxygen requirements of the human arterial intima in atherogenesis. In C. J. Miras, A. N. Howard, R. Paoletti (eds.), Progress in Biochemical Pharmacology, pp. 305−316. A. J. Phieberg, White Plains, N.Y.

Robertson, A. L., and P. A. Khairallah. 1973. Arterial endothelial permeability and vascular disease: The "trap door" effect. Exp. Mol. Pathol. 18:241–260.

Robertson, A. L. 1975. Effects of vasoactive agents on vascular smooth muscle. In S. Wolf and N. T. Werthessen (eds.), The Smooth Muscle of the Artery, pp. 243–253. Plenum Press, New York.

Romanul, F. C., and R. G. Bannister. 1962. Localized areas of high alkaline phosphatase activity in endothelium of arteries. Nature 195:611–612.

Rosen, L. A., and T. M. Hollis. 1973. Endothelial succinate utilization in atherosclerotic rabbits. Atherosclerosis 17:297–304.

Rosen, L. A., T. M. Hollis, and M. G. Sharma. 1974. Alterations in bovine endothelial histidine decarboxylase activity following exposure to shearing stress. Exp. Mol. Pathol. 20:329–343.

Scharfstein, H., W. H. Gutstein, and L. Lewis. 1963. Changes of boundary layer flow in model systems: Implications for initiation of endothelial injury. Circ. Res. 13:580–584.

Schwartz, S. M., and E. P. Benditt. 1972. Studies on aortic intima. I. Structure and permeability of rat thoracic aortic intima. Am. J. Pathol. 66:241–255.

Scott, R. F., E. S. Morrison, and M. Kroms. 1970. Effect of cold shock on respiration and glycolysis in swine arterial tissue. Am. J. Physiol. 219:1363–1365.

Shimamoto, T. 1963. The relationship of edematous reaction in arteries to atherosclerosis and thrombosis. J. Atherosclerosis Res. 3:87–102.

Sinapius, D. 1966. The regeneration of venous endothelium after experimental crushing. Virchows Arch. (Pathol. Anat.) 341:291–301.

Sinapius, D., and P. Rittmeyer. 1966. Experimental maceration and regeneration of the vein endothelium. Investigation on the vena jugularis externa of rabbits. Angiologica 3:349–359.

Somer, J. B., G. Evans, and C. J. Schwartz. 1972. Influence of experimental aortic coarctation on the pattern of aortic Evans blue uptake in vivo. Atherosclerosis 16:127–133.

Somer, J. B., and C. J. Schwartz. 1971. Focal ^{3}H-cholesterol uptake in the pig aorta. Atherosclerosis 13:293–304.

Stchelkounoff, I. 1936. L'intima des petites artères et des veines et de mesenchyme vasculaire. Arch. Anat. Microsc. Morphol. Exp. 32:139–194.

Stein, O., and Y. Stein. 1972. An electron microscope study of the transport of peroxidases in the endothelium of mouse aorta. Z. Zellforsch. Mickrosk. Anat. 133:211–222.

Stein, Y., and O. Stein. 1973. Lipid synthesis and degradation and lipoprotein transport in mammalian aorta. In CIBA Foundation Symposia No. 12, Atherogenesis: Initiating Factors, pp. 165–185. Associated Scientific Publishers, Amsterdam.

Stemerman, M. B. 1973. Thrombogenesis of the rabbit arterial plaque. An electron microscope study. Am. J. Pathol. 73:7–26.

Still, W. J. S., and P. R. Prosser. 1964. The reaction of aortic endothelium of the rabbit to hyperlipemia and colloidal thorium. J. Atherosclerosis Res. 4:517–526.

Sun, C. N., and J. J. Shidone. 1971. Comparison of ultrastructure of endothelial cells from normal canine abdominal aorta with that of cells on nylon velour silastic arterial prosthesis. Exp. Pathol. (Jena) 5:249–254.

Todd, A. S. 1958. Fibrinolysis autographs. Nature 181:495–496.

Todd, A. S. 1959. The histological localization of plasminogen activator. J. Pathol. Bacteriol. 78:281–283.

Todd, A. S. 1972. Endothelium and fibrinolysis. Atherosclerosis 15:137—140.

Ts'ao, C.-H. 1968. Myointimal cells as a possible source of replacement for endothelial cells in the rabbit. Circ. Res. 23:671—682.

Tsubohawa, Y. 1970. Studies on antithrombin activity in the human aortic intima, with special reference to its correlation to atherosclerotic changes. Jap. Circ. J. 34:615—616.

Verity, M. A., C. Su, and J. A. Bevan. 1972. Transmural and subcellular localization of monamine oxidase and catechol-*o*-methyl transferase in rabbit aorta. Biochem. Pharmacol. 21:193—201.

Warren, B. A. 1964. Fibrinolytic activity of vascular endothelium. Br. Med. Bull. 20:213—216.

Weibel, E. R., and G. E. Palade. 1964. New cytoplasmic components in arterial endothelia. J. Cell Biol. 21:101—112.

Whereat, A. F. 1967. Atherosclerosis and metabolic disorder in the arterial wall. Exp. Mol. Pathol. 7:233—247.

White, J. G. 1974. Current concepts of platelets, structural physiology and pathology. Human Pathol. 5:1—6.

Wolff, J. R., and T. Bär. 1972. "Seamless" endothelia in brain capillaries during development of the rat's cerebral cortex. Brain Res. 41:17—24.

Wright, H. P. 1972. Mitosis patterns in aortic endothelium. Atherosclerosis 15:93—100.

chapter 7

CONNECTIVE TISSUE

Zdenek Hruza

Nutrients, oxygen, water, and all other essential substances have to pass through the intercellular space on their way from the capillary to the cell, and all the metabolites have to be returned the same way either to the blood capillary or the lymphatic capillary. The hematoparenchymatous barrier consists of the capillary wall, intercellular material, and cell membranes; connective tissue is the major and perhaps most important part of this barrier.

The main function of connective tissue, as a part of the skeleton, cartilage, ligaments, vessels, and organs, is to preserve the structural integrity of the organism. It also preserves the microscopic structure of tissue, e.g., the spatial arrangement of cells, the relation of cells to each other and to the capillary, and the distance of the capillary from the cell. Among other things, connective tissue may help to keep the capillaries, or at least the lymphatic capillaries, open even if they are empty. It forms a barrier against infection and against spread of tumor cells (Grabowska, 1959; Vasiljev, 1961). Invasiveness of some bacteria is related to their content of collagenase, which degrades collagen (e.g., Clostridia), or of hyaluronidase, which depolymerizes the ground substance (e.g., Hemolytic streptococcus A and C). Changes of length and diameter of the microvessels with pressure are dependent on extravascular connective tissue. Peripheral vessels are stiffer than larger arteries because they derive their mechanical properties, in part, from the surrounding connective tissue (Gaehtgens, 1971).

There are many excellent reviews about connective tissue, among them a monograph by Chvapil (1967), reviews of special aspects by Harkness (1961), Gould (1968), Hall (1963), Asboe-Hansen (1963a), Ogston (1970), Catchpole (1973), and many others. Therefore only essential features are mentioned here, without references to every statement.

BIOCHEMISTRY OF CONNECTIVE TISSUE

The main components of connective tissue are collagen, elastin, and ground substance. Since elastin is not involved in the formation of the hematoparenchymatous barrier (except perhaps with respect to the permeability of the arterial wall), only collagen and ground substance are mentioned here.

Connective tissue, which originates from mesenchyme, is composed of cells and fibers embedded in the amorphous ground substance. The main connective tissue cell is the fibroblast which produces collagen and the macromolecular components of the ground substance. Other cells present in connective tissue are mast cells, plasma cells, histiocytes, neutrophils, lymphocytes, fat cells, and pigment cells.

Collagen Fibers

Native collagen fibers are formed by spontaneous polymerization and precise alignment of monomer collagen molecules, called tropocollagen. The intracellular form of the collagen monomer is called procollagen (Grant and Prockop, 1972). These polypeptides have α chains identical to the tropocollagen but the former are longer because of a "tailpiece" extending from the NH_2-terminal end of the molecules. In the normal course of events, these extensions are removed by an extracellular enzyme, procollagen peptidase, to form tropocollagen (Miller and Matukas, 1974).

The tropocollagen molecule consists of three polypeptide chains that are coiled into a rigid helical structure, containing 33% glycine, about 10% proline, 10% hydroxyproline, some hydroxylysine, and other amino acids. In most tissue collagens each tropocollagen molecule consists of two α_1 chains and one α_2 chain. Recent studies have provided evidence for the existence of at least four genetically distinct molecular types of collagen, termed types I to IV, each differing with respect to amino acid composition and sequence, as well as to the amount of hydroxylysine-linked carbohydrate (Miller and Matukas, 1974).

The most prominent cross striations in collagen fibrils are about 680 Å apart because of a specific alignment of the basic molecular units, i.e., tropocollagen. These units have the approximate dimension of a rod 3000 Å long and 15.0 Å wide. Connective tissues contain a wide spectrum of various sized aggregates in monomeric tropocollagen arranged in a characteristic manner. In tendon, all of the fibrillar units are arranged in parallel bundles. In skin most of them are oriented in the plane of the skin, and in cartilage the collagen is associated with mucopolysaccharides.

The solubility of the fibrils in a given tissue varies with age and other factors. The changes are attributable to covalent cross linking between collagen polypeptide chains. The covalent cross links arise from modified amino acids, especially from lysine. Once the collagen molecule exists in a polymerized fibrous form, cross linking occurs in a progressive fashion. The relative abundance of the different cross links varies markedly, depending on the tissue of origin of the collagen. These changes are under direct metabolic control, since major structural changes have been observed in pathologic conditions, such as diabetes, atherosclerosis, etc.

Since collagen is a structural protein, it is very important to understand how its structural stability is preserved. The primary stabilizing forces are, of course, the peptide bonds between the amino acids. These bonds are not susceptible to general proteolytic enzymes such as pepsin, trypsin, etc. However, these enzymes split the peptide bonds in the polar regions after denaturation, while collagenase splits the peptide bonds in the apolar region without denaturation. Hydrogen bridges are important stabilizing factors of the collagen molecule. These bonds are formed between the $>$ CO groups of the peptide bond of one chain and $-$NH$-$ groups of the peptide bond of the adjacent chain. Other, less important stabilizing forces are ionic bonds between the side chains of the polar amino acids, Van der Waals forces, steric rigidity of cyclic amino acids, hydrophobic contacts, and intermolecular stabilization by water molecules. The telopeptides are responsible for the solubility of procollagen within the cell.

Different properties of the collagen molecule can be measured by various means. The degree of aggregation of collagen is usually determined by stepwise extraction by aqueous NaCl and 0.5 M sodium citrate, pH 3.6. It has been demonstrated that newly formed collagen molecules are more easily extractable because they contain fewer cross links. Stronger, permanent bonds, mainly the covalent bonds connecting the α chains, cannot be dissolved in neutral buffers. Solubility in buffers or in dilute acids is often used as a criterion of the degree of stability of the collagen molecule. Swelling in dilute acids is another method of determining structural stability; less stable collagen, such as collagen from younger animals, swells more readily. Many techniques can be used to measure structural stability of the collagen fiber in tissues, such as tensile strength or dissolution of the fiber in urea or sodium perchlorate (e.g., contraction and relaxation, or time to break). Such techniques have been used in the determination of aging of animals and man. The most suitable technique, which can also be interpreted in biologic terms, is splitting of collagen with collagenase in animals (Hlavackova and Hruza, 1972) or human tissues (Hamlin and Kohn, 1972).

Synthesis of collagen takes place in the fibroblast, but formation and maturation of the collagen fiber is an extracellular process. In the process of synthesis, some proline residues undergo hydroxylation to form hydroxyproline. Turnover of mature collagen is very slow; its half-life is about 200 days in young rats and increases with age (Neuberger, Perrone, and Slack, 1951). The turnover of collagen is faster in some organs, as in liver, and slower in others, as in tendon.

Reticulin Fibers

Reticulin fibers are another component of connective tissue. Reticulin is similar to collagen, and many investigators believe that it is a precursor of collagen. The protein part of reticulin is identical with the protein part of collagen, but reticulin contains more carbohydrates than does collagen (4.25% against 0.55% in collagen); reticulin also contains 10% of bound fatty acids. Reticulin has stronger argyrophilia than collagen, but this does not necessarily mean that the protein part is different, since argyophilia depends on the quantity of ground substance and the manner of its association with the protein core of the fiber and not on the protein itself. Reticulin is not present in all tissues as is collagen; it is in basal membranes, around smooth and skeletal muscles, around glands and peripheral nerves, and in the kidney cortex, spleen, and lymph nodes. The whole concept of reticulin is controversial and there is still a disagreement as to whether it is collagen or not. A good summary of the properties of reticulin can be found in Chvapil (1967).

Ground Substance

Ground substance is an amorphous material containing high-molecular-weight polysaccharides called mucopolysaccharides (glycosaminoglycans). These compounds are large-molecular-weight heterologous polymers that consist, usually, of alternating units of an amino sugar and a uronic acid. These two six-carbon moieties form a disaccharide repeating unit. The hexosamine is often acetylated, and an ester sulfate group may be present. Proteoglycans are mucopolysaccharides bound by covalent links to protein (Jeanloz, 1970).

Hyaluronic acid ((1 → 4) O-β-D-glucopyranuronosyl-(1 → 3)-O-(2-acetamido-2-deoxy-β-D-glucopyranosyl)) has a tremendous capacity to bind water. One gram of hyaluronic acid is able to bind up to 0.5 liters of water. Tissues with high content of water contain high amounts of hyaluronic acid (e.g., vitreous humor, umbilical cord, synovial fluid, or sex skin). One molecule of hyaluronic acid weighing about 10 million daltons occupies a space of 1 μ^3. While collagen fibers are resistant to tension but not to compression, mucopolysaccharides filling the spaces between the collagen fibers are resistant to compression and are responsible for the elasticity of the tissues. It has been shown in a model system that collagen fibers, mucopolysaccharides, and water combine into an incompressible structure and that in vivo the fibers can prevent movement of fluid (e.g., vitreous humor). In the joints that contain no fibers, the fluid moves freely. In contrast to collagen, turnover of mucopolysacchaides is rapid The half-life of hyaluronic acid in the skin is 2.5–4 days; that of chondroitin sulfuric acid is 7–10 days.

These polysaccharides are synthesized in connective tissue cells that are capable of synthesizing uridine diphosphate derivatives of glucuronic acid, N-acetyl-glucosamine, and galactosamine. They are the precursors of heterologous polysaccharides, some of which become sulfated in the presence of $3'$-phospho-adenosine-$5'$-phosphosulfate (PAPS). A nondialyzable "serum sulfation factor" in normal sera is missing in hypophysectomized rats and reappears 6 hr after administration of growth hormone (Priest, 1967).

REGULATION OF CONNECTIVE TISSUE METABOLISM

Endogenous Factors

Enzymic Degradation of Collagen   Some bacteria (e.g., Clostridium) contain a collagenase that splits collagen into peptides. Similar enzymes, which, however, are not identical with the bacterial collagenase, have been found in the animal organism, e.g., a collagen-mucoproteinase from the pancreas that splits off mucin but does not split collagen into peptides. A collagenolytic enzyme has been found in the involuting uterus (Woessner, 1968; Montfort and Perez-Tamajo, 1975), in liver, pancreas, and oral cavity, and in inflammatory exudates (Menkin, 1956; Schaub, 1964; Goldstein, Patel, and Hauck, 1964). These enzymes are not active at physiologic pH. More recently, a collagenase that is active at neutral pH has been found in leukocytes (see Janoff in Volume III). Collagenase is activated by calcium ions and substances that contain SH-groups; on the other hand, EDTA, Fe^{++}, and Cu^{++} have an inhibitory action on this enzyme (McCroskery, Richard, and Harris, 1975).

Hyaluronidase   Hyaluronidase, originally isolated from bull testicles, causes spreading of dyes in the tissues. It degrades hyaluronic acid, chondroitin, and chondroitin-4 and -6 sulfates into oligosaccharides. Activators of hyaluronidase include pyrophosphate, cysteine, gelatine, protamine, and albumin. Some of the activators act by blocking the inhibitors. Besides some specific inhibitors, there are also nonspecific inhibitors that block hyaluronidase, e.g., serum (Herp, De Filippi, and Fabianek, 1968). Additional information on this subject can be found in the recent review by Harris and Krane (1974).

Endocrine Factors   As reviewed by Dougherty and Berliner (1968) and Asboe-Hansen (1963b), all hormones affecting connective tissue do so by their action on the fibroblasts, not on the structural elements already formed.

The inhibitory effect of glucocorticoids on formation of connective tissue has been extensively studied mainly because of their therapeutic effect on rheumatic joints. Cortisone acts on fibroblasts by decreasing the synthesis of both collagen fibers and glycosaminoglycans. It increases the degree of polymerization of hyaluronic acid, which brings relief to rheumatic joints because less hyaluronic acid with a higher degree of polymerization means less bound water and improved lubrication. Part of the relief caused by adrenal steroids may, perhaps, be explained by decreased capillary permeability and exudation, and inhibition of Menkin's leucotaxin, as suggested first by Ducommun and Mach (1950). As a corollary, the turnover of both hyaluronic acid and chondroitin sulfuric acid decreases after hydrocortisone treatment. According to Dougherty and Berliner (1968), the antiinflammatory effect of cortisone parallels its inhibition of growth of fibroblasts in tissue cultures. Since chondroitin sulfate provides the necessary matrix for collagen, its decreased synthesis after hydrocortisone slows down healing of wounds and reconstitution of cartilage matrix. The spreading capacity of dyes after hyaluronidase decreases upon cortisone therapy. In addition, the permeability of capillaries, which is increased by hyaluronidase, decreases after cortisone therapy. Mineralocorticoids counteract the inhibitory effect of glucocorticoids on wound healing and formation of the granulation tissue around foreign bodies. In addition, synthesis of hyaluronic acid and chondroitin sulfate decreases in diabetes and is restored after insulin therapy.

In hypothyroidism induced by thiouracil there is an increase of hyaluronic acid and a decrease of chondroitin sulfate in the tissues. Thyroxine restores both levels to normal (Schiller, Slover, and Dorfman, 1962). These effects may well be secondary to stimulation and increased secretion of TSH or exophthalmos stimulating factor, according to most researchers. After hypophysectomy, the amount of hyaluronic acid increases, chondroitin sulfate decreases, and growth hormone restores the level of chondroitin sulfate but not that of hyaluronic acid. When ACTH is given to hypophysectomized animals, chondroitin sulfate synthesis is normalized but that of hyaluronic acid increases further. Parathormone, besides its effect on calcium metabolism, dissolves collagen in the bones and also increases the output of mucoproteins in the urine. Estrogens increase the content of hyaluronic acid and water in the tissues (e.g., edema during phases of menstrual cycle), most apparently in the sex skin, and also increases incorporation of sulfate into different tissues. Spreading of fluid in tissues as well as capillary permeability increase after estrogens. Androgens are known to increase the formation of collagen fibers and their tensile strength. Some of the actions of these hormones may be related to the fact that they cause an increase in the water-rich phase and a decrease in the colloid-rich phase of ground substance (Gersh and Catchpole, 1960). An increase in the dense, colloid-rich phase occurs, on the other hand, during aging and after cortisone therapy.

Exogenous Factors

Nutritional deficiencies decrease the amount of connective tissue only as a result of a prolonged low-protein intake or starvation (Chvapil and Hruza, 1959). The decrease in the amount of collagen in nutritional deficiency is always small, not comparable to the losses of other proteins. Feeding with atherosclerosis-producing diets speeds up the physicochemical, age-related changes of collagen and increases collagen content in the lungs (Hruza and Chvapil, 1962).

Vitamin C is necessary for biosynthesis of collagen at the step of proline hydroxylation. In scurvy, formation of newly formed collagen is inhibited without changes in collagen already synthesized. Vitamin C is also necessary for synthesis of polysaccharides and incorporation of sulfate into acid mucopolysaccharides (Barnes, 1975).

It seems that hypoxia is a specific fibrogenic stimulus because optimal pO_2 tension for growth of fibroblasts is about 60 mm Hg, whereas the pO_2 of arterial blood is 95 mm Hg. In hypoxia, the collagen content of the lung (Loblich, 1965), as well as metabolism of mucopolysaccharides, increases. Collagen formation is common to all pathologic conditions in which the oxygen supply to the tissues is limited. At moderately low oxygen tensions, synthesis of collagen exceeds its degradation (Chvapil, Hurych, and Ehrlichova, 1968), whereas at high oxygen tensions the two processes are in equilibrium.

HEMATOPARENCHYMATOUS BARRIER

The Capillary

The older concepts of Zweifach (1961) appear to be still valid in light of new information obtained with the electron microscope. This technique delineated structures that could not be seen with the light microscope and that were only predicted on the basis of physiologic experiments. New data about the capillary wall have been reviewed by Majno (1965), Luft (1973), and Cotran (1967). The capillary consists of the endothelium, basement membrane, and adventitia. Closest to the blood is an endocapillary lining consisting probably of mucopolysaccharides; it is visualized in the electron microscope after fixation with ruthenium red (Luft, 1965). Endothelial cells make up the next layer. They are probably connected with intercellular cement as shown previously by Chambers and Zweifach (1947). This "cement" may be composed of mucopolysaccharides, but electron microscopic evidence concerning the nature of the cement is still uncertain. The basement membrane consists of collagen and ground substance. Connective tissue is interposed between the capillaries and organ cells. In addition, there is an incomplete sheet of pericytes around the capillary surrounded by ground substance. The presence of intercellular bridges in the endothelial cells of arterial endothelium has been demonstrated by Shimamoto and Numano (1969). The endothelial cells are 0.1–0.4 μ thick and contain micropinocytotic vesicles that are apparently important for the transcapillary exchange of macromolecular substances. The intercellular junctions, which were visualized by the electron microscope after fixation in glutaraldehyde-osmium, measure 120 Å according to Muir and Peters (1962) and are about 200 Å deep. The endocapillary layer (Fawcett, 1963; Wetzel, Wetzel, and Spitzer, 1966), which probably contains acid mucopolysaccharides, becomes thicker in venous congestion and after thermal injury (Cotran, 1967).

The outer layer of the endothelium is covered by a basement membrane 200–600 Å thick. It consists of fibrillar material embedded in an amorphous matrix. Collagen fibers are sometimes a part of the external surface of the basement membrane that also surrounds the pericytes. The basement membrane of the endothelium, intercellular junctions, endocapillary layer, and the basal membrane of the pericytes are in contact with each other. The ground substance of the basement membrane is partly condensed into very fine fibrillar material (Luft, 1965). Exchange of molecules between the plasma and interstitium has been reviewed by Crone (1972) and is discussed in detail elsewhere in this volume (see Chapter 8–10 and 19).

Besides histochemical evidence that the intercellular junction contains mucopolysaccharides, there is also a possibility that bivalent ions like Ca^{++} or Mg^{++} bind the endothelial cells together (Grand and Maddi, 1952). After injury, gaps are formed in the venular part of the capillary endothelium as demonstrated by electron microscopy (Cotran, 1967). This also happens after administration of histamine or serotonin, which allows for the passage of large particles. In addition, leucocytes also penetrate the intercellular junctions during inflammation, a process that again may increase the permeability of the capillary wall. Local destruction of the basement membrane is probably caused by hydrolytic enzymes (Cochrane and Aikin, 1966) that originate in the lysosomes of the leucocytes (see Janoff in Volume III for a recent review).

Basement Membranes

The term "basement membrane" originates with light microscopists and is promiscuously used with the terms "basal membrane" or "basal lamina" of the epithelial cells, which originated with the advent of the electron microscope (Martinez-Palomo, 1970). Most authors use the term "basement membrane" for the capillary and "basal membrane" for epithelial cells of organs.

The basement membrane, which consists of collagen fibers and ground substance, is obviously a structural support of the endothelial cells; it also acts as a guide for regenerating endothelium. According to Majno (1965), the basement membrane retains its guiding function after injury, similarly to Schwann cells in the Wallerian degeneration of the nerve. It also helps to stabilize the cell surface, which would bulge without this support. The basement membrane allows the passage of water while retaining larger particles, although this retention is not complete (Karnovsky, 1970). The amino acid analysis of glomerular basement membranes, which are usually isolated by sonication and differential centrifugation (Kefalides and Winzler, 1966; Spiro, 1970), suggests the presence of collagen because of their high hydroxyproline, hydroxylysine, and glycine content. However, a considerably larger amount of carbohydrate and a substantially higher number of polar amino acids are found here than in the fibrous proteins. An additional difference is the presence of cysteine, which is absent in interstitial collagen (Kefalides and Winzler, 1966). The biochemical structure of basement membranes has been investigated by two major groups. According to Kefalides (1972) the glomerular basement membrane appears to be composed of dissimilar glycoprotein subunits. One of the proteins is a type of collagen that is characterized by a high content of hydroxylysine and hydroxyproline and, unlike other mammalian collagen, contains cysteine. It also contains approximately 10% carbohydrate, mainly as glucosyl-galactose and to a small extent as galactose, linked O-glycosidically to hydroxylysine. The other subunit of the basement membrane is a noncollagenous polypeptide, rich in hexosamine, galactose, mannose, fucose, and sialic acid.

Spiro's (1970) hypothetical model pictures a specialized form of collagen, where disulfide bonds are assumed to be the major cross links, although other interchain bonds probably also exist. The carbohydrate exists either linked O-glycosidically to hydroxylysine, as a disaccharide, or as a polysaccharide, probably linked N-glycosidically to asparagine and containing hexosamine, galactose, mannose, fucose, and sialic acid.

Both groups of investigators believe that the carbohydrate residues affect the packing and the porosity of the polypeptide chains since the basement membranes do not possess the 640 Å periodicity characteristic of the fibrillar structure of collagen. The chemical composition of various basement membranes in specific tissues is qualitatively similar to that of the glomerulus. These membranes are rich in hydroxyproline, hydroxylysine, and glycine, indicating their collageneous nature, but differ quantitatively in their amino acid composition and in their carbohydrate content, depending on their embryologic origin and tissue localization. This suggests that their different functional roles may be related to these very differences. Experimental studies indicate that the antigen in basement membranes that gives rise to nephritogenic antisera is a glycoprotein, with an amino acid and a carbohydrate composition unlike that of the collagen component (Mohos and Skoza, 1969; Skoza and Mohos, 1974). Sensitive techniques revealed that the collagen fibers themselves seem to have a membrane that regulates the water content of the fiber. The permeability of this membrane may perhaps be influenced by glucocorticoids and aging (Smith, 1969).

Since the basement membrane retards migration of leucocytes in acute inflammation, it was thought that in diabetes, migration of leucocytes is slowed down owing to the thickening of the basement membrane. This change, it is speculated, may contribute to the increased sensitivity of diabetics to infection. Thickening of the basement membrane in diabetes was observed in all capillaries studied (skin, muscle, adipose tissue, pancreas, peripheral nerves, eyes, and kidneys) and was reported to increase from 930 Å to 1300 Å (Williamson, Vogler, and Kilo, 1971). The glomerular basement membrane that is the best analyzed has a different composition in diabetes in that the amount of hydroxylysine increases at the expense of lysine; this may cause differences in the formation of the peptide chains resulting in increased permeability of the glomerulus for proteins in diabetes (Spiro, 1973). The thickening of the basement membrane, according to some observations, precedes carbohydrate intolerance and diabetic retinopathy, but other reports imply that the reverse is true (for further discussion see Chick in Volume III). Thickening of the basement membrane also occurs in aging (Jordan and Perley, 1972) and in nephrosis, glomerulonephritis, and asthma but the pathophysiologic importance of this change is unknown. Formation of the collagen subunits of the basement membrane takes place within the cell, but cross linking of the subunits occurs outside the cell. Several enzymes and cofactors like iron, manganese, and ascorbic acid are necessary for the formation of the subunit.

TRANSPORT FUNCTION OF CONNECTIVE TISSUE

Experimental evidence indicates that there may be several types of flow through the connective tissue network. Among these are diffusional flow of water, bulk flow of solvents in general, and translational transport of macromolecules. According to Laurent (1972), diffusion of water is not affected to any great extent by the polysaccharide network, whereas bulk flow of solvents and transport of solutes, especially that of large molecules, is significantly inhibited by the presence of polysaccharides. In vivo, most tissues have less than 1% hyaluronic acid, which does not retard transport of albumin very much. In a 1% solution of hyaluronic acid, however, transport of albumin is decreased by 50%. Since cartilage may contain 10 times as much mucopolysaccharides, retardation of albumin transport in this tissue may be about 90%. In the connective tissue network, the rate of diffusion of asymmetric molecules suggests that they move along their long axis. While the translational movement of large spherical molecules is hampered in polysaccharide solutions (Laurent and Öbrink, 1972), the molecules can still rotate freely in the polymer network and carry out their chemical function. Laurent (1972) has advanced an interesting idea that may have some physiologic significance, namely, that some of the proteins (enzymes, etc.), by being excluded because of the presence of polysaccharides from connective tissue, are present in a greater concentration and are perhaps also more active in other tissue compartments.

The degree of aggregation of connective tissue can influence permeability of the interstitium; aging or application of cortisone cause a higher degree of aggregation, and hyaluronidase treatment or scurvy cause lowering of the degree of aggregation. Experiments in vitro have shown that higher concentrations of gels slow down diffusion; similarly, aggregation of connective tissue renders the tissue less permeable. In vivo, however, more aspects, in addition to aggregation of connective tissue, have to be taken into consideration if permeability from the capillary to the cell is studied, namely, hemodynamic factors, distance of the capillary to the cell, etc. Edema can be the consequence of hemodynamic changes or vascular damage. On the other hand, disintegration of ground substances in itself can make the interstitium more permeable and thus lead to edema (Zweifach, 1972). In inflammation, biologically active amines are released from certain cells into the extracellular compartment. These amines increase the permeability of the blood vessels, a process that can result in the further disaggregation of the connective tissue matrix (Catchpole, 1973).

Various models have been designed for measurement of permeability of connective tissue in vitro (Young, 1972; Wells, 1973). The technique of Day (1952) and that of Werle and Leusch (1952) uses as a measure the permeability of muscle fascia to saline solution under constant pressure. Hyaluronidase greatly increases the speed of flow through the membrane. The same happens in vivo if spreading of Evans blue is measured in the skin with hyaluronidase treatment. Hyaluronidase causes depolymerization of the mucopolysaccharides, which apprently play a major role in diffusion. Under normal conditions, the collagen fibers themselves are too far from each other to prevent diffusion although they may slow down fluid movement. In sclerotic processes (scars, cirrhosis), however, collagen fibers become aggregated to such an extent that they may become an obstacle to diffusion.

Polysaccharides slow down movement of water in the tissues significantly; the conductance of the corneal stroma to water increases 50-fold after removal of mucopolysaccharides (Hedbys and Mishima, 1962; Hedbys, 1963). During compression of tissue, water flow to the surrounding space is slow, owing to polysaccharides in the tissues, and so is the return of water after the compression is removed. This is perhaps the main reason for the resistance of tissues to pressure. Osmotic pressure in the macromolecular system is higher than would be expected from the molecular weight of each component separately. A solution of hyaluronic acid has an osmotic pressure 100 times higher than that which is theoretically calculated. Hyaluronidase does not have an effect on the interendothelial "cement" substance, only on interstitial connective tissue (Altschuler and Angevine, 1951). This finding seems to indicate that the cement substance has a composition that is different from that of the interstitial connective tissue and basal membrane.

CONNECTIVE TISSUE IN AGING

The main water-binding material in the extracellular space is hyaluronic acid; this substance is decreased with aging (Sobel and Hewlett, 1967). If there were a simple relationship between the amount of water and hyaluronic acid in the tissue, tissue water would decrease with aging as hyaluronic acid does. Since this is not the case, structural changes of hyaluronic acid with age have to be surmised. In older animals water is bound to less hyaluronic acid, and this may explain why these animals cannot retain as much water after a water load as young animals (Friedman and Friedman, 1957). Ma and Cowdry (1950) observed that the spreading reactions induced by hyaluronidase decrease in older animals, which again points to increased stability of ground substance in aging. Another reflection of this may be a slowdown of turnover in chondroitin sulfates with aging (Hauss, Junge-Hülsing, and Hollander, 1962).

It has been reported that the number of capillaries decreases during aging in the heart (Rakusan and Poupa, 1964), in fatty tissue (Pexieder, 1965), and in bones (Hruza and Wachtlova, 1969). The greatest decline is up to adulthood; the changes are less significant later on. The fragility of capillaries is also increased in old people (Bertolini, 1969). This does not necessarily mean that the capillaries work less efficiently, only that they are more vulnerable. Capillary flow in the muscles and skin, as measured by radioactive xenon, decreases during aging (Gosselin, 1971). Jones (1951) described a substantial decrease in the exchange of O_2 and CO_2 with age in man. His interpretation is that the main limitation to gas exchange is the decrease in regional blood flow with aging. Another factor, however, is that the thickness of the capillary basement membrane increases significantly during aging (Dohrmann and Herdson, 1969; Kilo, Vogler, and Williamson, 1972).

Changes in collagen and ground substance with aging have been studied and reviewed by many authors (Sobel, 1967, 1968; Sinex, 1968; Hruza, 1972). The old observation that aging is associated with fibrosis has been modified by recent and more detailed knowledge. The collagen fibers become thicker during development and aging, and the interstitial tissue contains less mucopolysaccharides, as demonstrated by chemical methods (Sobel, 1967, 1968) and by electron microscopy (Jackson, 1968). Several authors have shown a substantial decrease of acid mucopolysaccharides with aging. Stability of the collagen fibers is greatly increased during the aging as shown by the increase of tensile strength, decrease of solubility in buffers or acids, decrease of swelling in weak acids, smaller contraction, and less efficient relaxation in urea or sodium perchlorate, and greater resistance to collagenase. These changes are interpreted to be a consequence of formation of cross links in the tropocollagen chains. According to some workers, formation of cross links occurs under the influence of changes in body temperature (Verzár, 1957), by cross-linking agents (Bjorksten, 1958) or enzymic oxidation of lysine residues (Bornstein, Kang, and Piez, 1966). Lysyloxidase is probably the enzyme responsible for cross linking. This enzyme is activated by Cu^{++} ions, and inhibited by Zn^{++} ions in vitro (Chvapil and Walsh, 1972).

Another factor contributing to the increased stability of the collagen molecule during aging is the deposition of calcium salts (Freydberg-Lucas and Verzár, 1957); indeed, decalcified collagen fibers have properties resembling those of younger fibers, and their stability returns after recalcification (Hruza and Hlavackova, 1967). Changes in connective tissue structure with aging lead to slower turnover of collagen and ground substance and to alteration of their physiologic properties. The diffusion coefficients of gels "aging" in vitro decreases. There is convincing evidence that capillary permeability decreases during aging (Duran-Reynols, 1946; Bastai, 1955; Ries, 1961). It is also known that pulmonary diffusing capacity for gases decreases with age (Cohn, 1964). More recent evidence of changes in diffusion with aging has been reviewed by Sobel (1967, 1968). On the level of the cell surface it has been shown that in the aging erythrocyte, entry of water into the cell is slowed down and that resistance of the cell membrane to osmotic and mechanical injury is also decreased.

In spite of some conflicting evidence, it appears that transport from the blood to the cell is slowed during aging in most organs. This slowdown is caused by a decreased density of the capillaries, decreased regional blood flow, and increased stability of connective tissue. Owing to these deficiencies, aged tissues have to exist under a handicap, especially during conditions of stress when there are great demands on transport.

Despite great progress in the chemistry of connective tissue on the one hand and ultrastructural research on the other, these aspects are not yet well interfaced so as to present a unified picture of how transport of various substances from the blood to the tissue cell is accomplished under normal and pathologic circumstances, and how the connective tissue surrounding the blood vessels may participate in this regulation. This picture cannot be resolved until connective tissues from different sites (basement membrane, subendothelial layer, cement, interstitial connective tissue, etc.) are isolated, analyzed, and studied under in vitro conditions.

LITERATURE CITED

Altschuler, Ch. H., and D. M. Angevine. 1951. Acid mucopolysaccharides in degenerative diseases of connective tissue with special reference to serious inflammation. Am. J. Pathol. 27:141−156.
Asboe-Hansen, G. 1963a. Connective tissue. Ann. Rev. Physiol. 25:41−59.
Asboe-Hansen, G. 1963b. The hormonal control of connective tissue. In D. A. Hall (ed.), International Review of Connective Tissue Research 1, pp. 29−63. Academic Press, New York.
Barnes, M. J. 1975. Function of ascorbic acid in collagen metabolism. Ann. N.Y. Acad. Sci. 258:264−277.
Bastai, P. 1955. Die biologischen Grundlagen des Alterns. Z. Alternforsch. 9:211−219.
Bertolini, A. M. 1969. Gerontologic Metabolism. Charles C. Thomas, Springfield, Ill.
Bjorksten, J. 1958. A common molecular basis for the aging syndrome. J. Am. Geriat. Soc. 6:740−748.
Bornstein, P., A. H. Kang, and K. A. Piez. 1966. The nature and location of intramolecular links in collagen. Proc. Natl. Acad. Sci. U.S. 55:417−424.
Catchpole, H. R. 1973. Capillary permeability. III. Connective tissue. In B. W. Zweifach, L. Grant, and R. T. McCluskey (eds.), The inflammatory process, 2nd Ed., vol. 2, pp. 121−147. Academic Press, New York.
Chambers, R., and B. W. Zweifach. 1947. Intercellular cement and capillary permeability. Physiol. Rev. 27:436−463.

Chvapil, M. 1967. Physiology of Connective Tissue. Butterworth, London. 417 p.

Chvapil, M., and Z. Hruza. 1959. The influence of aging and undernutrition on chemical contractility and relaxation of collagen fibres in rats. Gerontologia 3:241–252.

Chvapil, M., J. Hurych, and E. Ehrlichova. 1968. The influence of various oxygen tensions upon proline hydroxylation and metabolism of collagenous and noncollagenous proteins in skin slices. Hoppe-Seylers. Z. Physiol. Chem. 349:211–217.

Chvapil, M., and D. Walsh. 1972. A new method to control collagen cross-linking by inhibiting lysyl-oxidase with zinc. In International Congress Serv. 264, Connective Tissue and Aging, pp. 226–228. Excerpta Medica, Amsterdam.

Cochrane, C. G., and B. S. Aikin. 1966. Polymorphonuclear leucocytes in immunologic reactions: The destruction of vascular basement membrane in vivo and in vitro. J. Exp. Med. 124:733–752.

Cohn, J. E. 1964. Age and the pulmonary diffusing capacity. In L. Cander and J. H. Moyer (eds.), Aging of the Lung, p. 311. Grune and Stratton, New York.

Cotran, R. S. 1967. The fine structure of the microvasculature in relation to normal and altered permeability. In E. B. Reeve and A. C. Guyton (eds.), Physical Bases of Circulatory Transport, pp. 249–275. W. B. Saunders, Philadelphia.

Crone, C. 1972. Exchange of molecules between plasma, interstitial tissue and lymph. Pflügers Arch. 338:S65–79.

Day, T. D. 1952. The permeability of interstitial connective tissue and the nature of the interfibrillary substance. J. Physiol. 117:1–8.

Dohrmann, G. J., and P. B. Herdson. 1969. Fine structural studies of capillaries in NZB-NZW mice. Exp. Mol. Pathol. 11:163–171.

Dougherty, T. G., and D. L. Berliner. 1968. The effects of hormones on connective tissue cells. In B. S. Gould (ed.), Biology of Collagen, Part A, pp. 367–394. Academic Press, New York.

Ducommun, P., and R. S. Mach. 1950. L'action de l'ACTH sur les adhérences dues à l'injection de talc dans la cavité peritonéale des rats. Sem. Hop. Paris 26:3170–3172.

Duran-Reynols, F. 1946. Age and infection. J. Gerontol. 1:358–373.

Fawcett, D. W. 1963. Comparative observations on the fine structure of blood capillaries. In J. L. Orbison and D. Smith (eds.), Peripheral Blood Vessels, pp. 17–44. Williams and Wilkins, Baltimore.

Freydberg-Lucas, V., and F. Verzár. 1957. Der Calciumstoffwechsel verschiedener Organen bei jungen und alten Tieren. Gerontologia 1:195–213.

Friedman, M., and L. Friedman. 1957. Salt and water balance in aging rats. Gerontologia 1:107–121.

Gaehtgens, A. L. 1971. Radial and longitudinal distensibility of arterial microvessels in the mesentery and their dependence on extravascular structures. Pflügers Arch. 330:227–289.

Gersh, I., and H. R. Catchpole. 1960. The nature of ground substance on connective tissue. Perspec. Biol. Med. 282–319.

Goldstein, E. R., Y. M. Patel, and J. C. Hauck. 1964. Collagenolytic activity of intact and necrotic connective tissue. Science 146:942–944.

Gosselin, R. E. 1971. Muscle blood flow and functional capillary density evaluated by isotope clearance. Pflüegers Arch. 322:197–216.

Gould, B. S. 1968. Biology of Collagen. Vol. 2, Part A, 434 p., Part B, 488 p. Academic Press, New York.

Grabowska, M. 1959. Collagen content of normal connective tissues, of tissue surrounding a tumor and of growing rat sarcoma. Nature 183:1186–1187.

Grand, C. G., and F. Maddi. 1952. The effects of various concentrations of calcium chloride on the intercellular cement of endothelial cells grown in vitro. Anat. Rec. 112:334–335.

Grant, M. E., and D. T. Prockop. 1972. The biosynthesis of collagen. New Engl. J. Med. 286:194–199, 242–249, 291–299.

Hall, D. A. 1963–1970. International Review of Connective Tissue Research. Vols. 1–5. Academic Press, New York.

Hamlin, C. R., and R. R. Kohn. 1972. Determination of human chronological age by study of a collagen sample. J. Exp. Gerontol. 7:377–378.

Harkness, R. D. 1961. Biological functions of collagen. Biol. Rev. 36:399–463.

Harris, E. D., and S. M. Krane. 1974. Collagenases. New Engl. J. Med. 291:557–562, 605–609, 652–660.

Hauss, W. H., G. Junge-Hülsing, and H. J. Hollander. 1962. Changes in metabolism of connective tissue associated with aging and arterio or atherosclerosis. J. Atheroscl. Res. 2:50–61.

Hedbys, B. O. 1963. Corneal resistance to flow of water after enzymatic digestion. Exp. Eye Res. 2:112–121.

Hedbys, B. O., and S. Mishima. 1962. The role of polysaccharides in corneal swelling. Exp. Eye Res. 1:262–275.

Herp, A., J. De Filippi, and J. Fabianek. 1968. The effect of serum hyaluronidase on acid polysaccharides and its action in cancer. Biochim. Biophys. Acta 158:150–153.

Hlavackova, V., and Z. Hruza. 1972. Differences in properties of newly formed collagen during aging and parabiosis. J. Gerontol. 27:178–182.

Hruza, Z. 1972. Aging of cells and molecules. In Handbuch der allgemeinen Pathologie, VI, 4, pp. 83–108. Springer Verlag, New York.

Hruza, Z., and M. Chvapil. 1962. Collagen characteristics in the skin, tail tendon and lungs in experimental atherosclerosis in the rat. Physiol. Bohemoslov. 11:423–429.

Hruza, Z., and V. Hlavackova. 1967. Effect of decalcification on collagen aging in rats. Gerontologia 13:246–252.

Hruza, Z., and M. Wachtlova. 1969. Diminution of bone blood flow and bone capillary network in rats during aging. J. Gerontol. 24:315–320.

Jackson, F. S. 1968. The morphogenesis of collagen. In B. S. Gould (ed.), Treatise on collagen. 2. Biology of collagen, Part B, pp. 1–67. Academic Press, New York.

Jeanloz, R. W. 1970. In W. Pipman, D. Horton, and A. Herp (eds.), The Carbohydrates, Vol. IIB, pp. 589–625. Academic Press, New York.

Jones, H. B. 1951. Molecular exchange and blood perfusion through tissue regions. Advan. Biol. Med. Phys. 2:53–77.

Jordan, S. W., and M. J. Perley. 1972. Microangiopathy in diabetes mellitus and aging. Arch. Pathol. 93:261–265.

Karnovsky, M. J. 1970. Morphology of capillaries with special reference to muscle capillaries. In C. Crone and N. A. Lassen (eds.), Capillary Permeability, pp. 341–350. Academic Press, New York.

Kefalides, N. A. 1972. Biochemical studies of the glomerular basement membrane in the normal kidney. In J. Hamburger, J. Crosnier, and M. H. Maxwell (eds.), Advances in Nephrology, Vol. 2, pp. 3–24. Year Book Publishers, Chicago.

Kefalides, N. A., and R. J. Winzler. 1966. The chemistry of glomerular basement membrane and its regulation to collagen. Biochemistry 5:702−712.
Kilo, C., N. Vogler, and J. R. Williamson. 1972. Muscle capillary basement membrane changes related to aging and diabetes mellitus. Diabetes 21:881−905.
Laurent, T. C. 1972. The ultrastructure and physico-chemical properties of interstitial connective tissue. Pflügers Arch. 336:S21−S33.
Laurent, T. C., and B. Öbrink. 1972. On the restriction of rotational diffusion of proteins in polymer networks. Eur. J. Biochem. 28:94−101.
Loblich, H. J. 1965. Der Einfluss des O_2-Mangels auf die Entwicklung der experimentalen Silicose. Beitr. Silicose-Forsch. S. Bd. Grundfragen Silicose-Forsch 6:155 (according to Chvapil, 1967).
Luft, J. H. 1965. The ultrastructural basis of capillary permeability. In B. W. Zweifach, L. Grant, and R. T. McCluskey (eds.), The Inflammatory Process, pp. 121−159. Academic Press, New York.
Luft, J. H. 1973. Capillary permeability. I. Structural considerations. In B. W. Zweifach, J. Grant, and R. T. McCluskey (eds.), The Inflammatory Process, 2nd Ed., Vol. 2, pp. 47−93. Academic Press, New York.
Ma, C. K., and E. V. Cowdry. 1950. Aging of elastic tissue in human skin. J. Gerontol. 5:203−210.
Majno, G. 1965. Ultrastructure of the vascular membrane. In W. F. Hamilton and P. Dow (eds.), Handbook of Physiology, Sect. 2, Circulation, Vol. 3, pp. 2293−2375. American Physiological Society, Washington, D.C.
Martinez-Palomo, A. 1970. The surface coats of animal cells. Int. Rev. Cytol. 29:29−75.
McCroskery, P. A., J. F. Richards, and E. D. Harris, Jr. 1975. Purification and characterization of collagenase extracted from rabbit tumors. Biochem. J. 152:131−142.
Menkin, V. 1956. Biochemical Mechanism of Inflammation, p. 195. Charles C. Thomas, Springfield, Ill. 439 p.
Miller, E. F., and V. J. Matukas. 1974. Biosynthesis of collagen. Fed. Proc. 33:1197−1204.
Mohos, S. C., and L. Skoza. 1969. Glomerular sialoprotein. Science 164:1519.
Montfort, I., and R. Perez-Tomajo. 1975. The distribution of collagenase in the rat uterus during postpartum involution. Conn. Tissue Res. 3:245−252.
Muir, A. R., and A. Peters. 1962. Quintuple-layered membrane junctions at terminal bars between endothelial cells. J. Cell. Biol. 12:443−448.
Neuberger, A., J. C. Perrone, and H. G. Slack. 1951. The relative metabolic inertia of tendon collagen in the rat. Biochem. J. 49:199−204.
Ogston, A. G. 1970. The biological functions of the glycosaminoglycans. In E. A. Balazs (ed.), Chemistry and Molecular Biology of the Intercellular Matrix, pp. 1231−1240. Academic Press, New York.
Pexieder, T. 1965. Age changes in vascularization of the adipose tissue in rats. Exp. Gerontol. 1:95−103.
Priest, R. A. 1967. Endocrine control of connective tissue metabolism. In B. M. Wagner (ed.), The Connective Tissue, pp. 50−60. Williams and Wilkins, Baltimore.
Rakusan, K., and O. Poupa. 1964. Capillaries and muscle fibres in the heart of old rats. Gerontologia 9:107−112.
Ries, W. 1961. Aging of the capillary system. Dtsch. Gesundheitswes. 16:580−585.

Schaub, M. C. 1964. Eigenschaften und intracellulare Verteilung eines Kollagenabbauenden Kathepsins. Helv. Physiolpharmac. Acta. 22:271–284.

Schiller, S., G. A. Slover, and A. Dorfman. 1962. Effect of thyroid gland on metabolism of acid mucopolysaccharides in skin. Biochim. Biophys. Acta 58:27–33.

Shimamoto, T., and F. Numano. 1969. An introduction to investigation of atherogenesis. *In* T. Schmamoto and F. Numano, Atherogenesis, pp. 5–27. Excerpta Medica Foundation, Amsterdam.

Sinex, F. M. 1968. The role of collagen in aging. *In* B. S. Gould (ed.), Treatise on Collagen, Vol. 2. Biology of collagen, Part B, pp. 410–448. Academic Press, New York.

Skoza, L., and S. C. Mohos. 1974. Enzymatic solubilization and separation of glomerular collagen and sialoprotein. Lab. Invest. 30:93–101.

Smith, D. J. 1969. The connective tissue fiber-water interface: physiological and pathological implications. J. Dental Res. 48, No. 5 (Suppl.):676–679.

Sobel, H. 1967. Aging on ground substance in connective tissue. *In* B. L. Strehler (ed.), Advances in Gerontological Research, Vol. 2, pp. 205–283. Academic Press, New York.

Sobel, H. 1968. Aging of connective tissue and molecular transport. Gerontologia 14:235–254.

Sobel, H., and M. J. Newlett. 1967. Effect of age on hyaluronic acid in heart of dogs. J. Gerontol. 22:196–198.

Spiro, R. G. 1970. Biochemistry of basement membranes. *In* E. A. Balazs (ed.), Chemistry and Molecular Biology of Intercellular Matrix, pp. 511–534. Academic Press, New York.

Spiro, R. G. 1973. Biochemistry of the renal glomerular basement membrane and its alterations in diabetes mellitus. New Engl. J. Med. 288:1337–1342.

Vasiljev, J. M. 1961. Soedinithelnaia tkan i opukhollevyi rost v eksperimente. Medgiz, Moskow.

Verzár, F. 1957. The aging of connective tissue. Gerontologia 1:363–378.

Wells, J. D. 1973. Salt activity and osmotic pressure in connective tissue. I. A study of solutions of dextran sulphate as a model system. Proc. Roy. Soc. Biol., London 183:399–419.

Werle, E., and G. Leusch. 1952. Ueber den Einfluss der Hyaluronidase auf die Wasserdurchlassigkeit von Bindegewebsmembranen. Klin. Wschr. 30:611–612.

Wetzel, M. G., B. K. Wetzel, and S. S. Spitzer. 1966. Ultrastructural localization of acid mucopolysaccharides in the mouse colon with iron-containing stains. J. Cell. Biol. 30:299–315.

Williamson, J. R., N. J. Vogler, and C. Kilo. 1971. Structural abnormalities in muscle capillary basement membrane in diabetes mellitus. Acta Diabetol. Lat. 8 (Suppl.):117–134.

Woessner, J. F. 1968. Biological mechanism of collagen resorption. *In* B. S. Gould (ed.), Treatise on Collagen, Vol. 2, Biology of collagen, Part B, pp. 253–330. Academic Press, New York.

Young, W. J. 1972. Dynamics of disolution of gas bubbles or pockets in tissue. J. Biochem. 5:321–332.

Zweifach, B. W. 1961. Functional Behavior of Microcirculation. Charles C. Thomas, Springfield, Ill.

Zweifach, B. W. 1972. Capillary filtration and mechanism of edema formation. Pflügers Arch. 336:S81–95.

BLOOD-TISSUE
EXCHANGE

chapter 8

INTRAVASCULAR AND TISSUE SPACE ONCOTIC AND HYDROSTATIC PRESSURES

Donald D. Stromberg and Curtis A. Wiederhielm

INTRAVASCULAR ONCOTIC PRESSURE

INTRAVASCULAR HYDROSTATIC PRESSURE

TISSUE SPACE HYDROSTATIC PRESSURE

TISSUE SPACE ONCOTIC PRESSURE

COMMENTS

Before the mid-nineteenth century the view was generally held that exchange processes between blood and tissues were mediated through an active process of secretion. A series of studies in Ludwig's laboratory during the years 1850–1861 led to the formulation of a filtration theory, in which the hypothesis was advanced that capillary hydrostatic pressure caused filtration of fluid and nutrients into the tissues. The simple filtration hypothesis was, however, inadequate to explain certain observations, e.g., the fact that extremely low lymph flows were observed from the resting limb. Clearly, other forces were acting in addition to the capillary hydrostatic pressure. One additional force that prevented excessive fluid shifts from the circulation to the tissues was identified by Starling in his classic paper (Starling, 1896). Starling postulated that a "balance of forces" acted across the capillary wall to maintain intravascular volume. The force resisting excessive transudation of fluid was the osmotic pressure generated by the plasma proteins. Measurements of the protein osmotic pressures conducted with a primitive membrane osmometer yielded values of 30–40 mm Hg, comparable to the indirect estimates of capillary pressures available at the time. It is a tribute to Starling's genius that he recognized the importance of the mechanism of dilution of extravascular proteins as a compensating factor, tending to limit large fluid shifts between the circulation and the tissues.

187

INTRAVASCULAR ONCOTIC PRESSURE

With the increasingly sophisticated technologic advances since Starling's experiments, the measurement of plasma protein oncotic pressure remains the most accurately measurable "force" acting across the capillary. The unexpectedly high pressures described by Starling have since been found to reflect bacterial degradation of the plasma protein due to the prolonged equilibration time of his osmometer. The modern membrane osmometer yields reliable determination from samples in a few minutes, even when minute quantities are involved (Hepp, 1936; Intaglietta and Zweifach, 1971; Friedman, 1973; Prather, Gaar, and Guyton, 1968; Wiederhielm, Lee, and Stromberg, 1973). Blood samples are readily accessible intermittently or continuously in experimental preparations or from patients. An underlying assumption is that the blood sample is representative of the blood in the capillaries, i.e., that the protein concentration in the samples is comparable to those of capillary blood. The validity of this assumption depends not only on the site of sampling but also on the method of obtaining the sample (Landis and Pappenheimer, 1963).

The protein oncotic pressure is operationally defined as that pressure required to balance the attractive forces of the proteins across a semipermeable membrane. Inherent in the concept of oncotic pressure is either fluid movement or the potential for fluid movement. In practice, osmometric pressures are determined at equilibration or, ideally, zero movement of fluid across the membrane in the measurement unit. In Starling's osmometer the measured pressure was the equilibrium height of solution in the manometer. In modern low-compliance osmometers, it is usually the equilibrium pressure developed in the reference solution compartment. The use of low-compliance pressure transducers and specific designs aimed at decreasing the overall compliance of the membrane chamber have made it possible to approach the ideal situation of zero fluid flux, and a rapid response time. It is, however, unlikely that any osmometer membrane accurately reflects capillary properties, which vary from tissue to tissue, and also in different portions of the capillary network.

Variations in plasma oncotic pressure are moderately wide. Intaglietta and Zweifach reported results from 266 rabbits followed over a period of 4 yr under conditions of constant habitat and diet (Zweifach and Intaglietta, 1971). Their reported average value of 16.5 mm Hg is lower than that usually given for normal man (24–26 mm Hg). It is on the low end of the spectrum of values given for other mammalian species (Landis and Pappenheimer, 1963). Recent studies of dehydration in experimental animals suggest a well-controlled plasma protein concentration during considerable shifts in extracellular fluid volume (Schultze, Kirsch, and Röcker, 1972). This observation suggests the existence of significant control mechanisms that may involve alterations in lymph flow.

INTRAVASCULAR HYDROSTATIC PRESSURE

As blood moves from the heart through the vascular system it undergoes a progressive decrease in pressure due to the resistance offered by the repeatedly branching, narrowing ramifications of the arterial system. Little pressure is lost in larger arteries, but the loss of pressure increases progressively in the smallest branches of the arterial tree, branches termed the resistance vessels. The first quantitative evaluation of the pressure profile in a microvascular bed was achieved by Landis's classic micropuncture technique in 1926 (Landis, 1926). In this study he demonstrated that the largest fraction of the pressure drop occurred between the terminal arteries and the arterial capillaries of the mesenteric microcirculation in frogs. Since the pressure drop was greatest across these vessels, changes in caliber of arterioles and their branches exerted the most profound influence on blood flow and hydrostatic pressure in capillaries. Landis also demonstrated that hydrostatic pressure in the arterial capillaries exceeded the colloid osmotic pressure of plasma proteins, while in the venous capillaries it was lower. This finding suggested a concept that arterial capillaries were a site of filtration, while venous capillaries reabsorbed fluid from the tissues. This basic concept is generally referred to as the "Starling hypothesis" of capillary filtration, but should more appropriately be titled the Starling—Landis hypothesis. Landis's initial studies in the frog mesentery were subsequently extended to the mesentery of other mammalian species (Landis, 1930*a*) and to the nailfold capillaries in man (Landis, 1930*b*). Landis's measurements in single capillaries were subsequently extended to a whole perfused organ by use of isogravimetric techniques (Pappenheimer and Soto-Rivera, 1948). The isogravimetric techniques yield indirect estimates of the average capillary hydrostatic pressure, and depend on maintaining arterial and venous pressures in the perfused organ at levels that lead to no net filtration or reabsorption, as evidenced by constant weight of the experimental preparation. Estimates for capillary blood pressure obtained by these methods generally yield lower mean capillary pressures than are found by direct puncture at the midcapillary. This difference may reflect a disproportionately greater exchange due to higher permeability and larger surface area at the venous end of the capillary network (Wiederhielm, 1968). The original micropuncture technique of Landis required use of micropipets of tip dimensions approaching those of mammalian capillaries. This large pipet size was essential to allow microscopic observation of a "null" point, at which dye barely entered the capillary from the micropipet. Microscopic vessels are difficult to puncture at best, and with large pipets like those used by Landis the puncture becomes an extraordinary feat. Also, measurements by this technique are by necessity intermittent and difficult to adapt for direct recording. A wide-ranging exploration of microvascular pressures in capillaries in other beds was made practical by development of an electronic feedback system adapted to the nulling technique of the Landis method, which provided a means for the use of micropipets with tip diameters less than 0.1 μ, and for increasing the frequency response of the system to 70 hz (Wiederhielm et al., 1964; Fox and Wiederhielm, 1973). Initial studies repeated Landis's measurements in frog microvessels and demonstrated pulsatile pressures extending throughout the capillary network. More recently, this method has been employed for a systematic survey of microvascular pressures in the wing web of the unanesthetized bat (Wiederhielm and Weston, 1973). Several laboratories are now using this active nulling system, or modifications thereof, in other microvascular systems, such as the kidney (Brenner, Troy, and Daugharty, 1972), skeletal muscle (Smäje, Zweifach, and Intaglietta, 1970), and brain (Stromberg and Fox, 1972).

Significant differences have been found in the pressure profile of these vascular beds, suggesting that the sites of controlled resistance may differ in different organs. Obviously, there is a need for much more data measured from as many sources as possible, using methods as direct as possible to indicate further the locus of microvascular control of hydrostatic pressure.

TISSUE SPACE HYDROSTATIC PRESSURE

The balance of forces across the capillary wall includes extravascular forces in addition to the capillary hydrostatic pressure and plasma protein osmotic pressure. Transcapillary exchange is determined by the pressure gradient acting across the capillary wall. The hydrostatic pressure in the tissues opposes filtration of fluids from the capillary (in concert with plasma oncotic pressure). It also likely plays a major role in movement of fluid into the lymphatic capillaries. Estimates of tissue space hydrostatic pressure magnitude have been hampered by a number of factors, however. These include primarily the very small dimensions of the spaces involved. There is, in fact, a question of whether sufficiently large fluid-filled spaces exist to allow meaningful measurements of hydrostatic pressure. It has been suggested that needle or pipet measurements necessarily involve significant tissue distortions that "create" spaces in which pressures are measured, and that not only the spaces but also the pressures measured in them are distortions and therefore differ from those existing under normal conditions (Guyton, 1963). This is the quintessence of the problem: How does one measure the pressure present in the "normal" state? No currently available techniques fully satisfy the requirement of normality. All are plagued by a kind of biologic uncertainty principle in that measurements distort the normal interstitium to a greater or lesser degree.

The most elegant and carefully controlled studies involving the hypodermic needle technique for measuring tissue pressure were the experiments done by McMaster (1946). In these studies, the smallest available hypodermic needles were inserted in tissues under microscopic observation to avoid injury to blood vessels and lymphatics. The pressure required to establish a minimal egress of fluid from the needle was considered to reflect an approximation of the tissue pressure and was found to average a few centimeters of water in mouse subcutaneous tissue. McMaster, however, refers to his measurements as "interstitial resistance," indicating his recognition of the limitation of this technique of measuring tissue pressure. Other studies utilizing hypodermic needle insertion in the skin and muscle of human subjects have yielded values of approximately the same magnitude (Wells, Youmans, and Miller, 1938).

The capsule technique developed by Guyton (1963) involved measurements of the pressure developed in the fluid space that forms inside an implanted hollow perforated plastic sphere or cylinder that was allowed to heal into the tissue for 4 or more weeks. An inherent assumption is that the fluid space in the capsule is representative of, and in direct communication with, the interstitial space fluid. The granulation tissue that develops around and inside the capsule during the "healing-in period" is, however, not representative of normal connective tissue. The pressures measured in these units were subatmospheric by about −5 mm Hg in a variety of tissues.

A wick technique developed by Scholander, Hargens, and Miller (1968) also yields subatmospheric pressures, but of smaller magnitude. This method involves placing a catheter through a relatively large trocar into a tissue. The tip of the catheter is filled with a porous material such as cotton thread and the catheter is connected to a pressure transducer filled with a solution such as physiologic saline. Besides the obvious trauma associated with inserting a relatively large catheter, the composition of the fluid in the wick is not identical to that of tissue fluid. Recent investigations of the wick method (Snashall et al., 1971) demonstrate that if wicks are soaked in hyaluronic acid solutions the recorded pressures become less negative and in many instances positive. Snashall et al. suggest that the apparent hydrostatic pressures recorded by the wick, and probably also by the subcutaneous capsules, are due to osmotic forces developed by the hyaluronic acid in the interstitial tissue.

Glass ultramicropipets using the servo nulling system have been used to measure pressures directly in the subcutaneous tissue on the bat wing. The crucial factor of these measurements was the demonstration that the wing web tissue fluid spaces were larger than the pipet tips. The technique demands careful pressure calibration and continuous checking of the zero-pressure reference level. Tissue pressure recordings by this method were very similar in magnitude to the resistances found by McMaster (Wiederhielm, 1969). In a few instances, subatmospheric pressures ranging from −0.1 to −1.7 mm Hg were recorded, but the average pressure for all determinations was 1.25 mm Hg.

It is difficult to reconcile fully the apparent differences between results obtained using pipets and needles with those obtained using the capsule or wick. One interpretation is that results from the capsule and wick techniques are influenced by more than the hydrostatic tissue space components. For example, part of the measured pressure may be oncotic in origin (Stromberg and Wieder-hielm, 1970). Further support for this interpretation is gained by the demonstration that tissue fluid oncotic pressure is substantial, as is discussed subsequently. It must be emphasized that the difference in results among techniques is largely one of degree. Future work will likely reveal factors previously overlooked and clarify aspects of these techniques that currently cloud our concepts of conditions in the normal tissue spaces. The current controversy is likely to be, at least in part, one of semantics, i.e., what distinguishes hydrostatic from oncotic pressure. This is clearly a critical area for future research and will require new inventive approaches.

TISSUE SPACE ONCOTIC PRESSURE

Several macromolecules contribute to tissue space oncotic pressure. Among these the plasma proteins are probably most easily conceptualized, since it is generally agreed that most capillary networks leak protein into the tissue spaces. This protein is continually returned to the circulation by way of the lymphatics. Changes in either leakage rate or the return rate will alter the amount of protein in the tissue space. The oncotic pressure exerted by the proteins is a function of their concentration, which is dependent not only on the protein leakage rate but also on the balance between fluid filtration and absorption by capillaries. Substantial amounts of plasma proteins are found in the interstitial space; tracer studies have indicated that as much as one-half of the total plasma protein pool is found extravascularly (Takeda, 1964). The calculated average plasma protein concentration in the interstitial fluid is on the order of 1.7–2.0%, yielding osmotic pressures of 4–5 mm Hg. It should be emphasized that the generally accepted concept that tissue fluid osmotic pressure is negligible is based on studies attempting to evaluate the average composition of capillary filtrate (Landis et al., 1932), in which venous pressure was elevated to 55–60 mm Hg for a considerable time. Other data that seemingly supported estimates for very low tissue fluid osmotic pressure appeared in the studies of Pappenheimer and Soto-Rivera (1948). However, in these studies, the isolated isogravimetric hind-limb preparation was perfused with hypooncotic blood (average plasma pressure, 15 mm Hg). Under both experimental circumstances, elevation of capillary filtration and virtual inhibition of reabsorption would occur, leading to dilution of tissue plasma proteins and low estimates for tissue osmotic pressure. The presence of plasma proteins in the interstitial space serves an important regulatory function in limiting excessive translocation of fluid from the circulation to the tissues. This mechanism was clearly identified by Starling in his classic paper (Starling, 1896),

> ". . . there must be a balance between the hydrostatic pressure of the blood in the capillaries and the osmotic attraction of the blood for the surrounding fluids. With increased capillary pressure, there must be increased transudation, until equilibrium is established at a somewhat higher point, when there

is more diluted fluid in tissue spaces, therefore higher absorbing force to balance the increased capillary pressures."

The importance of this mechanism and the factors discussed above have been emphasized in recent studies on capillary fluid exchange (Wiederhielm, 1967, 1968).

There are also substantial quantitites of other osmotically active macromolecules in the tissue spaces. The amounts and compositions of these macromolecules vary widely among tissues. Representative types include hyaluronic acid, chondroitin sulfates, elastin, and collagen. These high-molecular-weight substances probably exert their osmotic effect as much by their interaction with the plasma proteins as by a "direct" contribution to tissue space oncotic pressure. For example, by reducing interstitial fluid volume available to the proteins, these macromolecules may increase the effective concentration of the proteins and thereby increase the effective tissue fluid oncotic pressure. This concept is usually called the volume exclusion effect (Laurent, 1968). If this concept is valid, dilution may be a source of error in estimating the concentration of tissue space protein in extracted fluids (including lymph). This dilution of non-protein-containing fluid from interstitial space compartments occupied by mucopolysaccharides, and therefore not accessible to plasma proteins, would be flow dependent. In other words, direct sampling techniques by micropipet (Haljamäe and Fredén, 1970), or by similar methods, require careful assessment of the influence of the rate of fluid collection. Faster withdrawal rates may yield lower protein concentrations in the direct sampling techniques. Similar mechanisms may account for variations in lymph protein concentration. Those obtained at lower flow rates more nearly approximate concentrations of tissue space fluids. Recent estimates of tissue space protein concentrations obtained by assaying fluid from implanted wicks equilibrated in tissues have yielded protein concentrations corresponding to about 10 mm Hg oncotic pressure (Aukland and Fadnes, 1972; Aukland, 1973). This is in agreement with low flow rate lymph samples that yield protein concentrations more than half the concentration found in plasma (Staub, 1970). Similar values are obtained by calculations from isotope-labeled turnover measurements and by fluorometric techniques used from thin tissues to estimate protein concentrations in situ in tissue spaces (Hauck, 1969).

Direct measurements of the "swelling" pressure of tissue specimens have been carried out by placing excised rabbit skin samples on a membrane osmometer, yielding values of about 10 mm Hg (Wiederhielm, 1972). Similar skin specimen placed on membranes with large pores freely permeable to protein yielded pressures averaging 2 mm Hg, suggesting that the "swelling" pressure is of oncotic rather than hydrostatic origin. The swelling pressure of subcutaneous connective tissue has also been estimated in in vivo studies by implantation of membrane osmometers, using membranes with well-defined permeability characteristics (Stromberg and Wiederhielm, unpublished data). Using membranes impermeable to plasma proteins, pressures on the order of 10 mm Hg were recorded. When large-pore membranes with pore diameters on the order of 2,000 Å were used, which permit free passage into the reference chamber of plasma protein but retain mucopolysaccharides and other macromolecules, recorded pressures averaged between 1 and 2 mm Hg. This lends strong support to the concept that the pressures recorded in this manner are osmotic in nature rather than hydrostatic. The magnitude of pressures recorded in these in vitro and in vivo studies are similar to those predicted in a computer simulation study of capillary fluid dynamics (Wiederhielm, 1968). These values are also virtually identical to the oncotic pressure that would be exerted by the lymph of a 3.5% protein concentration (9.7 mm Hg). There is thus no reason to anticipate a significant gradient of osmotic pressure between interstitial fluid and lymph; the protein concentration in the interstitial free fluid spaces could be virtually identical to that of lymph. As predicted by Starling, the magnitude of this quantity would also be expected to change with variations in protein or fluid fluxes through the tissue spaces.

COMMENTS

Plasma protein oncotic pressure as determined by blood sampling and membrane osmometry is the most readily measurable and best defined quantity in the Starling–Landis relationship. It is subject to limited variations except in disease states. The intravascular hydrostatic pressure beyond the resistance vessels is a controlled variable with a significant influence on capillary fluid exchange. As measurements from different microvascular beds accumulate, significant differences have been found and there is reason to doubt the validity of extrapolating from one microvascular bed to another. Many tissues have yet to be studied. The question of interstitial hydrostatic pressure measurements will probably be subject to controversy and difficulty of interpretation for some time to come. Evidence is gradually accumulating that suggests that the concept of negative tissue pressures may be erroneous. Tissue fluid oncotic pressure represents an area in which further investigation is badly needed; the technical problems associated with collecting truly representative tissue fluid samples under normal conditions are formidable, but by means of ingenious methods such as those referred to previously, an ultimate answer to this problem may be provided. Ideally, a microosmometer of dimensions sufficiently small to be introduced into tissues without significant distortion could provide a direct measurement of tissue oncotic pressures. Technology has, however, not yet reached a point at which such an approach appears feasible.

LITERATURE CITED

Aukland, K., and H. O. Fadnes. 1972. Wick method for measuring interstitial fluid protein concentration. Acta Physiol. Scand. 84(4):26a (Abstr., Communications).

Aukland, K. 1973. Autoregulation of interstitial fluid volume. Scand. J. Clin. Lab. Invest. 31:247.

Brenner, B. M., J. L. Troy, and T. M. Daugharty. 1972. Pressures in cortical structures of the rat kidney. Am. J. Physiol. 222:246.

Fox, J. R., and C. A. Wiederhielm. 1973. Characteristics of the servocontrolled micropipet pressure system. Microvasc. Res. 5:324.

Friedman, J. J. 1973. A modified colloidal osmotic transducer for the determination of transcapillary fluid movement. Microvasc. Res. 5:222.

Guyton, A. C. 1963. A concept of negative interstitial pressure based on pressures in implanted perforated capsules. Circ. Res. 12:399.

Haljamäe, H., and H. Fredén. 1970. Comparative analysis of the protein content of local subcutaneous tissue fluid and plasma. Microvasc. Res. 2:163.

Hauck, V. G. 1969. Zur frage der existenz eines "gradient of vascular permeability" an der endstrombahn. Arch. fur Kreislaufforschung 59:197.

Hepp, O. 1936. Ein neues Onkometer zur Bestimmung des kolloidosmotischen Druckes mit gesteigerter Messgenauigkeit und vereinfachter Handhabung. Z. Ges. Exp. Med. 99:709.

Intaglietta, M., and B. W. Zweifach. 1971. Measurement of blood plasma colloid osmotic pressure. Microvasc. Res. 3:72.

Landis, E. M. 1926. The capillary pressure in frog mesentery as determined by microinjection. Am. J. Physiol. 75:548.

Landis, E. M. 1930a. The capillary blood pressure in mammalian mesentery as determined by the micro-injection method. Am. J. Physiol. 93:353.

Landis, E. M. 1930b. Micro-injection studies of capillary blood pressure in human skin. Heart 15:209.

Landis, E. M., L. Jonas, M. Angevine, and W. Erb. 1932. The passage of fluid and protein through the human capillary wall during venous congestion. J. Clin. Invest. 11:717.

Landis, E. M., and J. R. Pappenheimer. 1963. Exchange of substances through the capillary walls. In W. F. Hamilton and P. Dow (eds.), Handbook of Physiology, Sect. 2, Vol. II, Chap. 29, pp. 961–1034. American Physiological Society, Washington, D.C.

Laurent, T. C. 1968. The exclusion of macromolecules from polysaccharide media. In G. Quintarelli (ed.), The Chemical Physiology of Mucopolysaccharides, pp. 153–170. Little-Brown and Co., Boston.

McMaster, P. D. 1946. The pressure and interstitial resistance prevailing in the normal and edematous skin of animals and man. J. Exp. Med. 84:473.

Pappenheimer, J. R., and A. Soto-Rivera. 1948. Effective osmotic pressure of the plasma proteins and other quantities associated with the capillary circulation in the hindlimbs of cats and dogs. Am. J. Physiol. 152:471.

Prather, J. W., K. A. Gaar, Jr., and A. C. Guyton. 1968. Direct continuous recordings of plasma colloid osmotic pressure of whole blood. J. Appl. Physiol. 24:602.

Scholander, P. F., R. Hargens, and S. L. Miller. 1968. Negative pressure in the interstitial fluid of animals. Science 161(3839):321.

Schultze, G., K. Kirsch, and L. Röcker. 1972. Distribution and circulation of extracellular fluid and protein during different states of hydration in the cat. Pflügers Arch. 337:351.

Smäje, L., B. W. Zweifach, and M. Intaglietta. 1970. Micropressures and capillary filtration coefficients in single vessels of the cremaster muscle of the rat. Microvasc. Res. 2:96.

Snashall, P. D., J. Lucas, A. Guz, and M. A. Floyer. 1971. Measurement of interstitial 'fluid' pressure by means of a cotton wick in man and animals: An analysis of the origin of the pressure. Clin. Sci. 41:35.

Starling, E. H. 1896. On the absorption of fluids from the connective tissue spaces. J. Physiol. (London) 19:312.

Staub, N. C. 1970. The pathophysiology of pulmonary edema. Human Pathol. 1:419.

Stromberg, D. D., and J. R. Fox. 1972. Pressures in pial arterial microcirculation of the cat during changes in systemic arterial blood pressure. Circ. Res. 31:229.

Stromberg, D. A., and C. A. Wiederhielm. 1970. Effects of oncotic gradients and enzymes on negative pressures in implanted capsules. Am. J. Physiol. 219:928.

Takeda, Y. 1964. Metabolism and distribution of autologous and homologous albumin-I^{131} in the dog. Am. J. Physiol. 206:1223.

Wells, H. S., J. B. Youmans, and D. G. Miller, Jr. 1938. Tissue pressure (intracutaneous, subcutaneous, and intramuscular) as related to venous pressure, capillary filtration, and other factors. J. Clin. Invest. 17:489.

Wiederhielm, C. A., J. W. Woodbury, S. E. Kirk, and R. F. Rushmer. 1964. Pulsatile pressures in the microcirculation of frog's mesentery. Am. J. Physiol. 207:173.

Wiederhielm, C. A. 1967. Analysis of small vessel function. In E. B. Reeve and A. C. Guyton (eds.), Physical Basis of Circulatory Transport: Regulation and Exchange, pp. 313–326. W. B. Saunders, Philadelphia.

Wiederhielm, C. A. 1968. Dynamics of transcapillary fluid exchange. J. Gen. Physiol. 52:29.

Wiederhielm, C. A. 1969. The interstitial space and lymphatic pressures in the bat wing. In A. P. Fishman and H. Hecht (eds.), The Pulmonary Circulation and Interstitial Space, pp. 29–41. University of Chicago Press, Chicago.

Wiederhielm, C. A. 1972. The interstitial space. In Y. C. Fung, N. Perrone, and M. Anliker (eds.), Biomechanics: Its Foundations and Objectives, pp. 273–286. Prentice-Hall, Englewood Cliffs, N.J.

Wiederhielm, C. A., D. R. Lee, and D. D. Stromberg. 1973. A membrane osmometer for microliter samples. J. Appl. Physiol. 35:432.

Wiederhielm, C. A., and B. V. Weston. 1973. Microvascular, lymphatic and tissue pressures in the unanesthetized mammal. Am. J. Physiol. 225:992.

chapter 9

TRANSCAPILLARY EXCHANGE OF FLUID IN SINGLE MICROVESSELS

Marcos Intaglietta

EXPERIMENTAL BASIS FOR THE VALIDITY OF
STARLING'S HYPOTHESIS

PERMEABILITY PROPERTIES OF SINGLE CAPILLARIES

THE HYDRODYNAMIC CONDUCTIVITY OF SINGLE
VESSELS AND RATE OF EXCHANGE

THE CAPILLARY BARRIER VERSUS TISSUE BARRIER

TISSUE BLOOD FLOW AND EXCHANGE FLOW

STARLING'S HYPOTHESIS OF FLUID BALANCE
AND THE MICROSCOPIC EVIDENCE

The exchange of materials between blood and tissue comprises diffusive and convective processes that occur at the level of the microcirculation. The fact that materials of different molecular dimensions traverse the capillary barrier indicates that, functionally, this structure has the characteristics of a porous conduit. This property is in contrast with the need to maintain the intravascular volume of circulating fluid, since the concomitant pressure gradients could, in principle, determine the leakage of the circulating fluid through the porous wall. This problem does not occur in nature because of the presence of large-molecular-weight species that cannot pass through the capillary barrier, and thus give rise to an osmotic effect between intra-extravascular fluids. This effect diminishes the net hydrostatic pressure that causes filtration, and in the venous end of the microcirculation, is presumed to determine the reabsorption of fluid from the tissue into the intravascular compartment.

Supported by United States Public Health Service Grant HL 12493.

These phenomena determine the existence of two types of exchange fluxes through the capillary wall. One is a diffusive transport determined by concentration gradients, mediated by molecular size, lipid solubility, and the physical restriction imposed by the capillary barrier itself. In addition, there is a continuous flow of fluid through the capillary wall as a consequence of the interaction of hydraulic and osmotic forces. This convective exchange is essential for the maintenance of osmotic equilibrium in the tissue milieu, the facilitation of the movement of large molecules such as protein through the interstitium, and on a bodily scale for the regulation of blood volume. This convective flux of blood ultrafiltrate originates at the boundary between the blood and tissue, as a flow perpendicular to the intraluminal flow, and continues through the tissue gel as a combination of diffusive and percolative processes. Tissue perfusion can, therefore, be characterized by two fluid flows, namely, the convective or intravascular, and percolative or extravascular. These flows bear a precise relationship to each other, which is summarized by the concepts embodied in the so-called Starling hypothesis of fluid exchange (Starling, 1896).

The Starling hypothesis of fluid exchange is based on the concept that the balance of fluid between blood and tissue compartments is a consequence of the exchange that occurs at the level of blood capillaries, caused by the interaction of hydraulic and colloid osmotic pressures, and mediated by the permeability characteristics of the interface between blood and tissue. In the commonly accepted explanation of this process (Landis and Pappenheimer, 1963), blood enters the exchange vessels of the microcirculation at a comparatively high pressure, and owing to viscous losses, exits from the system at a lower pressure. The blood plasma colloid osmotic pressure is assumed to be straddled by these input and output hydraulic pressures, in such a fashion that outward filtration in the arterial (or high-pressure) portion of the network is balanced by absorption in the venous (or low-pressure) region.

Historically, the analyses of fluid exchange dealt primarily with the interplay of intravascular pressure and plasma colloid osmotic pressure neglecting extravascular factors. When Guyton (1963) presented data in support of a negative interstitial tissue pressure, attention was focused to the osmotic and hydrostatic pressures in the interstitial ground substance, and current theories attempt to include these extravascular factors. Thus the comprehensive analyses of fluid movement includes intravascular forces, the characteristics of the capillary barrier, the properties of the interstitial gel in which the blood capillaries lie, and what is essentially an extension of the interstitium, the microscopic beginning of the lymphatic system.

In terms of single vessels, as in the experiments of Landis (1927) and Zweifach and Intaglietta (1968), the Starling constitutive equation for blood–tissue fluid movement may be expressed in terms of fluid movement per unit area available for exchange and written as follows:

$$\dot{m} = K[P_c - \pi_{p\ell} - (P_t - \pi_t)].$$ (1)

In this equation, $\mathring{m}$ is the rate of fluid exchanged across the capillary wall. K is the filtration coefficient for single vessels; it is an operational term that includes the properties of the vessel barrier and those of the interstitial compartment. P_c is the capillary hydrostatic pressure, and P_t is the tissue fluid pressure. $\pi_{p\varrho}$ is the plasma colloid osmotic pressure, and π_t is that of the tissue fluid.

EXPERIMENTAL BASIS
FOR THE VALIDITY OF STARLING'S HYPOTHESIS

The validity of the Starling constitutive equation is ultimately based on whether the exchange system of the microcirculation has structurally and functionally the properties of an osmometer. A number of different approaches have been utilized to validate this concept. On the macroscopic level, the system has been studied in whole organs, where the different parameters of exchange and perfusion were deduced from the gain or loss of weight (or volume) of the organ (Pappenheimer, 1953), as a function of different arteriovenous hydrostatic pressure differences relative to flow (Folkow, 1961).

Pappenheimer and Soto-Rivera (1948) determined the relationships between arterial and venous pressure, blood flow, and plasma colloid osmotic pressure in an isolated hind limb. In this classical work, the limb was continuously weighed while both arterial and venous pressures were adjusted so as to maintain this weight constant. Recording the flow at which the preparation is at the control weight and repeating the experiment at different flow rates and AV pressure differentials, it was possible to extrapolate to zero flow and thus to determine the isogravimetric capillary pressure. At this condition the hydrostatic pressure in the blood capillaries balances all other colloid osmotic and tissue pressures so that the net flux is zero. This pressure corresponds to the "effective capillary pressure," determined by Zweifach and Intaglietta (1968) in single microvessels, since no correction has been made for the tissue factors in the Starling relationship.

The validation of the concept of fluid balance requires that the system be able both to filter and absorb fluid. A clear demonstration that absorption exists as a distinct phenomenon which is opposite to filtration was obtained by Pappenheimer and Soto-Rivera (1948) by elevating plasma colloid osmotic pressure. In these experiments the rate of decrease in weight reached a steady state comparable to the rate of increase caused by an increase in venous pressure. It should be considered that isogravimetric experiments represent perhaps the major evidence to validate the balance expressed by Starlings hypothesis, and therefore it is important to realize that the balance condition between compartments, as well as reproducible numerical values of the so-called isogravimetric capillary pressure, only obtain when a substantial amount of "free" water is available in the tissue. In practice, there seems to be no unequivocal way to determine whether the amount of free water in vivo and in situ is comparable to that under particular experimental conditions.

It should also be considered that in both in vivo and in situ conditions, plasma protein passes from blood into the tissue and is eventually collected by the lymphatics. In the absence of evidence for an active transport mechanism, it has been assumed that this process must take place through a system of pores of sufficiently large diameters to permit the passage of macromolecules. It is apparent that in the immediate vicinity of such large pores, the tissue fluid protein concentration must be similar to that of plasma, and therefore the exchange of fluid through these pores would be independent of osmotic effects. Given that the venular system constitutes this region of high permeability, the question of the location and magnitude of the process of absorption in vivo and in situ remains unanswered.

PERMEABILITY PROPERTIES OF SINGLE CAPILLARIES

The question of whether exchange in the microcirculation is governed by the factors that characterize an osmometer could, in principle, be resolved by establishing whether in the in situ and in vivo conditions the exchange of fluid in individual capillaries achieves a steady balance that can be related to that observed in the isogravimetric experiments. This analysis necessary for such a comparison requires in vivo microscopic data on the permeability characteristics of the barrier, the contribution of the interstitium, and the measurement of hydrostatic and colloid osmotic pressures in capillaries, as well as the rates at which fluids are exchanged between the different compartments.

The nature of the fluid exchange phenomena that take place in the capillary system are considered to be primarily determined by the characteristics of the vascular endothelium (rather than the surrounding medium). This cellular lining is relatively continuous, covers the entire intravascular compartment, and is presumed to have similar functional characteristics throughout the cardio-vascular system. The cell membranes are permeable to lipid-soluble materials, which traverse these cells by diffusion. Lipid-insoluble materials such as water, ions, and sugars pass through the barrier either by a different route or by a different mechanism.

Pappenheimer, Renkin, and Borrero (1951), Renkin (1954), Durbin, Frank, and Solomon (1966), and Solomon (1968) established the so-called pore theory, according to which pressure and concentration gradients cause hydrophilic materials to traverse the endothelial barrier through water-filled channels or pores. This concept provides the physical basis for the theory of molecular sieving, according to which the diffusion of molecules with dimensions comparable to the pore diameter is restricted, while molecules whose diameter is larger than the pore or slit are excluded.

The "pore" theory implies that the capillary wall has the operational properties of an ultrafiltration membrane. The validation of this concept has been attempted by several methods, and in particular, electron microscopists have sought for evidence of these structures given that macroscopic experiments suggest pore diameters of the order of 80–100 Å. To the present, capillary–tissue passages of this nature have not been clearly demonstrated, although given their size and hypothesized numbers, they should be visible. Chambers and Zweifach (1947) proposed that the pores be identified with the slits that exist between contiguous borders of cells, and suggested that the intercellular material provides the selective characteristics of a semipermeable membrane.

The relationship between pores and slits was validated by the electron microscopy work of Karnovsky (1967, 1970). In these experiments and similar experiments, a water-soluble tracer such as cytochrome C (M.W. 12,000) or horseradish peroxidase (M.W. 40,000) is injected intravenously; tissue samples are then stained with an electron-opaque substance that has an affinity for the tracer. Tissues studied by this method have shown tracers to be present in high concentration in the capillary lumen, in the interendothelial clefts, and also in vesicles in the endothelial cells.

Electron microscopy also revealed the presence of small membrane-lined vesicles containing water-soluble tracers inside of the endothelial cells. On this basis Bruns and Palade (1968a,b,) developed the concept of vesicular transport or cytopempsis. According to this theory, the vesicles begin as invaginations on the cell membrane, develop a neck, and become separated; once within the cytoplasm they move at random and they empty their contents when they again meet the cell boundary by a reversal of this procedure. The vesicular theory of transport, however, does not provide an explanation for molecular sieving, which has been characterized in detail by the work of Grotte (1956), Mayerson et al. (1960), and by Arturson, Groth, and Grotte (1972). On the basis of the way in which dextran fractions of different molecular sizes extravasate, these investigators were led to the conclusion that there must exist a distribution of pore sizes that extends to 700 Å in diameter. The "large-pore system" appears to be only in the proportion of 1/34,000 to the "small-pore system," is presumed to be located in the venous portion of the capillary system, and should account for the higher protein permeability of the venular segment of the microcirculation.

The arteriovenous gradient of permeability to water-soluble molecules, as well as the so-called gradient in hydrodynamic conductivity in the microcirculation, has been attributed primarily to differences in the physical properties of the endothelial barrier. Many venules do show an attenuated endothelium, which has been termed "fenestrae." These presumably constitute passages that allow the exchange of protein and high-molecular-weight dextrans.

On the basis of the preceding discussion, it is possible to summarize the available morphologic and functional data into an operational description of properties and mechanism of action of the capillary barrier. Inasmuch as hydrostatic and colloid osmotic pressures determine fluid motion through the barrier, hydrodynamic flow must be one of the mechanisms of transport of fluid according to the theory of irreversible thermodynamics of Kedem and

Katchalsky (1958). The site of this flow is through intercellular slits that in all probability constitute the so-called small pores. Vesicles and fenestrae, or endothelial windows, would appear to represent the large-pore system, and through this channel pass the proteins found in tissue and lymph.

THE HYDRODYNAMIC CONDUCTIVITY
OF SINGLE VESSELS AND RATE OF EXCHANGE

The measurement of capillary permeability to fluid, and more specifically, the rate at which fluid passes through the capillary wall under the influence of pressure and osmotic gradients, was pioneered by Landis (1927) through the development of the so-called microocclusion technique. (This methodology is discussed in Volume III.) In order to determine the capillary permeability to fluid, it is necessary to obtain, in addition to the data on the rate of exchange, the measurement of the hydraulic and colloid osmotic pressures that cause the observed exchange. Landis measured the pressure directly in the frog mesentery, by inserting a microcannula filled with a dye, and noting the pressure that had to be applied to the fluid in the micropipette in order to maintain the interface between capillary blood plasma and the dye at a constant position within the micropipette tip. In this study the plasma colloid osmotic pressure was assumed to be the hydrostatic pressure measured when fluid moved neither inward or outward. Combining these different factors yields the value of 0.006 μ/sec cm H_2O for the fluid permeability of frog mesenteric capillaries.

A different approach was utilized by Zweifach and Intaglietta (1968) based on the formulation of Starling's hypothesis [Eq. (1)]. In effect, if fluid exchange from a capillary is measured first under control conditions, and then again after the blood plasma colloid osmotic pressure has been changed, both the effective capillary pressure and capillary permeability can be determined simultaneously, if it is assumed that tissue effects are negligible. The value found for capillary permeability in the microcirculation of the rabbit omentum was 0.01 μ/sec cm H_2O. These studies validated the concept that the capillary barrier has the functional properties of an osmometer, however, they cast some doubt on the hypothesis that on a steady-state basis, exchange induced by interaction of hydrostatic and colloid osmotic forces is a balanced process by which arterial filtration is balanced by venous absorption. In fact, in the mesentery of frogs, cats, rats, and rabbits, Intaglietta and Zweifach (1966) found that more than 85% of the capillaries tested showed outward motion of fluid or filtration. In 15% of the capillaries studied by the microocclusion technique, red blood cells either remained stationary after occlusion or, in a few instances, their motion could actually be interpreted as due to absorption. This finding was true, irrespective of the anesthetic utilized. Similar results were reported by Brown and Landis (1947) in their study of the effect of local cooling on the capillary permeability in the frog mesentery. In the latter study, it was indicated that absorption could be observed as frequently as filtration only when the mesentery was cooled to −2 to +2°C temperature range. Svanes, Zweifach, and Intaglietta (1970), however, did not find a significant change in mammals when temperatures were reduced from 37°C to 20°C.

A possible explanation for this finding is that the visceral circulation, and thus the microcirculation of the mesentery and omentum, are atypical in that the venous outflow of these organs must traverse the liver, and therefore the corresponding venous outflow pressure is substantially higher than that of other microvascular networks, owing to the additional hydraulic resistance caused by the hepatic circulation. These considerations led Smaje, Zweifach, and Intaglietta (1970) to study the exchange process in single capillaries in rat cremaster muscle. It is important to realize that filtration was also found to be predominant through the capillary network of this tissue. Absorption was found to occur in small venules of the order of 12 μ diameter. It was not possible to determine whether the absorptive process continued in the larger venules because their large diameter precludes observation of the trajectory of single red blood cells.

In small experimental animals, such as the rat, Smaje et al. (1970) found that it was not practical to shift blood plasma colloid osmotic pressure and to measure this shift by means of systemic blood samples, since the process of sampling altered central blood pressure. This problem was circumvented by inducing changes of filtration rate in occluded capillaries by changing the colloid osmotic pressure of the bathing solution. The validity of this technique was corroborated by utilizing it to measure the filtration coefficient of capillaries in rabbit omentum. When applied to the capillaries in muscle, the method of osmotic transients in the bathing solution showed that the hydrodynamic filtration coefficient was of the order of 0.001 μ/sec cm H_2O, which is 10 times lower than the corresponding value for omentum and mesentery.

The magnitude and direction of fluid exchange becomes evident when the permeability of the capillary barrier to fluid is related to the local intravascular hydraulic and osmotic effects.

Comprehensive surveys of the distribution of microvascular pressure have recently become available through the development of the resistance servo nulling technique of Wiederhielm et al. (1964). Measurements have been reported for the omentum and mesentery of rabbits, cats, and dogs, and the rat cremaster muscle. A summary of these results is presented in Table 1, where it is also tabulated the corresponding colloid osmotic pressure, measured with the osmometer of Prather, Gaar, and Guyton (1968) which incorporates a membrane with a reflection coefficient of 1 for albumin.

It is significant to note that in these experiments, the hydraulic pressure was found to be consistently higher than the colloid osmotic pressure, with the

Table 1. Capillary parameters

	Mesentery frog	Omentum rabbit	Cremaster muscle rat
Diameter, μ	20.6	10.4	4.1
Length, μ	700	570	615
Hydraulic pressure, cm H_2O	5–25	25–38	22–38
Colloid osmotic pressure, cm H_2O	11.5	22.0	21.0
Filtration coefficient, μ/sec cm H_2O	0.006	0.005–0.025	0.001
Exchange/perfusion parameter, $R_{E/P}$	0.6×10^{-3}	3.6×10^{-3}	4×10^{-3}

exception of the venular capillaries in muscle. On the basis of this evidence, it is apparent that the Starling concept of fluid balance is not fulfilled in the conditions tested.

THE CAPILLARY BARRIER VERSUS TISSUE BARRIER

The fact that experimental data from single vessels do not support as a whole the concept of a balance between filtration and absorption in the exchange process requires careful scrutiny of the validity of the correspondence between the hydrodynamic conductivity of the capillary barrier measured by macroscopic experiments (which support the concept of balance) and that measured by microscopic techniques (which provide negative evidence).

A basic difference between the two approaches is that the experiments that provide data on the rate of exchange of fluid between blood and tissue in situ and in vivo only reveal the net effects that take place in terms of shifts in the volume of fluid contained in the capillary under study, but do not provide information on the actual pathway for this exchange process, or the source of the hydrodynamic resistance to exchange. In particular, it is not possible to decide on the basis of this type of experiment whether the measured permeability constant K is an intrinsic property of the endothelial barrier, or a property that derives from the structure of the connective tissue surrounding the capillaries.

A comparison between the two sources of resistance is made possible by analyzing the permeability properties of a capillary in terms of tube model, where all measured properties are a function of the wall, and in terms of a tunnel model, where the hydraulic exchange characteristics are determined by the properties of the medium in which the capillaries are imbedded.

The hydraulic permeability of connective tissue is defined as the ratio between the volumetric flow in a volume of tissue and the pressure gradient necessary to cause this flow. Data on the hydraulic permeability of tissue were obtained by Guyton, Scheel, and Murphree (1966), from measurements on the rate of fluid transfer between two capsules implanted in the subcutaneous tissue of the dog. The value reported was 18×10^{-10} ml cm/sec dyne. A lower value of the order of 0.45×10^{-10} ml cm/sec dyne can be deduced from the data reported by Winters and Kruger (1968). Recent measurements in our laboratories on the hydraulic conductivity of mesenteric membranes of known thickness (ranging from 30 to 150 μ) gave a value of the order of 2×10^{-10} ml cm/sec dyne.

A comparison between the two capillary models can be made by calculating the equivalent diameter of cylinder of connective tissue necessary to account for the measured values of capillary permeability. Assuming that tissue flux is described by Darcy's law, then the rate of fluid exchange observed in the intraluminal compartment is directly related to the flux through the tissue governed by the hydraulic permeability of connective tissue K_c and the pressure gradient in tissue ∇P_n, namely,

$$\overset{\circ}{m} = -K_c \nabla P_n. \tag{2}$$

The solution of Eq. (2) in terms of an axially symmetric tunnel where, at any given position, pressure in the surrounding medium changes radially, decaying from the net intraluminal value to that characteristic of the interstitial compartment is

$$\overset{\circ}{m} = \frac{K_c \Delta P_e}{\ln D_c/D_0} \tag{3}$$

where D_c is the capillary diameter, D_0 is the equivalent diameter of an equivalent tube of connective tissue, and ΔP_e is the net pressure difference across the tube wall.

Equating (1) and (3), and assuming that $\Delta P_e \cong (P_c - \pi_{p\ell} - P_t + \pi_t)$ we obtain

$$D_0 = D_c e^{\frac{2K_c}{KD_c}} \tag{4}$$

Substituting in Eq. (4) the values $K_c = 2 \times 10^{-10}$ ml cm/sec dyne, $K = 10^{-9}$ ml/sec dyne (Zweifach and Intaglietta, 1968), and $D_c = 8 \times 10^{-4}$ cm, we obtain the value of 500 for the exponent; consequently the equivalent radius of connective tissue is practically infinite, and therefore in mesentery and omentum, the rate of exchange is determined exclusively by the properties of the endothelial barrier.

These results validate the microocclusion method of Landis (1927) and Zweifach and Intaglietta (1968) for the determination of the coefficient of capillary permeability, and furthermore show that in two-dimensional tissues such as mesentery, omentum, and cremaster muscle, the capillaries can be considered as if they were imbedded in an infinite medium, where the exchange flows from different microvessels do not interact with each other. This result also shows that in these tissues the gradient of permeability, determined by the method of occluding arterial and venous portions of the same capillary in succession, provides the measurement of a property of the endothelial wall, rather than that of the conditions of the surrounding tissue.

The extension of these results to three-dimensional arrays of capillaries was studied by Intaglietta and de Plomb (1973). In this study it is shown that in very regular three-dimensional arrays of parallel, concurrent flow capillaries, in the absence of lymphatic drainage, where the hydraulic conductivity of the capillary wall and tissue are uniform and have the numerical values found experimentally, there exist hydrodynamic interactions between the exchange flows. As a consequence, the exchange properties of a three-dimensional organ (whose capillaries have the structural characteristics measured in two-dimensional structures) do not bear a one-to-one relationship to the exchange properties found in single vessels. In such a system exchange is influenced, among other factors, by intercapillary spacing, and the permeability of the extravascular compartment. The extent to which these findings affect the interpretation of data from two-dimensional structures has not yet been investigated.

A basic result, however, can be deduced even in the absence of the necessary three-dimensional data, namely, that absorption from the intravascular compartment into the intravascular venular system can occur only if there is no other route of exit for the fluid (which extravasates from the arterial exits in microcirculation), and furthermore it requires a venular capillary barrier with identical retention properties to the arterial counterpart. Given the evidence for the arterio-venous permeability gradient, and the existence of the terminal lymphatic network that presumably constitutes a low pressure system designed to absorb fluid, it is probable that even in three-dimensional organs constructed with capillaries with two-dimensional organ characteristics, the phenomenon of absorption does not obtain in the sense envisioned by Starling.

TISSUE BLOOD FLOW AND EXCHANGE FLOW

The fact that absorption is not readily demonstrable in experimental measurements in single capillaries requires the revision of some of the premises of the theories on homeostatic fluid balance, as well as the analysis of the extent to which this concept might violate existing quantitative knowledge on in situ and in vivo fluid exchange.

Our discussion, to this point, has focused on the fact that microscopic and macroscopic experiments validate the concept that the microcirculation has the operational properties of an osmometer, whose membrane has variable retention properties, but that there exists a fundamental discrepancy in terms of the balance between filtration and absorption.

The nature of this imbalance can be quantitatively analyzed by establishing the relative magnitude of tissue blood flow, and the corresponding exchange flow. As a first-order approximation, blood flow Q_B in any given microvascular segment can be assumed to follow Poiseuille's law, expressed by

$$Q_B = \frac{\pi D_c^4 \Delta P}{128 \mu L} \tag{5}$$

where L is the microvessel length, ΔP the pressure drop, and μ the viscosity of blood. Given the comparatively low hematocrit that is seen in in vivo observations of the peripheral vascular tree, in all probability the viscosity of blood in capillaries can be taken as that of blood at the corresponding hematocrit, without incurring large errors (i.e., errors of one order of magnitude). For simplicity, it also assumed that the viscosity is Newtonian.

The exchange flow from any given segment of the microvasculature can be calculated by rewriting Eq (1) as follows:

$$Q_E = \pi D_c L K \Delta P_e \tag{6}$$

where ΔP_e is the average net driving pressure for exchange, in the same terms utilized in Eq (3). Defining L as the length of a microvessel where only filtration occurs [in the paper of Intaglietta and de Plomb (1973) it is defined as the length over which both filtration and absorption occur], we can assume that in the absence of tissue effects, i.e., atmospheric tissue pressure and zero tissue colloid osmotic pressure, the relationship between ΔP and ΔP_c can be assumed to be

$$\Delta P = 2\Delta P_e \tag{7}$$

and, combining Eq. (5), (6), and (7), we obtain the perfusion exchange parameter:

$$R_{E/P} = 64 \frac{K \mu L_c^2}{D_c^3} . \tag{8}$$

This dimensionless parameter that relates in a simplified way to the factors that determine blood flow and exchange is a direct measure of the exchange flow relative to blood flow, and provides a measure of the dilution of plasma protein as a consequence of the exchange process. Furthermore, since this parameter is independent of pressure gradients, it provides an estimate of the rate of formation of lymph solely on the basis of the blood flow through a given structure. As an example, in the gastric circulation, it is a well-established fact that during digestion both blood flow and lymph increase, thus suggesting that, for this microcirculatory bed, the increased pressure drop across the exchange vessel (presumably caused by arteriolar vasodilation) causes an increased filtration. A similar situation is obtained in exercising skeletal muscle.

Table 1 summarizes pertinent microvascular data, including the $R_{E/P}$ parameter. As can be seen, when this parameter is calculated on the assumption of a microvasculature in which there is no absorption, it is of the order of 4×10^{-3}. This value is 4 times higher than that previously estimated by Intaglietta and dePlomb (1973), for a Starling-type balance capillary system, since in these conditions the average net driving pressure for exchange, as well as the length of the vessels over which the process takes place, are halved. In view of the finding by Intaglietta and Zweifach (1966) and Smaje et al. (1970) that absorption is not entirely non existent, but is present in approximately 15% of the tested capillaries, the perfusion exchange parameter should be corrected by this factor. A parameter R_{EP}^{*} can be defined to describe a microcirculatory bed in which a fraction α of the vessels absorb as follows:

$$R_{E/P}^{*} = (1 - \alpha)^2 \, R_{E/P}, \tag{9}$$

which gives a value of R_{EP}^{*} of the order of 3×10^{-3}. This value can be related to the systemic values of cardiac output and lymph flow. Thus, on the basis of a 5-liters/min cardiac output for man, we can deduce that lymph flow should be of the order of 15 ml/min, which is of the order of 3 blood volumes per day, and thus within the commonly accepted values for lymph flow.

STARLING'S HYPOTHESIS
OF FLUID BALANCE AND THE MICROSCOPIC EVIDENCE

The findings of Brown and Landis (1947), Intaglietta and Zweifach (1966), Zweifach and Intaglietta (1968), Svanes et al. (1970), and Smaje et al. (1970) suggest that the quantitative microscopic evidence for a balance between filtration and absorption cannot be as readily demonstrated as in the macroscopic experiments. In effect, the question arises whether the isogravimetric method does not, in fact, prove Starling's hypothesis of fluid balance, because it implicitly assumes that most organs and itssues are at the isogravimetric state, and thus the experimental conditions are adjusted in such a fashion that this state obtains, in the absence of lymph flow and in the presence of somewhat arbitrary and artificial venous pressures, which *determine* that the preparations are isogravimetric.

A number of critiques of the validity of the concept of a dynamic balance between filtration and absorption were recently put forward in a review by Intaglietta and Zweifach (1973). In this work it was pointed out that isolated preparations behave as osmometers in which there is a dynamic balance between filtration and absorption only when a substantial amount of fluid has filtered into the interstitium, and the venous outflow pressure has been set to a level presumed to correspond to the in vivo and in situ level.

The basic microscopic evidence that can be related to the mechanism of fluid balance is twofold: (1) the fact that the so-called microocclusion technique of

Landis shows that, in most capillaries, fluid is lost to the interstitium, and (2) that direct measurement of hydrostatic and colloid osmotic pressures show that the difference is primarily positive, in the sense that it causes filtration. The comparatively small value of the $R_{E/P}$ parameter furthermore indicates that there is no augmentation of the colloid osmotic effect in capillaries as a consequence of the exchange process. Therefore, it is licit to presume that in the intravital, in situ, microscopic experimental conditions, filtration is the predominant mode of exchange in mesentery, omentum, and the cremaster muscle.

The point must be raised that our findings could also be a consequence of the experimental conditions, such as exposure, surgery, and anesthesia. This matter was explored in terms of different anesthetic agents, as well as tests with vasodilators and vasoconstrictors, and in our estimation these preparations behave in a fashion as if similar to that which is presumed to obtain in situ.

A further point should be raised in terms of the forces that cause exchange. In the present treatment, we have assumed that extravascular factors of colloid and hydrostatic pressure are negligible. Considering the evidence for negative interstitial hydraulic pressure (Guyton, 1963; Scholander, Hargens, and Miller, 1968), and the possibility of comparatively high tissue colloid osmotic pressure due to the synergistic interaction of protein and interstitial hyaluronic acid suggested by Wiederhielm (1968), it is apparent that if these forces were to be included, the filtration mode would be even more pronounced. Furthermore, it must be also considered that the reabsorptive process is presumed to be due to osmotic effects that require a semipermeable membrane; however, it is precisely at the venous end of the microcirculation where the endothelium appears to lose its protein retention ability, thus causing further difficulties with the concept of absorptive balance.

The present discussion is based on microvascular data that suggest that if all of the exchange process were primarily filtrative, the net fluid efflux from the microcirculation would be of the order of 0.1% of the local blood flow. Given that this figure is of the order of lymph flow, it would seem that there is little or no excess fluid that would move from tissue to capillary. In the work of Landis and Pappenheimer (1963), where the hydraulic conductivity of the capillary barrier was deduced from CFC measurements, it was found that the maintenance of fluid balance in tissue required a comparatively large paracapillary flow, i.e., that flow which exits the arterial microcirculatory end reenters the venular segment as a consequence of the reabsorptive process. This paracapillary flow was envisioned to be of the order of 10 times the corresponding lymph flow, in such a fashion that if intracapillary flow is taken as unity (100%) then paracapillary flow is 1% and transcapillary flow or lymph flow is of the order of 0.1% of capillary flow.

Microvascular studies, on the other hand, indicate that the total filtration capacity of the microcirculation is of the order of 0.1% of the corresponding capillary flow. Since lymph flow is of the same order, then paracapillary flow must be only a fraction of 0.1% Furthermore, the study of pressure and permeability in the venular microcirculation suggests that the conditions for reabsorption, i.e., that the net effective capillary pressure be lower than the corresponding local plasma colloid osmotic pressure, might not be present.

Given the difficulty of demonstrating the balance of exchange at the microscopic level by means of reabsorption at the venous end of the microcirculation, and the fact that normal healthy tissue is not edematous, it is clear that a mechanism must exist for removing this excess of fluid from tissue, and this must be the lymphatic drainage. The validity of this concept is somewhat supported by the fact that on a systemic basis, if the whole microcirculation (with the exception of specialized organs such as the kidney) is geared to filter, lymph flow would be of the correct order of magnitude.

It is appropriate at this point to consider whether there are some special functions that can be served by a primarily filtering microcirculation. From the viewpoint of blood volume control, it would indicate that this is maintained through mechanisms that also include the lymphatic return. From the viewpoint of tissue homeostasis and tissue nutrition, considering that the amount of so-called "free water" (i.e., fluid which in tissue moves under the influence of pressure gradients) is estimated to be of the order of 0.1 liter in man, a tissue flux and thus lymph flow of the order of 15 ml/min indicates that the whole "free fluid" reservoir of the tissue can be exchanged in less than 10 min, thus providing an effective and active transport system for tissue materials that otherwise would move too slowly if diffusion were their only transport process.

In conclusion, the microscopic evidence for the balance of fluid exchange strongly suggests that this balance obtains, as a consequence of the lymphatic return, without a major involvement of an absorptive exchange in the venous microvasculature. A complete formulation of the exchange processes must, therefore, include the interstitium as well as the lymphatic return. In this manner, the microcirculation can be rigorously considered as an open system in which all inputs and outputs are accounted for. Furthermore, when the lymphatic circulation is included in the formulation of exchange, it becomes a relatively simpler problem to paragon this system with an osmometer, since both experimentally and theoretically, it becomes possible to specify exchange parameters, flows, and forces in fluid compartments, i.e., blood and lymph, without actual knowledge of the conditions in the tissue, where experiments cannot be carried out. A similar approach has been taken in the study of osmotic effects, where all measurements are made in compartments separated by membranes, but not within the membrane, where experiments are not possible.

Further developments in this field are, therefore, dependent on the quantitative characterization of exchange phenomena in the terminal lymphatics, and their relation to microvascular hemodynamics.

LITERATURE CITED

Arturson, G., F. Groth, and G. Grotte. 1972. The functional ultrastructure of the blood–lymph barrier. Computer analysis of data from dog heart–lymph experiments using theoretical models. Acta Physiol. Scand. Suppl. 374:1–30.

Brown, E., and E. M. Landis. 1947. Effect of local cooling on fluid movement, effective colloid osmotic pressure and capillary permeability in the frog mesentery. Am. J. Physiol. 149:302–315.

Bruns, R. R., and G. E. Palade. 1968a. Studies on blood capillaries. I. General organization of blood capillaries in muscle. J. Cell Biol. 37:244–276.

Bruns, R. R., and G. E. Palade. 1968b. Studies on blood capillaries. II. Transport of ferritin molecules across the wall of muscle capillaries. J. Cell Biol. 37: 277–99.

Chambers, R., and B. W. Zweifach. 1947. Intercellular cement and capillary permeability. Physiol. Rev. 27:436–463.

Durbin, R. P., H. Frank, and A. K. Solomon. 1956. Water flow through frog gastic mucosa. J. Gen. Physiol. 39:535–551.

Folkow, B. 1961. The comparative effects of angiotensin and Noradrenaline on consecutive vascular sections. Acta Physiol. Scand. 53:99–105.

Grotte, G. 1956. Passage of dextran molecules across the blood–lymph barrier. Acta Chir. Scand. 211:1–83.

Guyton, A. C. 1963. A concept of negative tissue interstitial pressure based on pressures in implanted perforated capsules. Circ. Res. 12:399–414.

Guyton, A. C., K. Scheel, and D. Murphree. 1966. Interstitial fluid pressure. III. Its effect on resistance to tissue fluid mobility. Circ. Res. 19:412–419.

Intaglietta, M., and B. W. Zweifach. 1966. Indirect method for the measurement of pressure in blood capillaries. Circ. Res. 19:199–208.

Intaglietta, M., and E. P. dePlomb. 1973. Fluid exchange in tunnel and tube capillaries. Microvasc. Res. 6:153–168.

Intaglietta, M., and B. W. Zweifach. 1973. Microcirculatory basis of fluid exchange. Advan. Biol. Med. Phys. 15:111–159.

Karnovsky, M. J. 1967. Ultrastructural basis of capillary permeability studied with peroxidase as a tracer. J. Cell. Biol. 35:213–236.

Karnovsky, M. J. 1970. Morphology of capillaries with special regard to muscle capillaries. In Alfred Benzon Symposium II on Capillary Permeability pp. 341–350. Munksgaard International, Copenhagen.

Kedem, O., and A. Katchalsky. 1958. Thermodynamic analysis of the permeability of biological membranes to non-electrolytes. Biochem. Biophys. Acta 27:229–246.

Landis, E. M. 1927. Micro-injection studies of capillary permeability. II. The relation between capillary pressure and the rate at which fluid passes through the walls of single capillaries. Am. J. Physiol. 82:217–238

Landis, E. M., and J. R. Pappenheimer. 1963. Exchange of substances through the capillary walls. In W. F. Hamilton and P. Dow (eds.), Handbook of Physiology, Section II, Circulation, Vol. 2, pp. 961–1034. American Physiological Society, Washington, D. C.

Mayerson, H. S., C. G. Wolfram, H. H. Shirley, and K. Wasserman. 1960. Regional differences in capillary permeability. Am. J. Physiol. 198:155–164.

Pappenheimer, J. R. 1953. Passage of molecules through capillary walls. Physiol. Rev. 33:387–423.

Pappenheimer, J. R., and A. Soto-Rivera. 1948. Effective osmotic pressure of the plasma proteins and other quantities associated with the capillary circulation in the hind limbs of cats and dogs. Am. J. Physiol. 152:471−491.

Pappenheimer, J. R., E. M. Renkin, and L. M. Borrero. 1951. Filtration, diffusion and molecular sieving through peripheral capillary membranes. Am. J. Physiol. 167:13−46.

Prather, J. W., K. A. Gaar, Jr., and A. C. Guyton. 1968. Direct continuous recording of plasma colloid osmotic pressure of whole blood. J. Appl. Physiol. 24:602−605.

Renkin, E. M. 1954. Filtration, diffusion and molecular sieving through porous cellulose membranes. J. Gen. Physiol. 38:225−243.

Scholander, P. F., A. R. Hargens, and S. L. Miller. 1968. Negative pressure in the interstitial fluid of animals. Science 161:321−328.

Smaje, L., B. W. Zweifach, and M. Intaglietta. 1970. Micropressure and capillary filtration coefficients in single vessels of the cremaster muscle of the rat. Microvasc. Res. 3:96−110.

Solomon, A. K. 1968. Characterization of biological membranes by equivalent pores. J. Gen. Physiol. 51:335S−364S.

Starling, E. H. 1896. On the absorption of fluids from the connective tissue spaces. J. Physiol. (London) 19:312−326.

Svanes, K., B. W. Zweifach, and M. Intaglietta. 1970. Effect of hypothermia on transcapillary fluid exchange. Am. J. Physiol. 29:740−741.

Wiederhielm, C. A. 1968. Dynamics of transcapillary fluid exchange J. Gen. Physiol. 52:Supplement 29S−61S.

Wiederhielm, C. A., J. W. Woodbury, S. Kirk, and R. F. Rushmer. 1964. Pulsatile pressure in the microcirculation of the frog's mesentery. Am. J. Phyiol. 207:173−176.

Winters, A. D., and S. Kruger. 1968. Drug effects on bulk flow through mesenteric membranes. Arch. Int. Pharmacodyn. 173:213−225.

Zweifach, B. W., and M. Intaglietta. 1968 Mechanics of fluid movement across single capillaries in the rabbit. Microvasc. Res. 1:83−101.

chapter 10

PASSAGE OF SUBSTANCES ACROSS THE WALLS OF BLOOD VESSELS: Kinetics and Mechanism

Emil Aschheim

The immediate environment of parenchymal cells of a complex multicellular organism is linked functionally to the various regulatory organs by means of the circulating blood. The relative constancy of this environment in the face of continuing metabolic activity of parenchymal cells and the varying functional load imposed by both internal and external demands imply modulation of transendothelial passage of various metabolites. This exchange can thus be broadly regarded as nutritive, even though it encompasses the passage of inorganic substances, such as univalent ions; it is a process that appears redundant in steady-state situations.

The permeability of blood vessels thus assumes a major significance, even though from the point of view of tissue nutrition it represents a relatively invariant attribute of the terminal vascular bed, changing somewhat under conditions of extreme vasodilation (Krogh, 1929) and increasing substantially only in inflammation (Lewis, 1916; Ramsdell, 1928). The dominant role of adequate tissue perfusion is also illustrated by macromolecules, which pass out of the blood vessels at rates proportional to blood flow at various stages of inflammation (Aschheim, 1964a, 1964b, 1965a, 1965b).

The considerable amount of work that went into the characterization of vascular permeability has resulted in a number of excellent reviews and discussions (Landis, 1934; Chambers and Zweifach, 1947; Pappenheimer, 1953; Wilhelm 1962; Landis and Pappenheimer, 1963; Rusznyák, Földi, and Szabó, 1967; Mellander and Johansson, 1968). A recent symposium surveys the major experimental approaches to the problem of vascular permeability (Crone and Lassen, 1970).

PERMEABILITY OF MEMBRANES

An attempt was made to keep the number of different formulations in this section to a minimum. The equations, often in simplified form, are largely limited to those that are frequently encountered in work on vascular permeability and are occasionally repeated to save the bothersome flipping of pages. For ease of back reference the symbols used by the various authors are retained. The prominence accorded diffusion reflects the majority opinion of the importance of this process to transendothelial transport.

Diffusional Limitation of Membrane Transport

Consider the system (Figure 1) where a dissolved substance tends to diffuse across the membrane M from compartment A to B under the influence of a concentration gradient. The magnitude of transport of the substance per unit time across the membrane will be smaller than what would obtain under identical conditions in the absence of the membrane. Except for an initial transient peak, this is true even in the optimal case when the substance diffuses faster in the body of the membrane than in compartments A and B.

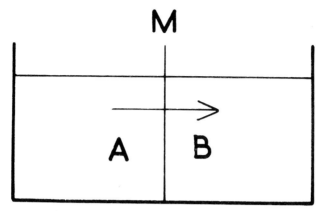

Figure 1. Rate of transport across membrane M is limited by the rate at which solute is brought by diffusion to one surface of the membrane and the rate at which it is removed from the other surface. If transport across the membrane were to exceed the diffusion rates in A and B, the activity gradient of the solute in the membrane would be reversed and oppose the macroscopic gradient.

This limitation occurs because the rate of transport across the membrane ultimately depends on the rate at which the substance diffuses from A toward one surface of the membrane and the rate at which it subsequently diffuses away from the other surface into the solution in B. This limitation applies to facilitated diffusion where transport across the "active patches" of the membrane may exceed by several orders of magnitude the rate of diffusion in the bulk solution (Wilbrandt and Rosenberg, 1961), and is probably responsible for the fact that no active "downhill" transport in a living system has so far been described.

Some Older and Newer Formulations

Traditionally, considerations of permeability begin with the first Fick equation for unidimensional diffusion,

$$\frac{dm}{dt} = -DA\frac{dc}{dx} \qquad (1)$$

where dm/dt represents the amount of mass transported per unit time. D is the diffusion coefficient, A is the area across which transport occurs, and dc/dx is the concentration gradient. This equation was developed by analogy from the then existing heat equation on the view that there ought to obtain a basic similarity between the flow of heat along a temperature gradient and flow of a substance along its concentration gradient. Dimensionally $(D) = L^2/T$ or in the cgs system, cm^2/sec. Didactically, it may be more palatable to multiply both the numerator and denominator by L to obtain L^3/LT since the unit of diffusion assumes then the meaning of a unit volume transported a unit distance in a unit time. In a more modern notation, Fick's first equation is sometimes given as $J = -D$ grad μ where the flux $J = dm/A\,dt$ and grad μ represents the gradient of activity of the substance. Since in biologic work the thickness of the membrane across which diffusion occurs was at best guessed, a modified Fick equation came into use. In the modified form

$$\frac{dm}{dt} = -PA\,(c_1 - c_2);\qquad(2)$$

the unknown thickness of the membrane has been absorbed into the permeability coefficient (i.e., $P = D/\Delta x$.) This equation has made possible the accumulation of a large number of comparative data on the permeability of cell membranes and is prominent in work on vascular permeability because of the belief that diffusion plays a major role in transendothelial exchange.

An equation analogous to Eq. (2) is

$$\frac{dV}{dt} = k'_w A(\Pi_0 - \Pi_i)\qquad(3)$$

where dV/dt refers to volume flow per unit time across an area A under the influence of the osmotic pressure difference $\Pi_0 - \Pi_i$, and where k'_w represents the permeability coefficient to water. The osmotic pressure is given by

$$\Pi = RTiC\qquad(4)$$

where R is the universal gas constant, T is the absolute temperature, C is the concentration of the solute, and i is the isotonic coefficient defined by

$$i = 1 + (n - 1)\alpha\qquad(5)$$

where n denotes the number of particles into which a solute molecule dissociates into and α represents the percent of molecules that dissociate. Combining Eqs. (3) and (4) yields

$$\frac{dV}{dt} = k_w\,A(C_0 - C_i)\qquad(6)$$

where RT and i are absorbed in k'_w to give k_w.

Equation (3) as well as the derived Eq. (6) are not quite correct in spite of their widespread use and the tremendous amount of data on the osmotic permeability of cell membranes obtained with their aid. The intuitive formulation of a linear relationship between the difference of osmotic pressures and rate of flow of water is demonstrably fallacious. For instance, when pure water diffuses across a perfectly semipermeable membrane into pure glycerol, the rate of flow according to Eq. (3) ought to be infinitely large (Ray, 1960).

Use of Eqs. (2) and (6) has led in the past to a number of conceptual difficulties. For instance, heavy water was found to permeate into various animal eggs in accordance with Eq. (2) like any ordinary solute. However, in the process it did not affect the volume of the eggs, contrary to Eq. (6), which holds reasonably well in the case of other solutes whenever they are added to the bathing solution in an equally high concentration (Prescott and Zeuthen, 1952). The reason for this anomalous behavior is that high permeability of these membranes to heavy water, a factor that does not enter into these formulations.

The turning point in modern discussions of the permeability of biologic membranes seems to coincide with the publications of O. Kedem and A. Katchalsky (Kedem and Katchalsky, 1958, 1961; Katchalsky and Kedem, 1962), who forcefully drew the attention of biologists to the ideas of Onsager (1931) first published some 30 years previously. In contrast to classical thermodynamics, the thermodynamics of irreversible processes does not deal with systems at equilibrium or close to it. Its conceptual and notational simplicity and clarity of exposition assured its rapid diffusion among biologists once the system succeeded in crossing interdisciplinary barriers (Denbigh, 1951; Spanner, 1964; Stein, 1967). The elegance and descriptive power of this approach are exemplified in Tosteson's discussion of the suggestion that transendothelial transport involves two paths, one through the intercellular clefts, and the other across the body of the endothelial cell (Tosteson, 1970).

The following describes only the rudiments of the system, mainly to illustrate how some baffling characteristics of membrane transport find a satisfactory resolution within its conceptual framework.

In general, it is reasoned, if one observes in a given system a flux across a membrane, one must assume that every force known to act in the system contributes to it. In line with this reasoning, a distinction is made between conjugate and nonconjugate forces. For example, a transmembrane chemical potential gradient of glucose is termed a conjugate force responsible for some part of the total flux of glucose. If in this system there exists also a transmembrane potential gradient of water, it is assumed a priori that it also contributes to the total flux of glucose. In relation to glucose transport, the chemical activity gradient of water is termed a nonconjugate force (it is a conjugate force in relation to the flux of water).

Next, the extent to which a given force contributes to a given flux is expressed by a phenomenologic coefficient, an entity that expresses the degree of coupling between the two.

Symbolically these relationships are given by

$$\begin{aligned}
J_1 &= L_{11}X_1 + L_{12}X_2 + \cdots L_{1n}X_n \\
J_2 &= L_{21}X_1 + L_{22}X_2 + \cdots L_{2n}X_n \\
J_n &= L_{n1}X_1 + L_{n2}X_2 + \cdots L_{nn}X_n
\end{aligned} \tag{7}$$

where J_1 is the total flux of substance 1, X_1 is its conjugate force. L_{11} is the coefficient that describes the extent to which X_1 contributes to J_1. In the second term of the first row X_2 is a nonconjugate force active in the system, and

L_{12} is the coupling coefficient that describes the extent to which X_2 contributes to J_1 and so on. When force X_i can be shown not to contribute to flux J_1, the coupling coefficient L_{1i} in the term $L_{1i}X_i$ is equated to zero. A major aspect of this development by Onsager is the demonstration that when forces and flows are expressed in appropriate units, the cross coefficients are identical, i.e., $L_{12} = L_{21}$. This identity is of such a fundamental nature that it has been hailed as a new law of nature. An example of how one goes about finding the appropriate units in which to express J and X is found in Spanner (1964).

Applied to transendothelial exchange, the formalism of Eq. (7) resolves the old controversy of whether a given substance crosses the endothelial membranes by virtue of its chemical or electrochemical potential gradient or whether it crosses by "bulk flow." The latter refers to the transport of a dissolved solute due to the flow of water. In terms of Eq. (7) both views are correct, since only one component of the total flux of a given substance is due to its conjugate force, i.e., its chemical or electrochemical potential gradient. The other contributions to the same total flux are due to the action of chemical or electrochemical potential gradients of other substances, and this includes water, the only other substance considered in this controversy.

Formally, this is expressed in Eq. (8), which is derived from Eq. (7) for the transport of a single solute and a solvent across the membrane:

$$J_v = L_p \Delta p + L_{pD} \Delta \Pi$$
$$J_D = L_{Dp} \Delta p + L_D \Delta \Pi \tag{8}$$

where J_v is volume flow, J_D is solute flow, Δ_p is the hydrostatic pressure difference acting across the membrane, and $\Delta \Pi$ is the osmotic pressure difference due to the unequal concentration of the solute on both sides of the membrane. When only osmotic forces are operative ($\Delta p = 0$), one obtains

$$J_v = L_{pD} \Delta \Pi \tag{9}$$
$$J_D = L_D \Delta \Pi$$

where L_D is the diffusional and L_{pD} the "solvent drag" coefficient of the membrane.

When only hydrostatic pressure acts across the membrane ($\Delta \Pi = 0$), the flows are given by

$$J_v = L_p \Delta p$$
$$J_D = L_{Dp} \Delta p \tag{10}$$

where L_p is the filtrational coefficient of the membrane and L_{Dp} is its "bulk flow" coefficient. The reflection or selectivity coefficient of the membrane is given by

$$\sigma = - \frac{L_{pD}}{L_p} \tag{11}$$

This coefficient describes the "leakiness" of a membrane to a given solute, a value of one denoting total impermeability (the membrane is ideally semipermeable), whereas a value of zero means that it does not restrict the passage of the solute relative to the solvent. The cross coefficients obey Onsager's law, i.e.,

$$L_{Dp} = L_{pD}. \tag{12}$$

An important feature of this derivation is the realization that an unambiguous characterization of the permeability of a membrane to a single solute and solvent requires the knowledge of three coefficients and not two as was implied in earlier derivations.

The formalism of thermodynamics of irreversible processes has also supplied a criterion by which active transport can be differentiated from passive transport—a hitherto baffling problem since no matter how many steps removed, an active "uphill" transport must be fed by energy provided by a "downhill" running process. According to this suggestion (Spanner, 1954), the only passive component of a given flux is that which is due to its conjugate force. All other components are, by definition, active. Although appealing, this distinction may meet with opposition when applied to transport across vascular membranes, which traditionally is viewed as passive. For instance, one would have to view that part of the total transendothelial transport of glucose that is due to the activity of hydraulic and osmotic pressure gradients established by other means as active.

Diffusional and Filtrational Fluxes of Water

An interesting aspect of the work of membrane permeability is that if one assumes with the majority of workers that osmosis is due to diffusion, one cannot readily account for the finding that osmotically induced flow of water may greatly exceed the diffusional flow, as measured with heavy water. This situation obtains in artificial (Mauro, 1957; Hays, 1970), epithelial (Hevesy, Hofer, and Krogh, 1935; Durbin, Frank, and Solomon, 1956; Hays and Leaf, 1962), and cell membranes (Prescott and Zeuthen, 1952), suggesting a basic common cause. The osmotically induced flow appears to be as large as the flow induced by an equivalent hydrostatic pressure gradient (Mauro, 1957; Durbin, 1960). At one extreme, this disparity has led to the conclusion that osmotic flow is not due to diffusion (Pappenheimer, 1953), and at the other to the denial of the presence of a hydraulic flow of water on the grounds that the presence of an osmotic gradient does not result in an observable correctly directed hydrostatic pressure gradient which alone could induce such a flow (Chinard, Vosburgh, and Enns, 1955).

According to a recent hypothesis, this phenomenon is due to the complex nature of the membranes, which may be composed of a dense layer that limits hydraulic flow and a parallel less dense layer that limits diffusional flow (Hays, 1970). This hypothesis is in accord with earlier views according to which pores in a membrane behave as if they were microscopic osmotic siphons.

In a system where a perfectly semipermeable membrane separates pure water from an osmotically active solution, the pores of the membrane must contain only water. Consequently, the effective chemical activity gradient of water between the water in the pores and the solution is established in a very short terminal segment of the pore, where it faces the solution. This segment is of molecular dimensions and is thus shorter than the length of the pore. The gradient is therefore steep and results in a correspondingly high rate of diffusion of water from the terminal segment of the pore into the solution (Ray, 1960; Ussing and Anderson, 1956).

Loss of water from this segment of the pore lowers the local hydrostatic pressure, and this leads to the establishment of a hydrostatic pressure gradient that extends along the entire length of the pore. The last link in the chain of causes and effects is a bulk inflow of water from the pore water compartment into the other end of the pore. This transfer of water is subject to factors that limit hydraulic flow along conduits, such as are incorporated in the Poiseuille formula. Reasonable as this suggestion seems, the concept of a chemical activity gradient of water in the terminal portion of a pore, the diameter of which is smaller than that of the solute molecules, may need clarification. Exclusion of solute molecules from the lumen of the pores may involve factors other than size, such as electrostatic repulsion.

In contrast to the high filtrational flow, purely diffusional transfer of water across the membrane is small. If in the system depicted above there is no osmotic gradient across the membrane, isotopic water added to one compartment will diffuse along the pores into the other compartment. However, the flux of the isotope will be proportional to its chemical activity gradient, which is less steep since it extends along the entire length of the pores.

Figure 2 presents a macroscopic model of an osmotic siphon. The tube connecting the two vessels corresponds to a single pore in the membrane. Its impermeability to solutes is assured by covering both ends with a semipermeable membrane. The tonicity of the solution contained in the tube is immaterial; for simplicity, the tube and one compartment may be considered filled with pure water.

The model exaggerates the differences in magnitude between osmotic and purely diffusional transfer of water because in the case of the latter the length of the tube very much reduces the concentration gradient of isotopic water added to one compartment.

The presence of discrete pores is not essential for this mechanism to operate; a sufficient requirement is a differential permeability of the membrane to solvent and solute. In the limiting case of an ideally semipermeable membrane, the solute is completely reflected at the surface of the membrane, whereas water is not. Provided the variables of the Poiseuille equation are kept constant, the higher the reflection coefficient of a membrane to a given solute, that is, the more it impedes its passage relative to water, the larger should be the difference between the diffusional and filtrational fluxes of water.

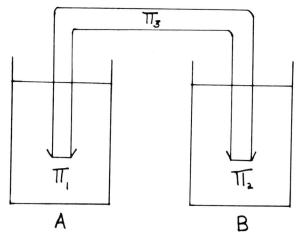

Figure 2. Osmotic siphon as a model of the interendothelial cleft. *A* is the intravascular and *B* the extravascular space and the tube is the interendothelial cleft. A perfectly semipermeable membrane covers the openings of the tube so as to exclude it from plasma proteins. If there is a difference in osmotic pressures between *A* and *B*, water will flow along the tube. If only *B* and the tube contain pure water, the activity gradients of the latter will extend across the interface where the solution contained in *A* is in contact with the contents of the tube; its steepness will result in a correspondingly large flow of water into *A*. The magnitude of Π_3 is immaterial as long as the volume of the siphon remains constant.

Vesicular Transport

Considerations of membrane transport in relation to vascular permeability would be deficient without discussion of pinocytotic vesicles first described by Palade (1960, 1961). These vesicles have a diameter of about 600 Å and occur in great numbers in the cytoplasm of a number of cell types, including vascular endothelium. Macromolecular substances like ferritin injected intravenously are found in such vesicles. Their participation in transport across the walls of blood vessels was considered unlikely because—in view of their size—large and small molecules would be expected to permeate with equal ease, which is not the case. However, the basement membrane may represent the major filtrational barrier that discriminates among molecules on the basis of size (Palade, 1961). (See Chapters 4 and 7 in this volume for further discussion.)

Pinocytotic vesicles move at random in the cytoplasm (Casley-Smith, 1963), their motion is Brownian, and their transit time across the cell is about 1 sec (Shea and Karnovsky, 1966; Shea, Karnovsky, and Bossert, 1969). If these structures also originate and terminate their existence at random at both surfaces of the cell, the net effect of vesicular transport will mimic diffusion, since it can only occur "downhill." The membrane in which this transport occurs could be kinetically characterized by an equivalent system of pores of an estimable radius, in spite of absence of phase continuity between the two compartments. On the other hand, recent work indicates that continuous transendothelial channels, the possible morphologic counterpart of the pores, may, in fact, exist (Simionescu,

Simionescu, and Palade, 1975). An important feature of this transport system is the complete control of diffusion by living processes, since it is likely that the rate of formation, movement, and dissolution of pinocytotic vesicles is subject to hormonal and metabolic influences. Experimental support for this view come from studies of a related membrane, the epithelium of the mesentery and peritoneum (Berndt and Gosselin, 1961, 1962; Gosselin, 1970). Transport of inorganic ions across these epithelia occurs "downhill," that is, in the direction of their electrochemical potential gradient, but is characterized by a Q_{10} that is substantially higher than 1.3, suggesting that the process is not a purely diffusional one.

EXPERIMENTAL APPROACHES

This section deals with selected techniques, including some that presently are enjoying relative popularity, by which various investigators approach the problem of blood–tissue exchange. Without exception, the methodologies described treat the blood–tissue barrier as if it were an entity of fixed and invariant properties. As a consequence, in spite of the sometimes considerable sophistication, these approaches completely bypass the intricately adaptive character of transendothelial transport. This applies also to compartmental analysis, even though this method treats the process phenomenologically and thus avoids the pitfalls that are associated with attempts to define the site of transport or assume its operative mechanism.

Although model building of necessity involves simplifications, in this instance it is felt that the most essential features of the system have been left out of consideration for the sake of tractability. This overall pessimistic evaluation of current approaches reflects the acute need of a calculus that would encompass the functional behavior of the terminal vascular bed; computer simulation may go a long way toward this goal.

The Starling Hypothesis

Published at the turn of the century, Starling's (1896) views on the forces that govern the movement of water across endothelial membranes have enjoyed a unique and preeminent place in the thinking of physiologists. According to Starling, water moves in and out of blood vessels solely as a result of the interplay of hydraulic and osmotic forces, and at equilibrium there is no net transfer of fluid. In its simplest form this hypothesis is presented by

$$P_i - P_o = \Pi_i - \Pi_o \tag{13}$$

where P_i and Π_i refer to the hydraulic and osmotic pressures, respectively, inside the capillary, and P_o and Π_o represent these pressures outside the capillary. A more modern and elegant formulation of these intractions includes also the reflection coefficient σ (Johnson, 1970).

It bears repeating that the intuitive view that volume flow is proportional to the difference of osmotic pressures (Johnson, 1970) is not correct and that the axiomatic acceptance of this formulation is probably because it has never been used to describe systems in which the magnitude of the osmotic gradient was large enough to reveal its limited applicability (Ray, 1960).

Starling's hypothesis is discussed more fully in Chapters 8 and 9 of this volume. In a simplified form it is incorporated in the transport hypothesis presented in the last section of this review.

Permeability of Single Capillaries

The Starling hypothesis was confirmed many times but never in a manner as direct as that involving investigations of single capillaries. Prominent is here the pioneering work of E. M. Landis (1934; Landis and Pappenheimer, 1963). Lately, more modern forms of his methodology, some involving computer simulation, have further confirmed the basic elements of the Starling hypothesis (Intaglietta, 1967; Wiederhielm, 1968; Zweifach and Intaglietta, 1968). The exchange between single capillaries and tissue fluid is dealt with in great detail in Chapter 9 of this volume. Here it is only appropriate to mention that we would be closer to reality were we to consider transport phenomenona between open and closed capillaries rather than the relations that obtain between the contents of a single capillary and tissue fluid (Aschheim, 1974). This view is amplified in a later section. It is conceptually simple and leads to the conclusion that the hydraulic pressure gradient need not exceed the osmotic pressure gradient for fluid to leave one capillary, circulate among parenchymal cells, and enter another capillary.

Blood Clearance Studies

Flexner and his co-workers studied blood–tissue exchange by following the blood concentration of tracer substances injected intravenously (Flexner, Cowie, and Vosburgh, 1948). They showed that small-molecular-weight substances like water, sodium, and chloride ions leave the circulation in an exponential manner. This process was expressed in the form

$$C_t - C_{eq} = (C_o - C_{eq})\, e^{-Rt/q} \tag{14}$$

where C_t is the tracer concentration in the blood at the time t, C_{eq} is the tracer concentration in the blood after it has equilibrated with extravascular fluid, C_o is the tracer concentration in the blood at zero time, e is the base of natural logarithms, R is the proportion of the substance in the plasma that escapes from the plasma into the extravascular fluid per unit time, t is time, and q is the proportion of the total amount of substance ("cold" and "hot") that is extravascular.

The experimental curves could be resolved into two exponential components (man) or were monoexponential (guinea pig). In the latter, the results indicated that 140% of plasma water exchanges every minute with extravascular water.

Since the figures for both chloride and sodium ions indicated a 60% exchange in 1 min, the authors concluded that vascular membranes are 2.3 times more permeable to water than to these ions. These authors also present a numerical argument to show that the large amount of fluxing chloride ions must cross the entire surface of the capillaries since transport across endothelial clefts would account for only 3% of the observed values (Flexner et al., 1948). The arguments on which this conclusion is based rest on the assumption that passage across capillary walls is exclusively due to diffusion.

The experimental model used by Flexner et al. has not enjoyed much popularity, mainly because the condition of instantaneous mixing of the tracer in the blood does not obtain. In addition, the values are global and neglect the fact that the permeability of vascular membranes of various organs varies widely. It has also been pointed out that C_t, C_o, and C_{eq} refer to the concentrations of the tracer in arterial rather than capillary plasma, which is the one that is subject to equilibrations. This is an important consideration in view of the existence of demonstrable concentration differences between the arterial and venous end of capillaries (Pappenheimer, Renkin, and Borrero, 1951).

Blood disappearance curves of macromolecules have also been studied. Investigations of the kinetics of disappearance of ^{131}I-labeled albumin from the intravascular compartment revealed that there exists a steady state between the mass of albumin in the blood and the mass of albumin in the extravascular space, since depending on the experimental situation there can occur a net shift of albumin in or out of the blood vessels. For instance, in the dog, following hemorrhage 50% of the albumin is replaced within 24 hr, most of it coming from the extravascular space by way of the lymphatic system (Wasserman, Joseph, and Mayerson, 1956).

In contrast to these studies, in short-term experiments, the exponential disappearance of macromolecular aggregates and other colloidal materials from the blood yields rate constants that characterize the sequestering capacity of the reticuloendothelial system (see, for instance, Biozzi et al., 1957).

Osmotic Transient Method

This method, underlying the now classical paper of Pappenheimer et al. (1951) involves the perfusion of an isolated limb, the weight of which is kept constant. Injection on the arterial side of a bolus of a test substance increases the osmotic pressure of the perfusing fluid, causing a transient withdrawal of fluid from the perfused limb. The resulting decrease of the weight of the limb is countered by lifting the end of an outflow tube that is connected to the draining vein. This maneuver increases the intracapillary hydraulic pressure and the magnitude of the change in pressure is taken as a measure of the osmotic force acting across the walls of the capillaries. Since increasing the venous pressure would diminish the rate of perfusion of the limb, the arterial pressure is also increased.

The computational background presented by Pappenheimer and his colleagues can be summarized as follows. The Fick equation is presented as

$$\frac{dm}{dt} = -D \; \frac{A}{\Delta x} \; \Delta C \tag{15}$$

where dm/dt is the amount of test substance transported across the capillaries, D is the diffusion coefficient, A is the actual area across which diffusion occurs, Δx is the thickness of the endothelial membrane, and ΔC is the transmural difference in the concentration of the test substance. Next, it is taken that the amount of substance lost from the blood corresponds to the product of blood flow and arteriovenous concentration difference, i.e.,

$$\frac{dm}{dt} = \dot{Q}(C_a - C_v). \tag{16}$$

Furthermore, when the isogravimetric state is maintained, it was assumed that the change of hydraulic pressure was equal to the osmotic force exerted by the test molecules. This gives

$$\Delta P = RT\Delta C \tag{17}$$

where R is the universal gas constant and T is the absolute temperature. Combining Eqs. (15)–(17), one obtains

$$\frac{A}{\Delta x} = \dot{Q}(C_a - C_v) \frac{RT}{D\Delta P} \tag{18}$$

where $A/\Delta x$ is the diffusion area per unit path length through the capillary walls. According to this equation, at constant blood flow and temperature, for any molecular species, the ratio of arteriovenous concentration difference to osmotic pressure should be constant throughout the duration of the osmotic transient. This prediction was confirmed experimentally. Determination of $A/\Delta x$ for various molecular species revealed that the diffusion area per unit path length decreases with increasing molecular weight, a phenomenon attributed mainly to steric hindrance. Extrapolation of these values to the molecular weight of water yielded $A/\Delta x$ for these molecules. All other values were then expressed in terms of the diffusion area per unit path length available to water.

Next, Pappenheimer et al. entered $A/\Delta x$ for water in the Poiseuille equation that describes flow through tubes,

$$\dot{Q}_f = \frac{\Delta P r^4 \pi}{8\eta l} \tag{19}$$

where $\dot{Q}_f$ is the filtrational flow induced by ΔP, the driving force, l is the length of the tube, r its radius, and η the visicosity of the filtrate, to obtain

$$\frac{\dot{Q}_f}{\Delta P} = \frac{A_f r^2}{\Delta x \, 8\eta} \tag{20}$$

where A_f is the total area of the pores available for filtration. In this derivation the assumptions made that the total surface area across which water diffuses is also available to filtrational transport. After substituting the appropriate values in Eq. (20) and solving for r, Pappenheimer et al. obtained the value $r = 30$ Å. Additional computations led to an estimate of about 2×10^9 such pores per cm^2 of endothelial surface.

A major criticism of this work is directed at the use of van't Hoff's formula [Eq. (17)] to calculate the osmotic pressure exerted by the test molecules. This equation can only be validly used when the reflection coefficient of the membrane equals one ($\sigma = 1$), that is, when the membrane is not permeable to the solute at all. Thus Eq. (17) should be replaced by

$$\Delta P = R T \Delta C \sigma . \tag{21}$$

The error involved could be large since work with artificial membranes permeable to water and solute revealed that the osmotic pressure calculated by means of van't Hoff's formula could exceed the observed hydrostatic pressure by several orders of magnitude (Grim, 1953). A later presentation deals with this criticism (Landis and Pappenheimer, 1963). Amended derivations have been published (Landis and Pappenheimer, 1963; Lifson, 1970).

Single Injection Method

This method, developed by Crone (1963a) and used extensively by a number of workers, is based on the work of Chinard and co-workers (Chinard and Enns, 1954; Chinard et al., 1955). It involves the injection into the circulation of an organ of a single bolus consisting of a mixture of the test substance, which is presumed to leave the circulation, and a reference substance, such as T-1824, which, because it is bound to serum albumin, can be assumed to be completely retained within the circulation during the short experimental period. The outflowing blood is collected serially and analyzed for both the test and reference substances, and the concentrations found are expressed as fractions of their respective concentration in the injectate.

If one assumes that the test substance leaves the circulation exclusively by diffusion, the following obtains:

$$\frac{\Delta m}{\Delta t} = PA \Delta C = \dot{Q}(C_a - C_v) = \dot{Q}(C_r - C_t) \tag{22}$$

where $\Delta m/\Delta t$ is the rate of loss of substance by diffusion, P is the coefficient of permeability, equal to the ratio of the diffusion coefficient of the substance to the thickness of the membrane across which it diffuses, i.e., $D/\Delta x$, A is the endothelial surface area, ΔC is the transmural concentration difference of the test substance, $\dot{Q}$ is the rate of blood flow, C_a and C_v are the arterial venous concentrations of the test substance, respectively, and C_r and C_t are the fractional concentrations of the reference and test substance, respectively. If the plasma concentration of the test substance decreases exponentially as blood flows along the capillary, ΔC, which is the most difficult quantity to determine, may be taken as approximately equal to the mean intracapillary concentration, i.e.,

$$\Delta C = \frac{C_r - C_t}{\ln (C_r/C_t)}. \tag{23}$$

Entering Eq. (23) in Eq. (22) and solving for P, Crone obtains

$$P = -\frac{\dot{Q}}{A} \ln (1-E), \tag{24}$$

where the extraction of the test substance is given by

$$E = \frac{C_r - C_t}{C_r} \tag{25}$$

In his use of the Fick equation, Crone defines A as the total area of the endothelial surface and this includes areas across which there is no transport at all.

Use of Eq. (24) is fraught with difficulties. Under experimental conditions in nonliving systems the size of the compartments that are separated by the membrane is not allowed to impose limitations on transport that could be wrongly regarded as residing in the membrane proper. In vivo there is no such assurance. When the extravascular compartment is small so that equilibration of a test substance across endothelial membranes is fast relative to the speed of sampling, the small amount transported and consequently the low value of P could be interpreted as due to the low permeability of the membrane. In a similar fashion, the permeability of endothelial membranes will be held accountable for low rates of passage in situations where there are additional barriers to transport in the extravascular spaces. Employment of Eq. (24) may thus lead to a false characterization of the membranes.

These remarks may apply to work on the permeability of the blood vessels of the brain (Crone, 1965; Fenstermacher, 1970), which allow the passage of glucose, a metabolic substrate, but are said to be impermeable to sucrose, a nonmetabolite. Since the molecular diameters of these substances differ only by about 2 Å, which hardly justifies the drastic differences in transport, an attempt was made to resolve the puzzle by postulating a facilitated transport of glucose across the endothelial membranes of the brain.

The active participation of endothelial cells in the transport of small molecules is not questioned, but the argument for such a differential facilitated transport would have carried more weight, had the possibility been more fully explored that the small interstitial space of the brain results in a very fast equilibration of sucrose and glucose across the endothelial membranes, and that the overall transport of glucose is large because of the continuous consumption of this substance by brain neurons. Work with insulin has also led to the additional conclusion that this hormone does not affect the transport of glucose in the brain. However, these experimental data may simply reflect the known lack of effect of insulin on the brain uptake of glucose. Application of the same methodology to the determination of the effect of insulin on transendothelial passage of glucose in a tissue in which insulin is known to affect the rate of uptake of this metabolite by parenchymal cells would by the same reasoning result in the conclusion that insulin increases the permeability of endothelial membranes to glucose.

Even when Eq. (24) is employed to determine the ratio of permeabilities of vascular membranes of the same organ to two substances, X and Y, the results may be equivocal (23). In this situation one obtains

$$\frac{P_X}{P_Y} = \frac{A_Y \ln (1 - E_X)}{A_X \ln (1 - E_Y)} \tag{26}$$

The permeability ratio is then obtained by assuming that $A_Y = A_X$ since both substances were tested on the same organ. However, if X crosses the walls of the arterioles, capillaries, and venules, and Y can only cross the walls of the venules, to take an extreme case, $A_X \gg A_Y$. The ratio of permeabilities obtained by regarding the vascular areas as identical is thus of doubtful usefulness.

A more serious objection to Eq. (24) is that it underestimates to an unknown degree the permeability of endothelial membranes, since materials can leave the circulation and return to it a number of times in a way that escapes this formulation. Calculations show that water molecules can diffuse a few dozen times in and out of a capillary during the time it takes the blood to flow along it (Landis and Pappenheimer, 1963), and this possibility may have been substantiated by some experimental observations. For instance, at low blood flows, when one injects intraarterially a mixture of labeled albumin and isotopic water, the two substances separate and, contrary to expectation, the isotopic water is the first to appear in the venous outflow (Chinard, 1970). In another study, monohydric alcohols appeared in the venous outflow earlier than the non-permeating reference substance (Chinard et al., 1969). Such a separation of injected materials results in a negative E [Eq. (25)] during the first part of the venous outflow. It is apparent that in this case a quantity of test molecules that entered the extravascular space by crossing the vascular barrier must have returned to the blood in order to appear on the venous side in front of the reference substance. In other words, some of the test molecules crossed the vascular membranes at least twice. However, in terms of Eq. (22), since C_v is larger, dm/dt and consequently P must be small. This internal inconsistency arises because Eq. (22) refers only to the net amount of substance that passes from the blood to the tissues; estimates of vascular permeability based on this formulation may thus grossly underestimate this property of the barrier.

Continuous Infusion Method

Developed by Renkin (1955, 1959, 1968), the method appears to yield best results when applied to substances such as K and Rb ions for which the parenchymal tissues constitute a very large sink. Renkin considers that because of loss of material from the circulation, the concentration of a substance along a capillary declines exponentially, i.e.,

$$C_v = C_a e^{-k} \qquad (27)$$

where C_v and C_a are the venous and arterial concentrations of the test substance, e is the base of natural logarithm, and the rate constant k is a function of permeability P, surface area S, and rate of blood flow $\dot{Q}$, i.e.,

$$k = \frac{PS}{\dot{Q}} \qquad (28)$$

Hence

$$\frac{PS}{\dot{Q}} = \ln \frac{C_a}{C_v} \qquad (29)$$

Furthermore, extraction E is defined as

$$E = \frac{C_a - C_v}{C_a - C_t} \qquad (30)$$

where C_t is the concentration just on the outside of the blood vessel. This is taken as zero because of the large intracellular sink. Entering Eq. (30) in Eq. (29) and solving for P shows that this derivation is identical to that of Crone [Eq. (24)], although the definition of E is not the same.

Assuming that loss of material from the capillary is exclusively due to diffusion, i.e.,

$$\dot{Q}(C_a - C_v) = \frac{\Delta m}{\Delta t} = PS\Delta C \qquad (31)$$

where ΔC is the transmural concentration difference, one obtains

$$\frac{PS}{\dot{Q}} = \frac{C_a - C_v}{\Delta C} \tag{32}$$

which, combined with Eq. (29), gives the transendothelial concentration difference:

$$\Delta C = \frac{(C_a - C_v)}{\ln (C_a/C_v)} \ . \tag{33}$$

The method of continuous infusion is subject to the same limitations that were mentioned in connection with the description of the single injection method, namely, the vexing problem of determining the transmural concentration difference, recirculation, effect of the functional size of the extravascular compartment, i.e., size of sink, presence of unstirred layers, and existence of other barriers to permeation. This last weakness, however, is being turned into a strength because the method may yield data regarding the relative contribution of the various barriers (capillary wall, interestitial material, cell membranes) to the total resistance to passage encountered by various materials (Renkin and Sheehan, 1970).

The product PS is sensitive to vasomotor activity and can vary eightfold from maximum nervous vasoconstriction to maximum metabolic vasodilation (Renkin, 1968). Stimulation of sympathetic nerves has yielded results suggestive of vasomotor control of precapillary sphincter activity (Renkin and Rosell, 1962). An unexplained finding is that conventional vasodilators not only fail to enhance, but actually on occasion reduce the blood–tissue equilibration of [86]Rb (Renkin, 1968). This observation may call for a reassessment of the basic assumption underlying the derivation of PS [Eq. (29)], i.e., that transendothelial transport is exclusively due to diffusion.

Clearance from Tissue Depots

Vascular permeability has also been studied by determining the rate at which substances injected into a tissue are removed from that site by the circulating blood. The rate of removal is a function of blood flow, vascular permeability, surface area of vessels that participate in the removal, mass of the injected substance, and the rate at which it is transported in the interstitial fluid. For ease of measurement, radioactive substances are usually employed. Clearance is described by Gosselin (1970):

$$\frac{\dot{M}}{M} = \frac{\dot{Q}}{\lambda} \ (1 - e^{-PS/Q}) \tag{34}$$

where $\dot{M}$ is the instantaneous rate of removal of the substance present in quantity M in the tissue, $\dot{Q}$ is the rate of blood flow (ml/g/unit time), λ is the tissue/blood partition coefficient (ml/g), and PS is the product of permeability and surface area. $\dot{M}/M$ is the rate of fractional removal equal to the slope of the line when $\lg M$ is plotted against time. Equation (34) is based on the derivation by Lassen and Trap-Jensen (1968). In the hands of Gosselin this methodology appears capable of partitioning the increase of blood flow that follows the application of vasodilators into an increase of capillary perfusion and increase in capillary surface area (1970), if one assumes that these substances do not affect vascular permeability.

In a somewhat similar approach (Strandell and Shepherd, 1968), PS was calculated from the basic equation of Renkin (1959),

$$PS = \dot{Q} \ln (1 - E) \tag{35}$$

where all symbols are as above and E is the extraction. The rate of blood flow $\dot{Q}$ was evaluated by following the rate of disappearance of ^{133}Xe injected into skeletal muscle together with the test substance, in this case ^{24}Na.

Since the disappearance of ^{133}Xe from the site followed a first-order kinetics, it could be described by

$$C_t = C_o e^{-kt} \tag{36}$$

where C_o and C_t is the radioactivity of the injected site at zero time and at time t, respectively, t is the elapsed time, and e is the base of natural logarithms. The rate constant k is given by

$$k = \frac{\dot{Q}}{V\lambda_{Xe}} \tag{37}$$

where $\dot{Q}$ is the rate of blood flow, V is the volume of the tissue, and λ_{Xe} is the partition coefficient of Xe between skeletal muscle and blood. Since the plot of the logarithm of tissue radioactivity against time yielded a straight line, the value of the half-time $t_{1/2}$ was read off the graph and used to calculate the rate constant k from

$$k = 2.3 \lg(2/t_{1/2\,Xe}) \tag{38}$$

Thus the rate of blood flow per 100 grams of muscle is given by Ingvar and Lassen (1962)

$$\dot{Q} = \frac{0.693\lambda_{Xe}100}{t_{1/2\,Xe}} . \tag{39}$$

In this manner the clearance of Xenon (Cl_{Xe}) from the muscle is taken as a measure of its blood flow. Finally since extraction E can be defined as Cl_{Na}/Cl_{Xe}, PS_{Na} can be obtained from

$$PS_{Na} = Cl_{Xe} \ln [1 - \frac{Cl_{Na}}{Cl_{Xe}}] \tag{40}$$

The clearance of ^{24}Na from the injection site was obtained in a manner similar to that described above for the clearance of ^{133}Xe, i.e.,

$$Cl_{Na} = \frac{0.693\lambda_{Na}100}{t_{1/2\,Na}} \tag{41}$$

This study has led to the important conclusion that the tissue clearance of radioactive sodium ions cannot be employed to measure blood flow, since at high rates of perfusion the removal of these ions from tissue depots becomes diffusion limited (Strandell and Shepherd, 1968).

Capillary Filtration Coefficient

In terms of Starling's hypothesis, net fluid extravasation will occur whenever the hydraulic pressure gradient across the walls of the capillaries exceeds the osmotic pressure gradient. Thus if one were to inflate an arm cuff to a pressure below diastolic, at first the outflow of blood from the arm would cease, but it would resume when the pressure in the distended capacitance vessels reached that in the cuff. Enclosing the part of the arm distal to the collecting cuff in a plethysmograph would register not only the initial rapid increase in volume due to the distension of the veins, but also a further slow increase due to filtration of fluid out of the blood vessels. Knowing the rate of this increase and the volume of the enclosed limb, one may express it per unit mass of tissue and relate it to the occlusion pressure, (Kitchin, 1963; Krogh, Landis, and Turner, 1932). The capillary filtration coefficient (CFC) is customarily expressed in milliliters of fluid filtered per minute per 100 grams of tissue per 1 mm Hg transmural pressure gradient. For example, it has been reported that, when skeletal muscle passes from rest to exercise, CFC increases from 0.015 to 0.04–0.05 (Cobbold et al., 1963).

This methodology has yielded important insights into the effects of vasomotor tone; it revealed a neurogenic component in the control of precapillary sphincter activity (Folkow and Mellander, 1960) and disclosed the fact that local metabolic factors can overcome sympathetic nervous influences (Cobbold et al., 1963). Importantly, simultaneous determinations of passage of solutes and water have disclosed an augmentation of transendothelial transport of solutes during induced fluid movement (Lundgren and Mellander, 1967), suggesting the participation of convection in addition to diffusion in this process.

Compartmental Analysis

The term capillary permeability is not a satisfactory one. For instance, "increased capillary permeability" is usually used to denote the extravasation of proteins, a process which, at least in the initial stages of inflammation, occurs in venules and not capillaries (Wilhelm, 1962). As mentioned in a later section, various areas of the circulatory tree may participate in the transport process depending on the molecular size of the solute. For this reason, it may be more appropriate to consider the intravascular and extravascular space as discrete, well-stirred compartments separated by a membrane more or less permeable to the studied substances. If cell membranes constitute another barrier to permeation, the model will consist of three distinct compartments. The permeability of the barrier can then be expressed by the noncommittal "transfer coefficient."

Compartmental volumes and transfer coefficients that are obtained by this methodology are functional in the sense that a kinetically determined volume of distribution may turn out to have no measurable physical dimensions. This may occur, for example, when a tracer becomes adsorbed onto fixed structural elements of an anatomically single compartment during the initial infusion and is desorbed during the subsequent washout period. If the rate of desorption is significantly lower than the rate at which the unadsorbed tracer leaves the compartment, desorption will kinetically mimic an additional parallel compartment of calculable physical dimensions and introduce what may be regarded as a phantom barrier.

Another seeming error may arise when a substance within a compartment binds or otherwise impedes the passage across the barrier of another tracer that by itself crosses the membrane unimpeded. Such interference may kinetically result in two compartments rather than one, as far as the otherwise freely permeable tracer is concerned, and provide a de facto characterization of the barrier. However, all such effects reflect what is actually happening to the test substance; compartmental analysis describes what a substance actually "sees" when it enters the circulation of an organ.

A lucid introductory reference to compartmental analysis is provided by Matthews (1971) and Atkins (1969). Especially valuable is the general solution for a three-compartment model by Skinner et al. (1959) since it enables the investigator to carve out any compartmental subset that he thinks describes his experimental model.

Analysis of washin or washout curves contributes to our understanding of tissue nutrition by establishing the number of compartments penetrated by a given substance, their volumes and rates of passage across the various intercompartmental barriers. Compartmental analysis of artificially perfused organs is predicated on the assumption that the various compartments are well mixed. This assumption has been made in studies involving fast introduction of substances into the blood of intact animals (Hamilton et al., 1932), but was later criticized (Sheppard et al., 1953; Sheppard, 1954, 1962; Zierler, 1963). In the main, it was argued that any exponential character of dilution curves is likely to be fortuitous because the distinct types of vascular architecture of various organs result in a spectrum of volume flows and transit times. However, these objections need not apply to washout curves obtained from a single perfused organ, in which the vascular bed supplies the nutritive demands of relatively uniform and functionally equivalent cells. In this situation, developmental strategy may call for averaging of the nutritive flux per cell, a function which may serve well by the randomization of the inflowing blood by the vascular bed. Similar evolutionary optimization of the heat-exchange function of the skin has probably contributed to the preservation of the random character of its vascular pattern, or even led to it. Thus it is felt that even if a randomizing vascular network were not the most likely configuration, it would have arisen as a result of developmental pressure both at the phylogenetic and ontogenetic plane. Kinetically, such a randomizing vascular network mimics the behavior of a well-stirred compartment. This view is in line with the manifest directive character of many organismic processes, a feature that has prompted the establishment of the principle of functional optimization as an evolutionary goal (Rosen, 1967). Sheppard recognized that a randomizing vascular labyrinth may in actuality be responsible for the kinetic behavior that also characterizes a well-stirred compartment, but considered such a coincidence unlikely (Sheppard, 1962).

These considerations indicate that the study of dilution curves of isolated organs may yield valid operational characterizations. Such descriptions may or may not correspond to visible anatomical features, but are correct in the sense that a given tissue presents simultaneously an array of functional aspects, each uniquely specific to a given constituent of the perfusing fluid. Unlike the other techniques described in this section, compartmental analysis is a vast topic. The nature of this review precludes any attempts at presenting its numerical aspects. Excellent introductory expositions are available (Atkins, 1969; Matthews, 1971).

Extravasation of Blood Proteins

The permeability of vascular membranes to macromolecules can best be studied in inflammation. Since blood proteins return to the circulation by way of lymphatics, which is a relatively slow process, study of their extravasation is not complicated by their reentrance via blood vessels.

The rate of accumulation in the skin of intravenously injected ^{131}I-labeled albumin (RISA) is a function of the permeability of the blood vessels at the time the determination is made, blood flow to the area, and blood level of the tracer. The blood flow to the inflamed site can be studied by determining the skin uptake of ^{86}Rb for which the intracellular compartment represents a sizeable sink relative to the total amount of ^{86}Rb injected (Sapirstein, 1958).

According to this method (Aschheim, 1964b, 1965a) a mixture of RISA and ^{86}Rb is injected through a jugular cannula into animals in which the inflammatory reaction had been proceeding for a known time, and 1 min later the heart is stopped by injecting a saturated solution of KCl by the same route. In analogy to renal clearance, removal of RISA can be defined in terms of milliliters of blood from which it is completely cleared by 1 g of dry skin in 1 min (Aschheim, 1965a).

Initially, protein extravasation is preceded by greater skin uptake of water (Aschheim and Zweifach, 1962). Following this, RISA begins to accumulate in the inflamed area at a rate that increases linearly with time, but after the peak is reached, the rate declines in an exponential fashion (Aschheim, 1965*b*). Relating clearance of RISA to the blood flow of the area, it was found that for any one stage of the inflammatory reaction, that is, for every given level of vascular permeability to protein, the skin uptake of RISA is linearly related to the blood flow (Aschheim and Zweifach, 1962; Aschheim, 1965*a*).

This methodology has made possible the characterization of the inflammatory state since experimental data could be interpreted in terms of changes of nutritional blood flow, intravascular blood plasma content, and minute rate of plasma extravasation throughout the course of xylene-induced reaction (Aschheim, 1965*a*).

FUNCTIONAL CHARACTERIZATIONS
OF THE TERMINAL VASCULAR BED

An acceptable hypothesis of blood–tissue exchange cannot contradict the various observational and experimental findings relating to the behaviour of the terminal vascular bed, nor can it address itself to only some of these. As shown in the previous section, the various approaches deal with transport as if it occurred across a membrane of well-defined characteristics and ignore the very attributes that make the system unique. This section describes those attributes about which there is little or no controversy regarding their reality.

Gradient of Permeability

Well established experimentally but neglected in theoretic treatments is the finding that there occurs a progressive reduction of the endothelial surface area available to transport of water-soluble molecules from the arterioles toward the venules, as the molecular weight of the substance increases (Chambers and Zweifach, 1947; Rous and Smith, 1931). This evidence suggests the existence of a continuum of pore sizes coupled with a differential distribution of these pores among the various vessels. Assuming, for instance, a normal distribution of pore sizes, arterioles would be characterized by smaller pores, capillaries by small and medium pores, and venules would exhibit the entire spectrum. The actual pore size profile of each type of vessel is unknown, but an old observation (Chambers and Zweifach, 1947) suggests that it is not a function of the anatomic structure of the wall, since manipulative reversal of blood flow so that it flows from the venules towards the arterioles also reverses the gradient of permeability, arterioles becoming the most permeable and venules the least. This finding points to humoral factors originating in the parenchyma of tissues, possibly of enzymic nature, as determinants of vascular porosity. In line with today's electron microscopic evidence (Karnovsky, 1968, 1970; Majno and Palade, 1961), these pores are identified with interendothelial clefts, but there is reason to believe that porosity should be ascribed to the basement membrane proper, since it is this structure, as discussed later on, which is traversed by various solutes.

The experimentally reached conclusion that pore sizes increase as one progresses from the arterioles toward the venules, coupled with the finding that they are modifiable by humoral factors, bears heavily on attempts to characterize vascular membranes of the terminal vascular bed in terms of the reflection coefficient σ (Fenstermacher, 1970; Gaby and Areekul, 1970; Johnson, 1970; Lifson, 1970; Pappenheimer, 1970a, 1970b; Tosteson, 1970; Vargas and Johnson, 1964).

As noted earlier, the simultaneous determination of the permeability of vascular barriers of an organ to two substances must take into account the difference in the surface area available to transport. Unless there is evidence to the contrary, the respective surface areas must be regarded as different. The permeability ratio should refer to a specified type of vessel, if it is to characterize the properties of its wall. It will be different for arterioles, capillaries, and venules (Wiederhielm, 1966; Intaglietta, 1967; Zweifach and Intaglietta, 1968). Estimates of membrane permeability tacitly imply that this property is spread uniformly over the substance of the membrane. However, perusal of the literature on vascular permeability reveals that estimates of the vascular surface area involved in transport are somehow always limited to capillaries, thus compounding the indeterminacy of the calculations.

Activity of Precapillary Sphincters

India ink injections have demonstrated that the number of open capillaries in exercising skeletal muscle may exceed by an order of magnitude the number open in the resting state (Krogh, 1929). The intermittent opening and closing of capillaries is due to the activity of precapillary sphincters (Zweifach, 1939). Each phase of the contraction relaxation cycle may last from 2 to 8 sec, the Q_{10} of this activity being 2.2 (Krogh, 1929). The modulating activity of precapillary sphincters affects transendothelial transport in a variety of ways. First, subject to the setting of the ceiling intracapillary hydraulic pressure by the smooth muscle activity of the arterioles and venules, it influences the relation between the transmural hydraulic and osmotic pressure gradients and thus determines the direction of water movement. Second, the average duration of each phase of the contraction—relaxation cycle in a given regional bed determines the number of capillaries that are open at any given time. The more open capillaries, the steeper the concentration gradients of blood-supplied metabolites owing to decreased average distance between open capillaries and parenchymal cells, the larger the surface area across which these metabolites pass out, and the greater the outward flux of water on which depends the magnitude of the "bulk-flow" component of metabolite flux. Analysis of the contribution of precapillary sphincter activity to water and metabolite transport suggests that it serves mainly the nutritional needs of parenchymal cells.

Restricted Diffusion

An important characteristic of vascular membranes is that they impede the passage of large molecules, as compared to small ones, more than would be expected on the basis of decreased diffusion coefficients. This finding has led to the conclusion that the total pore area available to transport of various solutes in a given tissue under identical conditions is not constant (Pappenheimer et al., 1951; Renkin, 1964). This phenomenon probably results from a combination of causes, of which the recognized ones are the arteriovenous permeability gradient, steric hindrance, and possibly molecular charge (Gaby and Areekul, 1970).

Regarding the first, early observational evidence based on the extravasation of intravenously injected dyes of graded molecular weights (Chambers and Zweifach, 1947; Landis, 1927; Rous and Smith, 1931) still stands unchallenged. If a substance is observed to cross the walls of the venules only, the combined pore area of the arterioles and capillaries, in addition to the small pores of the venules, does not contribute to this transport; consequently, the calculated permeability should be referred to the venules only. Because of its observational prominence, this effect should possibly have been accorded greater weight than it was given on the basis of a purely computational argument (Pappenheimer et al., 1951).

The second factor refers to steric hindrance, a concept according to which the chance of a permeant molecule striking the edge of a pore, and thus being prevented from entering it, increases as the molecular size approaches the dimensions of the pore. This mechanism is believed to be the major cause of restricted diffusion (Pappenheimer et al., 1951).

As to the third factor, the evidence that vascular membranes discriminate between molecules on the basis of their electric charge is scanty and is counterbalanced by experiments in which no such effect was found. For instance, studies involving the intravenous injection of labeled Na_2SO_4 indicate that both the anion and cation leave the intravascular compartment at the same rate in spite of differences in charge, sign, and valence.

The reality of restricted diffusion has been confirmed (Chambers and Zweifach, 1947; Renkin, 1964; Gaby and Areekul, 1970; Johnson, 1970; Mogensen, 1970; Pappenheimer, 1970a; Trap-Jensen and Lassen, 1970) and denied (Alvarez and Yudilevich, 1969; Crone, 1963b). Interestingly, confirmatory reports disregard the possibility that the observed effect could partly be accounted for by a shift of available pore area in the direction of the venules as the molecular size increases, and those who deny the reality of this phenomenon adopt an equally simplified view.

Permeability to Water- and Lipid-soluble Substances

The term lipid- and water-soluble when applied to a permeant substance is a relative one. It is expressed as a ratio of the distribution of the substance between olive oil and water at equilibrium, after it is shaken with a mixture of these solvents. For instance, in the ascending series of primary alcohols, the higher the molecular weight, the greater the influence of the lipid-soluble portion of the molecule and the greater the olive oil–water partition coefficient. In the context of research dealing with vascular permeability, the so-called lipid-soluble substances are still much more soluble in water than in oil.

As a rule, the passage of water-soluble substances out of the intravascular compartment is inversely related to their molecular weight. This is due to the decrease of the diffusion coefficient with increasing molecular weight and other restricting factors mentioned in the preceding section.

The observed decrease of transendothelial flux with increasing molecular weight does not obtain with lipid-soluble substances. In fact, if the increased molecular weight is associated with increasing lipid solubility, as in the ascending series of primary alcohols, permeability of vascular membranes increases with increasing molecular weight.

An excellent illustration of the differential behavior of water- and lipid-soluble substances is provided by the work of Renkin (1952) which demonstrates that urea when injected into the circulation of a perfused limb causes an osmotic withdrawal of water, but urethane, which has a larger molecular weight, does not. This difference can be accounted for by assuming that urethane equilibrates very fast across endothelial membranes. The olive oil/water partition coefficient of urea is 15/100,000, that of urethane 74/1000, and the molecular weight of the two substances is 60 and 89, respectively.

Experimental evidence of this type indicates that lipid-soluble substances can pass across areas of endothelial membranes that are not available to water-soluble substances. It is likely that this is due to their ability to dissolve in the outer lipid layers of endothelial cells. The lipid solubility of respiratory gases is believed to be responsible for their rapid equilibration between blood and tissues. As far as the permeability of water- and lipid-soluble substances is concerned, vascular membranes resemble cellular membranes (Collander and Barlund, 1933).

TRANSPORT OF MATERIALS
BETWEEN BLOOD AND TISSUE: A Unitary Hypothesis

Blood–tissue exchange emerges as a complex phenomenon that involves a hierarchy of interacting control mechanisms. At the level of the regional terminal vascular bed, smooth muscle activity determines arteriolar and vascular tone. At a lower level precapillary sphincters phasically control pressure and flow through capillaries. At the level of the endothelial sheet, transport appears to occur both across the interendothelial clefts and by way of pinocytotic vesicles. Since this presentation aims at an integrated picture, it may not be inappropriate to review the main features of a unitary hypothesis of blood–tissue exchange

(Aschheim, 1974). The hypothesis is a tentative one; it incorporates elements found scattered throughout the literature. Shift of emphasis from capillary–tissue fluid relationships to interactions between capillaries has led to a simplified reinterpretation of Starling's hypothesis and to a revised conception of nutritive exchange.

Pore Transport of Water

Electron microscopic evidence indicates that normally colloidal substances such as HgS are excluded from the interendothelial clefts. These spaces are occupied by a condensation of the ground substance, which forms a septum contiguous with the basement membrane. During inflammation the cells separate from each other and from the septum, and the colloidal material is able to enter the clefts but is prevented by the basement membrane from passing into the extravascular space (Majno and Palade, 1961). For this reason this membrane was thought to constitute the major permeability barrier of blood vessels (Palade, 1961).

Since the ground substance of the clefts normally excludes circulating plasma proteins, this space is accessible only to plasma ultrafiltrate. Consequently, the chemical activity gradient of water extends across the interface, where the ground substance of the cleft is in contact with blood plasma. The steepness of this gradient suggests the possibility that osmotic forces may induce large water flows into the capillaries. The actual steepness of the gradient is not known; among other factors, it will be influenced by the extent to which the ground substance of the clefts is impervious to plasma proteins.

In contrast, whenever capillary blood pressure is high enough to cause outward filtration, the driving gradient of hydraulic pressure extends along the entire cleft. This difference suggests that the structure of the interendothelial clefts biases the system in favor of resorption of water from extravascular spaces. This conclusion is in line with evidence according to which the pressure of fluid in the interstitial spaces is negative (Guyton, 1963; Guyton, Granger, and Taylor, 1971). It is possible, however, that during pronounced outward filtration endothelial cells separate somewhat, allowing blood plasma to enter the interendothelial spaces. The resulting increase in the steepness of the hydraulic pressure gradient could contribute to the overcoming of the osmotic pressure gradient.

These considerations account for the high permeability of endothelial membranes to water (Yudilevich and Alvarez, 1967; Yudilevich, 1970), are in line with the reported alteration of the geometry of interendothelial clefts not only in inflammation but also during filtrational distension of blood vessels (Landis, 1970), and may account for the bounding of one opening of the cleft only by the basement membrane in functional terms. Hopefully, the early observations of Landis, Majno, and Palade will be extended and the interendothelial clefts subjected to closer electron microscopic scrutiny.

Vesicular Transport of Water and Nutrients

Vesicular transport across the cell should result in the deposition of what may be regarded as the equivalent of a thin layer of blood plasma between the endothelial cell and the basement membrane. Since the latter is little permeable to blood proteins, these should quickly reach the same concentration on both sides of the cell. In contrast to these, small molecules and water should be able to cross the basement membrane to a varying extent. A flux of a given molecular species would then depend on its chemical or electrochemical potential gradient, as well as on the nature and magnitude of its interaction with both the membrane and other fluxing molecules. Onsager's theory is well suited to describing the various phenomena.

In all probability the flux of materials across the basement membrane exceeds that which is mediated by interendothelial clefts. This is suggested by the circumstance that the basement membrane presents a much larger surface area (total surface area of endothelial membrane less surface area occupied by the clefts) as well as by the fact that the length of the diffusion path across the basement membrane, which is about 500 Å wide, is shorter than the diffusion path along the clefts by approximately one order of magnitude (see Figure 3).

Changes in transmural hydraulic and osmotic gradients affect water transport along interendothelial clefts in an immediate and direct manner. In contrast, the vesicle-mediated transport is under cellular control, since the size, rate of

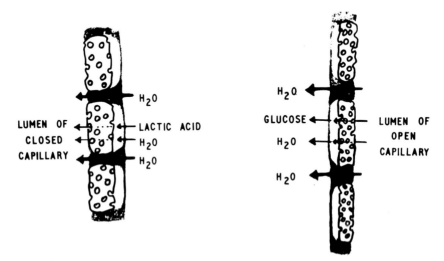

Figure 3. Random movement of Palade's vesicles in the cytoplasm equilibrates blood plasma with the liquid contained between the endothelial cells and basement membrane. Transport of water and metabolites by this means depends on intraplasmatic processes, whereas transport of water along interendothelial clefts does not. Heavy arrows indicate large flows.

formation, and rate of movement of Palade's vesicles can conceivably be influenced by metabolic and other factors. This mode of transport is only transiently affected by perturbations of osmotic and hydraulic forces.

Role of Precapillary Sphincters in Water and Metabolite Transport

Krogh's discovery of the intermittent closing and opening of capillaries, later shown to be due to phasic changes of tone of the then discovered precapillary sphincters (and sphincter-like vessels), appears to be crucial to the description of the process of blood–tissue exchange.

Since the blood pressure of open capillaries exceeds that of closed capillaries, a given microscopic tissue region is very likely characterized by a multitude of short-lived fugacity gradients of water, each extending from an open capillary to a neighboring closed one. Water that moves along these gradients flows among parenchymal cells and enters closed capillaries that act as sinks. This flow should carry (by "bulk flow") various solutes to and from capillary surfaces. This mode of transport and diffusion that occurs owing to concentration gradients that are established by cell metabolism may account for the overall traffic of solutes in intercapillary regions bounded by endothelial membranes. According to this view, blood contained in the capillaries tends to equilibrate with tissue fluid—as far as small molecules are concerned—by a combination of vesicular traffic, diffusion, and translational "bulk flow."

Since each phase of the relaxation–contraction cycle of precapillary sphincter activity lasts only 2–8 sec (Krogh, 1929), the contents of closed capillaries are swept into the general circulation probably before such equilibrations are completed. The intermittent activity of precapillary sphincters is thus responsible for both the phasic renewal of capillary blood and for the continuous abolition and establishment of intercapillary fugacity gradients of water. These two aspects represent the essential component of their nutritive function. (See Chapter 3 in this volume and Altura in Volume II for further discussion.)

As far as the function of precapillary sphincters is concerned, the picture presented above simplifies and modifies the Starling hypothesis, since one needs to consider only forces that are responsible for the movement of water between one capillary and another. The properties of the fluid between the capillaries are largely immaterial in this context.

This becomes clear when one considers a microscopic region of tissue of constant volume, containing two capillaries. The space between the capillaries bounded by capillary walls behaves in a manner analogous to an osmotic siphon, since it transmits water from one capillary to the other if the intracapillary hydraulic and osmotic forces are such as to result in a net fugacity gradient of water. The osmotic and hydraulic pressure of the intervening space is of no consequence as long as the total volume of the region is not altered.

In contrast to past considerations that focused only on relationships that obtain between a capillary and its surrounding fluid, the present view leads to the conclusion that capillary blood pressure does not have to exceed the oncotic pressure of blood plasma for water to filter out of a given capillary. Water may leave one capillary, flow past tissue cells, and enter another capillary as long as one capillary acts as a sink relative to the other as far as the chemical potential of water is concerned, irrespective of the properties of the intervening fluid, as long as the isovolumetric condition is maintained. According to this view, this exchange does not cease when the ceiling blood pressure of a given capillary network falls below the oncotic pressure of blood plasma, once the perturbation brought about by the shift of fluid from the tissue to the blood is over. This hypothesis may provide a satisfactory explanation of the observation discussed in the section concerning the single injection method, according to which at low flows (and presumably low pressure) an easily permeable substance appears on the venous side in front of the nonpermeating reference substance.

Physiologically, the constancy of tissue volume is assured by the relative paucity of interstitial tissue fluid due to the oncotic pressure difference between it and blood plasma. In pathologic conditions, as when blood proteins leak out of blood vessels and the osmotic pressure of the tissue fluid approaches that of blood plasma, maintenance of the isovolumetric condition is taken over by tissue fibrils and membranes that counter and progressively limit tissue distension.

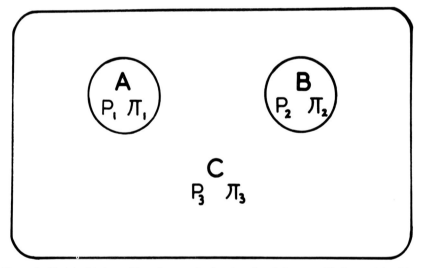

Figure 4. Model of intercapillary transport of water. A and B are capillaries contained in a tissue region of constant volume. The intercapillary space transmits water under the influence of both osmotic and hydraulic pressure differences established between the two capillaries. If, for simplicity, $\Pi_1 = \Pi_2$ but precapillary sphincter activity establishes a hydraulic pressure difference between A and B, water will flow from one capillary to the other. The hydraulic and osmotic pressures of the intervening space do not interfere with the intercapillary flow of water as long as its volume remains constant. This flow of water is responsible for the convective or "bulk-flow" component of solute transport.

Central and Local Control

The activity of precapillary sphincters is coupled to that of the arteriolar smooth muscle since the proportion of open capillaries appears to parallel the blood flow to the area. Since both systems seem to respond to the metabolic activity of parenchymal cells, locally produced metabolites, or perhaps their depletion, determine their function. However, experimental evidence indicates that pre-capillary sphincters and arteriolar smooth muscle also respond to sympathetic nervous influences (Folkow and Mellander, 1960; Renkin and Rosell, 1962). The dual nature of their control may reflect the fact that metabolite transport is intimately bound to flow of water in and out of blood vessels, a process that could on occasion compromise the regulation of blood volume. The basically nutritive character of precapillary sphincter activity is demonstrated by the finding that in extreme conditions local metabolic requirements override central constrictor influences (Cobbold et al., 1963), a phenomenon that parallels the vasodilation which follows intense peripheral vasoconstriction induced by hemorrhage (Chien, 1967).

Control of blood volume by the sympathetic nervous system appears to depend on the regulation of vascular resistances at the pre- and postcapillary levels. Heightened sympathetic tone increases arteriolar resistance more than venular resistance, causing a lowering of the ceiling blood pressure of the intervening vascular region (Mellander and Johansson, 1968). When the ceiling pressure falls below the oncotic pressure of blood plasma, excess water from the tissue region is mopped up. In this situation the cleft-mediated water transport figures prominently, since, unlike the vesicle-mediated transport, it does not depend on intraplasmatic processes. This Starling-type removal of water from a tissue region interferes transiently with the intercapillary movement of water induced by the activity of precapillary sphincters and to this extent only affects the convective component of solute transport. As mentioned earlier, no such interference should obtain in the absence of tissue volume changes.

The Hypothesis

The evidence and discussions presented in this section can be arranged in a meaningful and self-consistent manner if we consider that at the level of the terminal vascular bed there exist two separate and functionally distinct modes of transport.

The first deals mainly with water and serves the regulation of blood volume. The loci of passage are the interendothelial clefts, the forces involved are those originally described by Starling, and the controlling mechanism is the modulation of the pre- and postcapillary resistances by the autonomic nervous system.

The second mode of transport is nutritive in nature. It is concerned with the passage of substances of low molecular weight, such as might be involved in cell metabolism, and of water. This mode of transport consists of two distinct elements. The first consists of the equilibrating effect of peregrinations of Palade's vesicles, a mechanism that allows the overall magnitude of exchange to be regulated by cellular processes. Once outside the endothelial sheath these substances as well as the ones that are released from parenchymal cells are subjected to the combined action of diffusion and translational transport. The latter is believed to be due to water flows that arise between open and closed capillaries as a consequence of the intermittent operation of precapillary sphincters or sphincter-like vessels. In the absence of net water shifts between blood and tissue, this transport is not affected by conditions that obtain in the intercapillary regions.

LITERATURE CITED

Alvarez, O. A., and D. L. Yudilevich. 1969. Heart capillary permeability to lipid-insoluble molecules. J. Physiol. London 202:45–58.

Aschheim, E., and B. W. Zweifach. 1961. Kinetics of blood protein leakage in inflammation. Circ. Res. 9:349–357.

Aschheim, E., and B. W. Zweifach. 1962. Quantitative studies of protein and water shifts during inflammation. Am. J. Physiol. 202:554–558.

Aschheim, E. 1964a. Rate of protein extravasation in inflammation. Am. J. Physiol. 206:327–330.

Aschheim, E. 1964b. Determination of vascular permeability. Nature 201: 1291–1292.

Aschheim, E. 1965a. Kinetic characterization of the terminal vascular bed during inflammation. Am. J. Physiol. 208:270–274.

Aschheim, E. 1965b. Transendothelial passage of small and large molecules. Fed. Proc. 24:1104–1111.

Aschheim, E. 1974. Traffic of metabolites between blood and tissue. Microvasc. Res. 8:64–69.

Atkins, C. L. 1969. Multicompartment Models for Biological Systems. Methuen & Co., London.

Berndt, W. O., and R. E. Gosselin. 1961. Physiological factors influencing radiorubidium flux across isolated rabbit mesentery. Am. J. Physiol. 200: 454–458.

Berndt, W. O., and R. E. Gosselin. 1962. Differential changes in permeability of mesentery to rubidium and phosphate. Am. J. Physiol. 202:761–767.

Biozzi, G., B. Benacerraf, B. N. Halpern, and C. Stiffel. 1957. The competitive effect of certain celloids on the phagocytosis of other colloids by the cells of the recitulo-endothelial system and the phenomenon of phagocytic preference. Reticulo-Endothelial Society Bull. 3:3–7.

Casley-Smith, J. R. 1963. Pinocytotic vesicles: An explanation of some of the problems associated with the passage of particles into and through cells via these bodies. Med. Res. Council Memor. 1:58.

Chambers, R., and B. W. Zweifach. 1947. Intercellular cement and capillary permeability. Physiol. Rev. 27:436–463.

Chien, Shu. 1967. Role of the sympathetic nervous system in haemorrhage. Physiol. Rev. 47:214–288.

Chinard, F. P., and T. Enns. 1954. Transcapillary pulmonary exchange of water in the dog. Am. J. Physiol. 178:197–202.

Chinard, F. P., G. J. Vosburgh, and T. Enns. 1955. Transcapillary exchange of water and of other substances in certain organs of the dog. Am. J. Physiol. 183:221–234.

Chinard, F. P., C. N. Thaw, A. C. Delea, and W. Pearl. 1969. Intrarenal volumes of distribution and relative diffusion coefficients of monohydric alcohols. Circ. Res. 25:343–357.

Chinard, F. P. 1970. In discussion. In C. Crone and N. A. Lassen (eds.), Capillary Permeability, p. 106. Academic Press, New York.

Cobbold, A., B. Folkow, I. Kjellmer, and S. Mellander. 1963. Nervous and local chemical control of precapillary sphincters in skeletal muscle as measured by changes in filtration coefficient. Acta. Physiol. Scand. 57:180–192.

Collander, R., H. Bärlund. 1933. Permeabilitäts-studien an Chara Ceratophylla. Acta Bot. Fennica. 11:1–14.

Crone, C. 1963a. The permeability of capillaries in various organs as determined by the use of the "indicator diffusion" method. Acta Physiol. Scand. 58:292–305.

Crone, C. 1963b. Does "restricted diffusion" occur in muscle capillaries? Proc. Soc. Exp. Biol. Med. 112:453–455.

Crone, C. 1965. Facilitated transfer of glucose from blood into brain tissue. J. Physiol. London 181:103–113.

Crone, C., and N. A. Lassen, eds. 1970. Capillary Permeability. Academic Press, New York.

Denbigh, K. G. 1951. The Thermodynamics of the Steady State. Nethuen & Co., London.

Durbin, R. P., H. Frank, and A. K. Solomon. 1956. Water flow through frog gastric mucosa. J. Gen. Physiol. 39:535–551.

Durbin, R. P. 1960. Osmotic flow of water across permeable cellulose membranes. J. Gen. Physiol. 44:315–326.

Faber, J. J. 1970. The approximate contributions of each of the three cell layers of the rabbit placenta to the total resistance to diffusion. In C. Crone and N. A. Lassen (eds.), Capillary Permeability, pp. 372–393. Academic Press, New York.

Fenstermacher, J. D. 1970. The osmotic flow of water across the blood–brain barrier. In C. Crone and N. A. Lassen (eds.), Capillary Permeability, pp. 434–442. Academic Press, New York.

Flexner, L. B., D. B. Cowie, and G. J. Vosburgh. 1948. Studies of capillary permeability with tracer substances. Cold Spring Harbor Symp. Quant. Biol. 13:88–97.

Folkow, B., and S. Mellander. 1960. Aspects of the nervous control of the precapillary sphincters with regard to capillary exchange. Acta Physiol. Scand. 50(Supplement 1975):52–54.

Gaby, L., and S. Areekul. 1970. Reflection coefficients of neutral and sulphate-substituted dextran molecules in the capillaries of the isolated rabbit ear. In C. Crone and N. A. Lassen (eds.), Capillary Permeability, pp. 560–562. Academic Press, New York.

Gosselin, R. E., and W. O. Berndt. 1962. Diffusional transport of solutes through mesentery and peritoneum. J. Theoret. Biol. 3:487–495.

Gosselin, R. E. 1970. The tissue injection method for assessing capillary permeability. In C. Crone and N. A. Lassen (eds.), Capillary Permeability, pp. 218–227. Academic Press, New York.

Grim, E. 1953. Relation between pressure and concentration difference across membranes permeable to solute and solvent. Proc. Soc. Exp. Biol. Med. 83:195—200.

Guyton, A. C. 1963. A concept of negative interstitial pressure based on pressures in implanted perforated capsules. Circ. Res. 12:399—414.

Guyton, A. C., H. J. Granger, and A. E. Taylor. 1971. Interstitial fluid pressure. Physiol. Rev. 51:527—563.

Hamilton, W. F., J. Walker Moore, J. M. Kinsman, and R. G. Spurling. 1932. Studies on the circulation. 4. Further analysis of the injection method and of changes in haemodynamics under physiological and pathological conditions. Am. J. Physiol. 99:534—551.

Hays, R. M., and A. Leaf. 1962. Studies on the movement of water through the isolated toad bladder and its modification by vasopressin. J. Gen. Physiol. 45:905—919.

Hays, R. M. 1970. Do large pores exist in epithelial cell membranes? In C. Crone and N. A. Lassen (eds.), Capillary Permeability, pp. 509—519. Academic Press, New York.

Hevesy, G., E. Hofer, and S. Krogh. 1935. The permeability of the skin of frogs as determined by D_2O and H_2O. Skand. Arch. Physiol. 72:199—214.

Ingvar, D. H., and N. A. Lassen. 1962. Regional blood flow of the cerebral cortex determined by Krypton 85. Acta Physiol. Scand. 54:325—338.

Intaglietta, M. 1967. Evidence for a gradient of permeability in frog mesenteric capillaries. Bibl. Anat. 9:465—468.

Johnson, J. A. 1970. Reflection coefficients for non-electrolytes in the myocardium. In C. Crone and N. A. Lassen (eds.), Capillary Permeability, pp. 291—292. Academic Press, New York.

Karnovsky, M. J. 1968. The ultrastructural basis of transcapillary exchanges. J. Gen. Physiol. 52:64s—95s.

Karnovsky, M. J. 1970. Morphology of capillaries with special reference to muscle capillaries. In C. Crone and N. A. Lassen (eds.), Capillary Permeability, pp. 341—350. Academic Press, New York.

Katchalsky, A., and O. Kedem. 1962. Thermodynamics of flow processes in biological systems. Biophys. J. 2:53—78.

Kedem, O., and A. Katchalsky. 1958. Thermodynamic analysis of the permeability of biological membranes to non-electrolytes. Biochem. Biophys. Acta 27:229—246.

Kedem, O., and A. Katchalsky. 1961. A physical interpretation of the phenomenological coefficients of membrane permeability. J. Gen. Physiol. 45: 143—179.

Kitchin, A. H. 1963. Peripheral blood flow and capillary filtration rates. Br. Med. Bull. 19:155—160.

Krogh, A. 1929. Anatomy and Physiology of Capillaries. 2nd Ed. Yale University Press, New Haven, Conn.

Krogh, A., E. M. Landis, and A. H. Turner. 1932. The movement of fluid through the human capillary wall in relation to venous pressure and to the colloid osmotic pressure of the blood. J. Clin. Invest. 11:63—95.

Landis, E. M. 1927. Microinjection studies of capillary permeability. 2. The relation between capillary pressure and the rate at which fluid passes through the wall of single capillaries. Am. J. Physiol. 82:217—238.

Landis, E. M. 1934. Capillary pressure and capillary permeability. Physiol. Rev. 14:404—481.

Landis, E. M., and J. R. Pappenheimer. 1963. Exchange of substances through capillary walls. *In* W. F. Hamilton and P. Dow (eds.), Handbook of Physiology and Circulation II, Chapter 29, pp. 961–1034. American Physiological Society, Washington, D. C.

Landis, E. M. 1970. In discussion. *In* C. Crone and N. A. Lassen (eds.), Capillary Permeability, pp. 370–371. Academic Press, New York.

Lassen, N. A., and J. Trap-Jensen. 1968. Theoretical considerations on measurement of capillary diffusion capacity in skeletal muscle by the local clearance method. Scand. J. Clin. Lab. Invest. 21:108–115.

Lewis, P. A. 1916. The distribution of trypan red to the tissues and vessels of the eye as influenced by congestion and early inflammation. J. Exp. Med. 23: 669–676.

Lifson, N. 1970. Revised equations for the osmotic transient method. *In* C. Crone and N. A. Lassen (eds.), Capillary Permeability, pp. 302–305. Academic Press, New York.

Lundgren, O., and S. Mellander. 1967. Augmentation of tissue–blood transfer by transcapillary filtration and absorption. Acta Physiol. Scand. 70:26–41.

Majno, G., and G. E. Palade. 1961. Studies on inflammation. I. The effect of histamine and serotonin on vascular permeability: An electron microscopic study. J. Biophys. Biochem. Cytol. 11:571–605.

Matthews, C. M. E. 1971. Theoretical aspects of radioactive tracer studies. *In* E. H. Blecher and H. Vetter (eds.), Radioisotopes in Medical Diagnosis, pp. 236–257. Butterworth, Reading, Mass.

Mauro, A. 1957. Nature of solvent transfer in osmosis. Science 126:252–253.

Mellander, S., and B. Johansson. 1968. Control of resistance exchange and capacitance function in the peripheral circulation. Pharmacol. Rev. 20:117–196.

Mogensen, C. E. 1970. The permeability of the glomerular capillaries as studied by renal dextran clearance in normal and diabetic subjects. *In* C. Crone and N. A. Lassen (eds.), Capillary Permeability, pp. 530–543. Academic Press, New York.

Newman, E. V., M. Merrell, A. Genecin, C. Monge, W. R. Milnor, and W. P. McKeever. 1951. The dye solution method for describing central circulation. An analysis of factors shaping the time–concentration curves. Circulation 4:735–746.

Onsager, L. 1931. Reciprocal relations in irreversible processes. Phys. Rev. 37:405–426.

Palade, G. E. 1960. Transport in quanta across the endothelium of blood capillaries. Anat. Rec. 136:254.

Palade, G. E. 1961. Blood capillaries of the heart and other organs. Circulation 24:368–384.

Pappenheimer, J. R., E. M. Renkin, and L. M. Borrero. 1951. Filtration, diffusion and molecular sieving through peripheral capillary membranes. A contribution to the pore theory of capillary permeability. Am. J. Physiol. 167:13–46.

Pappenheimer, J. R. 1953. Passage of molecules through capillary walls. Physiol. Rev. 33:387–423.

Pappenheimer, J. R. 1970*a*. Osmotic reflection coefficient in capillary membranes. *In* C. Crone and N. A. Lassen (eds.), Capillary Permeability, pp. 278–286. Academic Press, New York.

Pappenheimer, J. R. 1970*b*. In discussion. *In* C. Crone and N. A. Lassen (eds.), Capillary Permeability, pp. 293–301. Academic Press, New York.

248   Aschheim

Prescott, D. M., and E. Zeuthen. 1952. Comparison of water diffusion and water filtration across cell surfaces. Acta Physiol. Scand. 28:77–94.

Ramsdell, S. G. 1928. The use of trypan blue to demonstrate the immediate skin reaction in rabbits and guinea pigs. J. Immunol. 15:305–311.

Ray, P. M. 1960. On the theory of osmotic water movement. Plant Physiol. 35:783–795.

Renkin, E. M. 1952. Capillary permeability to lipid soluble molecules. Am. J. Physiol. 168:538–545.

Renkin, E. N. 1955. Effect of blood flow on diffusion kinetics in isolated peripheral hindlegs of cats. Am. J. Physiol. 183:125–136.

Renkin, E. M. 1959. Transport of ^{42} potassium from blood to tissue in isolated mammalian skeletal muscle. Am. J. Physiol. 197:1205–1210.

Renkin, E. M., and S. Rosell. 1962. Independent sympathetic vasoconstrictor innervation of arterioles and precapillary sphincters. Acta Physiol. Scand. 54:381–384.

Renkin, E. M. 1964. Transport of large molecules across capillary walls. Physiologist 1:13–28.

Renkin, E. M. 1968. Transcapillary exchange in relation to capillary circulation. J. Gen. Physiol. 52:96s–107s.

Renkin, E. M., and R. M. Sheehan. 1970. Uptake of ^{42}K and ^{86}Rb in skeletal muscle from continuous arterial infusion. In C. Crone and N. A. Lassen (eds.), Capillary Permeability, pp. 310–318. Academic Press, New York.

Rosen, R. 1967. Optimality Principles in Biology. Plenum Press, New York.

Rous, P., and F. Smith. 1931. The gradient of vascular permeability. 3. The gradient along the capillaries and venules of frog skin. J. Exp. Med. 53:219–242.

Rusznyák, I., M. Földi, and G. Szabó. 1967. Lymphatics and Lymph Circulation. Physiology and Pathology. 2nd English Edition, Pergamon, New York.

Sapirstein, L. A. 1958. Regional blood flow by fractional distribution of indicators. Am. J. Physiol. 193:161–168.

Schafer, D. E., and Johnson, J. A. 1964. Permeability of mammalian heart capillaries to sucrose and inulin. Am. J. Physiol. 206:985–991.

Shea, S. M., and M. J. Karnovsky. 1966. Brownian motion: A theoretical explanation for the movement of vesicles across the endothelium. Nature 212:353–355.

Shea, S. M., M. J. Karnovsky, and W. H. Bossert. 1969. Vesicular transport across endothelium. Stimulation of a diffusion model. J. Theoret. Biol. 24:30–42.

Sheppard, C. W., R. R. Overman, W. S. Wilde, and W. C. Sangren. 1953. The disappearance of ^{42}K from the nonuniformly mixed circulation pool in dogs. Circ. Res. 1:284–297.

Sheppard, C. W. 1954. Mathematical considerations of indicator dilution techniques. Minn. Med. 37:93–104.

Sheppard, C. W. 1962. Basic principles of the tracer method. Wiley, New York. p. 202.

Simionescu, N., M. Simionescu, and G. E. Palade. 1975. Permeability of muscle capillaries to small heme-peptides. J. Cell. Biol. 64:586–607.

Skinner, S. M., R. E. Clark, N. Baker, and R. A. Shipley. 1959. Complete solution of the three-compartment model in steady state after single injection of radioactive tracer. Am. J. Physiol. 196:238–244.

Spanner, D. C. 1954. The active transport of water under temperature gradients. Soc. Exp. Biol. Symp. 8:76–93.

Spanner, D. C. 1964. An Introduction to Thermodynamics. Academic Press, New York.

Starling, E. M. 1896. On the absorption of fluid from the connective tissue spaces. J. Physiol. 19:312–326.

Stein, W. D. 1967. The Movement of Molecules Across Cell Membranes. Academic Press, New York.

Strandell, T., and J. T. Shepherd. 1968. The effect in humans of exercise on relationship between simultaneously measured ^{133}Xe and ^{24}Na clearance. Scand. J. Clin. Lab. Invest. 21:99–107.

Tosteson, D. C. 1970. In discussion. *In* C. Crone and N. A. Lassen (eds.), Capillary Permeability, pp. 658–664. Academic Press, New York.

Trap-Jensen, J., and N. A. Lassen. 1970. Capillary permeability for smaller hydrophilic tracers in exercising skeletal muscle in normal man and in patients with long term diabetes mellitus. *In* C. Crone and N. A. Lassen (eds.), Capillary Permeability, pp. 135–152. Academic Press, New York.

Ussing, H. H., and B. Anderson. 1956. The relations between solvent drag and active transport of ions. *In* Proceedings of the International Congress on Biochemistry, 3rd Congress, Brussels, 1955, pp. 434–440.

Vargas, F., and J. A. Johnson. 1964. An estimate of reflection coefficients for rabbit heart capillaries. J. Gen. Physiol. 47:667–677.

Wasserman, K., J. D. Joseph, and H. S. Mayerson. 1956. Kinetics of vascular and extravascular protein exchange in unbled and bled dogs. Am. J. Physiol. 184:175–182.

Wiederhielm, C. A. 1966. Transcapillary and interstitial transport phenomena in the mesentry. Fed. Proc. 25:1789.

Wiederhielm, C. A. 1968. Dynamics of transcapillary fluid exchange. J. Gen. Physiol. 52:29s–61s.

Wilbrandt, W., and T. Rosenberg. 1961. The concept of carrier transport and its corollaries in pharmacology. Pharmacol. Rev. 13:109–183.

Wilhelm, D. L. 1962. The mediation of increased vascular permeability in inflammation. Pharmacol. Rev. 14:251–280.

Yudilevich, D. L., and O. A. Alvarez. 1967. Water, sodium and thiourea transcapillary diffusion in the dog heart. Am. J. Physiol. 213:308–314.

Yudilevich, D. L. 1970. Serial barriers to blood–tissue transport studies by the single injection indicator diffusion technique. *In* C. Crone and N. A. Lassen (eds.), Capillary Permeability, pp. 115–128. Academic Press, New York.

Zierler, K. L. 1963. Theory of use of indicators to measure blood flow and extracellular volume and calculation of transcapillary movement of tracers. Circ. Res. 12:464–471.

Zweifach, B. W. 1939. The character and distribution of the blood capillaries. Anat. Rec. 73:475–495.

Zweifach, B. W., and M. Intaglietta. 1968. Mechanics of fluid movement across single capillaries in the rabbit. Microvasc. Res. 1:83–101.

BIOPHYSICAL ASPECTS
OF MICROCIRCULATION

chapter 11

INTRODUCTION TO BIOPHYSICAL ASPECTS OF MICROCIRCULATION

Yuan-Cheng Fung

The basic idea of biophysics is that the world of living and the world of nonliving are governed by the same laws of physics. The concept is probably correct. Modern success in molecular biology provides the most eloquent testimony to this concept. But since physicists cannot solve very complicated problems, it often appears that biology cannot be handled according to the basic principles of physics. This is true also in microcirculation. Many phenomena in microcirculation are so complex that empirical experimentation still is the only practical approach. Nevertheless, one strives to study the biophysical aspects for two reasons: (1) to understand and to unify the phenomena, (2) to simplify the design and the interpretation of experiments.

In the following chapters we consider biophysical aspects of microcirculation at the continuum level. The basic laws we use are the conservation of mass, the balance of forces, the balance of energy, the second law of thermodynamics, and Maxwell's equations. In addition, we need constitutive equations that describe the physical properties of the medium, such as the stress–strain-history law, Fick's law for diffusion, Starling's hypothesis for membrane, Hill's equation for skeletal muscle contraction (or the modified equations for the heart muscle and the smooth muscles), the equations describing excitable cells, and so on. With these basic laws the motion of the matter in the field can be determined under appropriate boundary conditions. The method we use is that of continuum mechanics. The objective is to understand the flow of blood, the motion of the red blood cells, the deformation of the blood vessels, the flow of water across the vessel wall and in the extravascular space, the pressure–flow relationship in specific organs, waves and transient phenomena in organ systems, the passive and active behavior of vascular smooth muscle, the nervous or myogenic control of blood flow, etc. For these problems the method of continuum mechanics offers a powerful tool for quantitative analysis.

Biophysics pervades every topic discussed in this book. What are singled out in the following chapters are relatively simple basic features of the microcirculation. The physical properties of the blood, the blood cells, and the blood vessels are discussed. The pressure flow relationship and the pulsatile flow in microcirculation are considered in some detail.

Although the principles of biophysics were promulgated by people such as Aristotle, Galileo, Hooke, Helmholtz, and Young, among others, detailed application to microcirculation is a relatively recent endeavor, and much is still in a tentative state. Many areas are yet untouched. It is easy to predict that important development is yet to come.

chapter 12

RED BLOOD CELLS AND THEIR DEFORMABILITY

Yuan-Cheng Fung

HUMAN RED CELL DIMENSIONS AND SHAPE

EXTREME-VALUE DISTRIBUTION

DEFORMABILITY OF THE RED CELLS

ESTIMATION OF THE ELASTIC PROPERTIES
OF RED CELL MEMBRANE

PHYSICAL THEORIES OF THE RED BLOOD CELL

BIBLIOGRAPHICAL NOTES

HUMAN RED CELL DIMENSIONS AND SHAPE

All evidences show that red blood cells (RBCs) are extremely deformable. They take on all kinds of odd shapes in the flowing blood in response to hydro-dynamic stresses acting on them. Yet when flow stops the red cells are seen as biconcave disks. In isotonic Eagle-albumin solution the shape of the red cell is remarkably regular and uniform. We speak of the red cell dimensions and shape in this static condition of equilibrium.

Although a most casual observation of the red cells in a microscope would tell us that they are biconcave disks, an accurate determination of their geometric parameters is not easy. The red cell thickness is comparable with the wavelength of visible light. The diffraction and interference of the light waves imposes serious complications on the measurement of cell dimensions. A rational approach is to describe the red cell geometry by an analytic expression with undetermined coefficients, calculate the image of such a body under a microscope according to the principles of physical optics, then compare the calculated image with the real, photographed image in order to determine the unknown

This work is supported by National Science Foundation Grant Eng-7519401 and GK 31160X and the USPHS NIH National Heart and Lung Institute through Grants HL 12494 and HL 17731.

coefficients. Such a program has been carried out by Evans and Fung (1972). They used an interference microscope to obtain a photograph of the phase shift of light that passes through the red cell in a microscope. They assumed the following formula to describe the thickness distribution of the red blood cell:

$$D(r) = [1 - (r/R_0)^2]^{1/2} [C_0 + C_2(r/R_0)^2 + C_4(r/R_0)^4]$$ (1)

where R_0 is the cell radius, r is the distance from the axis of symmetry, and C_0, C_2, C_4, and R_0 are numerical coefficients to be determined. The phase image corresponding to Eq. (1) is determined according to the principle of microscopic holography. The parameters C_0, C_2, C_4, and R_0 are determined by a numerical process of minimization of errors between the calculated and photographed images. It was possible in this way to determine the geometric dimensions of the red cell to within 0.02 μ. Hence a resolution of 0.5–1% for the cell radius and 1% for the cell thickness is achieved. The resolution of the cell surface area and cell volume are 2 and 3% respectively.

Results obtained by Evans and Fung (1972) for the red cells of a 30-yr-old male are shown in Tables 1 through 4. The cells were suspended in Eagle-albumin solution (Gregersen et al., 1967) at three different tonicities (osmolarity). At 300 mOsm the solution is considered isotonic. At 217 mOsm it is hypotonic. At 131 mOsm the red cells became spheres. In these tables the standard deviations of the samples are listed in order to show the spread of the statistical sample. The sample size was only 50 or 55.

Figure 1 shows the cross-sectional shape and other geometric data of the average RBC from Evans and Fung (1972). It is seen that the thickness is most sensitive to the environmental tonicity changes; the surface area is the least. It is remarkable that the average surface area of the cell remained constant during the initial stages of swelling (300–217 mOsm). The volume of the cell increases as the tonicity decreases. The χ^2 statistics data in Tables 1–4 show that the distribution of the maximum and minimum thickness and the volume are the closest to being normal for each tonicity. Since these geometric properties are functionally related, it is not possible for all of them to have normal distribution. For example, if the volume of a spherical cell is normally distributed, then the radius is not.

A more extensive collection of data based on the interferometric method named above was made by Tsang (1975). Figure 2 and Table 5 show the data from blood samples of 14 healthy subjects (graduate students and faculty from UCSD) with a total of 1,581 cells. Classification according to races, sexes, and ages showed no significant difference.

A comparison of the data obtained by the interferometric method with those of Ponder (1948) and others is given in Table 6. Unfortunately, there are so many variables that were not maintained constant that a meaningful comparison is impossible. For example, Ponder (1948) used autologous serum as the suspending medium and photographed the cells on edge to obtain a resolution of

Table 1. Statistics of 50 RBC at 300 mOsm, suspended in Eagle-albumin solution at pH 7.4. From Evans and Fung (1972)

	Diameter	Minimum thickness	Maximum thickness	Surface area	Volume
Average M_1	$7.82\ \mu$	$0.81\ \mu$	$2.58\ \mu$	$135\ (\mu)^2$	$94\ (\mu)^3$
Standard deviation σ	$\pm0.62\ \mu$	$\pm0.35\ \mu$	$\pm0.27\ \mu$	$\pm16\ (\mu)^2$	$\pm14\ (\mu)^3$
2nd mom. M_2	3.77×10^{-1}	1.20×10^{-1}	7.13×10^{-2}	2.46×10^2	2.02×10^2
3rd mom. M_3	2.19×10^{-1}	-2.51×10^{-3}	3.26×10^{-4}	3.58×10^3	2.11×10^3
4th mom. M_4	4.81×10^{-1}	3.22×10^{-2}	1.73×10^{-2}	2.16×10^5	1.59×10^5
Skewness G_1	0.97	-0.063	0.018	0.96	0.76
Kurtosis G_2	0.57	-0.70	0.58	0.75	1.11
χ^2 for 10 groups	35.1	10.2	8.2	22.1	18.7

Table 2. Statistics of 55 RBC at 217 mOsm. From Evans and Fung (1972)

	Diameter	Minimum thickness	Maximum thickness	Surface area	Volume
Average M_1	7.59 μ	2.10 μ	3.30 μ	135 $(\mu)^2$	116 $(\mu)^3$
Standard deviation σ	±0.52 μ	±0.39 μ	±0.39 μ	±13 $(\mu)^2$	±16 $(\mu)^3$
2nd mom. M_2	2.66×10^{-1}	1.56×10^{-1}	1.59×10^{-1}	1.57×10^2	2.40×10^3
3rd mom. M_3	5.54×10^{-1}	1.02×10^{-2}	1.45×10^{-2}	-5.76×10^1	-1.25×10^3
4th mom. M_4	3.96×10^{-1}	8.82×10^{-2}	5.26×10^{-2}	1.21×10^5	2.07×10^5
Skewness G_1	0.41	0.17	0.26	-0.03	-0.35
Kurtosis G_2	2.98	0.80	-0.62	2.21	0.78
χ^2 for 10 groups	18.6	4.0	7.2	10.0	6.37

Table 3. Statistics of RBC at 131 mOsm. From Evans and Fung (1972)

	Diameter	Surface area	Volume	Index of refraction difference
Average M_1	6.78 μ	145 $(\mu)^2$	164 $(\mu)^3$	0.0447
Standard deviation σ	±0.32 μ	±14 $(\mu)^2$	±23 $(\mu)^3$	±0.0043
2nd mom. M_2	1.01×10^{-1}	1.84×10^2	5.34×10^2	1.82×10^{-5}
3rd mom. M_3	2.83×10^{-3}	4.42×10^2	3.29×10^3	8.83×10^{-9}
4th mom. M_4	2.31×10^{-2}	7.83×10^4	6.77×10^5	9.60×10^{-10}
Skewness G_1	0.09	0.18	0.28	0.12
Kurtosis G_2	−0.68	−0.63	−0.56	0.02
χ^2 for 10 groups	18.5	15.9	14.2	10.5

260   Fung

Table 4. Shape coefficients for the average RBC.
From Evans and Fung (1972)

Tonicity (mO)	R_0 (μ)	C_0 (μ)	C_2 (μ)	C_4 (μ)
300	3.91	0.81	7.83	−4.39
217	3.80	2.10	7.58	−5.59
131	3.39	6.78	0.0	0.0

about 0.25 μ for the dimensions of the cell. Canham and Burton (1968) also used the method of photographing a red cell hanging on edge in a sessile drop. Evans and Fung (1972) used Eagle-albumin solution. Tsang (1975) used Tris-buffered Ringer's solution. A comprehensive study to evaluate the influence of these parameters on the red cell geometry is needed, but has not yet been done. Older data obtained by many authors prior to 1948 can be found in Ponder (1948).

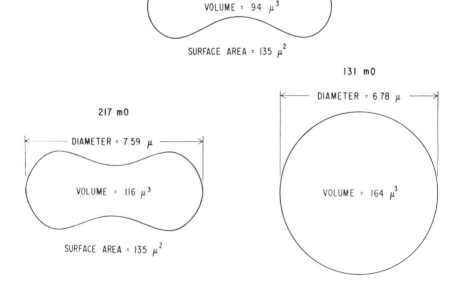

Figure 1. Scaled cross-sectional shape of the average RBC and other geometrical data of Evans. From Evans and Fung (1972), reprinted by permission.

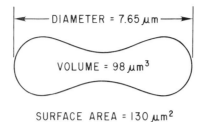

SURFACE AREA = 130 μm²

Figure 2. The average human red cell. From Tsang (1975), 14 subjects, N = 1581. Reprinted by permission.

EXTREME-VALUE DISTRIBUTION

One of the most dramatic features of microcirculation when it is observed in vivo is the unsteadiness of the flow. The red cells are seen to flow off and on, sometimes crowded together, sometimes with space far in between. This is principally due to the pulsation of the heart. But there are stochastic features superposed on the pulsatile flow. To analyze the stochastic features, it is necessary to know the statistical distribution of the dimensions of blood vessels, erythrocytes, leucocytes, and other cellular bodies, and the branching pattern of the small blood vessels. Since the largest resistance to flow in a capillary blood vessel comes from the largest cells, it is meaningful to ask the question: How large is the largest red blood cell in a blood sample? The answer obviously depends on the size of the sample, but cannot be obtained reliably by the ordinary procedure of adding a multiple of standard deviation to the mean. To assess the extreme velue in a large sample, one has to use the statistical distribution of extreme values. The theory of statistics of extremes is a well-developed subject. E. J. Gumbel (1954, 1958) has consolidated the theory in a book. He made many applications of the theory to such problems as the

Table 5. The geometric parameters of human red blood cells. Statistics of pooled data from 14 subjects; sample size N = 1581

	Diameter (μ)	Minimum thickness (μ)	Maximum thickness (μ)	Surface area (μ^2)	Volume (μ^3)	Sphericity index
Mean $\bar{X}$	7.65	1.44	2.84	129.95	97.91	0.792
Std. error of mean	0.02	±0.01	±0.01	±0.40	±0.41	±0.001
Std. dev. σ	0.67	0.47	0.46	15.86	16.16	0.055
Min. value	5.77	0.01	1.49	86.32	47.82	0.505
Max. value	10.09	3.89	4.54	205.42	167.69	0.909
Skewness G_1	0.26	0.46	0.52	0.53	0.30	−1.13
Kurtosis G_2	1.95	1.26	0.24	0.90	0.30	3.27

From Tsang, 1975.

Table 6. Comparison of normal red blood cell geometric data[a] in the literature

Source	Diameter (μ)	Minimum thickness (μ)	Maximum thickness (μ)	Surface area (μ^2)	Volume (μ^3)	Sphericity index	Sample size
Ponder (1948)	8.50 ± 0.41	1.02 ± 0.08	2.40 ± 0.13	152.0	112.0	0.74	5 subjects, 50–100 cells each
Houchin, Munn, and Parnell (1958)	8.28		1.71^b	134.0	82.0	0.69	2,177 cells
Canham and Burton (1968)	8.07 ± 0.55			138.1 ± 17.4	107.5 ± 16.8	0.783 ± 0.026	7 subjects excluding newborn, 1,016 cells
Chien, Usami, Dellenback, and Bryant (1971)	8.40		1.6^b	152.0	90.0	0.64	At least 6 individuals
Evans and Fung (1972)	7.82 ± 0.62	0.81 ± 0.35	2.58 ± 0.27	135 ± 16	94 ± 14	0.742	1 subject, 50 cells
Tsang and Fung (1975)	7.65 ± 0.67	1.44 ± 0.47	2.84 ± 0.46	129.95 ± 15.86	97.91 ± 16.16	0.792 ± 0.055	14 subjects, 1,581 cells

[a]Values listed are mean ± standard deviation whenever available.
[b]Thickness of RBC was measured from side view of rouleaux and, hence, represented mean thickness.

prediction of flood and drought, rain and snow, fatigue strength of metals, gust loading on aircraft, quality control in industry, oldest age in a population, etc. His method has been used by Chen and Fung (1973) to study the red blood cells.

The method may be briefly described as follows: Take a random sample of blood consisting of, say, 100 red cells. By visual observation under an interference microscope, select and measure the diameter of several, say, 5, largest red cells. Rank the cells according to their diameter; then we know the largest diameter in 100 cells, the second largest diameter, the third largest diameter, etc. Throw away this sample; take another sample of 100 red cells, and repeat the process. In the end we obtain a set of data on the largest diameter in every 100, the second largest in every 100, etc. From this set of data we can determine the ordered statistics, and predict the probable largest diameter in a large sample of, say, 10^9 cells.

It is fortunate that the asymptotic formula for the distribution of the largest among n independent observations turns out to be the same for a variety of initial distributions of the *exponential type,* which includes the exponential, the Laplace, the Poisson, the normal, the chi-square distribution, the so-called logistic distribution, and the logarithmically transformed normal distribution. In these distributions the variates are unlimited toward the right, and the probability functions $F(x)$ converge with increasing x toward unity at least as quickly as an exponential function. The distribution of the diameter of red cells is most likely of the exponential type (past publications usually claim it to be approximately normal; see, for example, Ponder, 1930; Houchin, Munn, and Parnell, 1958; Canham and Burton, 1968), and hence we have great confidence in the validity of the extreme distribution. This was found to be the case by Chen and Fung (1973).

According to Gumbel (1954), the probability that the largest value in a sample of size n will be equal to or less than a certain value x is given by

$$F(x) = e^{-e^{-y}} \tag{2}$$

where

$$y = \alpha(x - u) \tag{3}$$

and α, u, are parameters depending on n. The probability density function corresponding to Eq. (2) is

$$\Phi(x) = \alpha e^{-y - e^{-y}}. \tag{4}$$

The parameter u is the *mode,* and is the most probable value of x. The inverse of the parameter α is a measure of dispersion, called the *Gumbel slope.* These parameters are determined by the following formulas:

$$\frac{1}{\alpha} = \frac{S\sqrt{6}}{\pi} \tag{5}$$

$$u = \bar{x} - \frac{0.57722}{\alpha} \tag{6}$$

where $\bar{x}$ is the mean and S is the standard deviation of the extreme variate. The variable y is dimensionless and is called the *reduced largest value*. For a continuous variate there is a probability $1 - F(x)$ for an extreme value to be equal to or exceeded by x. Its reciprocal

$$T(x) = \frac{1}{1 - F(x)} \qquad (7)$$

is called the *return period,* and is the number of observations required so that, on the average, there is one observation equalling or exceeding x.

Gumbel (1954, 1958) has reduced the procedure of testing the goodness of fit of the mathematical formula to any specific set of observed data, as well as the evaluation of parameters α and u, to a simple graphical method. He constructed a probability paper for extreme values in which the reduced largest value y, the cumulative probability $F(x)$, and the return period $T(x)$, are labeled on the abscissa while the variate x is labeled linearly on the ordinate. (Such graph paper is made available in King, 1971) The entire set of n observed largest values is plotted to this paper in the following manner: List all the data points in order of their magnitude, x_1 being the smallest, x_m the mth, x_n the largest. Plot x_m against a cumulative probability

$$\bar{F}_m = \frac{m}{n + 1} \qquad . \qquad (8)$$

If the theoretical formula (2) applies, the data plotted should be dispersed about a straight line,

$$x = u + \frac{y}{\alpha}. \qquad (9)$$

The intercept and the slope of the fitted straight line give us the parameters u and α. Having this straight line, we can find the expected largest value corresponding to any desired large return period T from the reduced variate:

$$y = \log_e T(x). \qquad (10)$$

Chen and Fung (1973) used the method of superresolution of microscopic holograph (Evans and Fung, 1972) discussed in the first section of this paper to obtain the dimensions of the red cells.

The experimental results of four subjects in the age range of 22–29 yr are summarized in Table 7. A typical extreme-value plot for subject DV is shown in Figure 3. Within the 95% confidence limit it can be seen that the distribution of the largest diameter follows the theoretical asymptote for the exponential type of initial distribution. The Gumbel slope is relatively constant for all the subjects. When compared to the study of normal blood samples, the large cells have a larger surface area and volume, the minimum thickness is higher, the maximum thickness remains approximately the same, and the sphericity is lower. A correlation study shows that for the most probable largest cell in a sample of size n, the cell surface area and the minimum thickness are proportional to the cell diameter. The maximum thickness seems independent of the

Table 7. Distribution of diameter, area, volume, maximum thickness, minimum thickness, sphericity index of the cells with the largest diameter in samples of size 100 cells each. From Chen and Fung (1973)

Subject	PC	JP	DV	MY
Sex	M	M	M	M
No. of samples	55	36	35	37
Mode (μ) of largest diameter	9.083	9.372	9.386	9.168
Gumbel slope $(1/\alpha)$ of largest diameter	0.5204	0.5255	0.4548	0.5314
Area	175.34	184.42	182.00	178.01
(μ^2) ±SD	±20.21	±20.29	±14.25	±20.37
Volume	119.87	129.08	132.38	130.03
(μ^3) ±SD	±17.45	±17.37	±16.81	±19.64
Maximum thickness	2.367	2.449	2.456	2.510
(μ) ±SD	±0.281	±0.217	±0.249	±0.229
Minimum thickness	0.751	1.086	0.9716	1.0281
(μ) ±SD	±0.358	±0.318	±0.2815	±0.314
Sphericity index	0.6711	0.6703	0.6907	0.6979

cell diameter. The sphericity index decreases with increasing cell diameter. There is no correlation between cell volume and cell diameter for the largest cell.

Figure 4 shows a comparison between a mean cell from Evans and Fung (1972) and an extreme cell from Chen and Fung (1973). The difference in cell shape is quite evident.

If we predict the size of the largest cell in a population of 10^8 cells, then for subject PC we obtain an impressive value of 15.66–17.06 μ for its diameter, as compared with the mean value of 7.65 μ; i.e., the largest cell's diameter is more than twice that of the average.

The same technique can be used to study the smallest red cell in a given sample, but there seems to be no reason to do so. However, a study of the smallest cross section of a blood vessel may have meaning. We can think of many biological variables whose extreme values are of interest. The method deserves to be widely known.

DEFORMABILITY OF THE RED CELLS

In flowing through capillary blood vessels the red cells are so highly deformed that they give an impression of great flexibility. See Figure 5. The order of magnitude of the stresses that correspond to such a large deformation may be estimated as follows. Assume that a capillary 500 μ long contains 50 RBC and has a pressure drop of 2 cm H_2O. Then the pressure drop is about 0.04 g/cm^2 per RBC. Imagine that the RBC is deformed into the form of a cylindrical plug with an end area of 25 μ^2 and a lateral area of 90 μ^2. The axial thrust 0.04 × 25 ×

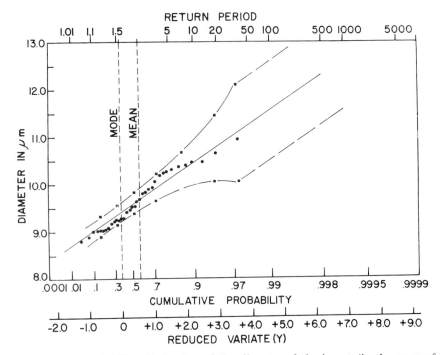

Figure 3. The probability distribution of the diameter of the largest (in the sense of diameter) red blood cell in sample batches of 100 cells each from healthy male graduate students.

10^{-8} g is resisted by the shear force of $\tau \times 90 \times 10^{-8}$ acting on the lateral area. Then the shear stress τ is of the order of $0.04 \times 25/90 = 0.01$ g/cm^2, or 10 dynes/cm^2. Such a small stress field is sufficient to induce a deformation with a stretch ratio of the order of 200% in some places on the cell membrane. This stress level may be compared with the "critical shear stress" of about 420 dynes/cm^2, which Fry (1968, 1969) has shown to be causing changes in the endothelial cells. It may also be compared with the "shearing" stress of about 50–1,020 dynes/cm^2 acting at the interface between a leucocyte and an endo-

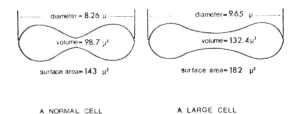

Figure 4. Comparison between a normal red blood cell from Evans and Fung (1972) and an extreme cell from Chen and Fung (1973).

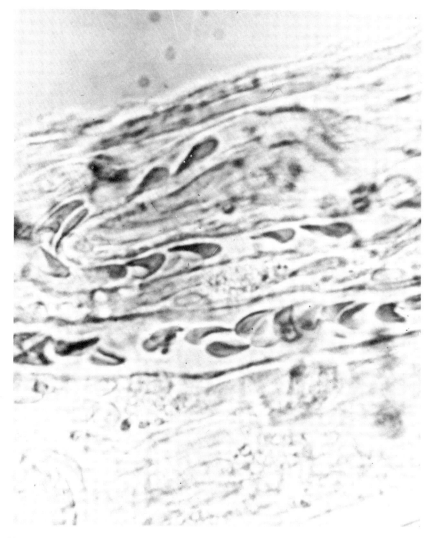

Figure 5. A photograph of the blood flow in the capillary blood vessels in the mesentery of a dog, showing the deformation of the red cells. Courtesy of Dr. Ted Bond.

thelium when the leucocyte is adhering to or rolling on the endothelium of a venule (Schmid-Schönbein, Fung, and Zweifach, 1975).

Red cell deformation can be demonstrated also in Couette flow and in Poiseuille flow (Schmid-Schönbein and Wells, 1969; Hochmuth, Marple, and Sutera, 1970). In fact, one of the successful calculations of the viscosity of the hemoglobin solution inside the RBC was made by Dintenfass (1968) under the assumption that the cell membrane behaves as a liquid–liquid interface, with surface tension but no resistence to bending. He calculated the viscosity of the RBC contents to be about 6 cp. Experiments by Cokelet and Meiselman (1968) and Schmidt-Nielsen and Taylor (1968) on red cell contents, obtained by fracturing the cells and removing the cell membrane, yielded about the same value. Thus one might infer that the red cell does behave mechanically more or less like a liquid droplet.

There are other ways to demonstrate the deformability of red cells; some can yield an estimate of the elastic constants of the cell membrane. Hochmuth, Mohandas, and Blackshear (1970) observed the motion and stretching of a red cell that is tethered to a glass slide and subjected to a fluid flow over the slide. By computing the shear stress due to viscosity and the deformation of the cell, they arrived at certain modulus of elasticity of the membrane (see the estimation of the elastic properties of the membrane, below). Gregersen et al. (1967) forced blood to flow through the pores of a sheet of polycarbonate sieves and showed that human red cell can flow through a circular cylindrical tube with a diameter as small as 2.9 μ. If the red cells were forced to flow through tubes less than 2.9 μ in diameter, substantial hemolysis occurs.

The basic reason for the great deformability of the red cells is that they are flaccid. In mathematical terms, Fung (1966) showed that the biconcave geometry of the red cells endows them the capability to take on an infinite variety of transformations that are *isochoric* (equal volume), and *applicable* (a term in the theory of differential geometry indicating a deformation without changing the length of elements in any direction anywhere). For a cell with membranes as thin as 30–100 Å the bending stress would be very small. If bending stresses are neglected, an isochoric and applicable transformation induces no stress in the cell membrane at all. The contents of the red cell being liquid (or liquid crystal) implies that in slow deformation there is no resistance to changing from one configuration to another isochoric, applicable configuration. Resistance to deformation will be encountered only if the boundary conditions are such that the RBC has to deform into a nonapplicable shape (for example, in a very small capillary blood vessel with diameter smaller than that of the RBC). In those "off-design" conditions the cell membrane would be stressed.

In this light we observe that many regular geometric shapes such as a sphere, an ellipsoid, a circular cylinder, etc., do not enjoy many isochoric applicable transformations. A sphere cannot deform isochorically without stretching its surface somewhere. If a spherical cell is forced to deform, its cell membrane would be stressed. Thus even if we do not know how the biconcave shape of the RBC comes about, we do know that it has tremendous advantage: it endows great flexibility to the red cells to enable them to flow through large and small blood vessels with virtually no stress in the cell membrane. Thus with the biconcave geometry, nature made red cells strong by making them flexible.

ESTIMATION OF THE ELASTIC PROPERTIES OF RED CELL MEMBRANE

The outstanding feature of the red cell membrane is that it is capable of large deformation with little change in surface area. This fact has been observed for a long time and elaborated by Ponder (1948). The data shown in the first section of this chapter tell us that the red cell membrane is not unstretchable, but that even when the cell is sphered in a hypotonic solution the increase of surface area is only 7.5% of the normal.

A second remarkable feature is that the shape of the red cell at equilibrium in a hydrostatic field is extremely regular. Stress and strain history experienced by the red cell does not seem to affect the regular cell shape in equilibrium. This suggests that the cell membrane may be considered elastic.

Based on these observations, several stress–strain relationships for the red cell membrane have been proposed. It was shown by Fung and Tong (1968) that for a two-dimensional generalized plane-stress field in an isotropic incompressible material, under the general assumption that the stress is an analytic function of the strain, the most general stress–strain relationship may be put in the form

$$\sigma_1 = \frac{E}{1 - \nu^2} \; (e_1 + \nu e_2) \tag{11}$$

$$\sigma_2 = \frac{E}{1 - \nu^2} \; (e_2 + \nu e_1)$$

where E and ν are elastic constants that are functions of the strain invariants,

$$e_1 + e_2, \quad e_1 e_2, \tag{12}$$

σ_1, σ_2 are the principal stresses referred to the principal coordinate axes x_1, x_2; and e_1, e_2, are the principal finite strain components. Equation (11), although it has the appearance of the familiar linear law, is actually nonlinear since E and ν do not remain constant.

There are several alternative ways to define the strain tensor. If Green's strains are used, then the principal strains can be expressed in terms of the principal stretch ratios λ_1, λ_2:

$$e_1 = \tfrac{1}{2} (\lambda_1^2 - 1), \quad e_2 = \tfrac{1}{2} (\lambda_2^2 - 1) \tag{13}$$

where λ_1 is the quotient of the changed length of an element in the principal direction (corresponding to the principal strain e_1) divided by the original, relaxed length of that element; λ_2 is the stretch ratio corresponding to e_2.

If the membrane can be distorted, λ_1 and λ_2 can assume arbitrary numbers. If the area cannot be changed, then $\lambda_1 \lambda_2 = 1$. If the membrane material is incompressible, then $\lambda_1 \lambda_2 \lambda_3 = 1$, where λ_3 denotes the stretch ratio of elements in the direction perpendicular to the membrane. It follows that if the area of an incompressible membrane cannot change, then the thickness of the membrane must remain constant, $\lambda_3 = 1$. The reverse is also true. Since the red cell membrane changes its area very little in ordinary deformation, we conclude that its membrane thickness does not change when the cell deforms (except possibly when hemolysis is approached).

The quasilinear form, Eq. (11), is convenient because there exists a large stock of classical solutions in the linearized theory of elasticity, which might be applicable to the red cell problem. The linearized solutions, each valid in a small area, may be joined to obtain a valid solution of the whole cell. But, in order explicitly to express the idea that the red cell membrane can be stretched but cannot change its area easily, it is better to put the stress–strain relation in a different form. Skalak et al. (1973) proposed the following:

$$\sigma_1 = \frac{\lambda_1}{\lambda_2} \left[\frac{B}{2} (\lambda_1^2 - 1) + \frac{C}{2} \lambda_2^2 I_2 \right]$$

$$\sigma_2 = \frac{\lambda_2}{\lambda_1} \left[\frac{B}{2} (\lambda_2^2 - 1) + \frac{C}{2} \lambda_1^2 I_2 \right] \tag{14}$$

$$I_1 = \lambda_1^2 + \lambda_2^2 - 2$$

$$I_2 = \lambda_1^2 \lambda_2^2 - 1$$

where σ_1, σ_2 are the principal stress components, and B and C are constants. Here I_2 is clearly related to the areal strain. If C is much larger than B, then the areal stiffness is much larger than the stiffness against uniaxial stretching.

The first estimate of the elastic modulus of the red cell membrane was given by Katchalsky et al. (1960) based on sphering experiments in a hypotonic solution. The estimated value of the elastic modulus during the spherical phase of the cell and just before hemolysis is 3.1×10^7 dynes/cm^2 (as corrected by Skalak et al., 1973). The general range of this estimate was confirmed by Rand and Burton (1964) based on experiments in which red cells were sucked into micropipettes of the order of $2\ \mu$ in diameter. Rand and Burton gave the range of the moduli 7.3×10^6 to 3.0×10^8 dynes/cm^2. More recently, Hochmuth and Mohandas (1972) have reported experiments in which red blood cells adhering to a glass surface were elongated due to shearing stress applied by the flow of the suspending fluid over the cells. Their estimate of the modulus of elasticity is of the order of 10^4 dynes/cm^2. In another type of test in which the deformed cells were allowed to recover their natural shape, Hoeber and Hochmuth (1970) gave a value 7.2×10^5 dynes/cm^2. Skalak et al. (1973) observed that the elongation in sphering and pipette experiments that give the higher estimates is about 8%; that in the uniaxial tests giving the lowest modulus is 40–60%. They therefore suggest that the lower values are appropriate for the constant B, the higher values are appropriate for the constant C. If the thickness of the cell membrane is assumed to be 50 Å, then $B = 10^4$ dynes/cm^2 and $h = 50$ Å gives a value $hB = 0.005$ dynes/cm, whereas $C = 10^7$ dynes/cm^2 and $h = 50$ Å gives $hC = 5$ dynes/cm.

Evans (1973b) has analyzed the deformation of the red blood cell under the very simple hypothesis that there is no area change of the membrane. He has shown by micropipette experiments that hemolysis may result if area change exceeds 3.5%. Evans (1974), Evans and La Celle (1975), Evans and Simon (1975), and Evans and Hochmuth (1976a,b) have studied the visoelasticity and viscoplasticity of the red cell membrane, and determined the breaking strength of the membrane, as well as the bending moments.

PHYSICAL THEORIES OF THE RED BLOOD CELL

One of the most remarkable features of the red blood cells is the regularity of their geometry in hydrostatic equilibrium. On the one hand, we may say that this is the way nature makes red cells. We are impressed, but not surprised, because we see great regularity in many things in the biologic world. But scientiest are forever asking the question of whether there are other bases for this regular biconcave shape. Could this be due to nonuniformity in surface tension between the cell membrane and the surrounding solution? Could the electric charge on the cell, or the electric doublet layer (corresponding to the membrane potential) be responsible for the biconcave geometry? How do the mosaic theory and the theory of fluid-like cell membrane explain the red cell mechanical properties? Could there be some special molecular structure of the cell membrane, or some mathematical minimization principles that could explain this geometric property?

These questions have led to several interesting investigations, each adding some new understanding to the behavior of the red cell, but the complete answer is probably yet to come.

Fung and Tong (1968) presented a rigorous mathematical solution of the sphering of a red cell under the assumptions that the red cell is a fluid-filled shell and that it can swell into a perfect sphere in an appropriate hypotonic medium. That a red cell can sphere is a well-known fact (see the first section of this chapter). Fung and Tong's idea is that not all fluid-filled shells can become spheres under an internal pressure (e.g., a pair of rubber gloves cannot), therefore the capability to sphere tells us something about the structure of the membrane. They assumed that the cell membrane is elastic, obeying a stress–strain law given in the Eq. (11). They assumed that a surface tension (due to the membrane–fluid interface) acts on the membrane. Electric forces are ignored. They determined the cell geometry as a function of the internal pressure and reached the conclusion that if a red cell can sphere, then the parameter $(1 - \nu)(pa - 2\gamma)/(2Eh)$ cannot be a constant throughout the sphered cell. Here E and ν are the elastic constants of Eq. (11), h is the cell membrane thickness, p is the internal pressure of the cell, a is the radius of the sphered red cell, and γ is the surface tension. Moreover, if the ratio of the diameter of the sphered cell to that of the equator of the normal biconcave cell is less than unity (according to experiments of Evans and Fung, 1972, this ratio is 0.867 for human red cell), then near the equator the surface tension γ must be greater than $pa/2$, whereas near the axis of symmetry the reverse must be true. Therefore a nonuniform surface tension would be required, with surface tension reduced near the poles (i.e., the dimples). The numerical value of γ required, however, is very small, of the order of 0.04 dynes/cm, if p is of the order of 0.23 cm H_2O as estimated by Rand and Burton (1964).

This calculation is unsatisfying because the resulting requirement is so stringent, although Murphy's (1965) discovery that cholesterol in the red cell is concentrated around the equator does lend support to the possibility that a nonuniform distribution of elasticity and surface tension does exist.

Skalak et al. (1973) repeated the calculation with the elasticity law given in Eq. (14). They started with a cell that was biconcave in shape with a thickness distribution described by Eq. (1) when the internal pressure is zero, and then calculated the cell deformation when the internal pressure was gradually increased. The surface tension was neglected. In the limiting case in which $B = 0$, they showed that a biconcave cell can always be deformed into a sphere, (but not isochoric, see section above on the estimation of membrane elastic properties). If $B > 0$, the cell gradually bulges out with increasing internal pressure p. If $C \gg B$ and p is sufficiently high, the cell approaches a spherical shape.

Since in hypotonic sphering of a red cell whether the cell becomes an exact sphere or not is of no great concern, the analysis of Skalak et al. (1973) is convincing. They have replaced the stringent requirements of Fung and Tong (1968) by removing the condition of perfect sphere as the end point of the sphering process.

So far the effect of electric charges on the red cell has been neglected. If electricity is responsible for the biconcave shape, one might be able to explain the regularity in geometry with greater ease. Lopez, Duck, and Hunt (1968) first presented a calculation in which the red blood cell is regarded as a perfectly conducting liquid droplet, and the surrounding fluid (plasma) as an insulator. They set out to compute the equilibrium shape of such a drop in its own electric field, and found that, besides spheres, the biconcave cell is a solution. Lew (1970, 1972), on the other hand, considered the cell membrane as an insulating layer carrying fixed charges at fixed sites and enveloped by conducting fluids on both sides. The ions in the plasma and in the cell form a doublet layer at the membrane. Lew (1972) showed that such a membrane would exhibit elastic resistance to stretching and bending (i.e., the elasticity of the membrane has an electric origin). Since ions are free to move in the fluids, the strength of the doublet layer depends on the geometry of the membrane. Through Maxwell's equation, he determined the charge distribution and the equilibrium shape of the cell. He was able to show that a whole family of cell shapes from biconcave to sphere evolves as internal pressure is changed.

Much earlier, there is a theory by Hartridge (1919) which says that the shape of the red cell is a compromise between a sphere and a disk which is peculiarly adapted to a rapid and even diffusion of gas from its periphery toward its interior. Ponder (1925) elaborated on this idea and showed that the biconcave surface is a surface of equivelocity-potential to a ring, so that if diffusing molecules were started off simultaneously at the membrane, they would all reach the ring at the same time. These theories show that the biconcave shape is good for more than one reason.

An interesting mathematical theory was given by Canham (1970), who showed that if the integral

$$I = \pi D \int_0^a \left(\frac{1}{R_1^2} + \frac{1}{R_2^2} \right) \, x \, dx,$$

where D and a are constants, and

$$\frac{1}{R_1} = \frac{y''}{(1 + y'^2)^{3/2}}, \qquad \frac{1}{R_2} = \frac{y'}{x(1 + y'^2)^{1/2}},$$

is minimized with respect to the class of curves

$$y(x) = B \left\{ (C^4 + 4A^2 x^2)^{1/2} - A^2 - x^2 \right\}^{1/2}$$

by varying the constants B, A, and C, subjected to the side conditions of appropriate constant volume and area, the solution turns out to look very much like the red blood cell. Canham explained the integral I as the strain energy of bending of the cell membrane. Therefore his theory identifies the normal red cell geometry with the minimization of the bending strain energy of the cell membrane.

Cahham's identification of the integral I as the bending energy is based on an analogy with a result in the theory of elastic plates, and is valid only if the cell is a flat plate when it is unstrained. It is not valid if the unstrained cell is a curved surface.

If we think of the cell membrane as composed of a continuum of isotropic homogeneous elastic material so hat the same constitutive equation applies for bending as for stretching (as in the ordinary theory of plates and shells), then Canham's neglect of the stretching energy versus the bending energy is unacceptable. For a shell made of an isotropic material the relative importance of bending versus stretching was discussed by Fung (1966). It can be shown that in deforming a thin plate of diameter 8 μ and wall thickness 100 Å into a biconcave shell like a red cell, the strain energy for stretching is so much larger than that for bending that the latter is completely negligible.

Nevertheless, Brailsford and Bull (1973) succeeded in constructing a "membrane" model that does exactly what Canham's theory needs. They took a number of U-shaped staples, inserted the legs of three staples into a short length of small plastic tubing to produce a joint that is rigid with respect to bending but free to rotate. Proceeding from one leg to another, a complete network of hexagonal pattern can be constructed. If such a network is made into a sphere with every hexagon regular, the completed sphere can be gently collapsed into a flat circular disk. Such a model resists bending. It does not resist stretching unless the hexagons are regular and the stretching load is uniform in every direction. When Brailsford and Bull (1973) wrapped a spherical shell made of such a "membrane" in a piece of Saran wrap (a thin, clear, plastic sheet) and sucked out the air gradually, the shell deformed gradually into an ellipsoid, a biconcave cell, and finally, flat disk. Reinflation reversed the sequence.

Such an interesting invention cannot fail to rouse speculation that the real red cell membrane is made this way (Bull and Brailsford, 1973). In continuum mechanics, there is a theory of micropolar material (theory of couplestress, the Cosserat theory) that can account for a membrane with the properties postulated by Canham (1970) and constructed by Bull and Brailsford (1973). Further development in this direction can be expected.

Finally, the recent advent of the fluid lipid–globular protein mosaic model of cell membrane by Lenard and Singer (1966, 1968), Wallach and Zahler (1966), Glaser et al. (1970), and Singer (1971) and others, would certainly influence the theories on red cells. In exactly which way, however, remains to be seen. For a most stimulating article on this subject, see Singer (1973).

Evans (1973a,b, 1974), Evans and La Celle (1975), Evans and Simon (1975), and Evans and Hochmuth (1975a,b) have constructed a cell membrane theory consistent with Singer's concept, but relying on the protein substructure under the lipid layer for elasticity and plasticity of the membrane. They were able to obtain the estimates of a full set of elastic, viscoelastic, and viscoplastic constants, as well as the failure strength of the cell membrane.

BIBLIOGRAPHICAL NOTES

The discussion of red blood cells and their deformability presented above is extremely brief and does not do justice to the literature. Therefore, in the bibliography below, selected additional references are presented on topics that are passed over lightly or even omitted in the text. In this selection, preference is given to review articles where a large bibliography can be found. This is done in the interest of brevity.

Hemolysis of red blood cells occurs when the deformation becomes too great. Phenomena that occur at hemolysis are discussed in papers by Baker (1964), Blackshear et al. (1965), Blackshear (1972), Kochen (1966), Ponder (1937, 1948).

The geometry of red cells and other cells in the blood and blood-forming organs is presented in the following references: Bessis (1956), Brånemark and Lindström (1963), Guest et al. (1963), and Teitel (1965).

The way a red cell acquires its shape at its birth is discussed in Simpson and Kling (1967).

For osmotic equilibrium, see Dick and Lowenstein (1958).

A large literature exists on the electric charges on red blood cells. Some account relevant to the topics discussed in this chapter is given in Elul (1967), Jan and Chien (1973), Jay and Burton (1969).

Further references on the deformability of red blood cells are given in Miller, Chien, and Usami (1972), and Moffatt and Harris (1971), Bull (1972). Hochmuth et al. (1973), Rand (1967), Singer (1972), Singer and Nicolson (1972), and Skalak (1973).

LITERATURE CITED

Baker, R. F. 1964. The fine structure of stromalytic forms produced by osmotic hemolysis of red blood cells. J. Ultrastruct. Res. 11:494–507.

Bessis, M. 1956. Cytology of the Blood and Blood-Forming Organs. Grune and Stratton, New York.

Blackshear, P. L., Jr. 1972. Mechanical hemolysis in flowing blood. In Y. C. Fung, N. Perrone, and M. Anliker (eds.), Biomechanics: Its Foundations and Objectives. Prentice-Hall, Englewood Cliffs, N.J.

Blackshear, P. L., Jr., F. D. Dorman, and J. H. Steinbach. 1965. Some mechanical effects that influence hemolysis. Trans. Am. Soc. Artif. Int. Org. 11: 112–117.

Brånemark, P. I., and J. Lindström. 1963. Shape of circulating blood corpuscles. Biorheology 1:139–142.

Brailsford, J. D., and B. S. Bull. 1973. The red cell—A macromodel simulating the hypotonic sphere isotonic disk transformation. J. Theoret. Biol. 39: 325–332.

Bull, B. S. 1972. Red cell biconcavity and deformation—a macromodel based on flow chamber observation. Nouv. Rev. Francaise Hematol. 12:835–844.

Bull, B. S., and J. D. Brailsford. 1973. A new method of measuring the deformability of the red cell membrane. Blood 45:581–586.

Canham, P. B. 1970. The minimum energy of bending as a possible explanation of the biconcave shape of the human red blood cell. J. Theoret. Biol. 26: 61–81.

Canham, P. B., and A. C. Burton. 1968. Distribution of size and shape in populations of normal human red cells. Circ. Res. 22:405–422.

Chen, P., and Y. C. Fung. 1973. Extreme value statistics of human red blood cells. Microvasc. Res. 6:32–43.

Cokelet, G. R., and H. J. Meiselman. 1968. Rheological comparison of hemoglobin solutions and erythrocyte suspensions. Science 162:275–277.

Dick, D. A. T., and L. M. Lowenstein. 1958. Osmotic equilibrian in human erythrocytes by immersion refractometry. Proc. Roy. Soc. London, Ser. B 149:241–256.

Dintenfass, L. 1968. Internal viscosity of the red cell and a blood viscosity equation. Nature 219:956–958.

Elul, R. 1967. Fixed charges in the cell membrane. J. Physiol. (London) 189: 351–365.

Evans, E. A. 1973. A new material concept for the red cell membrane. Biophys. J. 13:926–940.

276   Fung

Evans, E. A. (1973b). New membrane concept applied to the analysis of fluid shear- and micropipette-deformed red blood cells. Biophys. J. 13:941–954.

Evans, E. A. 1974. Bending resistance and chemically induced moments in membrane bilayers. Biophys. J. 14:923–931.

Evans, E., and Y. C. Fung. 1972. Improved measurements of the erythrocytes geometry. Microvasc. Res. 4:335–347.

Evans, E. A., and P. L. La Celle. 1975. Intrinsic material properties of the erythrocyte membrane indicated by mechanical analysis of deformation. Blood 45:29–43.

Evans, E. A., and S. Simon. 1975. Mechanics of bilayer membrane. J. Colloid Interface Sci. 51:266–271.

Evans, E. A., and R. M. Hochmuth. 1976a. Membrane viscoelasticity. Biophys. J. 16:1–12.

Evans, E. A., and R. M. Hochmuth. 1976. Membrane viscoplastic flow. Biophys. J. 16:13–26.

Fry, D. L. 1968. Acute vascular endothelial changes associated with increased blood velocity gradients. Circ. Res. 22:165–197.

Fry, D. L. 1969. Certain histological and chemical responses of the vascular interface to acutely induced mechanical stress in the aorta of the dog. Circ. Res. 24:93–108.

Fung, Y. C. 1966. Theoretical considerations of the elasticity of red cell and small blood vessels. Fed. Proc. 25:1761–1772.

Fung, Y. C., and P. Tong. 1968. Theory of the sphering of red blood cells. Biophys. J. 8:175–198.

Glaser, M., H. Simpkins, S. J. Singer, M. Sheetz, and S. I. Chan. 1970. On the interactions of lipids and proteins in the red blood cell membrane. Proc. Nat. Acad. Sci. U.S. 65:721–728.

Gregersen, M. I., C. A. Bryant, W. E. Hammerle, S. Usami, and S. Chien. 1967. Flow characteristics of human erythrocytes through polycarbonate sieves. Science 157:825–827.

Guest, M. M., T. P. Bond, R. G. Cooper, and J. R. Derrick. 1963. Red blood cells: Change in shape in capillaries. Science 142:1319–1321.

Gumbel, E. J. 1954. Statistical theory of extreme value and some practical applications. National Bureau of Standards. Applied Math. Series 33, pp. 1–51. Superintendent of Documents, Washington, D.C.

Gumbel, E. J. 1958. Statistics of Extremes. Columbia University Press, New York.

Hartridge, H. 1919. Shape of red blood cells. J. Physiol. 53:lxxxi, (Abstr.).

Hochmuth, R. M., R. N. Marple, and S. P. Sutera. 1970. Capillarly blood flow. 1. Erythrocyte deformation in glass capillaries. Microvasc. Res. 2:409–419.

Hochmuth, R. M., and N. Mohandas. 1972. Uniaxial loading of the red-cell membranes. J. Biomech. 5:501–510.

Hochmuth, R. M., N. Mohandas, and R. L. Blackshear, Jr. 1973. Measurement of the elastic modulus for red cell membrane using a fluid mechanical technique. Biophys. J. 13:747–762.

Hoeber, T. W., and R. M. Hochmuth. 1970. Measurement of red blood cell modulus of elasticity by in-vitro and model cell experiments. Trans. ASME, Ser. D., J. Basic Eng. 92:604.

Houchin, D. W., J. I. Munn, and B. L. Parnell. 1958. A method for the measurement of red cell dimensions and calculation of mean corpuscular volume and surface area. Blood 13:1185–1191.

Jan, K. M., and S. Chien. Role of surface electric charge in red blood cell interactions. J. Gen. Physiol. 61:638–654.

Jay, A. W. L., and A. C. Burton. 1969. Direct measurement of potential difference across the human red blood cell membrane. Biophys. J. 9:115–121.

Katchalsky, A., O. Kedem, C. Klibanshy, and A. De Vries. 1960. Rheological considerations of haemolysing red blood cell. In A. L. Copley and Ct. Stainsby (eds.), Flow Properties of Blood and other Biological Systems, pp. 155–171. Pergamon Press, New York.

Kochen, J. A. 1966. Visco-elastic properties of the red cell membrane. In Proceedings of the First International Conference on Hemorheology, Iceland. Pergamon Press, New York.

Lenard, J., and S. J. Singer. 1966. Protein conformation in cell membrane preparations. Proc. Natl. Acad. Sci. U.S.A. 56:1828–1835.

Lenard, J., and S. J. Singer. 1968. Structure of membranes: Reaction of red cell membranes to phospholipase C. Science 159:738–739.

Lew, H. S. 1970. Effect of membrane potential on the mechanical equilibrium of biological membrane. J. Biomech. 3:569–582.

Lew, H. S. 1972. Electro-tension and torque in biological membranes modeled as a dipole sheet in fluid conductors. J. Biomech. 5:399–408.

Lopez, L. I. M. Duck, and W. A. Hunt. 1968. On the shape of the erythrocyte. Biophys. J. 8:1228–1235.

Miller, L. H., S. Chien, and S. Usami. 1972. Decreased deformability of *Plasmodium Coatneyi* infected red cells and its possible relation to cerebral malaria. Am. J. Trop. Med. Hyg. 21:133–137.

Moffatt, E. A., and E. H. Harris. 1971. The effect of the contents of the human red blood cell on its deformability. Paper No. 71-WA/BHF-1. American Society of Mechanical Engineers.

Murphy, J. R. 1965. Erythrocyte metabolism. VI. Cell shape and the location of cholesterol in the erythrocyte membrane. J. Lab. Clin. Med. 5:756–774.

Ponder, E. 1925. The inhibitory effect of blood serum on hemolysis. Proc. Roy Soc. London Ser. B. 98:484–493; Quart. J. Exp. Physiol. 15:235; Quart. J. Exp. Physiol. 16:173.

Ponder, E. 1930. Measurement of diameter of erythrocytes. V. the relation of diameter to thickness. Quart. J. Exp. Physiol. 20:29–39.

Ponder, E. 1937. The physical structure of the red cell membrane with special reference to its shape. Trans. Faraday Soc. 33:947.

Ponder, E. 1948. Hemolysis and Related Phenomena. Grune & Stratton, New York.

Rand, R. P. 1967. Some biophysical considerations of the red cell membrane. Fed. Proc. 26:1780–1784.

Rand, R. P., and A. C. Burton. 1964. Mechanical properties of the red cell membrane I. Membrane stiffness and intracellular pressure, II. Viscoelastic breakdown of the membrane. I, Biophys. J. 4:115–135; II, Biophys. J. 4:303–316.

Schmidt-Nielsen, K., and C. R. Taylor. 1968. Red blood cells: Why or why not? Science 162:274–275.

Schmid-Schönbein, G. W., Y. C. Fung, and B. W. Zweifach. 1975. Vascular Endothelium-Leukocyte Interaction: Sticking Shear Force in Venules. Circulation Research, 36:173–184.

Schmid-Schönbein, H., and R. E. Wells. 1969. Fluid drop-like transition of erythrocytes under shear. Science 165:288–291.

Simpson, C. F., and J. M. Kling. 1967. The mechanism of denucleation in circulating erythroblasts. J. Cell Biol. 35:237–245.

Singer, S. J. 1971. *In* L. I. Rothfield (ed.), Structure and Function of Biological Membranes, p. 145. Academic Press, New York.

Singer, S. J. 1972. A fluid lipid-globular protein mosaic model of membrane structure. Ann. N.Y. Acad. Sci. 195:16–23.

Singer, S. J. 1973. Architecture and topography of biological membranes. Hosp. Practice 8:81–90.

Singer, S. H., and G. L. Nicolson. 1972. The fluid mosaic model of the structure of cell membranes. Science 175:720–731.

Skalak, R. 1973. Modeling the mechanical behavior of red blood cells. Biorheology 10:229–238.

Skalak, R., A. Tozeren, R. P. Zarda, and S. Chien. 1973. Strain energy function of red blood cell membranes. Biophys. J. 13:245–264.

Teitel, P. 1965. Disk-sphere transformation and plasticity alteration of red blood cells. Nature 204:409–410.

Tsang, W. C. O. 1975. The size and shape of human red blood cells. M. S. Thesis. University of California, San Diego.

Wallach, D. F. H., and P. H. Zahler. 1966. Protein fonformation in cellular membranes. Proc. Natl. Acad. Sci. U.S. 56:1552–1559.

chapter 13

RHEOLOGY OF
BLOOD IN MICROVESSELS

Yuan-Cheng Fung

THE CONCEPT OF BLOOD VISCOSITY

The Newtonian concept of viscosity is related to a constitutive equation that relates stress with strain rate for an isotropic incompressible fluid:

$$\sigma_{ij} = -p\delta_{ij} + 2\mu \, \dot{e}_{ij} \tag{1}$$

$$\dot{e}_{ij} = \frac{1}{2}\left(\frac{\partial u_i}{\partial x_j} + \frac{\partial u_j}{\partial x_i}\right), \quad \dot{e}_{ii} = 0. \tag{2}$$

Here σ_{ij} is the stress tensor, $\dot{e}_{ij}$ is the strain-rate tensor, u_i is the velocity component, δ_{ij} is the isotropic tensor or Kronecker delta, p is the hydrostatic pressure, and μ is a constant called the *coefficient of viscosity;* the indices i, j range over 1, 2, 3, and the components of the tensors and vectors are referred to a set of rectangular Cartesian coordinates x_1, x_2, x_3. A fluid obeying Eqs. (1)

This work is supported by National Science Foundation Grant Eng-7519401 and the USPHS NIH National Heart and Lung Institute through Grant HL 12494 and HL 17731.

and (2), with a constant μ, is called an isotropic, incompressible, *Newtonian fluid.*

The question arises whether blood obeys Eq. (1). The answer is that it does not. When experimental results of blood flow in long circular cylindrical tubes or in a Couette-flow viscometer (concentric rotating cylinders) are reduced, it is found that they do not fit Eq. (1); but they do fit reasonably well a constitutive equation that is similar to Eq. (1), in which μ is not a constant, but varies with the strain rate. An illustration is shown in Figure 1. Thus blood is said to be *non-Newtonian.* Similar experiments do verify, however, that normal plasma alone is Newtonian. Therefore the non-Newtonian feature of whole blood comes from the cellular bodies in the blood.

Red blood cells have finite size, can form aggregates, and can be hardened by artificial means. The non-Newtonian features of the whole blood depend, therefore, on the hematocrit, the size of the aggregates, the size of the blood vessel or testing equipment, the hardness of the cells, the viscosity of the plasma, and, if any, the abnormality of the plasma and the blood cells.

If the blood vessel (or a test equipment) is very large compared with the red blood cells, then blood may be regarded as a homogeneous fluid in such a vessel.

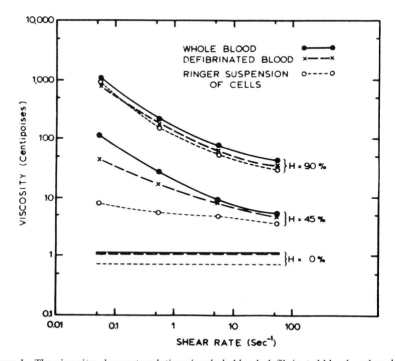

Figure 1. The viscosity–shear-rate relations in whole blood, defibrinated blood, and washed cells in Ringer at 0, 45, and 90% red cell concentrations. From Chien, Usami, Taylor, Lundberg, and Gregersen, J. Appl. Physiol. 21:81–87, 1966; reprinted with permission.

In a shear flow at high strain rate in such a large vessel, the red blood cells deform and elongate in the direction of the streamlines. Then the coefficient μ tends to a constant. In other words, at a high shear strain rate (say, when $\dot{\gamma} >$ 100 sec^{-1}) blood behaves as if it were a linear viscous fluid with a constant coefficient of viscosity. Even then, the cell concentration may be stratified in the vessel, and the coefficient of viscosity may vary with the location in the flow field.

If the strain rate decreases to zero, it is conceivable that the entire body of blood may become one large aggregate. In that case one may expect that blood will exhibit the behavior of a plastic solid with a finite yield stress. Below the yield point it will behave like an elastic solid, beyond the yield point it flows as a viscous fluid. This is an attractive idea, but the experimental evidences are still debated.

An empirical formula often quoted for blood viscosity in a large vessel is the so-called Casson's equation (Casson, 1958). We may express it in the following form: Within a moderate range of shear strain rate (a range to be discussed below), the constitutive equation of blood may be given by Eq. (1), with the coefficient of viscosity μ given by the expression

$$\mu = \frac{[(\tau_y)^{\frac{1}{2}} + b\,(\dot{\gamma})^{\frac{1}{2}}]^2}{\dot{\gamma}} \tag{3}$$

where τ_y and b are constants that depend on the hematocrit and other factors named above. For a general, three-dimensional flow, $\dot{\gamma}$ may be interpreted as the square root of the second invariant of the strain-rate tensor,

$$\dot{\gamma} = 2\,(\dot{e}_{ij}\,\dot{e}_{ij})^{\frac{1}{2}}. \tag{4}$$

The summation convention is used in this formula: a repeated index means summation over its range, 1, 2, and 3. With Eq. (3) substituted for μ, Eq. (1) describes the constitutive equation of whole blood. The constant τ_y is interpreted as a yield stress, which is of the order of 0.05 dynes/cm^2 (Cokelet, 1963; Merrill et al., 1963; Charm and Kurland, 1962, 1974). The constants τ_y and b depend on hematocrit, cell aggregate size, temperature, etc.

In a simple shear flow, in which the only nonvanishing velocity component is u_1 and the only nonvanishing component of the strain-rate tensor is $\dot{e}_{12} = \frac{1}{2}$ $(\partial u_1/\partial x_2)$, Eqs. (1)–(4) can be greatly simplified. Let us write x_2 as y, u_1 as u, σ_{12} as τ, and $2\dot{e}_{12}$ as $\dot{\gamma}$. Then Eq. (1) becomes

$$\tau = \mu\dot{\gamma} \tag{5}$$

whereas the Casson equation becomes

$$(\tau)^{\frac{1}{2}} = (\tau_y)^{\frac{1}{2}} + b(\dot{\gamma})^{\frac{1}{2}}. \tag{6}$$

These simpler, more familiar equations, however, are not sufficient for application to the analysis of more complex, three-dimensional blood-flow problems.

For the latter purposes, a generalization, such as those embodied in Eqs. (1)–(4), is necessary.

Equation (3) is not valid when $\dot{\gamma} = 0$. To how small a value of $\dot{\gamma}$ Eq. (3) remains a reasonable representation is a point of debate in the literature. See Cokelet (1972), Chien et al. (1967a,b), and Chien (1972).

The transition from Eq. (3) to the Newtonian equation, μ = constant, depends on the hematocrit H (the volume fraction of red blood cells in whole blood). For a normal blood with a low hematocrit $H = 8.25\%$, μ appears to be constant over the entire range of shear rate from 0.1 to 1,000 $\sec^{-1}$. When $H = 18\%$, the blood appears to be Newtonian when $\dot{\gamma} > 600 \sec^{-1}$, but obeys Eq. (3) for smaller $\dot{\gamma}$. For higher H the transition point increases to $\dot{\gamma} \cong 700 \sec^{-1}$. See Cokelet (1972, p. 76).

An excellent review by Cokelet (1972) discusses the problems of measurement of blood viscosity, the nonlinear features, and the parameters that influence the viscosity. A comprehensive book by Dintenfass (1971) presents data on pathologic changes in plasma and blood rheology. Chien (1972) presents a cogent review of the blood rheology from the point of view of its microscopic structure. Charm and Kurland (1972, 1974) offer extensive reviews of blood rheology. These reviews are clear and concise, and quite up-to-date. There is no need to repeat their contents here. We turn, therefore, to the question of relevance of such measurements to microcirculation.

The question of relevance arises because Eq. (1) is a concept of macroscopic continuum, and is applicable only to those problems in which the characteristic dimensions are so large that the fine structure of the fluid is completely hidden. A characteristic dimension of the fine structure of blood is the diameter of the red blood cell. The dimension of the viscometer is much larger than that of the red cell; hence Eq. (1) is applicable to viscometry of the blood. The diameter of the aorta is much larger than that of the red cell; Hence Eq. (1) again is applicable. For blood flow in a large blood vessel, the only region where the homogeneous continuum concept may be questioned is at the interface with the wall. In the immediate neighborhood of the wall, the interaction between the blood and the wall necessarily causes rotation, translation, and deformation of the red blood cells. A thorough analysis of the boundary conditions between the blood and the wall must consider the motion of individual blood cells, and therefore, must forego the homogeneous fluid concept.

Turning our attention to the capillary blood bessels, we notice that their diameter is about the same as that of the red blood cell. To a capillary blood vessel, the red cells are not small; they are large; they have to deform and squeeze in order to pass. A red cell interacts with the wall of a capillary very differently from the way it interacts with the wall of a viscometer. This difference accounts for the difficulty in applying the viscometric data to the analysis of microcirculation.

If blood cannot be represented by a homogeneous Newtonian or nonNew-tonian fluid of the usual kind, is there a way to describe it as a homogeneous fluid with a more complex property? The answer is ambiguous. In continuum mechanics, there is a theory of "couple stress" and "micropolar" material, which generalizes the constitutive equation to include materials not describable in ordinary terms. There are a number of proponents (Cowin, 1968; Valanis and Sun, 1969; Kline and Allen, 1970; Ariman, Turk, and Sylvester, 1973) who believe that blood can be described by the micropolar theory. They show that the micropolar theory can predict the Fahraeus–Lindqvist effect (see below) without explicitly considering the distribution of hematocrit. The hematocrit becomes a hidden variable in this theory. However, there are three difficulties to this approach: (1) To determine the large number of material constants in the constitutive equation of a micropolar fluid requires extensive and refined experi-ments that have not been performed. (2) How to determine the appropriate boundary conditions at the blood–endothelium interface is a task of such obvious difficulty that no definitive experiments have been proposed. (3) In principle, a micropolar theory can hold only in large blood vessels, although it is in the microvessels that an acute demand exists to account for the rotation and the nonuniform distribution of red blood cells. In the narrow, capillary blood vessels whose diameter is comparable with that of the red cells the micropolar theory is useless.

In conclusion, it is seen that there are circumstances in which it is necessary to regard the cellular bodies as individual entities in microcirculation. This approach requires more detailed analyses, but also reveals more details about blood flow. This last approach is used by most investigators in microcirculation.

APPARENT VISCOSITY AND RELATIVE VISCOSITY

The difficulty mentioned at the end of the preceding section makes the rheology of blood in microcirculation a very distinctive subject. It is different from the ordinary macroscopic rheology. Some details are discussed in subsequent sec-tions. In the present section we consider two intermediate terms that are introduced to help organize experimental data, namely, the *apparent viscosity* and the *relative viscosity*. To explain their meaning, consider a flow through a circular cylindrical tube. If the fluid is Newtonian and the flow is laminar, we have the Hagen–Poiseuille formula,

$$\frac{\Delta p}{\Delta L} = \frac{8\mu}{\pi a^4} \dot{Q} \tag{7}$$

where Δp is the pressure drop in a length ΔL, μ is the coefficient of viscosity of the fluid, a is the radius of the tube, and $\dot{Q}$ is the volume rate of flow. Now if we let blood flow through this tube, we can measure $\Delta p/\Delta L$ and $\dot{Q}$, and use Eq. (7)

to calculate a coefficient μ. The μ so computed is defined as the *apparent coefficient of viscosity for the circular cylindrical tube,* and is denoted by μ_{app}. If μ_0 denotes the viscosity of plasma, then the ratio μ_{app}/μ_0 is defined as the *relative viscosity,* and denoted by μ_r. Note that the unit of apparent viscosity is (force·sec/area), or poise, whereas the relative viscosity is dimensionless.

The concept of relative viscosity can be generalized to an organ system. To measure the relative viscosity of blood in such a system we perfuse it with plasma and measure the pressure drop Δp corresponding to a certain flow $\dot{Q}$. We then perfuse the same system with whole blood and again measure the pressure drop at the same flow. The ratio $\Delta p/\dot{Q}$ for the whole blood divided by $\Delta p/\dot{Q}$ for the plasma is the *relative viscosity* μ_r.

Note that the concept of apparent viscosity can be extended to any flow regime, including turbulent flow, as long as we can compute it from a formula that is known to work for a homogeneous Newtonian fluid. On the other hand, the relative viscosity can be extended to any flow system, even if we do not know its structural geometry and elasticity, as long as flow and pressure can be measured. Neither μ_{app} nor μ_r needs to be constant. They are functions of all the dimensionless parameters defining the kinematic and dynamic similarities, and, if the system is nonlinear, of pressure p and the flow $\dot{Q}$.

There are as many definitions for apparent viscosities as there are good formulas for well-defined problems. Examples are Stokes flow around a falling sphere, channel flow, flow through an orifice, flow in a cylindrical tube.

It is clear that apparent and relative viscosities are not intrinsic properties of the blood; they are properties of the blood, the blood vessels, and the data reduction procedure.

Examples of blood flow in single tubes are discussed in Chapter 16 of this volume.

Another example is the blood flow through the network of capillary blood vessels of the pulmonary alveolar septa (sheets), for which a theory was presented by Fung and Sobin (1969). With dimensional analysis it can be shown that the pressure gradient in an alveolar sheet at a small Reynolds number (10^{-4} to 10^{-2}) can be presented in the form

$$\text{grad } p = -\frac{\mu U}{h^2} k\left(\frac{w}{h}\right) f\left(S, \frac{h}{\epsilon}, \frac{\epsilon}{a}, \theta, N_R \cdots\right) \tag{8}$$

where p is pressure, μ is the apparent coefficient of viscosity, U is the mean velocity of flow, h is the sheet thickness, k is a dimensionless function of the ratio of width of the sheet, w, to the sheet thickness h, and f is the so-called geometric friction factor, which is a dimensionless number defined by the *vascular-space–tissue ratio* S (the percentage of area, in a plane view of the pulmonary alveolar sheet, occupied by the capillary blood vessels) the thickness-to-postal-diameter ratio h/ϵ, the ratio of post diameter, ϵ, to interpostal distance,

a, the direction of flow θ, the Reynolds number $N_R = \rho\, Uh/\mu$, and whatever other dimensionless parameters defining the configuration of the flow. The function k is defined by the flow of a homogeneous Newtonian fluid in a vessel with a rectangular cross section, and is well known in fluid mechanics (Purday, 1949). When $h/w < 0.2$, it is given by the equation

$$k \doteq 12\left(1 - 0.630\frac{h}{w}\right)^{-1}. \tag{9}$$

The function f has been analyzed by Lee (1969) for flow of a homogeneous viscous fluid in a lung alveolar model at low Reynolds number ($N_R \ll 1$). In adopting Lee's result to our experiment, we must decide to which factor we shall attribute the effects of cellular bodies, as represented by the hematocrit, the ration of the cell diameter to the sheet thickness, the elasticity of the red blood cells, etc. In Yen and Fung (1973), f is defined for the plasma (a Newtonian fluid in normal blood), and all effects of red cells are included in the apparent coefficient of viscosity μ.

This rather complex example is quoted here to show that (1) the definition of apparent viscosity is not unique and (2) it may not be simple. The selection of each particular definition depends on how useful it is for the purpose at hand, and how much light it throws on the problem. To complete the example, we may quote Yen and Fung (1973), who experimented on a scale model of the pulmonary alveolar sheet, with the red blood cells simulated by soft gelatin pellets and with the plasma simulated by a silicone fluid. Their results show that the pressure–flow relationship is quite linear, and that for $h/\epsilon < 4$, the relative viscosity is a function of the hematocrit (Hct):

$$\mu_{\text{relative}} = 1 + a\,\text{Hct} + b\,\text{Hct}^2. \tag{10}$$

Thus the apparent viscosity is

$$\mu_{\text{blood in alv}} = \mu_{\text{plasma}}\,(1 + a\,\text{Hct} + b\,\text{Hct}^2). \tag{11}$$

These relations are illustrated in Figure 2, where the values of the constants a and b are listed.

DIFFERENCE BETWEEN FLOW OF
BLOOD IN LARGE BLOOD VESSELS AND THAT IN MICROVESSELS

The introduction of the apparent viscosity and relative viscosity satisfies the needs for organizing experimental data and for practical clinical applications. It remains to understand these coefficients. It is obvious that if we know how these coefficients depend on the red blood cells, capillary blood vessels, plasma, and other factors, and if we can estimate their values theoretically or empirically, then circulatory physiology can be related to these factors, and many phenomena would be understood at a more basic level. This objective has not been

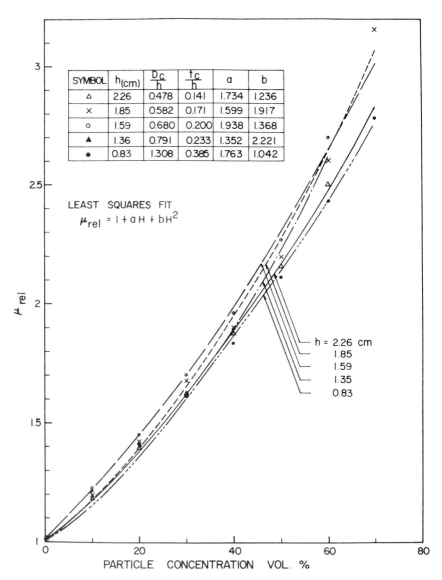

Figure 2. The relative viscosity of a simulated whole blood (gelatin pellets in silicone oil) in a pulmonary alveolar model. Here D_c is the diameter of the red cell, h is the thickness of the alveolar sheet, t_c is the thickness of the red blood cell, and a and b are constants in Eq. (8). The model is so large that h is in centimeters although in a real lung h is only a few microns. From Yen and Fung (1973); reprinted with permission.

achieved yet. It is, however, worthwhile to discuss the general biophysical considerations in this direction.

We may begin by asking whether there is a fundamental difference between hemodynamics of large blood vessels and hemodynamics of capillaries, other than the obvious differences in size. The answer is yes, and is basically a matter of balance of forces. When Newton's law is applied to a fluid, the equation of motion obtained is

Density X acceleration = divergence of shear stresses − gradient of pressure. (12)

The three terms in this equation are not always of equal importance. For pulsatile blood flow in the large blood vessels, the inertia and pressure forces predominate and the shear stress term is sometimes negligible. For pulsatile blood flow in the capillaries the convective inertia is negligible and the shear and pressure terms balance each other. In either of these extreme cases the mathematical problem is considerably simplified because one of these three terms can be treated in an approximate manner. The case in the middle, in which the inertia, pressure, and shear terms are equally important, occurs at the level of terminal arteries and small venous tributaries, for which the mathematical problem is truly difficult.

The basic consequence of the difference in the relative magnitudes of the inertial, shear, and pressure forces in arteries and capillaries is exhibited by the equations governing the pulsatile flow in these vessels. (See Chapter 17). When the equations of motion are combined with the equations describing the conservation of mass and energy, the resulting mathematical expression for pulsatile flow in arteries is reducible to a wave equation—mathematically the same kind of equation that governs the vibrations in pianos and organs. On the other hand, the pulsatile flow in capillaries is reduced to a diffusion equation—the kind that governs the diffusion of mass in a fluid or conduction of heat in a solid. Many features of capillary blood flow differ from those of arterial flow because of this difference. Let us name two examples: (1) Arterial waves can be propagated without much attenuation. In fact, with certain conditions of tapering and reflection at the terminals, the wave amplitude can increase downstream. In contrast to this, oscillations in capillary blood flow are generally attenuated in the direction of propagation in a manner with which we are familiar in case of conduction of heat. (2) If a large vein is subjected to a transmural pressure that is positive at the entry of flow but is negative at the exit end where the vein can be collapsed, a self-excited oscillation may occur. Such an oscillation, known as flutter, is well known in the Starling resistor—a thin-walled rubber tube used by Starling (1918) in his first heart–lung preparation. In capillaries such flutter has not been observed. Experiments with water flowing through a penrose tubing show high-frequency oscillations in a flow at large Reynolds number (>100). However, experiments with the same tubing with a highly viscous fluid flowing through it so that the Reynolds number of flow was as small as that in the capillaries (<0.01) do not show self-excited flutter, even though the tube was buckled under external pressure.

The parameter that gives a measure of the relative importance of the inertia force versus the viscous force is the Reynold number:

$$\text{Reynold number} = R_n = \frac{VL\rho}{\mu} = \frac{VL}{v} \tag{13}$$

where V is a characteristic velocity, L is a characteristic length, ρ is the fluid density, μ is the fluid viscosity, and $v = \mu/\rho$ is the kinematic viscosity of the fluid. In the case of blood flow in arteries we may take V to be the mean speed of flow, L to be the tube diameter. If Reynolds number is greater than 1, the inertia force dominates; if it is less than 1, the viscosity force dominates. The most useful way to deduce the meaning of the Reynolds number is to reduce the Navier–Stokes equation into a dimensionless form. On the other hand, a qualitative, heuristic derivation may be useful: In a flow the convective acceleration arises from terms such as $u(\partial u/\partial x)$; the inertia force per unit volume is, therefore, $\rho u(\partial u/\partial x)$. The shear stress arises from terms such as $\mu(\partial u/\partial y)$. The viscous force per unit volume is, therefore, $(\partial/\partial y)[\mu(\partial u/\partial y)]$. The order of magnitude of these terms is, respectively,

$$\text{inertia force:} \quad \rho V^2/L,$$
$$\text{viscous force:} \quad \mu V/L^2.$$

The ratio is

$$\frac{\text{inertia force}}{\text{viscous force}} = \frac{\rho V^2/L}{\mu V/L^2} = \frac{\rho VL}{\mu} = \text{Reynolds number.} \tag{14}$$

For blood flow in human arteries, the Reynolds number is about 2,500 in the aorta, 10 in the terminal arteries, 0.03 in the arterioles, 0.0001–0.01 in the capillaries, 0.01 in venules, 10 in small veins, and 2,100 in the venae cavae. It is about 2,000 in pulmonary artery, and 10^{-2} to 10^{-4} in pulmonary capillaries. Thus Reynolds number varies over a wide range in our circulation system; microcirculation, however, is mostly concerned with low-Reynolds-number flow.

For flow with Reynolds number less than 1, it is expected that the pressure drop in a vascular system will be proportional to the viscosity of the fluid and the rate of flow. If the Reynolds number is greater than 1, then the pressure drop should consist of two terms: one proportional to the product $\eta \dot{Q}$ representing friction loss along the wall, another proportional to velocity squared or $\dot{Q}^2$, representing pressure loss due to convection turbulence, secondary flow, perturbation at branching points, sharp curvature, local constriction, etc. That such must be the case was pointed out a long time ago by the English physician and physicist, Thomas Young, in 1808. Young made use of theoretical reasoning and model testing data on rivers, hydraulic channels, and tubings to make some remarkably accurate predictions about microcirculation.

But Young's teaching had been forgotten (in physiology), and when Benis et al. (1973) showed that in the perfusion of isolated hindpaw of the dog, the pressure drop is best represented by the expression

$$\Delta p = A\mu\dot{Q} + B\dot{Q}^2 \tag{15}$$

many objections were raised. It is true that the hindpaw is a complex organ and the experiments of Benis et al. (1973) leave a number of questions unanswered, but in principle Eq. (15) should be valid, because in hindpaw the Reynolds number of the flow is not limited to less than 1.

THE FAHRAEUS–LINDQVIST EFFECT

On the arterial side blood flows from a larger blood vessel into smaller blood vessels. Two phenomena affect the apparent viscosity in this case;

1. The hematocrit changes when the blood enters into the smaller vessel.
2. The cell deformation varies with the tube diameter, so that the resistance to the motion of individual cells changes.

It is useful to consider these phenomena in some detail.

Fahraeus (1929) pointed out that when blood of a constant hematocrit is allowed to flow from a large feed reservoir into a small tube, the hematocrit in the tube decreases as the tube diameter decreases. Fahraeus observed this trend for human blood in tubes down to 50 μ diameter. Barbee and Cokelet (1971), by an extensive series of experiment on human blood, showed that the trend continues down to 29-μ tubes.

As to the resistance to blood flow in small blood vessels, Fahraeus and Lindqvist (1931) showed that at high flow rates where the pressure drop is proportional to the flow rate, the calculated apparent viscosity of the human blood decreases as the tube diameter decreases from 500 to 50 μ. Barbee and Cokelet (1971) showed that the Fahraeus–Lindqvist effect can be explained by the Fahraeus effect when the tube diameter is 29 μ or larger (mean diameter of human red cells is about 7.6 μ; see Chapter 12). In other words, if one measures the apparent viscosity of blood in a large tube (say, 1 mm diameter) as a function of the hematocrit, then the data can be used to compute the apparent viscosity of the same blood in a smaller tube, provided that the actual hematocrit in the smaller tube be used. This is an important finding, because it not only extends the usefulness of the apparent viscosity measurements, but also furnishes insight into the mechanism of flow resistance.

One of the greatest unknowns today in blood rheology in microvessels is the hematocrit distribution in various vessels. It is well known that the hematocrit decreases as blood flows from arteries to arterioles and capillaries, but quantitative information is lacking. It is not easy to measure local hematocrit in vivo. If the hematocrit distribution were known, the Fahraeus–Cokelet explanation would enable us to calculate the apparent viscosity in microvessels.

Incidentally, there is no mystery in blood's changing hematocrit along its path. If a stagnant pool of plasma is annexed to a given vessel, the hematocrit in that vessel would have been decreased! For the same reason, the average velocity of red cells can be different from that of the plasma in a given vessel without violating the conservation of mass.

Why does the hematocrit decrease in small blood vessels? One of the explanations is the existence of a *cell-free layer* at the wall. Another explanation is the *oriented nature* of red cells in a shear flow. To explain the first effect, we note that when blood flows down a vessel of diameter equal to several cell diameters (in vivo or in models) there is a thin region near the wall in which the concentration of red cells falls significantly. This is the cell-free layer, or plasma layer. It is the "stagnation pool" hinted at in the preceding paragraph; therefore, its existence reduces the hematocrit. The smaller the vessel, the larger is the proportion of the volume of the cell-free layer, and the lower is the hematocrit. Furthermore, if a small side branch of a vessel draws blood from the vessel mainly from the cell-free layer, the hematocrit in the side branch will be smaller. This is usually referred to as *plasma skimming*.

To explain the second effect, we note that when the blood flows in a tube the red cells have a preferred orientation in which the faces of the red cell are aligned with the flow direction. If a small side branch having a diameter about the same size as that of the red cell draws blood from the tube (such as a small capillary branching from a small artery), the *entry condition* into the small branch is affected by the orientation of the red cells. If the entry section is aligned with the red cells it will be easier for the cells to enter. If the entry is perpendicular to the cells more cells will skim over the small branch and do not enter, and the hematocrit will be decreased.

When there is a cell-free layer at the wall, the viscous stress will be reduced because the viscosity of the plasma is smaller than that of the whole blood. We have seen (Figure 1) that the apparent viscosity of blood increases with hematocrit. When the hematocrit is concentrated toward the core of the blood vessel, blood arranges its viscosity in such a way that the viscosity is the least where the shear gradient is the largest (near the wall), whereas at the core the viscosity is high but the shear gradient is very small. In a tubular flow the wall region far outweighs the core region, and the apparent viscosity of the tube flow is reduced. The smaller the tube, the greater is the portion of the cell-free layer, the lower is the hematocrit, and the lower is the apparent viscosity. This argument holds until the tube becomes so small that the red cells have to move in single file and to severely deform themselves in order to pass through.

THE FLOW OF SUSPENSIONS IN FAIRLY NARROW RIGID TUBES

Mason and Goldsmith (1969) conducted an exhaustive series of experiments with suspensions of variously shaped particles, which may be rigid, or deformable, or merely viscous immiscible droplets, flowing through straight rigid pipes. Their results provide the best insight to the cell-free layer mentioned in the preceding section.

For a suspension of neutrally buoyant rigid spheres, the explanation of the cell-free layer is primarily geometric, in that the center of the spheres must be at least a radius away from the wall. At very low Reynolds number, whether there is any dynamic effect tending to force spheres away from the wall is still unknown. Isolated rigid spheres in Poiseuille flow can be shown to experience no net radial force; they rotate, but continue to travel in straight lines; thus they cannot create a cell-free layer.

When inertia force is not negligible, rigid spheres in a Poiseuille flow do, in general, experience a radial force. They exhibit a *tubular pinch effect* demonstrated both experimentally and theoretically by Segré and Silberberg (1962), in which particles near the wall move towards the axis, and particles near the axis move towards the wall. This effect is probably unimportant in arterioles or capillaries where the Reynolds number is much less than 1. Similar results are obtained for suspensions of rigid rods and disks. There is no overall radial motion unless inertial effect is important.

When the particles in suspension are deformable, Mason and Goldsmith (1969) found that they do experience a net radial hydrodynamic force even at very low Reynolds numbers, and tend to migrate towards the tube axis. The mechanism of this phenomenon is obscure. A full theoretical analysis is not yet available.

ANALYSIS OF SINGLE-FILE FLOW OF BLOOD CELLS IN VERY NARROW CAPILLARY BLOOD VESSELS

In flowing through very small blood vessels, the red cells deform a great deal. Would the tight squeeze cause a lot of friction, thus inducing a large pressure drop in the capillaries?

It is recognized that in flowing blood the red cells never come to solid-to-solid contact with the endothelium of the blood vessel; there always seems to be a fluid layer in between. The thicker the fluid layer, the smaller would be the shear strain rate, and the viscous stress would be reduced. On the other hand, suppose the thickness of the fluid layer is fixed; then, is there any trick to reduce the shear strain on the vessel wall (endothelium) and thereby reduce the resistance on the blood? The answer is yes, by forcing the fluid in the layer in such a way as to reduce the slope of the velocity profile on the vessel wall. This is a hydrodynamic effect used in engineering, in the lubrication of journal bearings. Lighthill (1968, 1972) pointed out that such an effect can be expected from a red cell squeezing through a tight capillary vessel. The theory is called a "lubrication layer" theory, the effect is due to a "leak-back" flow in the gap between the cell and the vessel wall. The mathematical theory would have to fit the elastic deformation of the endothelium and the red cells. Lighthill (1968) worked out the principal features of the lubrication layer without really solving the red cell problem. Fitz-Gerald (1969a, 1969b, 1972) elaborated on the theory, and deduced many results that are in agreement with experimental observations. But a theory in which the red cell is analyzed as a cell, with membrane characteristics as described in Chapter 12 (in the section, "Physical Theories of the Red Blood Cell") and the contents as a liquid, has not yet been worked out.

Since the effect of a lubrication layer on each red cell is localized, it is expected that the resistance to blood flow in narrow capillaries will increase with increasing local hematocrit. Experiments by Jay, Rowlands, and Skibo (1972), however, showed that the relative viscosity of blood tends to be independent of the hematocrit for human blood flowing in glass tubes of 4–15 μ diameter. Earlier, such a phenomenon was also described by Prothero and Burton (1961, 1962). Jay et al. (1972) believed that this is a direct contradiction to the Lighthill–Fitz-Gerald theory. Chien (1972) points out, however, that theoretical analysis by Skalak, Chen, and Chien (1972) showed that when the spacing between the red cells is small, the plasma trapped between the cells move with the cell. Hence when the hematocrit is sufficiently high, the cell-plasma core moves almost like a rigid body, and the apparent viscosity will be independent of the hematocrit. Furthermore, the size of the core depends on the deformation of the red cell. One can estimate the size of the red cell core from the experimental results of Hochmuth, Marple, and Sutera (1970). It is seen that the core is quite small in very tight capillaries. Chien (1972) contends that the results of Jay et al. (1972) can be understood from these effects. More extensive experimentation is surely necessary to obtain a clearer picture on this point.

THEORETICAL ANALYSIS

The dynamics of red cells in a capillary blood vessel is difficult to analyze. From the point of view of mechanics, it is expedient to study the plasma around the red cells. It is fortunate that normal plasma is Newtonian, so that its motion is governed by Navier–Stokes equations that can be analyzed with confidence. For example, considerable details are known about the entry flow when plasma enters from a large vessel into a small branch of capillary blood vessel. It is shown (Lew and Fung, 1969, 1970b) that near the entry section the radial velocity can be as large as 30% of the mean axial velocity. Further downstream from the entry section the velocity profile is a parabola, as was pointed out long ago by Poiseuille. The convergence to the Poiseuille profile is rather rapid at Reynolds numbers much below 1. At a distance about 0.65 times the diameter of the tube from the entry section, the deviation from Poiseuille profile is already less than 1%. This distance, 0.65D, is a characteristic distance for the viscous fluid to readjust itself to the parabolic profile after it is disturbed in some way; it has a more or less general significance. For example, consider a capillary tube with several pellets. If the distance between the pellets is as large as 1.3 diameter of the tube, the velocity profile at the midpoint between the pellets will be almost Poiseuillean: The deviation would be less than 1%.

A detailed analysis of a flow of rigid spheres down the center of a narrow tube is presented by Wang and Skalak (1969). Among other things the analysis shows that the pressure drop required for a given volume flow rate increases when the ratio of the diameters of the sphere (b) and the tube (a) increases. But even when b/a = 0.9 and the spheres are touching the pressure drop is only about 2.0 times that required by the same flow with plasma only, without spheres. However, the apparent viscosity of whole blood is at least 2.5 times that of plasma, so the Fahraeus–Lindqvist effect is still operating even when b/a is as large as 0.9. The numerical methods of Wang and Skalak break down above b/a = 0.9, because of the very high pressure encountered in the thin lubrication layer between the cell and the tube wall.

Lee and Fung (1969) presented experimental data on local pressure distribution on the tube wall when a simulated red cell (made of thin-walled rubber membrane filled with a viscous fluid) flows in a circular cylindrical tube. Expressed in terms of pressure drop along the tube wall, the profile of resistance for a series of sparsely spaced red cells is shown in Figure 3. Although the red cell geometry and the flow Reynolds number were simulated in this experiment, the rubber membrane cannot simulate the stress–strain relationship of the red cell membrane. The model cells were not as deformable as the real cells.

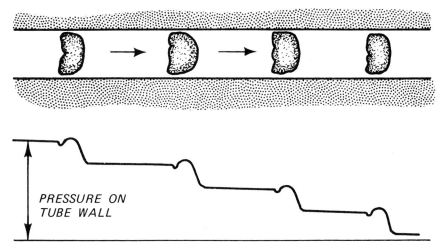

Figure 3. Pressure distribution measured on the wall of a circular cylindrical tube in which a silicone fluid containing a series of red cell models flows. The red cell models are made of thin-walled latex rubber and filled with liquid. From Lee and Fung (1969); reprinted with permission.

The truly important task for theoretical investigations of the future is to compute the deformation of a red cell in passing through capillaries. Many approximate calculations have been done (see Lighthill, 1968; Fitz-Gerald, 1969*a,b,* 1972; Lopez et al., 1968), but none has solved the complete boundary-value problem, with conditions satisfied on the entire red cell, including the elastic equilibrium of the cell membrane. The problem has not been attacked seriously, probably because the constitutive equation of the cell membrane was not known for certain; but recent suggestions as discussed in Chapter 12 are very convincing, and a serious analysis would be worthwhile.

Experimental evidence on red cell deformation in microcirculation is being rapidly accumulated. Chien (1972) and Goldsmith and Skalak (1975) have systematically reviewed these results. Generally speaking, the faster the flow, the larger the viscosity of the plasma, the more flexible the red cells, and the smaller the tube, the larger would be the deformation of the red cells. Red cell deformation virtually always reduces the apparent viscosity of the blood in the capillaries.

BIBLIOGRAPHICAL NOTES

Limitation of space does not permit us to go into the details of history of the subject and the very extensive literature. See books by Copley and Stainsby, (1960), Charm and Kurland (1974), Dintenfass (1971), and Scott Blair (1974).

The boundary condition of blood at the endothelial surface of the blood vessel, or at the solid wall in a viscometer, has great theoretical and practical significance. It affects the flow and the red cell distribution. See Bennett, (1967), Brandt and Bugliarello (1966), Bugliarello, Kapur, and Hsiao (1965), and the articles on micropolar theory.

List of articles related to Fahraeus effect and the apparent viscosity in capillaries should include Braasch and Jennet (1968), Cokelet (1963), Haynes (1960, 1962), Whitmore (1968), Whittaker and Winton (1933). Somewhat earlier than Fahraeus and Lindqvist's work on extracorporeal blood experiment, Bingham and Green, working on paints (1919), had reported a similar effect. For a brief history of this problem, see Scott Blair (1974).

For a review of the mathematical theory of capillary flow see Aroesty and Gross (1970), Gross and Aroesty (1972), and Goldsmith and Skalak (1975).

So far we have considered blood as a fluid whose property does not change with time. The constitutive equation is assumed to be *invariant* with respect to time—it does not contain time explicitly as a parameter. But blood is a dynamic fluid: the red cells can aggregate and disaggregate, and the process may depend on the shear strain rate. Following a sudden change in shear rate, the red cells take time to settle down to a new course. Thus Huang et al. (1973) describe blood as a *thixotropic* fluid. Huang, King, and Copley (1973) measured blood motion over a shear rate range from 1,000 down to 0.0009 sec^{-1}. They concluded that between 50 and 1000 sec^{-1} the blood exhibits nearly Newtonian behavior. Between 10^{-2} and 50 sec^{-1} the blood is thixotropic. Its viscosity depends on the time of shearing. In shear rates less than 10^{-2}, they describe blood as a solid. Huang (1972) derived an expression for blood thixotrophy on the basis of irreversible thermodynamics.

White blood cells tend to stick to the blood vessel endothelium. Measurements of the force of interaction between leucocytes and vascular endothelium are given by Atherton and Born (1972), and Schmid-Schönbein, Fung, and Zweifach (1975).

An excellent review of the whole field is given by Caro, Pedly, and Seed (1974). Motion of particles is discussed by Chaffey, Brenner and Mason (1965). The viscosity of hemoglobin solution and interior of red cells is given by Cokelet and Meiselman (1968), and Dintenfass (1968a,b). The stochastic feature of red cell motion in microvessels is discussed by Fung (1973), who explains, in particular, why the hematocrit in capillary blood vessels is so very non-uniform. Microscopic observation of red cell deformation in flow is presented by Goldsmith (1971). Gregersen (1967) and Gregersen et al. (1967) discuss flow through polycarbonate sieves. Johnson and Wayland (1967) present in vivo measurements of red cell velocities in capillaries. Schmid-Schönbein et al. (1968, 1969) discuss cell deformability and blood viscosity, whereas Skalak (1972) and Skalak (1973) present mathematical theories. The subject is obviously being pursued vigorously.

LITERATURE CITED

Ariman, T., M. A. Turk, and N. D. Sylvester. 1973, 1974. On steady and pulsatile flow of blood. Int. J. Eng. Sci. 11:905−930; 12:273−293.

Aroesty, J., and J. F. Gross. 1970. Convection and diffusion in the microcirculation. Microvasc. Res. 2:247−267.

Atherton, A., and G. V. R. Born. 1972. Quantitative investigations of the adhesiveness of circulating polymorphonuclear leucocytes to blood vessel walls. J. Physiol. 222:447−474.

Barbee, J. H., and G. R. Cokelet. 1971. The Fahraeus effect. Microvasc. Res. 3:1−21.

Benis, A. M., S. Chien, S. Usami, and K. M. Jan. 1973. Inertial pressure losses in perfused hindlimb: a reinterpretation of the results of Whittaker and Winton. J. Appl. Physiol. 34:383−389.

Bennett, L. 1967. Red cell slip at a wall in vitro. Science 155:1554−1555.

Bingham, E. C., and H. Green. 1919. Quoted from Scott Blair (1974), p. 53.

Braasch, D., and W. Jennett. 1968. Erythrozyten flexibilität, Hämokonzentration and Reibungswiderstand in Glascapillaren mit Durchmessern zwischen 6 bis 50μ. Pflügers Arch. Physiol. 302:245−254.

Brandt, A., and G. Bugliarello. 1966. Concentration redistribution phenomena in shear flow of nomolayers of suspended particles. Trans. Soc. Rheol. 10: 229−251.

Bugliarello, G., C. Kapur, and G. Hsiao. 1965. The profile viscosity and other characteristics of blood flow in a nonuniform shear field. *In* A. L. Copley (ed.), Proceedings of the Fourth International Rheology Conference, Vol. 4, pp. 351—370. Interscience, New York.

Caro, C. G., T. J. Pedley, and W. A. Sead. 1974. Mechanics of the Circulation. *In* A. C. Guyton (ed.), *Cardiovascular Physiology*, MTP International Review of Science, Physiology Ser. 1, Vol. 1, pp. 1—48. Univ. Park Press, Baltimore.

Casson, M. 1958. A flow equation for pigment-oil suspensions of the printing ink type. *In* C. C. Mills (ed.), Rheology of Disperse System, pp. 84—104. Pergamon Press, Oxford.

Chaffey, C. E., H. Brenner, and S. G. Mason. 1965. Particle motions in sheared suspensions. XVII Rheological Acta, 4:56, 4:64—72; Correction, 6:100 (1967).

Charm, S. E., and G. S. Kurland. 1962. The flow behavior and shear stress-shear rate characteristics of canine blood. Am. J. Physiol. 203:417—421.

Charm, S. E., and G. S. Kurland. 1972. Blood Rheology. *In* D. H. Bergel (ed.), Cardiovascular Fluid Dynamics, Chap. 15, pp. 158—204. Academic Press, New York.

Charm, S. E., and G. S. Kurland. 1974. Blood Flow and Microcirculation. John Wiley, New York.

Chien, S. 1972. Present state of blood rheology. *In* Hemodilution: Theoretical Basis and Clinical Application, International Symposium Rottach-Egern, 1971, pp. 1—45. S. Karger, Basel.

Chien, S., S. Usami, R. T. Dellenback, and M. I. Gregersen. 1967*a*. Blood viscosity: Influence of erythrocyte aggregation. Science 157:829—831.

Chien, S., S. Usami, R. T. Dellenback, and M. I. Gregersen. 1967*b*. Blood viscosity: Influence of erythrocyte deformation. Science 157:827—829.

Cokelet, G. R. 1963. Comments on the Fahraeus—Lindqvist effect. Biorheology 4:123—126.

Cokelet, G. R. 1972. The rheology of human blood. *In* Y. O. Fung, N. Perrone, and M. Anliker (eds.), Biomechanics: Its Foundations and Objectives. Prentice-Hall, Englewood Cliffs, N.J.

Cokelet, G. R., and H. J. Meiselman. 1968. Rheological comparison of hemoglobin solutions and erythrocyte suspensions. Science 162:275—277.

Copley, A. L., and G. Stainsby (eds.). 1960. Flow Properties of Blood and Other Biological Systems. Pergamon Press, New York.

Cowin, S. C. 1968. Polar fluids. Phys. Fluids 11:1919—1927.

Dintenfass, L. 1968a. Blood viscosity, internal fluidity of the red cell, dynamic coagulation, and the critical capillary radius as factors in physiology and pathology or circulation and microcirculation. Med. J. Australia 1:688—696.

Dintenfass, L. 1968*b*. Internal viscosity of the red cell and a blood viscosity equation. Nature 219:956—958.

Dintenfass, L. 1971. Blood Microrheology: Viscosity Factors in Blood Flow, Ischaemia and Thrombosis. Appleton-Century-Crofts, New York.

Fahraeus, R. 1929. The suspension stability of the blood. Physiol. Rev. 9:241—274.

Fahraeus, R., and T. Lindqvist. 1931. The viscosity of the blood in narrow capillary tubes. Am. J. Physiol. 96:562—568.

Fitz-Gerald, J. M. 1969*a*. Mechanics of red-cell motion through very narrow capillaries. Proc. Roy. Soc. London B, 174:193—227.

Fitz-Gerald, J. M. 1969*b*. Implications of a theory of erythrocyte motion in narrow capillaries. J. Appl. Physiol. 27:912—918.

Fitz-Gerald, J. M. 1972. The mechanics of capillary blood flow. *In* D. H. Bergel (ed.), Cardiovascular Fluid Dynamics, Vol. 2, Chap. 16, pp. 205–241. Academic Press, New York.

Fung, Y. C. 1973. Stochastic flow in capillary blood vessels. Microvasc. Res. 5:34–48.

Fung, Y. C., and S. Sobin. 1969. Theory of sheet flow in the lung alveoli. J. Appl. Physiol. 26:472–488.

Goldsmith, H. L. 1971. Deformation of human red cells in tube flow. Biorheology 7:235–242.

Goldsmith, H. L., and R. Skalak. 1975. Hemodynamics. Ann. Rev. Fluid Mech. 7:213–247.

Gregersen, M. I. 1967. Factors regulating blood viscosity: Relation to problems of the microcirculation. Colloque International, Les Concepts de Claude Bernard sur le Milieu, pp. 231–244. Intérieur, Masson et cie, Paris.

Gregersen, M. I., C. A. Bryant, W. E. Hammerle, S. Usami, and S. Chien. 1967. Flow characteristics of human erythrocytes through polycarbonate sieves. Science 157:825–827.

Gross, J. F., and J. Aroesty. 1972. Mathematical models of capillary flow: A critical review. Biorheology 9:225–264.

Haynes, R. H. 1960. Physical basis of the dependence of blood viscosity on tube radius. Am. J. Physiol. 198:1193–1200.

Haynes, R. H. 1962. The viscosity of erythrocyte suspensions. Biophys. J. 2:95–103.

Hochmuth, R. M., R. N. Marple, and S. P. Sutera. 1970. Capillary blood flow: I. Erythrocyte deformation in glass capillaries. Microvasc. Res. 2:409–419.

Huang, C. R. 1972. A thermodynamic approach to generalized rheological equation of state for time-dependent and time-independent non-Newtonian fluids. Chem. Eng. J. 3:100–104.

Huang, C. R., R. G. King, and A. L. Copley. 1973. Rheogoniometric studies of whole human blood at shear rates down to 0.0009 sec^{-1}. Part II. Mathematical Interpretation. Biorheology 10:23–28.

Hyman, W. A., and R. Skalak. 1972. Viscous flow of a suspension of liquid drops in a cylindrical tube. Appl. Sci. Res. 26:27–51.

Jay, A. W. C., S. Rowlands, and L. Skibo. 1972. The resistance to blood flow in capillaries. Can. J. Physiol. Pharmacol. 5:1007–1013.

Johnson, P. C., and H. Wayland. 1967. Regulation of blood flow in single capillaries. Am. J. Physiol. 212:1405–1415.

Kline, K. A., and S. J. Allen. 1970. Non steady flows of fluids with microstructure. Phys. Fluids 13:263–270.

Lee, J. S. 1969. Slow viscous flow in a lung alveolar model. J. Biomech. 2:187–198.

Lee, J. S., and Y. C. Fung. 1969. Modeling experiments of a single red blood cell moving in a capillary blood vessel. Microvasc. Res. 1:221–243.

Lew, H. S., and Y. C. Fung. 1969. The motion of the plasma between the red blood cells in the bolus flow. Biorheology 6:109–119.

Lew, H. S., and Y. C. Fung. 1970a. Plug effect of erythrocytes in capillary blood vessels. Biophysic. J. 10:80–99.

Lew, H. S., and Y. C. Fung. 1970b. Entry flow into blood vessels at arbitrary Reynolds number. J. Biomech. 3:23–38.

Lighthill, M. J. 1968. Pressure-forcing of tightly fitting pellets along fluid-filled elastic tubes. J. Fluid Mech. 34:113–143.

Lighthill, M. J. 1972. Physiological fluid dynamics: A survey. J. Fluid Mech. 52:475–497.

Lopez, L., I. M. Duck, and W. A. Hunt. 1968. On the shape of the erythrocyte. Biophysical J. 8:1228–1235.

Mason, S. G., and H. L. Goldsmith. 1969. The flow behavior of particulate suspensions. In G. E. W. Wolstenholme and J. Knight (eds.), Circulatory and Respiratory Mass Transport, A Ciba Foundation Symposium, p. 105. Churchill, London.

Merrill, E. W., E. R. Gilliland, G. R. Cokelet, H. Shin, A. Britten, and R. E. Wells. 1963. Rheology of blood and flow in the microcirculation. J. Appl. Physiol. 18:255–260.

Prothero, J., and A. C. Burton. 1961, 1962. The physics of blood flow in capillaries. Biophys. J. 1:565–579, 2:199–212, 2:213–222.

Purday, H. F. 1949. An Introduction to the Mechanics of Viscous Flow. Dover, New York.

Schmid-Schönbein, H., P. Gaethgens, and H. Hirsch. 1968. On the shear rate dependence of red cell aggregation in vitro. J. Clin. Invest. 47:1447–1454.

Schmid-Schönbein, H., R. E. Wells, and J. Goldstone. 1969. Influence of deformability of human red cells upon blood viscosity. Circ. Res. 25:131–143.

Schmid-Schönbein, G., Y. C. Fung, and B. Zweifach. 1975. Vascular endothelium-leucocyte interaction: Sticking shear force in venules. Circ. Res. 36: 173–184.

Scott Blair, G. W. 1974. An Introduction to Biorheology. Elsevier, New York.

Segré, G., and A. Silberberg. 1962. Behavior of macroscopic rigid spheres in Poiseuille flow. J. Fluid Mech. 14:136–157.

Skalak, R. 1972. Mechanics of the microcirculation. In Y. C. Fung, N. Perrone, and M. Anliker (eds.), Biomechanics: Its Foundations and Objectives, pp. 457–500. Prentice-Hall, Englewood Cliffs, N. J.

Skalak, R., P. H. Chen, and S. Chien. 1972. Effect of hematocrit and rouleaux on apparent viscosity in capillaries. Biorheology 9:67–82.

Skalak, R. 1973. Modelling the mechanical behavior of red blood cells. Biorheology, 10:229–238.

Starling, E. H. 1918. The Linacre lecture of the law of the heart. London, Longmans, Green.

Valanis, K. C., and C. T. Sun. 1969. Poiseuille flow of a fluid with couple stress with applications to blood flow. Biorheology 6:85–97.

Wang, H., and R. Skalak. 1969. Viscous flow in a cylindrical tube containing a line of spherical particles. J. Fluid Mech. 38:75–96.

Whitmore, R. L. 1968. Rheology of the Circulation. Pergamon Press, Oxford.

Whittaker, S. R. F., and F. R. Winton. 1933. The apparent viscosity of blood flowing in the isolated hindlimb of the dog, and its variation with corpuscular concentration. J. Physiol. 78:339–369.

Yen, R. T., and Y. C. Fung. 1973. Model experiments on apparent blood viscosity and hematocrit in pulmonary alveoli. J. Appl. Physiol. 35:510–517.

Young, T. 1808. The Croonian Lecture. On the functions of the heart and arteries. Phil. Trans. 99:31. Hydraulic investigations, subservient to an intended Croonian lecture on the motion of the blood. Phil. Trans. of the Roy. Soc. London 98:164–186.

chapter 14

RHEOLOGY
OF BLOOD VESSELS

Yuan-Cheng Fung

RHEOLOGY OF LARGE ARTERIES

NONLINEAR VISCOELASTIC FEATURES OF ARTERIES AND THEIR
VARIATION ALONG THE ARTERIAL TREE

RHEOLOGY OF MATERIAL SURROUNDING CAPILLARIES

CAPILLARY SYSTEM TOPOLOGY AND COMPLIANCE

CAPILLARY PATENCY

ACTIVE STATE OF VASCULAR SMOOTH MUSCLE

BIBLIOGRAPHICAL NOTES

Blood flows in deformable vessels. As the interacting stresses change, the blood
vessels deform, thus changing the boundary conditions and the flow. It is
therefore necessary to know the rheology of the blood vessels in order to
understand the flow of blood. The word rheology was coined by Bingham from
the Greek ρελ (flow) to denote the mechanics of deformable bodies. It is used
most frequently in connection with fluids, but it is equally applicable to solids.

Large arteries and veins are viscoelastic. As a rough approximation, however,
they may be regarded as perfectly elastic, but with a nonlinear stress–strain
relationship. If the conditions of loading are such that the time-dependent aspect
of the stress–strain relationship can be revealed, then the viscoelastic features
can be seen. If we suddenly stretch a segment of blood vessel and then hold the
stretch constant, the stress is seen to decrease with time. This is called *stress
relaxation under a constant strain*. Over a long period of time an artery may
relax 20 or 30% of its tension under a step strain. On the other hand, if we load
a segment of artery with a constant tensile load, the segment will continue to

This work is supported by National Science Foundation Grant ENG-75-19401 and the
United States Public Health Service, National Institutes of Health National Heart and Lung
Institute through Grant HL 12494 and HL 17731.

299

increase its length. This is called *creep under a constant load*. Finally, if we impose a cyclic change of stress in the material, the strain will change cyclically but not exactly in phase with stress. If we stretch a segment of blood vessel at a constant rate and then reverse the motion at the same rate, the stress in loading will be somewhat different from that in unloading. This is called *hysteresis*. Blood vessels exhibit all of these viscoelastic features.

It is well known that arteries generally become stiffer (having a higher Young's modulus) as they become smaller along the arterial tree. This is usually due to an increasing wall-to-radius ratio and an increasing content of collagen. But the smallest capillary blood vessels in the mesentery are known to be so rigid that a change of internal pressure in the range of 100 mm Hg induces only an almost undetectable change in diameter ($< 0.5\ \mu$). This high rigidity of a capillary is attributable to the support the vessel receives from the surrounding tissue. It is therefore necessary to study the rheology of the surrounding tissue in order to understand the behavior of capillary blood vessels.

On the other hand, there are small blood vessels that do not receive much support from the surrounding tissue. A typical example is the capillaries in the pulmonary alveoli, which are separated from the air by a wall less than 1 μ thick. These vessels are expected to be distensible.

In the present chapter we summarize briefly what we know of the rheology of soft tissues relevant to microcirculation. This includes both the larger blood vessels and other tissues in which capillary blood vessels are imbedded.

RHEOLOGY OF LARGE ARTERIES

Large blood vessels are well-structured tissues whose mechanical property has been investigated by many authors. For the elastic property and for references to the literature, see the excellent reviews by Bergel (1972) and by Patel and Vaishnav (1972). Only the most salient features are presented below.

Blood vessel wall material may be considered incompressible. The question of compressibility arises not only because the blood vessel walls are about as compressible as water, but also because water can be expressed through the surface of the tissue when it is stressed. One asks whether in a physiologic condition such a loss or gain of water accompanied by stressing is significant or not. A crude study by Carew, Vaishnav, and Patel (1968) showed that the latter is insignificant in the sense that (1) the bulk modulus is several thousand times that of the shear modulus, and (2) the Poisson's ratio that may be computed for an incremental stress–strain law about a physiologic condition is approximately 0.5. With this kind of ratios, the assumption of incompressibility is justified in the mathematical analysis of certain physiologic problems such as the problem of arterial wave propagation.

One of the most useful form of stress–strain relationship is the *incremental law about some initial stressed state*. We consider an elastic body stressed in a certain steady-state manner, then perturb it slightly to incur some small changes in stress and strain. The superposed small changes are called the *incremental changes*. For sufficiently small incremental stresses and strains, they are related by a linear relationship, which is a great advantage. The disadvantage of such a linear incremental law is that it changes with the initial state. Every time a different initial state is examined, a new set of incremental elastic moduli would have to be determined.

Consider a segment of circular cylindrical vessel subjected to a steady internal pressure p and longitudinal force F, at which state the midwall radius of the vessel is R, the length of the segment is L, and the thickness of the wall is h. Now consider a small perturbation of this steady state so that R, L, h, p, and F are changed to $R + \Delta R$, $L + \Delta L$, $h + \Delta h$, $p + \Delta p$, $F + \Delta F$. Then we define the incremental strains

$$e_\theta = \frac{\Delta R}{R}, \qquad e_z = \frac{\Delta L}{L}, \qquad e_r = \frac{\Delta h}{h}, \tag{1}$$

and the incremental stresses

$$P_\theta = \Delta \left[p \left(\frac{R}{h} - \frac{1}{2} \right) \right] \cong \left(\frac{R}{h} - \frac{1}{2} \right) \Delta p + \frac{2p\Delta R}{h} + \frac{pR\Delta L}{Lh},$$

$$P_z = \Delta \left[\frac{p}{2} \left(\frac{R}{h} - 1 \right) + \frac{F}{2\pi RLh} \right] \tag{2}$$

$$\cong \left(\frac{R}{2h} - \frac{1}{2} \right) \Delta p + \frac{p\Delta R}{h} + \frac{\Delta F}{2\pi Rh} + \left(\frac{pR}{2Lh} + \frac{F}{2\pi RLh} \right) \Delta L$$

$$p_r = \Delta \left[-\frac{p}{2} \right] \cong -\frac{1}{2} \Delta p .$$

In deriving Eq. (2) the fact that the vessel wall is incompressible is used, so that $e_\theta + e_z + e_r = 0$, and Δh can be expressed in terms of R and ΔL. According to the general theory of elasticity, and under the assumption that the blood vessel has an orthotropic symmetry, the incremental stress–strain relationship can be written in the following matrix form:

$$\begin{bmatrix} e_\theta \\ e_z \\ e_r \end{bmatrix} = \begin{bmatrix} C_{\theta\theta} & -C_{\theta z} & -C_{\theta r} \\ -C_{z\theta} & C_{zz} & -C_{zr} \\ -C_{r\theta} & -C_{rz} & C_{rr} \end{bmatrix} \begin{bmatrix} P_\theta \\ P_z \\ P_r \end{bmatrix} \tag{3}$$

On assing the Onsager principle for the symmetry of the C_{ij} matrix, and using the condition of incompressibility, it can be shown that of the nine constants C_{ij}, only three are independent (Patel and Vaishnav, 1972). The inverses of $C_{\theta\theta}$, C_{zz}, and C_{rr} are the incremental Young's moduli for appropriate uniaxial incremental load:

$$E_\theta = \frac{1}{C_{\theta\theta}}, \qquad E_z = \frac{1}{C_{zz}}, \qquad E_r = \frac{1}{C_{rr}}. \tag{4}$$

Some other combinations have the meaning of Poisson's ratio:

$$\nu_{\theta z} = \frac{C_{\theta z}}{C_{zz}}, \qquad \nu_{zr} = \frac{C_{zr}}{C_{rr}}, \qquad \nu_{r\theta} = \frac{C_{r\theta}}{C_{\theta\theta}}$$

$$\nu_{z\theta} = \frac{C_{z\theta}}{C_{\theta\theta}}, \qquad \nu_{rz} = \frac{C_{rz}}{C_{zz}}, \qquad \nu_{\theta r} = \frac{C_{\theta r}}{C_{rr}}.$$

(5)

Note that $\nu_{ij} \neq \nu_{ji}$.

These equations are applicable also to small sinusoidal perturbations of an initially static stress state. If the stress and strain are represented by complex variable in terms of $e^{i\omega t}$, then the coefficients C_{ij} are complex-valued.

Figure 1 shows the results of Patel, Janicki, and Carew (1969) from in vivo static experiments. Table 1 shows the results of Patel and Vaishnav (1972) on in

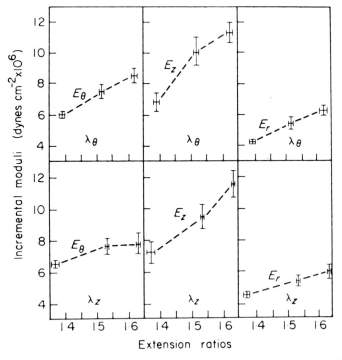

Figure 1. Incremental elastic moduli versus extension ratios. E_θ, circumferential modulus; E_z longitudinal modulus; E_r, radial modulus; λ_θ, circumferential extension ratio; λ_z, longitudinal extension ration. Horizontal and vertical bars indicate the standard error of the mean for each of the groups. In the upper panels the moduli are plotted versus the mean λ_θ for each of three groups; the corresponding values of λ_z (from left to right) are 1.45 ± 0.04 SE, 1.56 ± 0.02 and 1.51 ± 0.02. In the lower panels the moduli are plotted versus λ_z; the corresponding values of λ_θ for each of these groups (left to right) are 1.46 ± 0.02, 1.58 ± 0.02 and 1.48 = 0.02. From Patel et al., 1969; reprinted by permission.

vitro harmonic-oscillation tests. Both refer to middle descending thoracic aorta of dogs. For Table 1, the mean pressure was 148 cm H_2O; the initial strain was around stretch ratios $\lambda_\theta = 1.53$ and $\lambda_z = 1.51$. The values of static coefficients (0 frequency) from the same dogs are also included in the table for comparison.

For a more complete description of the nonlinear constitutive equation, Patel and Vaishnav (1972) ignored the history-dependent features of the arteries and treated them as perfectly elastic. Again limiting their treatment to a cylindrical vessel subjected to symmetric loading, they expressed the strain-energy function in the form of a polynomial of the Green's strain components:

$$a = \overline{\gamma}_\theta = \tfrac{1}{2}(\lambda_\theta^2 - 1), \quad b = \overline{\gamma}_z = \tfrac{1}{2}(\lambda_z^2 - 1), \quad c = \overline{\gamma}_r = \tfrac{1}{2}(\lambda_r^2 - 1). \quad (6a)$$

Here λ_θ, λ_z, λ_r are the *stretch ratios* defined by the equations

$$\lambda_\theta = \frac{R}{R_0}, \quad \lambda_z = \frac{L}{L_0}, \quad \lambda_r = \frac{h}{h_0}, \quad (6b)$$

where R, L, h are the mean radius, length, and wall thickness of the vessel, and R_0, L_0, h_0 are the corresponding values in the unstressed, relaxed state. From the strain-energy function, stress can be obtained by differentiation in the usual manner. Patel and Vaishnav (1972) considered polynomials of third and fourth order, introduced the condition of incompressibility, and showed that it suffices to write

$$W = Aa^2 + Bab + Cb^2 + Da^3 + Ea^2 b + Fab^2 + Gb^3 + Ha^4 + Ia^3 b + Ja^2 b^2 + Kab^3 + Lb^4 \quad (7)$$

Table 1. Patel and Vaishnav's results from the middle descending thoracic aorta of six dogs

Frequency (Hz)	E_θ (dynes cm^{-2} × 10^6)		E_z (dynes cm^{-2} × 10^6)		E_r (dynes cm^{-2} × 10^6)	
	E_θ'	E_θ''	E_z'	E_z''	E_r'	E_r''
0.0	7.38	0.0	6.72	0.0	4.58	0.0
0.5	9.13	0.06	9.96	0.95	6.25	0.59
1.0	9.18	0.10	10.11	0.96	6.31	0.59
2.0	9.30	0.12	10.25	0.95	6.36	0.65
3.0	9.47	0.18	10.19	0.96	6.44	0.69
4.0	9.39	0.32	10.11	1.00	6.28	0.77
5.0	9.50	0.29	10.18	1.04	6.46	0.81

E_θ, E_z and E_r are the complex incremental viscoelastic moduli in the θ, z, and r directions; E_θ, E_z, and E_r' are the real parts of the complex moduli representing the elastic coefficients and E_θ'', E_z'', and E_r'' are the imaginary parts related to the viscous coefficients. From Patel and Vaishnav (1972), p. 39.

where $A, B, \ldots, L$ are material constants. If the material were transversely isotropic in the θ, z surface, then

$$A = C, \quad E = F, \quad D = G, \quad H = L, \quad I = K. \tag{8}$$

Thus the second-order theory would need only two constants, the third-order theory four constants, and the fourth-order theory seven constants.

Patel and Vaishnav (1972) and their associates experimented in vitro on four dogs (average weight, 28 kg) in the range of λ_θ from 1.10 to 1.65, λ_z from 1.47 to 1.53, and maximum values of $S_\theta - S_r, S_z - S_r$ at 2.13×10^6 and 1.47×10^6 dynes/cm^2, respectively. For the three-constant theory [keeping the first three terms in Eq. (7)] they obtained the following average values (mean $\pm$ SEM) in units of dynes/cm$^2 \times 10^6$:

$$A = 0.372(\pm 0.030), \quad B = 0.219(\pm 0.019), \quad C = 0.288(\pm 0.038).$$

For the seven-constants theory [keeping the first seven terms in Eq. (7)], they obtained (mean $\pm$ SEM)

$$\begin{aligned}
&A = 0.412(\pm 0.066), \quad B = -0.067(\pm 0.131), \quad C = 0.191(\pm 0.059), \\
&D = -0.055(\pm 0.036), \quad E = 0.162(\pm 0.051), \quad F = 0.179(\pm 0.103), \\
&G = 0.099(\pm 0.08)
\end{aligned}$$

where the units are (dynes/cm$^2 \times 10^6$). The 12-constant theory was also tried and found to fit the data still better, but the marginal improvement in the quality of fit was not judged to be of sufficient importance to recommend the use of the 12-constant theory.

Other investigators of arterial elasticity favor exponential stress–strain relationship. See Gou (1970). The recent work by Ayorinde, Kobayashi, and Merati (1975) is especially refined and notable.

NONLINEAR VISCOELASTIC FEATURES OF ARTERIES AND THEIR VARIATION ALONG THE ARTERIAL TREE

In the preceding section we listed a polynomial strain-energy function to represent the nonlinear elasticity of the arteries when the viscous features are ignored. Experiments show, however, that arteries are not elastic. If we stretch a segment of an artery at a specific strain rate to a specified strain, and then unload at the same strain rate, the stress–strain curves of the loading and unloading do not coincide (see Figure 2). Fung (1967, 1972) pointed out an interesting fact that the loading and unloading curves, although different, change but little with the strain rate over a wide range, from 0.001 to 1.0 length/sec. Therefore, for such ordinary strain rate the stress can be regarded as a unique function of the strain in a loading process. In other words, an approximate elastic law may be used for the loading process. If the slope of the stress–strain

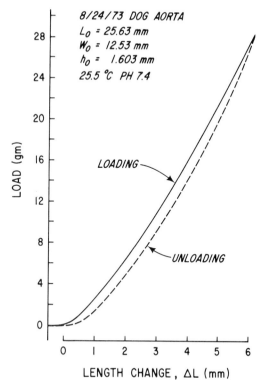

Figure 2. A typical stress–strain curve of a longitudinal segment of middle thoracic aorta of the dog. Stretch rate 0.5 mm/sec, 0.02 length/sec. From Tanaka and Fung (1973); reprinted with permission.

curve in uniaxial tension is plotted against the stress, it is a horizontal straight line if the material obeys Hooke's law. Figure 3 shows a collection of such plots for loading at constant rate. The stress is defined here in the Lagrangian sense: load divided by the original cross sectional area in the natural, relaxed state. It is seen that above $T > 200$ g/cm^2, the slope $dT/d\lambda$ varies approximately linearly with the stretch ratio λ(changed length divided by the original length); hence T is an exponential function of λ. The variation of the exponent along the arterial tree is clearly seen from Figure 4.

For stress relaxation after a step change in strain, it was shown by Tanaka and Fung (1973) that the relaxation function can be normalized (for $T > 200$ g/cm^2) in the sense that the stress response to a step change in strain can be expressed in the form

$$T(t,\lambda) = G(t) * T^{(e)}(\lambda) \qquad (9)$$

where $G(t)$ is a function of time and $T^{(e)}(\lambda)$ is a function of the stretch ratio λ.

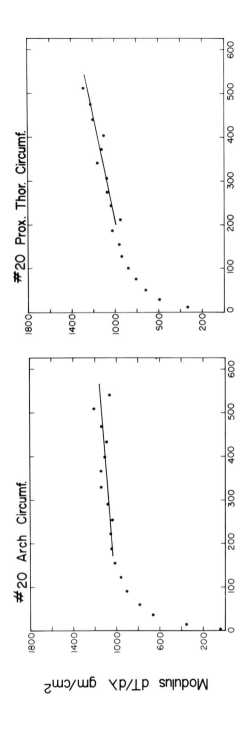

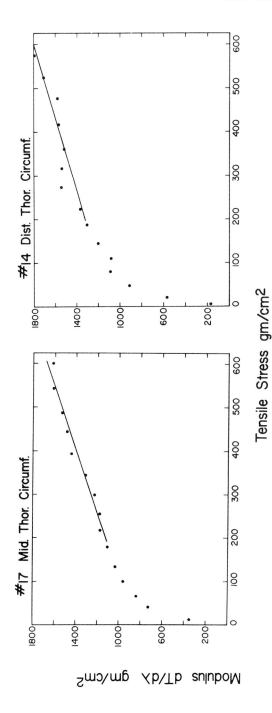

Figure 3. Plot of the Young's modulus (tangent modulus), $dT/d\lambda$, versus the tensile stress (T) in the specimens in a loading process. The straight line represents the equation $dT/d\lambda = \alpha T + E_0$. From Tanaka and Fung (1973); reprinted with permission.

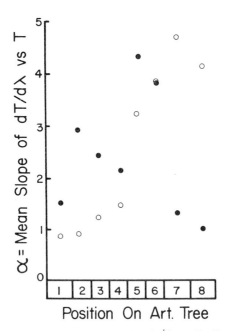

Position On Art. Tree

Figure 4. Variation of the constant α in the equation $dT/d\lambda = \alpha T + E_0$ along the aortic tree Open circles, longitudinal segments. Filled circles, circumferential segments. Numbers of positions on aortic tree are 1, arch; 2, proximal thoracic; 3, midthoracic; 4, distal thoracic; 5, proximal abdominal; 6, distal abdominal; 7, external iliac; 8, femoral artery. From Tanaka and Fung (1973); reprinted with permission.

The form of $G(t)$, called the *reduced relaxation function,* is shown in Figure 5. It is seen that considerable changes occur in $G(t)$ along the arterial tree.

The normalizability of the relaxation function is interpreted by Fung (1972) to mean that the material is governed by a quasilinear viscoelasticity law, Eq. (9), even when an arbitrary program of loading is imposed on the specimen. In that case $\lambda(t)$ is a function of time, and the ∗ symbol in Eq. (9) would represent an operation of convolution, namely,

$$T(t,\lambda) = \int_{-\infty}^{t} G(t-\tau)\frac{dT^{(e)}[\lambda(\tau)]}{d\lambda}\frac{d\lambda(\tau)}{d\tau}\,d\tau. \qquad (10)$$

The insensitivity of the stress and strain relationship to the strain rate in loading and unloading is explained by Fung (1972) as an evidence for a very broad and flat relaxation spectrum, $S(\tau)$, in the following expression:

$$G(t) = \frac{1}{A}\left[1 + \int_{0}^{\infty} S(\tau)e^{-t/\tau}\,d\tau\right], \qquad (11)$$

Where A is a normalization factor. In Tanaka and Fung (1973), it is shown that an adequate spectrum is

$$S(t) = \frac{C}{\tau} \quad \text{for } \tau_1 \leqslant \tau \leqslant \tau_2$$

$$= 0 \quad \text{for } \tau < \tau_1, \quad \tau > \tau_2$$

(12)

where τ_1, τ_2 are two constants and C is a normalization constant.

We consider the broad relaxation spectrum and the insensitivity of hysteresis to strain rate important. It justifies the assumption of pseudoelasticity, and the use of pseudo-strain-energy function to derive the stress–strain relationship in a loading process. But it is a subject of controversy. Whoever has looked for the effect of strain rate on the stress–strain relationship of living tissues has found it. The point is that it is remarkably uniform over a wide range of rates. McElhaney (1966), in his study of the dynamic response of muscles, shows a strain-rate effect on the stress–strain curve that amounts to about a 2.5-fold increase in stress at any given strain when the strain rate was varied from 0.001 to 1,000 sec-1, an increase of 10^6-fold. This is surely to be considered as an evidence of insensitivity. Van Brocklin and Ellis (1965), in their study of tendons, stated that there is no strain-rate effect when the rate is small, but the effect becomes significant when the rate is high. Collins and Hu (1972) who used explosive methods to impose high strain rate ($\dot{\epsilon}$) on to human aortic tissue, obtained the result

$$\sigma = (0.28 + 0.18\,\dot{\epsilon})(e^{12\epsilon} - 1) \quad \text{for } \dot{\epsilon} < 3.5 \text{ sec}^{-1}.$$

Bauer and Pasch (1971), working with rat tail artery, said that the dynamic Young's modulus is independent of frequency from 0.01 to 10 Hz, but the loss coefficient does vary with frequency. All these do not give a uniform picture, but it is clear that these tissues cannot be represented by a Maxwell model or a Voigt model. Our suggestion of a continuous relaxation spectrum (an assemblage of an infinite number of Maxwell and Voigt oscillators) does seem logical. The idea is indeed anticipated by aeronautical engineers in their concept of "structural" damping (Neubert, 1963), and by physicists Wagner (1913), Becker and Föppl (1928) and Becker and Döring (1939) in electromagnetic hysteresis. We also found that long before we proposed the quasilinear viscoelasticity embodied in Eqs. (14)–(16), Guth, Wack, and Anthony (1946) had already proposed it for rubbery materials.

The insensitivity of the hysteresis loop in cyclic loading to frequency is a remarkable feature of living tissues. From ultrasound experiments, it is known that energy dissipation per cycle seems to change no more than a factor of 2 or 3 when the frequency changes from 1,000 to 10^{-8} Hz. See critical reviews and extensive summaries by Fry and Dunn (1962) and Dunn, Edmonds, and Fry (1969), especially with regard to the curve of α/f versus $\log/f$, where f represents frequency and α the attenuation per unit distance, so that α/f is the attenuation per cycle. Dunn et al. (1969) show that α/f is virtually constant with respect to $\log/f$. Note, of course, that the amplitude of stress fluctuations is

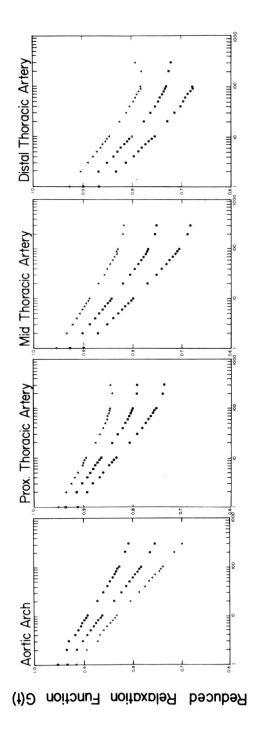

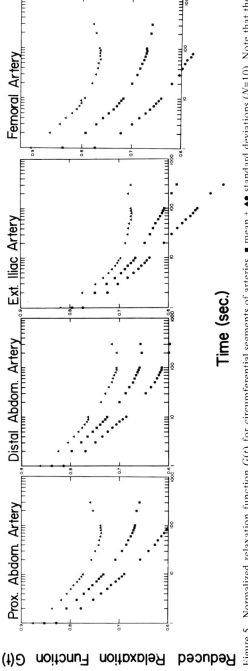

Figure 5. Normalized relaxation function $G(t)$ for circumferential segments of arteries. ■ mean ± ▲● standard deviations (N=10). Note that the vertical coordinates range over 0.6–1.0 in the upper panels; but they are from 0.6 to 0.9 in the lower panels. $G(t)$ is dimensionless. From Tanaka and Fung (1973); reprinted with permission.

very small in the ultrasound experiments, whereas in our experiments the range of stress variation in each cycle is very large (from near zero to upper ranges of physiologic stress). Nevertheless, it is interesting to observe this uniform behavior in a frequency range from nearly static condition to several hundred thousand cycles per second. Translated to the language of relaxation spectrum presented in Eq. (12), the ultrasound experiments suggest that the lower limit of relaxation time, τ_1, is very small for most living tissues, perhaps in the range of 10^{-8} sec.

Our view, if it continues to be supported by future experiments, does offer a great simplification. But since such a simplification is only an approximation, we shall always be on the lookout for improvements or further simplifications.

RHEOLOGY OF MATERIAL SURROUNDING CAPILLARIES

To understand the elastic behavior of the capillary blood vessels we must know the mechanical properties of the surrounding medium. Now, all capillary blood vessels do not have the same geometric relation with respect to their surrounding. A capillary blood vessel in the mesentery, for example, is surrounded by a gel substance. The distances between the capillaries are large, and the size of the gel is very large compared with the diameter of the capillary blood vessel. In this case the capillary may be considered as buried in an infinite medium. On the other hand, the capillary blood vessel in the lung is bounded by a thin layer of endothelial cells, epithelial cells, and interstitium with a total thickness of less than 1 μ. On the other side of the membrane is air. Such a capillary vessel does not receive the same kind of support from its surrounding as that in the mesentery.

To assess the support a capillary blood vessel in the mesentery receives from the surrounding gel, the assumption is made that the mechanical property of the gel is the same as that of the entire mesentery membrane. This is based on the observation that the mesenteric membrane is composed of amorphous material with a thickness of the order of 30 μ bounded by two layers of mesothelial cells each about 2 μ thick. At the interface there are basement membranes of varying thickness (300–500 Å) that blend with the connective tissue matrix. The stress–strain relation of such a membrane therefore roughly represents that of the connective tissue in the membrane. Experiments can be done on those avascular parts of the mesentery, in which only the smallest capillaries exist, which should not affect the overall mechanical properties of the membrane.

The mesentery shows a nonlinear viscoelastic behavior somewhat similar to that of the arteries. The stress–strain curve obtained in loading at constant strain rate is more truly exponential; it is independent of strain rate over a wide range (see Figure 6). The relaxation function can be normalized as in Eq. (9). The quasilinear viscoelastic relationship Eq. (10) holds. See Fung (1967, 1972) and

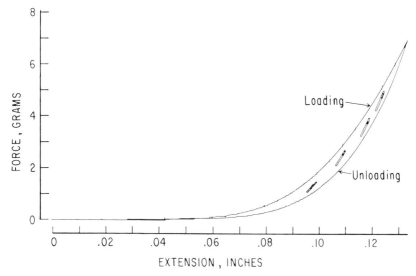

Figure 6. Stress–strain relations of the mesentery of the rabbit. From Fung (1967); reprinted with permission.

Chen and Fung (1973). The results of a torsion test (Fung, Zweifach, and Intaglietta, 1966) are also consistent with these observations.

For the mesentery, ureter, and muscles, the tangent-modulus-versus-tension curves for loading after preconditioning may be represented by the following equation in the tensile stress range $T_a \leqslant T \leqslant T_b$:

$$\frac{dT}{d\lambda} = \alpha(T + \beta). \tag{13}$$

An integration of this equation yields the relation (Fung, 1967)

$$T = (T^* + \beta)e^{\alpha(\lambda - \lambda^*)} - \beta \tag{14}$$

for λ in the range λ_a, λ_b that corresponds with T_a, T_b. This solution satisfies the condition

$$T = T^* \quad \text{when} \quad \lambda = \lambda^* \tag{15}$$

where T^*, λ^* is a point on the stress–stretch curve. According to Eq. (14), T does not go to zero when $\lambda = 1$ as it should if $\lambda = 1$ corresponds to the natural state (unstretched, stress-free state); but this is all right if $T_a > 0$, $\lambda_a > 1$, so that Eq. (13) and (14) are bounded away from the resting state.

The exponential type of stress–strain relationship can be generalized to two and three dimensions. For example, the extensive experimental results of Lanir and Fung (1974) on the rabbit skin can be fitted by the following stress–strain relationship (Tong and Fung, 1976):

$$\sigma_1 = \frac{\partial W}{\partial e_1}, \qquad \sigma_2 = \frac{\partial W}{\partial e_2}, \qquad (16)$$

where e_1, e_2 are the finite strain components corresponding to the stretch ratios λ_1, λ_2, respectively:

$$e_1 = \tfrac{1}{2}(\lambda_1^2 - 1), \qquad e_2 = \tfrac{1}{2}(\lambda_2^2 - 1), \qquad (17)$$

and W is the two-dimensional strain-energy function,

$$W = \tfrac{1}{2}(\alpha_1 e_1^2 + 2\alpha_4 e_1 e_2 + \alpha_1 e_2^2)$$
$$+ \tfrac{1}{2}C \exp\left[a_1 e_1^2 + a_2 e_2^2 + 2a_4 e_1 e_2 + e_1 e_2 (\beta_1 + \beta_2 e_2)\right]. \quad (18)$$

The constants α_1, α_4, c, a_1, a_2, a_4, β_1, β_2 must be determined experimentally. A typical set of values is

$$\alpha_1 = 13.8, \qquad \alpha_4 = 7.8,$$

$$a_1 = 3.904, \qquad a_2 = 11.28, \qquad a_4 = -13.97,$$
$$\beta_1 = 24.85, \qquad \beta_2 = 32.77, \qquad c = 0.0164. \qquad (19)$$

The skin was taken from rabbit's abdomen. The directions 1 and 2 refer, respectively, to longitudinal and tranverse directions. Since W is exponential, the stresses σ_1, σ_2 are exponential functions of the strains e_1, e_2. The experiments were done on the skin with the third dimension free, so that $\sigma_3 = 0$. The specimens were stretched only in the x_1, x_2 directions. The shear stresses τ_{12}, τ_{23}, τ_{31} were zero. The skin was considered incompressible, so that $\lambda_1 \lambda_2 \lambda_3 = 1$. Swelling of the skin existed, and was a function of the fluid environment and time after excision; however, with respect to stress loading at any given time, the assumption of incompressibility is acceptable.

Many other forms of strain-energy function have been proposed, the most popular one being a polynomial. It is often found that the degree of the polynomial has to be quite high and the number of needed empirical constants is, therefore, quite large.

Correspondingly, many other types of stress–strain relationship have been proposed. Nonlinear power laws of one kind or another have been used to describe the length–tension relations of simple elongation experiments. (See a review of literature in Fung, 1972.) But the present author prefers the exponential law, for the following reason. No matter how nonlinear the constitutive equation is, the equation of equilibrium is always linear when it is expressed in terms of Cauchy stresses. Hence a substitution of a stress–strain relationship of the exponential type into the equation of equilibrium will result in an equation in which the exponential function will be cancelled out throughout, yielding a relatively simple equation. Since the exponential function is the only function whose derivative is the same function, it is uniquely qualified for this purpose. The advantage of an exponential stress—strain law is the simplicity in theoretical analysis. Its shortcoming is the nonlinear fashion in which the empirical constants [such as α, β, in Eq. (14) and a_1, a_2, etc. in Eq. (18)] enter into the stress—strain relationship. This nonlinearity makes the ordinary method of least squares inoperative in the determination of these constants, and, as a consequence, statistical methods are difficult to apply. For example, we found that Eq. (18) can be used to fit the experimental results of the skin. For each run there is no difficulty in determining a set of constants that gives a good fit. But an attempt to optimize these constants so that a large number of test runs might be said to have been fitted statistically was not successful. We feel that this might not necessarily be the fault of the exponential function, but is a consequence of the rapidly rising stress with increasing strain when the strain is large.

With a nonlinear constitutive equation to describe the material surrounding the capillaries in the mesentery, Fung (1966) showed that practically all of the elastic rigidity (dp/dR) of the capillary blood vessels in the mesentery is derived from the surrounding gel.

CAPILLARY SYSTEM TOPOLOGY AND COMPLIANCE

For a proper analysis of the capillary system, three pieces of information must be known:

1. The topology of the capillary system.
2. The boundary conditions.
3. The compliance of the blood vessels.

The topology of the capillary bed varies from tissue to tissue. The long, circular, cylindrical tube systems of the mesentery and the muscles are well known. Capillaries in other organs may be quite different. Figure 7 shows a capillary network in the lung of the cat. These capillaries are organized into tightly knit sheets. Blood flow in the pulmonary alveolar sheets has little resemblance to Poiseuille flow in long tubes (Fung and Sobin, 1972a,b; Sobin et al., 1972).

The dependence of flow on topology and boundary conditions is modulated by the compliance of the capillaries. Capillaries in connective tissues and muscles are relatively rigid. It is well known that the change in capillary lumen diameter in the mesentery is not measurable in an ordinary optical microscope (with a sensitivity about $0.5~\mu$) when the static pressure in the vessel is varied over the physiologic range. In contrast to this, the thickness of the pulmonary alveolar sheet is quite compliant. Figure 8 shows the variation of the thickness of the alveolar sheets of the cat's lung with respect to the transmural pressure (local

316   Fung

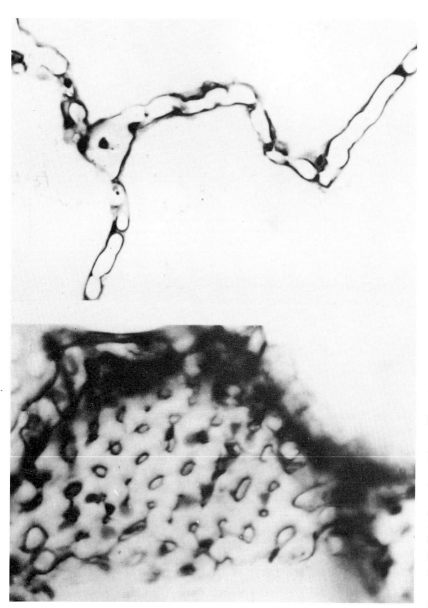

Figure 7. (*Left*) A plane view of the capillary blood vessels in the lung of the cat. (*Right*) A cross-sectional view of the same. These vessels form alveolar "sheets."

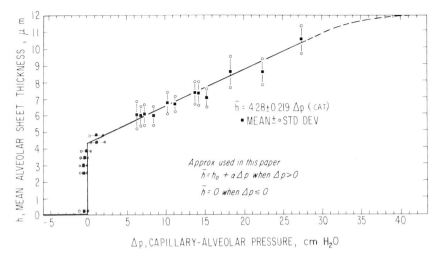

Figure 8. The dependence of the thickness of the pulmonary alveolar sheet of the cat on the transmural pressure (local pressure of blood minus the alveolar gas pressure). From Sobin et al. (1972); reprinted with permission.

pressure of blood minus the alveolar gas pressure), obtained by Sobin et al. (1972). When the transmural pressure is positive the thickness increases linearly with increasing pressure according to the formula

$$h = h_0 + \alpha \Delta p. \tag{20}$$

When the transmural pressure is negative, it is a good approximation to take the thickness h as zero. The compliance coefficient α depends on the degree of inflation of the lung. For a cat with a transpulmonary pressure (TPP) of 15 cm H_2O, α was found (Sobin et al., 1972) to be 0.22 μ per cm H_2O pressure; hence at Δp of 25 cm H_2O the thickness would have increased 5.5 μ from its value at $\Delta p = 0$. Values of α for dog are estimated to be 0.079 μ/cm H_2O at a TPP of 25 cm H_2O, 0.122 μ/cm H_2O at TPP of 10 cm H_2O, and 0.172 μ/cm H_2O at TPP of 5 cm H_2O (see Fung and Sobin, 1972a,b; data estimated from Glazier et al., 1967; and Permutt et al., 1968). The linear relationship given in Eq. (15) ceases to be vaild when Δp is too large, say, greater than 25 cm H_2O. At high values of Δp compliance becomes quite small.

On the other hand, the capillary dimension in the plane of the pulmonary alveolar membrane is essentially independent of the blood pressure; it depends mainly on the degree of inflation of the lung. Therefore, for the pulmonary capillaries one must distinguish compliance in the direction perpendicular to the sheet (which is large with respect to the blood pressure) from that in directions parallel to the sheet (which is small with respect to the blood pressure). Thus, to understand the elasticity of the capillary blood vessels in the lung one must not think of them as round tubes. They are organized into a sheet the thickness of which increases with blood pressure, but the area does not.

The principal cause for these differences in compliances is the differences in the amount of tissue surrounding the capillaries. The capillaries of the mesentery are embedded in a gel-like medium that contributes practically all of the rigidity to the capillary. The capillaries in the pulmonary alveolar sheets are organized as a two-dimensional structure that shows a combination of two features: In the plane of the membrane, each capillary is bounded by the "posts" whose interstitial spaces are filled with fluids, proteins, elastin, and collagen fibers (Sobin et al., 1972). These posts lend support to the capillaries in the plane of the interalveolar septa so that the capillary width is practically unaffected by the blood pressure. However, in the direction perpendicular to the sheet, the alveolar–capillary membrane has no surrounding tissue to support it; therefore, under a transmural pressure the membrane will deflect. These membranes are stretched because the lung is inflated. The tension in the membranes makes them deflect linearly with respect to the transmural pressure. The dispersed posts make the linear reaction localized. The linear relation (15) is a consequence of this situation.

CAPILLARY PATENCY

The basic idea that the mesenteric capillaries derive their rigidity from the surrounding gel tissue may be more figuratively expressed by saying that mechanically the mesenteric capillaries are tunnels in gels. Once this idea is developed, it naturally follows that such a capillary will not collapse when the entire tissue is subjected to a hydrostatic pressure, for the same reason that the Simplon tunnel can exist thousands of feet under the Alps. This is most probably the reason why capillaries remain patent in muscles even though contraction induces compressive stress in a direction perpendicular to the muscle bundle.

Patency of the capillaries is of course of great importance to the circulation system. The metabolic needs of a tissue can be answered only if blood flow can reach the tissue. Fortunately, in most tissues the capillaries are surrounded by a substantial amount of materials that provide the needed rigidity. In this regard the patency of capillaries in muscles is of special interest, because muscles contract and generate tension along their length. In many muscle bundles the longitudinal tension acting on a spindle-shaped muscle can create a considerable lateral compression in the circumferential direction. The pressure so generated can conceivably close down those capillaries that are parallel to the muscle fibers, but fortunately the surrounding material usually manages to keep the capillaries open.

If the configuration of the muscle bundle is such that no lateral pressure is generated when the muscle contracts, then by virtue of the constancy of volume of the tissue, the cross-sectional area of these capillary blood vessels that are parallel to the muscle fibers will be increased together with the cross section of the muscle bundle. At the same time, the lengths of the capillaries are shortened with the muscle. Therefore, if active control by sphincters were absent, the hemodynamic resistance of these capillaries would be decreased when the muscle shortens. Since the resistance to flow in a capillary is directly proportional to its length and inversely proportional to the fourth power of the radius, it follows that the percentage reduction of resistance is exactly three times the percentage reduction in length. Thus the resistance will be halved if the muscle shortens by 17%. This is seen as follows. Suppose the length shortens by 1%; then the cross-sectional area is increased by 1%, the radius will be increased by $\frac{1}{2}$%, and its fourth power, by 2%. The resistance is changed therefore, by 2 + 1 = 3%. In a general way this is well known. Observations of such dilatation of the capillaries and increase of flow in frog and mamalian muscles were reported by Krogh as early as 1918 (see Krogh, 1922, p. 61).

For those capillaries that lie in a direction perpendicular to the muscle fibers, and for feeding arterioles and venules, the opposite is true; the resistance therein will be raised by contraction. The total length of these transverse vessels is 3 or 4 times shorter than the total length of those vessels parallel to the muscle fibers, (Krogh, 1922).

Recently, Tillmanns et al. (1975) reported in vivo high-speed microcinematography of blood flow in the beating turtle and dog heart. They found that the diameters of the coronary arterioles, capillaries, and venules in the turtle ventricle all declined about 34% during systole. Similar results were obtained in the dog. The capillaries do not close in systole. The reduction of vessel diameter may be interpreted in terms of a balance between the lateral compression (due to increased ventricular pressure) and the support from surrounding tissues. The coronary capillaries are essentially parallel with muscle fibers (Bassingthwaite, Yipintsoi, and Harvey (1974).

ACTIVE STATE OF VASCULAR SMOOTH MUSCLE

No discussion of the rheology of blood vessels can be complete without considering the active state of the vascular smooth muscles. The active contraction of the muscles controls the diameter of the blood vessels. A vascular smooth muscle can respond to stimulation by nerves, drugs, electric pulses, and mechanical stretching. The last named response is known as the Bayliss phenomenon: that a muscle begins to contract when stretched, and relaxes when released—a phenomenon familiar to children who play with earthworms. Vascular smooth muscle can also maintain a "tone"—a certain constant value of active tension—which is extremely important in the control of the circulatory system (see Volume II for full discussion).

In the opinion of the present writer, our knowledge about the mechanics of the vascular smooth muscles is incomplete. The relationship between tension, length, and velocity of contraction is not precisely known—not well enough to serve as a basis for a general analysis of circulation. Future research on the control of circulation, including the problem of hypertension, must be centered around the determination of the mechanical properties of the vascular smooth muscles.

BIBLIOGRAPHICAL NOTES

The literature on the rheology of blood vessels and tissues surrounding blood vessels is very extensive. In the brief space above, we have reviewed only a few salient points. Other important material can be found in the following: Anliker (1972) discusses the damping of high frequency elastic waves in the arteries in in vivo experiments. Azuma and Hasegawa (1971) Azuma, Hasegawa, and Matsuda (1970), and Fischer and Llaurado (1966, 1967) discuss the structure (the contents of the collagen, elastin, smooth muscle and their structures) of the arteries and veins and its correlation with the viscoelastic properties of the arteries and veins. Baez, Lampart, and Baez (1960) present a remarkable paper about the mechanical property of the arterioles and metarterioles in the meso-appendix of the rat. Bergel (1961a, 1961b, 1964, 1972) and Bergel and Schultiz (1971) in a series of papers, have treated and reviewed both static and dynamic properties of the arteries. Blatz, Chu, and Wayland (1969) and Chu, Frasher, and Wayland (1972) present the nonlinear stress–strain relationship for the mesentery of the cat, and propose a power law. They also compare the differences between in vivo and in vitro properties. Buchthal and Kaiser (1951) give an extensive treatment of muscle. Dobrin and Rovick (1969) and Dobrin and Doyle (1970) deal with features of smooth muscles in arteries. Frank (1920) presents an excellent review of early data on blood vessel elasticity. Frasher (1966) discusses structure and function of the arteries, as well as the testing equipment. Fung (1973a, 1973b,) proposes mathematical formulations for the stress–strain law for solid soft tissues and membranous structures, such as the lung. Viscoelasticity of the arteries is discussed by Gow and Taylor (1968), Gow (1972), and Hardung (1953); inhomogeneity and anisotropy are discussed by Hardung (1964). A classic paper on collagen elasticity is given by Harkness (1961). Kenner's (1967) paper is an extensive review. Laszt (1968), Lee, Frasher, and Fung (1967), McDonald (1968), Patel, de Freitas, Greenfield, and Fry (1963), Peterson, Jensen, and Parnell (1960), and Remington (1955) present data on arteries. Remington's paper (1957) is a conference proceeding containing many interesting articles. Roy (1882), Roach and Burton (1957), Taylor (1964), Wetterer and Kenner (1968, and Wiederhielm (1965) are other well-known classics in this field.

This list is by no means exhaustive. Further references can be found from the articles named above.

LITERATURE CITED

Anliker, M. 1972. Toward a nontraumatic study of the circulatory system. *In* Y. C. Fung, N. Perrone, and M. Anliker (eds.), Biomechanics: Its Foundations and Objectives, Chap. 15, pp. 337–379. Prentice-Hall, Englewood Cliffs, N.J.

Ayorinde, O. A., A. S. Kobayashi, and J. K. Merati. 1975. Finite elasticity analysis of unanesthetized and anesthetized aorta (Abstract). *In* 1975 ASME Symposium on Biomechanics. American Society of Mechanical Engineers, New York.

Azuma, T. and M. Hasegawa. 1971. A rheological approach to the architecture of arterial walls. Japan J. Physiol. 21:27–47.

Azuma, T., M. Hasegawa, and T. Matsuda. 1970. Rheological properties of large arteries. *In* S. Onogi (ed.), Proceedings of the Fifth International Congress on Rheology, pp. 129–141. University of Tokyo Press, Tokyo, and University Park Press, Baltimore.

Baez, S. H., H. Lamport, and A. Baez. 1960. Pressure effects in living microscopic vessels. *In* A. Copley and G. Stainsby (eds.), Flow Properties of Blood and other Biological Systems, pp. 122–36. Pergamon, London.

Bassingthwaighte, J. B., T. Yipintsoi, and R. B. Harvey. 1974. Microvasculature of the dog left ventricular myocardium. Microvasc. Res. 7:229–249.

Bauer, R. D., and T. Pasch. 1971. The quasistatic and dynamic circumferential elastic modulus of the rat tail artery studied at various wall stresses and tones of the vascular smooth muscle. Pflügers Arch. 330:335–346.

Becker, E., and O. Föppl., 1928. Forsch. aus dem Geb. Ingenieurwesens V. D. I., No. 304.

Becker, E., and W. Döring. 1939. Ferromagnetismus, Chap. 19. Springer-Verlag, Berlin.

Bergel, D. H. 1961*a*. The static elastic properties of the arterial wall. J. Physiol. 156:445–457.

Bergel, D. H. 1961. The dynamic elastic properties of the arterial wall. J. Physiol. 156:458–469.

Bergel, D. H. 1964. Arterial viscoelasticity. *In* E. O. Attinger (ed.) Pulsatile Blood Flow. McGraw-Hill, New York.

Bergel, D. H. 1972. The properties of blood vessels. *In* Y. C. Fung, N. Perrone, and M. Anliker (eds.), Biomechanics: Its Foundations and Objectives, Chap. 5, pp. 105–140. Prentice-Hall, Englewood Cliffs, N.J.

Bergel, D. H., and D. L. Schultiz. 1971. Arterial elasticity and fluid dynamics. *In* J. A. V. Butler and D. Noble (eds.), Progress in Biophysics and Molecular Biology, Vol. 22. Pergamon Press, Oxford.

Blatz, P. J., B. M. Chu, H. Wayland. 1969. On the mechanical behavior of elastic animal tissue. Trans. Soc. Rheol. 13:83–102.

Buchthal, F., and E. Kaiser. 1951. The Rheology of the Cross Striated Muscle Fibre with Particular Reference to Isotonic Conditions. Copenhagen: Det Kongelige Danske Videnskabernes Selskab, Dan. Biol. Medd., 21, No. 7. 318 p.

Carew, T. E., R. N. Vaishnav, and D. J. Patel. 1968. Compressibility of the arterial wall. Circ. Res. 23:61–68.

322   Fung

Chen, Y. L., and Y. C. Fung. 1973. *1973 Biomechanics Symposium,* ASME Pub. No. AMD-2, pp. 9–10. American Society of Mechanical Engineers, New York.

Chu, B. M., W. G. Frasher, and H. Wayland. 1972. Hysteretic behavior of soft living aminal tissue. Ann. Biomed. Eng. 1:182–203.

Collins, R., and W. C. Hu. 1972. J. Biomechanics 5:333–337.

Dobrin, P. B., and A. A. Rovick. 1969. Influence of vascular smooth muscle on contractile mechanics and elasticity of arteries. Am. J. Physiol. 217:1644–1651.

Dobrin, P. G., and J. M. Doyle. 1970. Vascular smooth muscle and the anistropy of dog carotid artery. Circ. Res. 27:105–119.

Dunn, F., P. D. Edmonds, and W. J. Fry. 1969. *In* H. P. Schwan (ed.), Biological Engineering, p. 205. McGraw-Hill, New York.

Fischer, G. M., and J. G. Llaurado. 1966. Collagen and elastic content in canine arteries selected from functionally different vascular beds. Circ. Res. 19:394–399.

Fischer, G. M., and J. G. Llaurado. 1967. Connective tissue composition of canine arteries. Effects of renal hypertension. Arch. Pathol. 84:95–98.

Frank, O. 1920. Die Elastizität der Blutgefässe. Z. Biol. 71:255–272.

Frasher, W. G. 1966. What is known about the physiology of large blood vessels. *In* Y. C. Fung (ed.), Biomechanics. American Society of Mechanical Engineers, New York.

Fry, W. J., and F. Dunn. 1962. *In* W. L. Nastuck (ed.), Physical Techniques in Biological Research, Vol. IV, pp. 251–394. Academic Press, New York.

Fung, Y. C. 1966. Theoretical considerations of the elasticity of red cells and small blood vessels. Fed. Proc. 25:176.

Fung, Y. C. 1967. Elasticity of soft tissues in simple elongation. Am. J. Physiol. 213:1532–1544.

Fung, Y. C. 1972. Stress–strain-history relations of soft tissues in simple elongation. *In* Y. C. Fung (ed.), Biomechanics: Its Foundations and Objectives, pp. 181–208. Prentice-Hall, Englewood Cliffs, N.J.

Fung, Y. C. 1973. Biorheology of soft tissues. Biorheology 10:139–155.

Fung, Y. C. 1973. A theory of elasticity of the lung. J. Appl. Mech. APM-R:1–7.

Fung, Y. C., B. W. Zweifach, and M. Intaglietta. 1966. Elastic environment of the capillary bed. Circ. Res. 19:441–461.

Fung, Y. C., and S. S. Sobin 1972a. Elasticity of the pulmonary alveolar sheet. Circ. Res. 30:451–469.

Fung, Y. C., and S. S. Sobin. 1972b. Pulmonary alveolar blood flow. Circ. Res. 30:470–490.

Glazier, J. B., J. M. B. Hughes, J. E. Maloney, and J. B. West. 1967. Vertical gradient of alveolar size in lungs of dogs frozen intact. J. Appl. Physiol. 23(5):694–705.

Gou, P. F. 1970. Strain-energy function for biological tissues J. Biomech. 3:547–550.

Gow, B. S., and M. G. Taylor. Measurement of viscoelastic properties of arteries in the living dog. Circ. Res. 23:111–122.

Gow, B. S. 1972. The influence of vascular muscle on the viscoelastic properties of blood vessels. *In* D. H. Bergel (ed.), Cardiovascular Fluid Dynamics, Vol. 2, Chap. 12, pp. 66–110. Academic Press, New York.

Guth, E., P. E. Wack, and R. L. Anthony. 1946. J. Appl. Physics 17:347–351.

Hardung, V. 1953. Vergleichende Messungen der dynamischen Elastizität and Viskosität von Blutgefässen, Kautschuk and synthetischen Elastomeren. Helv. Physiol. Pharmacol. Acta 11:194–211.

Hardung, V. 1964. Significance of anisotropy and inhomogeneity in the determination of the elasticity of blood vessels. Angiologica 1:185–196.

Harkness, R. D. 1961. Biological functions of collagen. Biol. Rev. 36:199–463.

Johnson, P. C. 1974. The microcirculation, and local and humoral control of the circulation. In A. Guyton (ed.), Cardiovascular Physiology, MTP Intern. Rev. of Science, Physiol Ser. 1, Vol. 1. pp. 163–195. University Park Press, Baltimore.

Kenner, T. 1967. Neue Gesichtspunkte and Experimente zur Beschreibung and Messung der Arterienelastizität. Archiv für Kreislaufforschung. 54:68–139. Dr. Dietrisch Steinkopf Verlag, Darmstadt.

Krogh, A. 1922, 1929, 1959. The Anatomy and Physiology of Capillaries. With a new Introduction and Preface by E. M. Landis. 1st Ed., 1922. 2nd Ed., 1929. Reprint of 2nd Ed., 1959. Hafner, New York.

Lanir, Y., and Y. C. Fung. 1974. Two-dimensional mechanical properties of rabbit skin. I. Experimental System. II. Experimental results. J. Biomech. 7:29–34; 7:171–182.

Laszt, L. 1968. Untersuchungen über die elastischen Eigenschaften der Blutgefässe in Ruhe-und im Kontraktionszustand. Angiologica 5:14–27.

Lee, J. S., W. G. Frasher, and Y. C. Fung. 1967. Two-dimensional finite deformation experiments on Dog's Arteries and Veins. Report No. AFOSR 67-1980. University of California, San Diego.

McDonald, D. A. 1968. Regional pulse-wave velocity in the arterial tree. J. Appl. Physiol. 24:73–78.

McElhaney, J. H. 1966. J. Appl. Physiol. 21:1231–1236.

Neubert, H. K. P. 1963. Aeronautical Quarterly 14:187–197.

Patel, D. J., F. M. de Freitas, J. C. Greenfield, Jr., and D. L. Fry. 1963. Relationship of radius to pressure along the aorta in living dogs. J. Appl. Physiol. 18:1111–1117.

Patel, D. J., J. S. Janicki, and T. E. Carew. 1969. Static anisotropic elastic properties of the aorta in living dogs. Circ. Res., 25:765–779.

Patel, D. J., and R. N. Vaishnav. 1972. The rheology of large blood vessels. In D. H. Bergel (ed.), Cardiovascular Fluid Dynamics, Vol. 2, Chap. 11, pp. 2–65. Academic Press, New York.

Permutt, S., P. Caldini, A. Maseri, W. H. Palmer, W. H. T. Sasamori, and K. Zierler 1968. Recruitment versus distensibility in the pulmonary vascular bed. In A. Fishman and H. Hecht (eds.), The Pulmonary Circulation and Interstitial Space, pp. 375–387. University of Chicago Press, Chicago.

Peterson, L. H., R. E. Jensen, and J. Parnell. 1960. Mechanical properties of arteries in vivo. Circ. Res. 8:622–639.

Remington, J. W. 1955. Hysteresis loop behavior of the aorta and other extensible tissues. Am. J. Physiol. 180:83–95.

Remington, J. W. (ed.). 1957. Tissue Elasticity. Conference Proceeding, Dartmouth, 1955. American Physiological Society, Washington, D.C.

Roach, M. R., and A. C. Burton. 1957. The reason for the shape of the distensibility curves of arteries. Can. J. Biochem. Physiol. 35:681–690.

Roy, C. S. 1882. The elastic properties of the arterial wall. J. Physiol. 3:125–159.

Sobin, S. S., Y. C. Fung, H. M. Tremer, and T. H. Rosenquist. 1972. Elasticity of the pulmonary alveolar microvascular sheet in the cat. Circ. Res. 30:440–450.

Tanaka, T., and Y. C. Fung. 1973. Elastic and inelastic properties of the canine aorta and their variation along the aortic tree. J. Biomech. 7:357–370.

Taylor, M. G. 1964. Wave travel in arteries and design of the cardiovascular system. *In* E. O. Attinger (ed.), Pulsatile Blood Flow. McGraw-Hill, New York.

Tickner, E. G., and A. H. Sacks. 1967. A theory for the static elastic behaviour of blood vessels. Biorheology, 4:151—168.

Tillmanns, H., S. Ikeda, H. Hansen, J. S. M. Sarma, and R. J. Bing. 1975. Microcirculation in the ventricle of the dog and turtle. (Abstract). 1st World Congress for Microcirculation. Toronto, Canada.

Tong, P., and Y. C. Fung 1976. The stress-strain relationship for the skin. J. Biomechanics. In press.

Van Brocklin, J. D., and D. Ellis. 1965. A study of the mechanical behavior of toe extensor tendons under applied stress. Arch. Physical Medicine and Rehabilitation 46:369—375.

Wagner, K. W. 1913. Ann. der Physik 40:817—855.

Wetterer E., and T. Kenner. 1968. Grundlagen der Dynamik des Arterienpulses. Springer-Verlag, New York. 379 p.

Wiederhielm, C. A. 1965. Distensibility characteristics of small blood vessels. Fed. Proc. 24:1075—1084.

Yin, F. C. P., and Y. C. Fung. 1971. Mechanical properties of isolated mammalian ureteral segments. Am. J. Physiol. 221:1484—1493.

Zatzman, M., R. W. Stacy, J. Randall, and A. Eberstein. 1954. Time course of stress relaxation in isolated arterial segments. Am. J. Physiol. 177:299—302.

chapter 15

VISCOSITY
In Vitro
versus In Vivo

William I. Rosenblum

WHAT SHEAR RATE IS RELEVANT TO IN VIVO PHENOMENA

DO IN VITRO MEASUREMENTS OF VISCOSITY ASSIST
IN THE PREDICTION OF FLOW IN VIVO

INFLUENCE OF VISCOSITY ON RELATIVE MOVEMENTS
OF RED CELLS AND PLASMA IN VIVO

INFLUENCE OF VISCOSITY AS MEASURED IN VITRO
ON SHAPE OF VELOCITY PROFILE IN VIVO

COMMENTS

Elsewhere in this treatise, the sections on blood viscosity and disease makes clear in a very practical way the reasons for accepting as true the hypothesis that blood viscosity is an important determinant of blood flow. Indeed, if Poiseuillian laws of fluid mechanics are the basis of in vivo flow behavior, then flow must, of course, be a function of viscosity. However, in the microcirculation (let us say in vessels of under 100 μ i.d.), flow may be affected by other laws, in addition to, or in place of, those of Poiseuille. For example if laminar flow is absent, or if vessels admit only a single row of red blood cells (RBC), then other laws may take effect. In addition, one must remember that blood is a suspension of RBC, rather than a solution, and the concentration and flexibility of the RBC, as well as their tendency to aggregate, also alter the flow (Gregerson et al., 1970; Chien et al., 1970a, 1970b). Some of these factors may be more important in the microcirculation than in vitro; for example, erythrocyte rigidity may cause a finite rise in viscosity measured in vitro but an infinite "rise" (i.e., complete stoppage of flow) in a portion of the vascular bed where all orifices have dimensions smaller than that of the RBC. In this regard it must be remembered that RBC, in general, are larger than capillaries, and that RBC deformation is required for passage of RBC through the capillaries. Furthermore, before extrapolating in vitro observations to in vivo situations, it must be remembered that some of the factors determining viscosity may change as the blood passes through the microcirculation. Hematocrit, for example, is not identical at all points in the microcirculation of a given animal and its exact value at a given point in the microcirculation may remain unknown. Thus it may be impossible precisely to replicate in vivo conditions during an in vitro measurement. For all of these reasons, and in spite of the relationship between viscosity and blood flow as apparently manifest in disease states, there has arisen a question concerning the importance of in vitro determinations in predicting blood flow. The following section reviews the experimental data relating in vitro measurements to a variety of microvascular alterations observed in vivo.

WHAT SHEAR RATE IS RELEVANT TO IN VIVO PHENOMENA?

The viscosity of blood is not fixed, but rises as shear rate falls below a certain critical level. For normal blood this level is about $100 \ sec^{-1}$ (Whitmore, 1968; Merrill, 1969). Therefore, in recent years, many workers have stressed the importance of knowing the shear rate at which an in vitro viscosity measurement is made. For a blood vessel of any given size, shear rate falls as the rate of blood flow diminishes. With the development of instruments for measuring viscosity at low shear rates analogous to very low flow rates through the microcirculation, there has been an emphasis on the particular relevance of these measurements to in vivo phenomena. The impression has been given that low shear rates were the rule in the microcirculation, and that measurements were not relevant to in vivo conditions if they were made at shear rates higher than the critical level referred to above (Wells, Denton, and Merrill, 1961; Schrier et al., 1970; Kontros et al., 1970). Unfortunately, this view is not correct, because the average shear rate in the microcirculation actually exceeds the "critical" level below which large rises in viscosity are seen. Thus, for almost all vascular beds for which we have relevant velocity or flow data, the shear rate near the wall exceeds $100 \ sec^{-1}$ (Haynes and Burton, 1959; Berman, 1965; Bloch, 1968; Whitmore, 1968; Rosenblum, 1969). In fact, as recent communications indicate, even when some literature values for flow and shear rate are reduced by a factor of 10, the shear rates may reach $800 \ sec^{-1}$ at the capillary wall and $500 \ sec^{-1}$ at the arteriole wall (Hyman, 1971). It is true that shear rates fall as one moves from the vessel wall toward the center of the blood stream. Thus the average shear rate across the stream will be less than the shear rates just alluded to. Nevertheless, it is clear that within the microcirculation, as well as in the larger vessels, shear rate often exceeds $100 \ sec^{-1}$. This fact has recently been acknowledged even by one of the workers who originally emphasized the importance of low shear rates during in vitro measurements (Merrill, 1969).

Although it is erroneous to dismiss as unphysiologic viscosity measurements made at high shear rates, and although high shear rates are often found in the microcirculation, measurements at low shear rates are also of physiologic interest. Lower shear rates are present near the center of some vessels and during conditions of low flow, for example, across the entire vessel during development of or recovery from, stopflow conditions. Such conditions are often observed in the microcirculation in vessels displaying intermittent flow. Even during apparently continuous and rapid flow there may, in fact, be periodic reductions in flow, and hence in shear rate, since blood flow in the microcirculation is actually pulsatile, diminishing during the diastolic portion of each cardiac cycle and accelerating again during systole (Hugues, 1953; Bloch, 1968; Rosenblum, 1969; Intaglietta, Richardson, and Thompkins, 1971).

In addition to the periodic or episodic appearance of low flow and low shear in almost any vascular bed, there are also vascular beds with comparatively low basal or average flow rates. Measurements of RBC velocity in vivo indicate that the microvasculature of the conjunctiva and the inner ear are characterized by low flow (Perlman and Kimura, 1961; Wells and Edgerton, 1967). The observations of the inner ear were made under rather hypotensive conditions, however (Perlman and Kimura, 1961), and the low RBC velocities observed there may simply reflect the abnormally low blood pressures (Rosenblum, 1970). In any case, the low RBC velocity in conjunctiva or inner ear should not generate conclusions about microvascular shear rates generally, since velocity values in these beds are up to 10 times smaller than those reported elsewhere.

DO IN VITRO MEASUREMENTS OF
VISCOSITY ASSIST IN THE PREDICTION OF FLOW IN VIVO?

Irrespective of the shear rate employed during in vitro measurement, several workers have reported a discrepancy between the rate of blood flow measured in vivo and blood flow predicted from viscosity values obtained through in vitro examination of the blood in question. Often this discrepancy is expressed by comparing the viscosity measured in vitro (Skovborg, Nielsen, and Schlichtkrull, 1968; Schrier et al., 1970; Benis et al., 1970), with the value of "apparent" viscosity, calculated from pressure flow curves in vivo. Several groups have shown that large changes in blood viscosity (in vitro) lead to surprisingly small changes in flow, so that in vivo "viscosity" appears to be relatively little changed even when in vitro viscosity is greatly changed (Bollinger and Luthay, 1968; Skovberg et al., 1968; Braasch and Jenett, 1968; Djojosugito et al., 1970; Baeckstrom et al., 1971).

Among the explanations for these data has been the finding in model systems that in true capillaries there is a relatively low resistance with a total blood viscosity that is relatively independent of hematocrit and approaches plasma alone (Rowlands and Skibo, 1971). On the other hand, several investigations demonstrate that alterations in hematocrit profoundly affect flow in vivo just as one would expect from the strong relationship between hematocrit and viscosity in vitro (Whitmore, 1968; Merrill, 1969), and that in a model system hematocrit did influence capillary flow (Tickner, 1972).

For vessels down to 20 μ i.d., several workers have invoked the Fahreaus–Lindquist (1931) effect to explain an unexpectedly low viscosity. This "effect," however, is really a restatement of the fact that in narrow tubes viscosity appears unexpectedly low as judged by pressure–flow curves for these tubes. Recently, the actual explanation for this effect appears to have been elucidated and with it at least a partial basis for some of the surprisingly low viscosities found from in vivo experiments. It has now been shown that within capillaries less than 100 μ i.d., the hematocrit is reduced when compared with that in either the feeding reservoir or draining container (Barbee and Cokelet, 1971a, 1971b). When the actual intra-"capillary" hematocrit is utilized in calculating the resistance term of the Poiseuille equation, the equation accurately predicts the pressure–flow relationship in the tubes (Barbee and Cokelet, 1971b). In short, the "unexpected" aspect of the drop in viscosity, described as the Fahreaus–Lindquist phenomenon, then disappears, and the viscosity is exactly that expected at the corrected hematocrit. Thus it may be that pressure–flow curves through a vascular bed, since they include flow through the microcirculation, are modified by a reduction of hematocrit in the smaller vessels, so that the apparent viscosity for the entire bed appears lower than that obtained when blood from feeding arteries or veins is examined in vitro. In fact, it is well known that organ hematocrits are less than large vessel hematocrits (Whitmore, 1968; Rosenblum, 1972a). Many people seem to have difficulty in understanding where the "excess" RBC "go" if they do not enter the microvessel. The answer is that they do not "go" anywhere. They do enter the vessel, passing through in reduced concentration but at an accelerated rate, so that at equilibrium, the hematocrit in the large "reservoir" and the large "drain" are similar and greater than the hematocrit in the intervening microvessels. In bringing this result about, the linear velocity of the RBC passing through the microvessels must be faster than that of the plasma. This is indeed the case (Whitmore, 1968; Rosenblum, 1972a) and is referred to again, below, in a slightly different context. Meanwhile, this phenomenon, and the Fahreaus–Lindquist effect that may depend on it, provides a basis for understanding why in vivo flow rates may exceed those predicted from in vitro viscosity measurements.

Benis, Usami, and Chien (1972) have provided an alternative explanation for the apparent discrepancy between in vitro viscosity levels and those calculated from pressure–flow curves in perfused vascular beds. They concluded that an apparently low in vivo viscosity is not the result of the Fahreaus–Lindquist phenomenon, but is merely the result of a failure to take into account inertial losses when calculating flow resistances. In their own experiments, they found that by applying this correction for inertial losses, the apparent viscosity of blood in vivo was elevated to levels consistent with in vitro observations, and they stated that the Fahraeus–Lindquist effect was not important in determining overall pressure loss in a complex vascular bed (the perfused canine hindpaw). They did leave open the possibility that the Fahraeus–Lindquist effect was still important in local microcirculatory dynamics. In this context it should be reiterated that the Fahraeus–Lindquist effect is demonstrated by experiments with single tubes of microcirculatory dimensions. The existence of the phenomenon and its dependence on hematocrit changes in the microvessels and on differential linear velocities of RBC and plasma, are not called into question by experiments in which pressure–flow analysis is carried out on an entire limb or organ whose vascular bed includes many vessels of larger size, leading to and from the microcirculation proper. Thus it is possible that the Fahraeus–Lindquist effect may diminish apparent viscosity in some experimental situations and play a lesser role in others, depending upon the relative significance of the microcirculation in the experimental design.

In any event it is apparent that viscosity is a determinant of flow in vivo, through both the micro- and "macro"-circulations. The preceding paragraphs indicate that changes in flow may sometimes be smaller than expected from in vitro measurements of altered viscosity, but that such discrepancies can be explained either by a failure to take into account inertial losses in the calculation of resistance to flow, or by the Fahraeus–Lindquist effect and/or reduction of hematocrit within the microcirculation. It is also possible that altering the viscosity of blood will have a surprisingly small effect on flow in vivo if the organ in question is capable of making compensatory circulatory adjustments, such as vasodilation or recruitment of previously closed channels during hyperviscous states (Segel and Bishop, 1967; Murray, Karp, and Nadel, 1969). Under such circumstances, there is, of course, still a relationship between viscosity and flow, but the relationship is obscured by the compensatory alterations in the volume of the vascular bed. It is certainly incorrect to conclude, as some workers have done, that with the possible exception of flow in certain microvessels, viscosity is not a significant determinant of flow (Baeckstrom et al., 1971; Djojosugito et al., 1970).

INFLUENCE OF VISCOSITY ON
RELATIVE MOVEMENTS OF RED CELLS AND PLASMA IN VIVO

In addition to a relationship between in vitro viscosity levels and flow rate, certain other effects may be demonstrated in vivo after in vitro detection of an altered blood viscosity. For example, when blood viscosity was elevated by any one of three methods, the normal difference between RBC velocity and plasma velocity was apparently increased (Whitmore, 1968; Rosenblum, 1972a). In our earlier discussion of the Fahraeus–Lindquist effect we alluded to the fact that, in the microcirculation, the linear velocity of RBC may exceed that of plasma with a resultant drop in organ hematocrit as compared to hematocrit in large vessels

(Whitmore, 1968; Rosenblum, 1972). We have recently found that elevations of viscosity are associated with a prolonged plasma transit time in the absence of a decreased RBC velocity (Rosenblum, 1970, 1971, 1972a, 1972b). This seems best explained by assuming the following sequence of events. The axial migration of RBC is accelerated by the increased viscosity (Whitmore, 1968; Goldsmith, 1970), so that a greater proportion of RBC are located near the center of the lumen where velocities are highest (Whitmore, 1968); in addition, plasma skimming is increased when axial migration is enhanced, so that an increasing proportion of plasma is skimmed of the periphery of the moving column of blood into side branches, leading to a passage of the skimmed plasma through vessels with a longer average path length or a higher overall resistance (Whitmore, 1968; Rosenblum, 1972a). Thus increased axial migration of RBC and increased plasma skimming may contribute separately, as well as cooperatively, to the differential effect of elevated viscosity on the velocities of plasma and RBC. If enhanced plasma skimming does contribute to the observed phenomena, then one would expect higher RBC velocities in capillaries with higher hematocrits. Such an observation has, in fact, been made (Johnson, 1971).

INFLUENCE OF VISCOSITY AS MEASURED IN VITRO ON SHAPE OF VELOCITY PROFILE IN VIVO

Beside the effects of increased viscosity on axial migration, plasma skimming and the differential velocity of plasma and RBC, increased viscosity can alter the velocity profile within a given microvessel. This has been suggested by measurements at different hematocrits of RBC velocity at multiple points across the blood stream moving through glass tubes (Gaehtgens, Meiselman, and Wayland, 1970). This in vitro observation appears to have been confirmed by in vivo measurements of RBC velocity at the center of the stream (V_c) and near the vessel wall (V_w). The ratio of V_w to V_c was used to estimate the velocity profile and it was found (Rosenblum, 1972c) that this ratio became greater at high blood viscosities (i.e., velocity profile became blunter). In the same study it was found that when elevated plasma viscosity was counteracted by a reduced hematocrit, so that the overall blood viscosity remained within normal limits, the ratio V_w/V_c became smaller (i.e., the velocity profile became less blunt or more parabolic). Anemic blood with a normal plasma viscosity gave the smallest ratios of V_w/V_c (i.e., the most "pointy" velocity profiles). These measurements (Rosenblum, 1972c) not only provide evidence of an effect of blood viscosity on the velocity profile, but also provide almost unique published data confirming the presence of a velocity profile within microvessels. Heretofore, simultaneous velocity measurements at multiple points across the blood stream had been confined almost solely to glass tubes (Gaehtgens et al., 1970).

   In view of the agreement between in vivo data of Rosenblum (1972c) cited above and the in vitro data concerning the influence of hematocrit on the shape of velocity profiles, it is disconcerting to find that the in vitro data has not been challenged by Baker and Wayland (1974). The in vitro measurements were made using an indirect method for monitoring red cell velocity. The method employs photocells to detect changes in optical density, and Baker and Wayland have shown that the technique gives erroneous results. When they "correct" these results they find that the velocity profile remains absolutely parabolic and is not influenced by hematocrit, or by changes in shear rate, even over a very wide range of values for either of the latter parameters. Why then do the data of Rosenblum (1972c) suggest that alterations in viscosity can, in fact, alter the shape of the velocity profile? At present, one can only suggest possible explanations for the discrepancy.

First of all, Rosenblum's (1972c) data do, in fact, suggest a *relative* constancy of the velocity profile over a wide range of shear rates, and it was only on further analysis of the data that subgroups appeared with a profile that was related to viscosity. It may be that the indirect technique for measuring red cell velocity (Baker and Wayland, 1974) is not as sensitive as the direct cinematographic method employed by Rosenblum (1972c) and hence was not able to detect the effects of hematocrit (i.e., viscosity) on the profile. Baker and Wayland (1974) did confirm some of their findings by employing high-speed cinematography, but only performed the latter studies at an extremely low hematocrit (6%).

Secondly, Baker and Wayland (1974) report constancy of velocity profile for tubes greater than 40 μ i.d. The vessels examined by Rosenblum (1972c) had a smaller average diameter, so that the tube diameter more closely approached the diameter of the red cells. This may account for the fact that the ratio of centerline velocity to wall velocity, indicated by Rosenblum's data, suggests a velocity profile that was not only affected by viscosity but that was much blunter than a parabola under most flow conditions.

Third, Rosenblum's measurements were made in vivo where pulsatile flow is an important characteristic of the microcirculation, the pulse being generated by each beat of the heart (Rosenblum, 1969). The in vitro measurements made by Baker and Wayland (1974) were performed under conditions of steady flow. During pulsatile flow, shear rate is near its nadir twice during each cycle, and viscosity is correspondingly increased. This could conceivably alter the rheologic phenomena described by Baker and Wayland (1974) under steady-state conditions. Indeed, Singh, Scearse, and Coulter (1974) have reported that the apparent viscosity of blood is greatly increased under conditions of pulsatile flow, even with pulse frequency as low as 36 cycles per minute, and that the effect on viscosity becomes progressively greater as the pulse frequency increases. This effect was related by Singh et al. (1974), at least in part, to the yield stress of the blood. Whatever the explanation, their concluding paragraph may provide an important key to understanding the discrepancies between Rosenblum's in vivo data, and the in vitro data of Baker and Wayland (1974).

Singh et al. (1974) suggest "that the non-Newtonian properties of blood may play a more important role in pulsatile situations than is generally realized."

COMMENTS

We may summarize the available data relating in vitro blood viscosity determinations to microcirculatory events by stating that alterations in viscosity demonstrated in vitro can be related to changes in flow and flow patterns in minute blood vessels. This fact is manifest by the patterns of disease that accompany high-viscosity states as discussed elsewhere (see Rosenblum in Volume III). It is also manifest in experimental investigations of flow and viscosity. Where changes in the viscosity level as measured in vitro are accompanied by relatively little change in flow, it is possible that viscosity in vivo has also changed relatively little. This may be because of a change in hematocrit within the microvasculature. It is also possible that initial alterations in flow did occur and resulted in homeostatic compensations such as vasodilation, which counteract the effects of the altered viscosity. In addition, departures from expected or predicted alterations in flow may occur because shear rates used to measure viscosity in vitro are not applicable to in vivo conditions. In this regard it should be kept in mind that high shear rates often characterize flow in microvessels, so undue emphasis should not be given to measurements at extremely low rates of shear, although these rates may also be found in vivo. Apparent discrepancies between flow rates predicted on the basis of in vitro viscosity measurements and those actually found in vivo may also be caused by a failure to take into account inertial forces when calculating in vivo flow resistances. Finally, beside affecting overall flow, viscosity levels determined in vitro can be related to the degree of axial migration of RBC within small blood vessels, to the degree of plasma skimming within the microvasculature, and to the shape of the velocity profile within individual microvessels. When extrapolating from in vitro measurements to the situation in vivo, caution is required, not only when different methods of examination are employed, but also when the pulsatile characteristics of in vivo flow are not mimicked by the in vitro model.

LITERATURE CITED

Baeckstrom, P., B. Folkow, E. Kendrick, B. Lofving, and B. Oberg. 1971. Effects of vasoconstriction on blood viscosity in vivo. Acta Physiol. Scand. 81: 376–385.

Baker, M., and H. Wayland. 1974. On-line volume flow rate and velocity profile measurement for blood in microvessels. Microvasc. Res. 7:131–143.

Barbee, J. H., and G. R. Cokelet. 1971a. The Fahraeus effect. Microvasc. Res. 3:6–17.

Barbee, J. H., and G. R. Cokelet. 1971b. Prediction of blood flow in tubes with diameters as small as 29 μ. Microvasc. Res. 3:17–22.

Benis, A. M., P. Taveres, F. Mortara, and A. Lockhart. 1970. Effect of hematocrit on pressure flow relations for perfused isolated lobes of canine lungs. Pflügers Arch. 314:347–360.

Benis, A. M. U. Usami, and S. Chien. 1972. Evaluation of viscous and inertial pressure losses in isolated tissue with a simple mathematical model. Microvasc. Res. 4:81–93.

Berman, H. J. 1965. Rheological properties of the microvasculature. Bibl. Anat. 7:29–34.

Bloch, E. H. 1968. High speed cinephotography of the microvascular system. In A. L. Copley (ed.), Hemorheology–Proceedings of the First International Conference, pp. 655–667. Pergamon Press, New York.

Bollinger, A., and E. Luthy. 1968. Blood viscosity and blood flow in the human forearm Helv. Med. Acta 34:255–264.

Braasch, D., and W. Jenett. 1968. Erythrocytenflexibilität, Hamonkonzentration und Reibungswiderstand in Glascapillaren mit Durchemessern zwischen 6 bis 50 μ. Pflügers Arch. 302:245–254.

Chien, S., S. Usami, R. J. Dellenbock, and M. I. Gregersen. 1970a. Blood viscosity: Influences of erythrocyte deformation. Science 157:827–829.

Chien, S., S. Usomi, R. J. Dellenbock, M. I. Gregersen, L. B. Narruvga, and M. M. Girest. 1970b. Blood viscosity: Influence of erythrocyte aggregation. Science 157:829–831.

Djojosugito, A. M., B. Folkow, B. Oberg, and S. White. 1970. A comparison of blood viscosity measured in vitro and in a vascular bed. Acta Physiol. Scand. 78:70–88.

Fahraeus, R., and R. Lindquist. 1931. The viscosity of the blood in narrow capillary tubes. Am. J. Physiol. 96:562–568.

Gaehtgens, P., H. J. Meiselman, and H. Wayland. 1970. Velocity profiles of human blood at normal and reduced hematocrit in glass tubes up to 130 μ diameter. Microvasc. Res. 2:13–23.

Goldsmith, H. L. 1970. Motion of particles in a flowing system. In F. Koller et al. (eds.), Vascular Factors and Thrombosis, pp. 91–110. Suppl 40 to Thrombosis et Diathesis Haemorrhagic. Schattauer, New York.

Gregersen, M. I., C. Bryant, W. E. Hammerle, S. Usami, and S. Chien. 1970. Characteristics of human erythrocytes through polycarbonate sieves. Science 157:825–857.

Haynes, R. H., and A. C. Burton. 1959. Role of the non-Newtonian behavior of blood in hemodynamics. Am. J. Physiol. 197:943–950.

Hugues, J. 1953. Contribution a l'étude des facturs vasculaires et sanguins dans l'hemostase spontanée. Arch. Int. Physiol. Biochim. 61 (suppl):565.

Hyman, W. A. (and reply by Whitmore). 1971. Rheology and hemodynamics. Biorrheology 8:103–104.

Intaglietta, M., D. R. Richardson, and W. R. Tompkins. 1971. Blood pressure flow and elastic properties in microvessels of cat omentum. Am. J. Physiol. 221:922–929.

Johnson, P. C. 1971. Red cell separation in the mesenteric capillary network. Am. J. Physiol. 221:99–104.

Kontros, S. B., J. G. Bodenbender, J. Craenen, and D. M. Hosier. 1970. Hyperviscosity in congenital heart disease. J. Pediatr. 76:214–221.

Merrill, E. W. 1969. Rheology of blood. Physiol. Rev. 49:863–888.

Murray, J. F., R. B. Karp, and J. A. Nadel. 1969. Viscosity effects on pressure flow relations and vascular resistance in dog's lungs. J. Appl. Physiol. 27: 336—341.

Perlman, H. B., and R. Kimura. 1961. Cochlear blood flow in acoustic trauma. Acta Oto. Larying. 54:99—110.

Rosenblum, W. I. 1969. Erythrocyte velocity and a velocity pulse in minute blood vessels on the surface of the mouse brain. Circ. Res. 24:887—892.

Rosenblum, W. I. 1970. The differential effect of elevated blood viscosity on plasma and erythrocyte flow in the cerebral microcirculation of the mouse. Microvasc. Res. 2:399—408.

Rosenblum, W. I. 1971. Erythrocyte velocity and fluorescein transit time in the cerebral microcirculation of macroglobulinemic mice. Differential effect of a hyperviscosity syndrome on the passage of erythrocytes and plasma. Microvasc. Res. 3:288—296.

Rosenblum, W. I. 1972a. Can plasma skimming or inconstancy of regional hematocrit introduce serious errors in regional cerebral blood flow measurements or their interpretation? Stroke 3:248—254.

Rosenblum, W. I. 1972b. Erythrocyte velocity and fluorescein transit time through the cerebral microcirculation in experimental polycythemia. J. Neuropathol. Exp. Neurol. 31:126—131.

Rosenblum, W. I. 1972c. Ratio of red cells velocities near the vessel wall to velocities at the vessel center in cerebral microcirculation, and an apparent effect of blood viscosity on this ratio. Microvasc. Res. 4:98—101.

Rowlands, S., and L. Skibo. 1971. Erythrocyte flow in tubes of capillary size. Can. J. Physiol. Pharmacol. 49:373—374.

Schrier, R. W., K. M. McDonald, R. E. Wells, and D. P. Lauler. 1970. Influence of hematocrit and colloid on whole blood viscosity during volume expansion. Am. J. Physiol. 218:340—353.

Segel, N., and T. M. Bishop. 1967. Circulatory studies on polycythemia vera at rest and during exercise. Clin. Sci. 32:527—549.

Singh, M., R. W. Scearse, and N. A. Coulter, Jr. 1974. Flow and frequency dependent viscosity of blood and blood—dextran mixtures. Microvasc. Res. 7:268—273.

Skovborg, F., A. V. Nielsen, and J. Schlichtkrull. 1968. Blood viscosity and vascular flow rate. Scand. J. Clin. Lab. Invest. 21:83—88.

Tickner, E. 1972. Concentration effects on viscosity of blood flow through capillaries. Microvasc. Res. 4:102—104.

Wells, R. E., R. Denton, and E. W. Merrill. 1961. Measurement of viscosity of biologic fluids by cone plate viscometer. J. Lab. Clin. Med. 57:646—655.

Wells, R., and H. Edgerton. 1967. Blood flow in the microcirculation of the conjunctival vessels of man. Angiology 18:699—704.

Whitmore, R. L. 1968. Rheology of the Circulation. Pergamon Press, New York.

chapter 16

PRESSURE-FLOW RELATIONSHIPS OF SINGLE VESSELS AND ORGANS

Jen-shih Lee

FULLY DEVELOPED FLOW IN A CIRCULAR TUBE

PRESSURE DROP OF BLOOD FLOW IN GLASS TUBES

FACTORS AFFECTING THE PRESSURE–FLOW RELATIONSHIP OF SINGLE VESSELS WITH DIAMETERS MUCH LARGER THAN THAT OF THE RED BLOOD CELLS

DISTRIBUTION OF PRESSURE AND FLOW IN THE MESENTERIC MICROCIRCULATION

MODEL OF MESENTERIC VASCULAR NETWORK

FLOW IN PULMONARY MICROVASCULATURE

EFFECT OF BIFURCATION ON HEMATOCRIT DISTRIBUTION AND PRESSURE LOSS

PRESSURE–FLOW RELATIONSHIP OF AN ORGAN

FULLY DEVELOPED FLOW IN A CIRCULAR TUBE

Let us consider the blood flow in a long, straight, circular tube of diameter d. The flow is incompressible, steady state, and fully developed such that any disturbance generated at the entrance is not present in the flow. For these conditions, the flow is axisymmetric and the velocity in the radial direction is zero. By balancing the momentum in the radial direction, one can show that the hydrostatic pressure p is constant across the cross section of the tube. (For such a simple flow, the normal strain rate vanishes. Thus the normal stress is equal to

Research supported by PHS, NHLI Grants HL 11747, 14517, and 16812.

the hydrostatic pressure.) However, because of the variation in axial velocity u in the radial direction, the total pressure head, given by

$$p_t = p(z) + \frac{1}{2}\rho u^2(r),\tag{1}$$

is a function of the radial coordinate r and the axial one z. The density of the fluid is designated ρ. Balancing the forces in the axial direction for any concentric column of length L in the tube leads to the following identity:

$$\pi r^2 (p_1 - p_2) = 2\pi r L \tau \tag{2}$$

where τ is the shear stress acting in the direction opposite to the flow, p_1 the hydrostatic pressure at the front surface of the column, and p_2 that at the back surface. As shown by Eq. (2), τ is a linear function of the radius.

If the fluid is Newtonian with a viscosity η, the Poiseuille pressure–flow relationship is given by

$$\frac{p_1 - p_2}{L} = \eta \frac{128\,Q}{\pi d^4} \tag{3}$$

where Q is the flow rate. Since the shear rate at the wall, γ_w, can be calculated as

$$\gamma_w = \frac{32\,Q}{\pi d^3},\tag{4}$$

Eq. (2) and (3) can be transformed to

$$\tau_w = (p_1 - p_2)\frac{d}{4L} = \eta\gamma_w,\tag{5}$$

which is Newton's law of friction. τ_w is the shear at the wall.

Many investigators have used the above equations to reduce the data on the rheologic properties of blood. Since the total flow rate and the pressure difference across a capillary viscometer can be readily measured, one can generalize Eq. (4) to define a pseudo shear rate at the wall for the blood as

$$\gamma_w^* = \frac{32\,Q}{\pi d^3}.\tag{6}$$

We use the adjective pseudo to indicate that γ_w^* is close to the value of true shear rate at the wall. In particular, $\gamma_w^* = \gamma_w$ if the blood is Newtonian. If the flowing fluid obeys Casson's equation (see the following section of this paper) the value of γ_w^* for Merrill's experimental data of blood ($H = 39\%$) is 15%, 6%, and 2% smaller than γ_w when $\gamma_w = 1, 10,$ and 100 sec^{-1}, respectively.

Replacing γ_w in Eq. (5) by γ_w^*, one defines an apparent viscosity, η^*, according to this generalized form:

$$\tau_w = (p_1 - p_2)\frac{d}{4L} = \eta^*\gamma_w^*.\tag{7}$$

In this version, η^* may be a function of γ_w^* and other physical parameters of the blood. Since γ_w^* is not exactly the shear rate, Eq. (7) is only an approximate version of the stress–strain relationship.

PRESSURE DROP OF BLOOD FLOW IN GLASS TUBES

Several questions may be raised in using the above generalization for analyzing the pressure–flow relationship of blood flowing in single vessels. In the first place, what important parameters of the blood must be considered in the generalized version of the pressure–flow relationship? Second, is there a simple master equation that specifies the relationship for blood flow in various sizes of vessels? As such a generalization is based on the assumption that the blood may be treated as a homogeneous fluid, one may ask, because of the finite size of the red blood cells, what the limit is on the vessel size above which the assumption is valid (Cokelet, 1972)?

There are no satisfactory answers for these questions, owing to a lack of detailed information on the velocity profile and hematocrit distribution in microvascular flows. From his extensive study on blood flow in a 811-μ glass capillary, Barbee (1971) showed that, for a given pseudo shear rate, the logarithm of the shear stress is linearly proportional to the hematocrit of the feed reservoir, H. See Figure 1. As a result, it was suggested that

$$\tau_w = A\, e^{BH} \tag{8}$$

where A and B are functions of $\gamma_w{}^*$. For Eq. (8) to be applicable to plasma, a Newtonian fluid with a viscosity η_p, one finds $A = \eta_p \gamma_w{}^*$. The value of B was found to decrease as $\gamma_w{}^*$ increased. With a slight modification of the function B given by Barbee (1971), the shear stress at the wall can be calculated from the following equations:

$$\tau_w = \gamma_w{}^* \, \eta_p e^{5.8H(\gamma_w{}^*)^{-0.15}} \mid \quad 3 \leqslant \gamma_w{}^* < 150 \ \text{sec}^{-1}$$

$$= \gamma_w{}^* \, \eta_p e^{H[\,2.0\,+\,18.5(\ln \gamma_w{}^*)^{-2}\,]} \quad 150 \leqslant \gamma_w{}^* \leqslant 800 \ \text{sec}^{-1}. \tag{9}$$

This relationship between τ_w and $\gamma_w{}^*$ and Barbee's experimental data for an 811-μ tube are plotted in Figure 2. Other functions have been used satisfactorily by Merrill et al. (1965) and Meiselman, Frasher, and Wayland (1972) in fitting their own data.

For $\gamma_w{}^* < 3$, the following approximate version of Casson's equation was used:

$$\tau_w{}^{1/2} = \tau_y{}^{1/2} + [(1 + 2.5H + 7.35H^2)\, \eta_p \gamma_w{}^*]^{1/2} \tag{10}$$

where the yield stress τ_y for a blood hematocrit of 40% is typically 0.04 dynes/cm^2 (Merrill, 1969). For very large shear rate, the blood behaves like a Newtonian fluid.

For smaller vessels, the viscosity calculated from the feed hematocrit, H_F, was higher than the measured value (Fahraeus and Lindquist, 1931). They showed that the change in viscosity may be due to the reduction of hematocrit

338   Lee

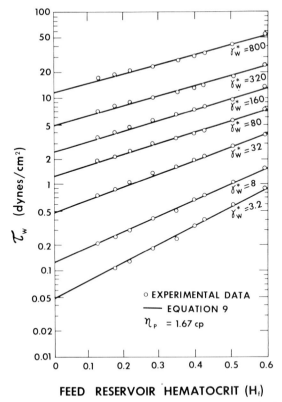

FEED RESERVOIR HEMATOCRIT (H$_f$)

Figure 1. Semi-log plot of the shear stress at the wall, τ_w, versus the hematocrit H_f at constant shear rate γ_w^* for 811-μ tube. Notice the linear relationship in this plot. The solid lines were computed from Eq. (9). Courtesy of Barbee (1971); reprinted by permission.

in the capillaries. Let H_T be the hematocrit in the capillary, obtained by stopping the flow and centrifuging the whole capillary. The tube hematocrit equals the feed hematocrit for an 811-μ tube. The correlation of the ratio H_T/H_F with H_F for human blood flowing in various sizes of capillary is given in Figure 3 (Barbee and Cokelet, 1971a), and is expressed by

$$H_T/H_F = a + bH_F \tag{11}$$

where, for human blood, the two dimensionless parameters a and b are functions of the diameter ratio of the red blood cell and the capillary. This relationship, independent of flow rate, is also valid for cat blood (Jendrucko and Lee, 1973). However, matching the ratio of erythrocyte diameter d_c to capillary diameter for the cat blood with the ratio for the human blood does not result in the same a and b. This observation suggests that a and b may depend also on dimensionless parameters related to the shape and elasticity of the red blood cells.

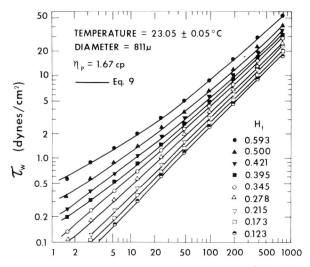

Figure 2. The shear stress τ_w versus the pseudo shear rate $\gamma_w{}^*$ for blood of various hematocrit flowing in a $811\text{-}\mu$ tube. The solid curves were computed from Eq. (9). Courtesy of Barbee (1971); reprinted by permission.

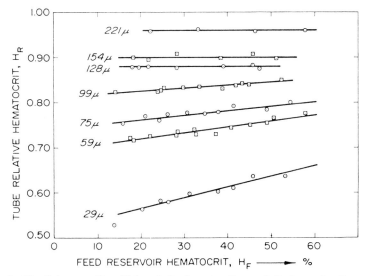

Figure 3. The Fahraeus effect. Tube relative hematocrit was plotted as a function of tube diameter and feed-reservoir hematocrit. Lines are least-squares-fitted straight lines. Reprinted with permission of Barbee and Cokelet (1971a) and Journal of Microvascular Research (Academic Press).

However, working with the same type of blood, one may still regard a and b as functions of the ratio d_c/d.

Barbee and Cokelet (1971a) showed that if the value of H_T was used for H in Eq. (9), the predicted viscosity agreed with the measured value for capillary sizes ranging from 29 to 811 μ. An example of this agreement is illustrated in Figure 4 for a 29-μ capillary.

This remarkable finding suggests that two average quantities, the tube hematocrit and the pseudo shear rate, play a very important role in determining the pressure drop in single vessels. Recent findings by Cokelet (personal communication) indicate that Eq. (9) is valid down to 8-μ capillaries if the tube hematocrit is used. On the other hand, if the tubes are even smaller, so that their diameter is smaller than that of the cellular bodies, an entirely new picture evolves. In such small tubes neither the Fahraeus–Lindquist (1931) effect, nor the Fahraeus (1929) effect, continues to hold. This is discussed in Chapter 13 in this volume.

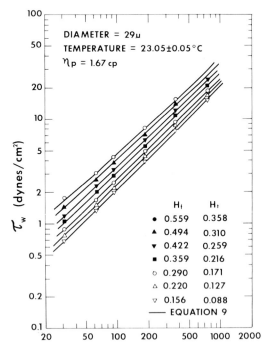

Figure 4. The flow behavior of blood in a 29-μ-diameter tube. The listed value of the feed reservoir hematocrit and tube hematocrit were both measured experimentally. The solid lines were computed from Eq. (9) with the tube hematocrit. Reprinted by permission of Barbee and Cokelet (1971b) and Journal of Microvascular Research (Academic Press).

FACTORS AFFECTING THE PRESSURE–FLOW RELATIONSHIP OF SINGLE VESSELS WITH DIAMETER MUCH LARGER THAN THAT OF THE RED BLOOD CELLS

Let us briefly review the law of resistance for turbulent flow, flow in curved and tapered tubes, and flow in tubes of various cross-sectional shapes for a Newtonian fluid. Most of the results discussed here have been well established in fluid mechanics (Schlichting, 1968). Similar studies done on blood flow are quoted to substantiate our discussion.

Let us define the Reynolds number, Re, as

$$Re = \frac{\rho \bar{u} d}{\eta} \qquad (12)$$

where the average velocity $\bar{u}$ is equal to $4Q/(\pi d^2)$. As established by Reynolds, when Re is smaller than 2,300, the fully developed flow is laminar. Above this critical number, 2,300, the flow is turbulent. More recent investigations reveal that in the range of 2,300–2,600, the flow alternates in time between laminar and turbulent. Above 2,600, the flow is fully turbulent. Transition from laminar to turbulent is accompanied by a noticeable change in the law of resistance, which is commonly expressed as

$$\frac{p_1 - p_2}{L} = \frac{\lambda}{d} \frac{\rho \bar{u}^2}{2} \qquad (13)$$

where λ is a dimensionless number. For laminar flow, Eq. (13) is equivalent to a λ given by

$$\lambda = 64/Re. \qquad (14)$$

For turbulent flow, Blasius (1913) established the following empirical law:

$$\lambda = (100/Re)^{1/4}. \qquad (15)$$

Because most of the rheologic measurements of blood have been made at low Reynolds numbers, it is not clear whether one critical Reynolds number is sufficient to define the transition for laminar to turbulent flow and Eq. (15) is valid for turbulent blood flow. In blood there is a microscale, the RBC diameter, which may be comparable to the microscale of incipient turbulence, the Tollmien wave. The interference may change the ordinary result obtained on homogeneous fluid. However, Hershey and Gupta (1968) have shown that the critical Reynolds number for blood is in the range of 2,150–2,300.

Experiments done on tapered capillaries by Merrill et al. (1965) showed that local pressure gradient in a nonuniform tube could be considered as that in a uniform tube of the same diameter and same flow. The angles of taper used in their experiments ranged from 0.3° to 2°. On the other hand, for a medium Reynolds number flow (e.g., 600) through a divergent or convergent channel with a taper of $10°$, the nonlinear inertia effect could alter considerably the flow resistance (Millsaps and Pohlhausen, 1953).

For tubes of noncircular cross section, it is convenient to introduce a hydraulic diameter d_h, defined by

$$d_h = 4A/C \tag{16}$$

where A denotes the cross-sectional area of the tube and C its wetted perimeter. If the tube is circular, d_h is its diameter. The law of resistance, Eq. (13), can be generalized to

$$\frac{p_1 - p_2}{L} = k \frac{\lambda}{d_h} \frac{\rho \bar{u}^2}{2} \tag{17}$$

where k is a dimensionless shape factor and λ is the resistance factor for a circular tube with a diameter d_h. If the cross section is elliptical with a ratio of major axis to minor axis of 1.2, then $k = 0.984$. If the ratio is increased to 1.5, k drops to 0.924. For tubes of square cross section, the parameter k is 0.891. On the other hand, for turbulent flow, the measurements of the pressure drop for pipes of rectangular, triangular, and square cross section are well represented by the law for a circular tube, i.e., $k = 1$.

The preceding considerations concerning tube flow are valid only for a straight tube. In curved tubes there exists a secondary flow, because the particles near the axis, which have a higher velocity, are acted upon by larger centrifugal forces than the slower particles near the walls. The characteristic dimensionless parameter that determines the influence of the curvature in the laminar case is the Dean number (Dean, 1927):

$$D = \frac{1}{2} Re \sqrt{0.5 d/r_c} \tag{18}$$

where r_c is the radius of curvature of the circular tube. Measurements done on Newtonian fluid by White (1929) and Adler (1934) can be fitted best by the formula

$$k = 0.37 D^{0.36} \tag{19}$$

when the Dean number lies in the range $20(k = 1.1)$ to $500(k = 3.5)$. The value of k is unity when $D < 10$. Working with hollow plastic fibers, Merrill et al. (1965) found no discernible effects of curvature existed for a suspension of red cells in plasma. It is estimated from their data that the Dean number employed in the experiment was smaller than 5.

White has found that flow in curved tube is more stable than flow in straight tubes. For example, the Reynolds number must be higher than 9,000 for the turbulence to be persistent throughout the length of the tube when the curvature is $1/15$ ($= 0.5 d/r_c$). Even with a relatively small curvature of $1/50$, streamlined flow is maintained up to 6,000, twice the critical Reynolds number of a straight tube. White's experimental data for turbulent flow in a curved tube can be fitted by this formula (White, 1932):

$$k = 1.0 + 0.075\ Re^{1/4}(0.5d/r_c)^{1/2}. \tag{20}$$

Note that the Dean number no longer serves as the characteristic dimensionless variable.

The laws of resistance presented previously are valid only for steady flow. The nature of pulsatile flow, which has been observed in microvessels, may affect the rheology of the blood, the transition from laminar to turbulent flow, and the interaction between the blood and the wall of microvessels. For more detailed information the reader is referred to Chapter 17 in this volume.

In preparing the blood for in vitro experiments, it is likely that the concentrations of various constituents of the blood are altered. For example, a change in the concentration of fibrinogen could affect considerably the rheology of the blood at low shear rate. A critical discussion of this area is given in Chapter 15 of this volume by Rosenblum.

All the formulas presented above are valid only in blood vessels whose diameter d is considerably larger than that of the red and white blood cells, d_c. For smaller tubes the diameter ratio d/d_c becomes an important factor. Rheology of blood when d/d_c is of the order of 1 or smaller is discussed in Chapter 13.

DISTRIBUTION OF PRESSURE
AND FLOW IN THE MESENTERIC MICROCIRCULATION

To relate the pressure—flow relationship of a single vessel to that of a vascular bed, we examine the distribution of pressure, flow, and associated parameters in the mesenteric microcirculation. This information may be used as a guide for selecting an appropriate law of resistance and for constructing a simple, but realistic vascular model.

In Table 1, the vessels in the mesenteric vascular bed of the cat are classified into seven generations. Their approximate ranges of diameter are given in the second column. Based on a total flow rate of 20 cm^3/min, the average velocity in the first and last generation was calculated and is shown in the third column. The velocity ranges in the arterioles, capillaries, and venules were taken from Gaehtgens, Meiselman, and Wayland's (1970) measurement of erythrocyte velocity. In some microvessels, the flow may be intermittent. Sometimes, the flow reverses its flowing direction. By assuming a uniform viscosity, $\eta^* = 4$ cp, and using only one significant digit, the Reynolds number for each vessel generation was tabulated in column four. The largest kinetic energy density, $\frac{1}{2}\rho\bar{u}^2$, in the vascular bed is in the mesenteric artery and is about 200 dyne-cm/cm^3. This energy density is equivalent to a pressure head of 0.2 cm H$_2$O, negligible in comparison with the pressure head in the mesenteric artery. Using Eq. (6),

Table 1. Distribution of flow, pressure, and associated parameters in the mesenteric vascular network of a cat

Vessel type	Diameter d (μ)	Velocity[a] u (cm/sec)	Reynolds[b,c] number, Re	Pseudo shear[c] rate, γ_w^* (1/sec)	Pressure p (cm H_2O)	Compliance C^d (%/cm H_2O)
Mesenteric artery	1500	20	80	1000	130–190	0.1–0.3
Arteriole 1	31–60	1–2	<0.3	<3000	80–130	1–2
Arteriole 2	10–30	0.5–1.2	<0.06	<3000	40–90	0–0.5
Capillary	7.5	0.1–0.4	<0.008	<4000	35–60	0
Venule 2	10–30	0.2–1	<0.05	<4000	25–55	0–0.5
Venule 1	31–60	1	<0.2	<1300	20–45	1–2
Portal vein	3500	4	40	90	18	0.4–1

[a] The average velocities for the first and last generation were computed with a flow rate of 20 cm³/min. The mesenteric artery is usually branched into about 10 terminal arteries, which further branch into some 150 arterial branches.

[b] The viscosity η^* was taken as 4 cp in computing the Reynolds number.

[c] Because of the occurrence of the intermittent flow in the microvessels, the value given here may represent the upper limit of the shear rate.

[d] The compliance, percentage change in diameter for a pressure increase of 1 cm H_2O, of the venules was assumed to be similar to the correspondent arterioles.

pseudo shear rates were determined, as presented in the fifth column. Because of the possibility of on—off flow in the microvessel, the lower limit of the shear rate may be zero.

The distribution of pressure in these vessels measured by Zweifach (1975a) is given in the sixth column. If there is a redistribution of pressure in the vascular bed, the vessel size and hence the flow resistance change. Thus the compliance can play an important role in determining the pressure—flow relationship of the vascular bed. The value of the compliance, the percentage change of vessel diameter per 1 cm H_2O pressure increase, for each generation is listed in the last column. Part of the results were derived from Baez's work (Baez, Lamport, and Baez, 1960).

Although the information given in Table 1 may be used to construct a vascular network of parallel arrangement, where vessels branch into identical daughter vessels, the pressure—flow relation of this model may be oversimplified from the point of view of the real vascular system. To illustrate the irregular nature of blood flow and the arrangement of the vascular network, the distribution of the red cell velocity and opacity in the mesenteric membrane of cat as mapped by Johnson is reproduced in Figure 5. The left-hand panel of the figure shows the network together with the local measurement of the velocity and opacity. The right-hand panel indicates their changes versus the capillary position in the branching network starting from the arterial side. The velocity, measured by the two-slit photometric method, represents the average value derived from a record of 4—5 min. This velocity is related to the flow rate in the microvessel. The product of the opacity and the dimension of a microvessel is a measure of the hematocrit in that microvessel.

From Table 1, one sees that Reynolds number is small for the mesenteric circulation. The inertia effects discussed in the preceding section of this paper may not have a significant influence on the pressure—flow relation. However, when a passive bed is perfused with plasma, the Reynolds number is drastically enlarged because of the higher flow rate and lower viscosity. In some situations the Reynolds number in the artery can reach a value of 4,000. Then the turbulence, curvature, and taper of the tube will enhance the pressure loss in the vascular bed.

Recently, Zweifach (1975a,b) made an extensive analysis of the pressure distribution in the terminal vascular bed in cat mesentery. The pressure in almost 500 microvessels organized according to their size is shown in Figure 6. These arterioles and venules were separated into six groups whose diameter variation was ±5 μ from their average value. Although the measurements exhibited large standard variations, the distribution of the mean pressure for one vessel size showed a well-defined trend. The greatest reduction in the mean pressure occurred during transport of the blood through the vessels (10—40 μ) lumped as the arteriolar—precapillary portion of the network. The decline in pressure in

346   Lee

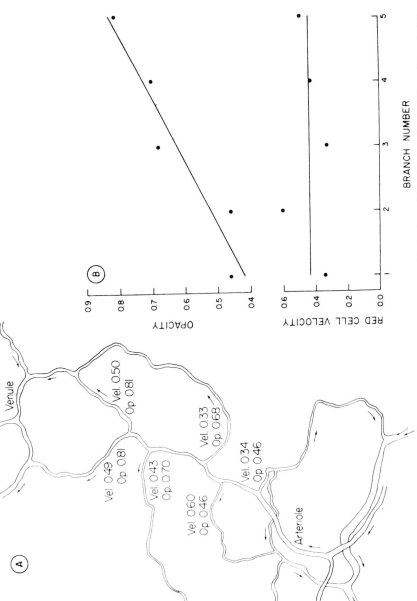

Figure 5. (A) *Left-hand panel*, velocity (Vel) and opacity (Op) in capillaries branching from a thoroughfare channel. (B) *Right-hand panel*, plot of velocity and opacity versus position of capillary in the branching network beginning on arterial side. Note systematic increase in opacity in more distal capillaries. Reprinted by permission of Johnson (1971), The American

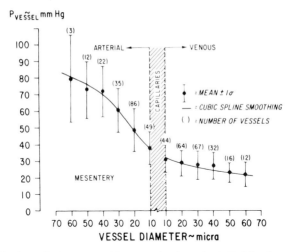

Figure 6. Distribution of micropressure in normotensive cats plotted for the range of vessels between 60-μ arterioles and 60-μ venules. The mean and standard deviation were computed for ± 5-μ intervals about each abscissa point. The smoothed line is the best fit of the distribution of mean pressure. From Zweifach (1975a). Reprinted by permission of the author and the American Heart Association, Inc.

larger arterioles was much more gradual. For true capillaries and vessels in the venous network, the pressure reduction was the least.

One step closer to establish the in vivo pressure–flow relationship of single vessels, Zweifach used two microprobes to measure the pressure along un-branched microvessels. The distribution of pressure gradient is reproduced in Figure 7. In the larger arterioles and venules (40–70 μ wide), the probe separation L was at least 1–2 mm. In vessels narrower than 35 μ, the pressure drop between the probes can be measured accurately across a length as small as 200–250 μ. The pressure gradient dp/dL along the length of the larger arterioles (>30 μ) was quite small (average 0.1–0.2 cm $H_2O/100$ μ). In 18–20-μ terminal arterioles, the pressure gradient increased (0.3–0.4 cm $H_2O/100$ μ). Depending on the diameter and the flow, the pressure gradient in the capillaries ranged from 0.6 to 1.2 cm $H_2O/100$ μ. The gradient in the venules was usually smaller than that in the arterioles of similar size.

MODEL OF MESENTERIC VASCULAR NETWORK

The construction of simple but realistic models of the arrangement of the arterioles, capillaries, and venules has proved useful for the analysis of the distribution of blood flow and its regulation within the microcirculation. Most model studies consider a parallel arrangement, which is not substantiated by direct microscopic observations. In addition, because the flow resistance is inversely proportional to the fourth power of the diameter, a slight change in

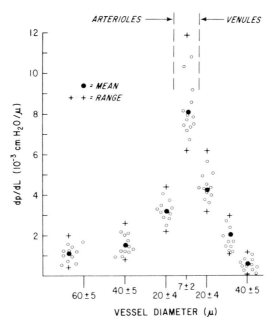

Figure 7. The pressure gradient along unbranched microvessels measured by two micro-probes. Values indicated cover a diameter range of ±5 μ for each of the categories listed except for capillaries in which the range is ±2 μ. From Zweifach (1975a). Reprinted by permission of the author and the American Heart Association, Inc.

diameter of the daughter vessel, say 10%, can alter the flow resistance by 46%. The semiregular network consisting of branches of uniform length and diameter, as proposed by Renkin (1964), is subject to similar criticism and may be oversimplified for the study of the pressure–flow relation of an organ.

From experimental studies, a microvascular network built from interlocking thoroughfare channels was first recognized by Chambers and Zweifach (1944). In 1972 Frasher and Wayland described a repeating module in the cat mesentery that was defined at a level of branching prior to the chain of thoroughfare channels (Figure 8). The average area of the module and the diameter and length of the microvessels forming the module were given in their paper.

To provide data on the flow distribution in such a module, we recently developed a microscopic indicator dilution method for the measurement of the mean transit time (MTT) in selected microvessels of cat mesentery (Nellis and Lee, 1974). Since the indicator was injected into the mesenteric artery, the MTT is a measure of the flow from the injection site to the measurement site. In 90 measurements, we found that the MTT ranged from 2 to 7.5 sec for arterioles (average value, 3.9 sec) and from 3 to 10 sec for venules (average 5.7 sec). In contrast, the distribution of the difference in MTT between an arteriole and the adjacent venule is much narrower with a range of 1–3 sec (average 2.1 sec).

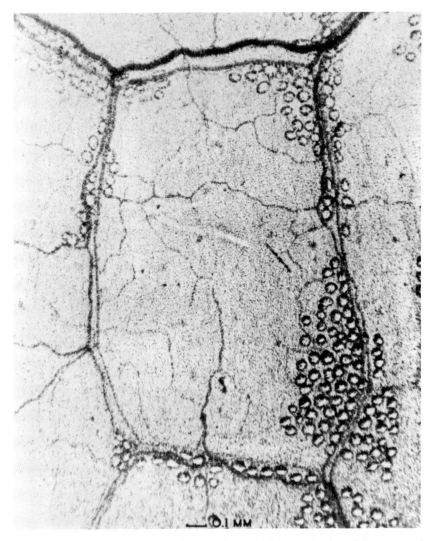

Figure 8. Single-frame photograph of a repeating modular organization of the mesenteric microcirculation. Note the vein-to-vein and artery-to-artery continuity at each apex representing an external branch. Reprinted by permission of Frasher and Wayland (1972) and Journal of Microvascular Research (Academic Press).

To associate our experimental MTT results with a simple vascular network, a repeating modular organization, which combines the essence of Renkin's and Frasher and Wayland's models, was constructed and sketched in Figure 9. This model is also known as a ladder network. In this figure, the arterioles are indicated by the white and the venules by the shaded channels. The area of the

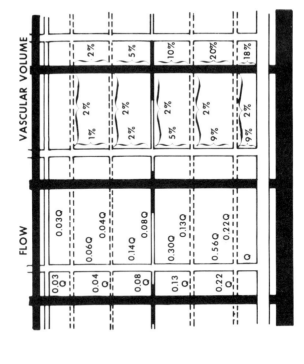

DISTRIBUTION OF FLOW AND VOLUME WITH EQUAL VOLUME FOR THE CAPILLARY SEGMENTS

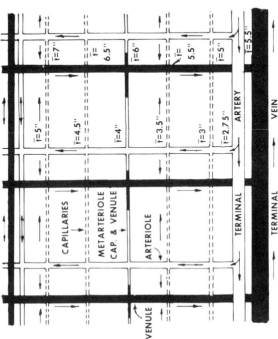

DISTRIBUTION OF MEAN TRANSIT TIME IN A REPEATING MODULAR NETWORK

Figure 9. The distribution of the mean transit time in a repeating network (*left-hand panel*) as suggested from a microvascular indicator dilution study. The computed distribution of the flow and the vascular volume were sketched in the right-hand panel. Reprinted by permission of Lee and Nellis and Academic Press. (From Lee and Nellis, 1974.)

basic module is represented by the rectangle with the vein and the venules at its sides.

At the top of the figure, the arterioles are connected to each other. So are the venules. A bidirectional arrow is used there to indicate an uncertainty in the direction of blood flow. The loop so formed was first recognized by Frasher and Wayland (1972) and was also seen in our preparation of the cat mesentery. A shorter distance between the arteriole and venule symbolizes that they are physically adjacent to each other. The four sets of broken lines (each of them representing a group of capillaries that may be connected to the arterioles in a distributed fashion) and an additional flow channel (consisting of a metarteriole, capillaries, and a venule) form the pathways connecting the arterioles and the venules. The directions of flow in these modules are indicated by the arrows. When the terminal artery and vein are replaced by an arteriole and a venule, respectively, the module represents those in the central part of the mesenteric membrane.

As suggested from our experimental results, the distribution of MTT in this ladder network is given in the left-hand panel of Figure 9. Note the adverse distribution of MTT along the direction of venous flow. This adverse distribution was observed in our experiments. Based on the conservation of mass at the trifurcation or junction of the network, a relation between the flow and MTT there could be derived. With the additional assumption of equal volume for the five capillary groups, the distributions of flow and volume in this ladder network were determined and are presented in the right-hand panel of Figure 9 (Lee and Nellis, 1974). The calculated results are expressed in percentage of the total volume and the fraction of flow. It was found that the volume of all five capillary segments is 20% of the total volume. This small percentage agrees qualitatively with the value calculated from Frasher and Wayland's measurements (1972). Because of the long delay time to the fifth group of capillaries, its flow is only 3% of the total flow (or one-seventh of the flow to the first group of capillaries). This calculation suggests a high shunt flow through the first group.

In this approach, the distribution of pressure is not considered. Theoretically, for a given pressure–flow relationship, we may adjust the cross-sectional area of the vessel and its length (our calculation specifies their product) to conform to a measured pressure distribution.

To integrate the pressure–flow relation of single vessels with that of a repeating module in the cat mesentery, Lipowsky and Zweifach (1974) employed a network analysis to compute the distribution of pressure and its gradient in a single module. In their analysis, the blood flow is considered to be Poiseuillian. The arteriolar pressure at the boundary vessels of the module was set as 61 cm H_2O whereas the venous pressure as 21 cm H_2O. Comparison with the in vivo measurements of pressure distribution (Figure 6) shows that the theoretical results exhibited a smaller pressure decline for larger vessels and a sharper one for vessels of capillary size. In like manner, the computed pressure gradient was smaller for larger vessels than the in vivo results given in Figure 7 and 4–6 times higher for vessels of capillary size.

These disparities between the theoretical computation and the in vivo measurement were attributed to three factors not accounted in the theory: (1) the narrow constriction in the arteriolar–precapillary branches, (2) the bifurcation effect, and (3) the non-Newtonian behavior of the blood. It is also probable that the disparities are due to the assumption of a constant input or output pressure at the boundary vessels. Under this condition there would not be any shunt flow along the peripheral vessels. As a result, the pressure gradient along the peripheral vessels of the module is reduced and the pressure drop across the capillary network is increased.

FLOW IN PULMONARY MICROVASCULATURE

The blood flow in the pulmonary alveolar septa has been modeled by Fung and Sobin (1969) as a sheet flow. The structure of the sheet is shown in Figure 7 of Chapter 14. It is formed by two membranes interconnected by many posts. The blood flows in between the membranes and around the posts. Let the mean flow in the sheet be specified by a velocity vector v, which is related to the gradient of the local blood pressure $\bar{p}$ by

$$v = \frac{h^{-2}}{\eta f} \text{ grad } \bar{p} \tag{21}$$

where η is the viscosity of the blood, $\bar{h}$ the thickness of the sheet, and f a friction parameter dependent on the post arrangement (Lee and Elsaden, 1969). The conservation of mass in the sheet flow requires that

$$\text{div } v \, \bar{h} = 0. \tag{22}$$

When $\bar{p} > p_{\text{alv}}$, where p_{alv} is the alveolar pressure, the thickness of the sheet (Sobin et al., 1972) is related to the pressure by

$$\bar{h} = h_0 + \alpha \, (\bar{p} - p_{\text{alv}}) \tag{23}$$

where h_0 and α are constants. At zero or negative transmural pressure, $\bar{p} - p_{\text{alv}} < 0$, $\bar{h} = 0$. By taking η, α, h_0, p_{alv}, and f as constants, the substitution of Eq. (21) and (23) results in

$$\nabla^2 h^{-4} = \nabla^2 \, (\bar{p} - p_{\text{alv}}) = 0. \tag{24}$$

Thus, with appropriate boundary conditions on $\bar{h}$ or the transmural pressure, their distributions in a given alveolar sheet can be computed and are illustrated in a special example in the lower panel of Figure 10. In this panel, the left-hand sketch shows the distribution of the sheet thickness, the middle one the contour of constant pressure, and the right-hand one the streamline of the flow. Because the difference in pressure between two adjacent contours is constant, the denser distribution of the contours near the venous end of the sheet indicates a

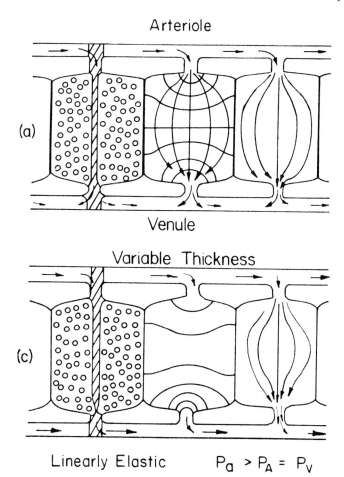

Arteriole
Venule
Variable Thickness

(a)

(c)

Linearly Elastic $P_a > P_A = P_V$

Figure 10. The variation of the average sheet thickness, pressure distribution (contour of constant pressure), and the streamlines computed from Eq. (23) with given sheet dimension and boundary conditions. *Top panel,* the case of rigid alveolar sheet. *Lower panel,* the case of a distensible sheet specified by a linear relationship between the thickness and pressure. Reprinted by permission of Fung and Sobin (1969) and Journal of Applied Physiology (American Physiological Society).

significant pressure drop there. The top sketch of the figure illustrates the situation if the sheet were rigid.

From the general theory, Fung and Sobin (1972a) calculated the flow per alveolar sheet, Q, as

$$Q = \frac{SA}{4\eta f L \alpha}(h_a{}^4 - h_v{}^4) \qquad (25)$$

where h_a and h_v are the sheet thicknesses of the vascular space in the alveolar septum at the arteriole and venule, respectively. L is the average length of the streamline in the sheet, S the vascular space tissue ratio (on the order 0.9), and A is the sheet area.

Using the h_0 and α values from Glazier et al. (1967), Fung and Sobin (1972a) computed from Eq. (25) the pressure–flow relationship and resistance of flow for an alveolar sheet at a constant venular pressure of 3 cm H_2O and a pleural pressure of 0. The alveolar pressure was set at 7, 17, and 23 cm H_2O. The computed results, together with the experimental data by Roos et al. (1961), are plotted in Figure 11. It can be seen that a reasonable agreement between the theory and the experiment is obtained.

For the same variation in the arteriolar and venular pressure, $dp_\text{ven} = dp_\text{art}$, Fung and Sobin (1972b) computed the ratio of changes in the flow Eq. (25) as

$$\frac{\partial Q}{\partial P_\text{ven}} \bigg/ \frac{\partial Q}{\partial P_\text{art}} = \left(\frac{h_v}{h_a}\right)^3. \qquad (26)$$

If the value of h_v^3 for a given p_ven is much smaller than h_a^3, the equation above implies that a change in venous pressure has little effect on the flow compared

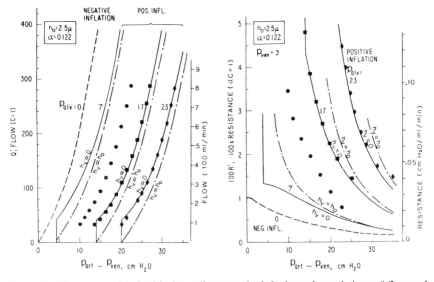

Figure 11. Curves associated with the ordinate to the left show the variations of flow and resistance with pressure heat, $P_\text{art} - P_\text{ven}$, at a constant venular pressure of 3 cm H_2O. The alveolar pressures are 23, 17, and 7 cm H_2O for positive inflation, with pleural pressure equal to 0. For negative inflation, P_alv is 0, while pleural pressure is negative. Q' is the flow when $C=1$ and $R'=\alpha R$ in units of $(\mu)^4$ and $(\mu)^{-3}$, respectively. Points associated with the ordinate to the right correspond to experimental data by Roos et al. on dogs with left atrium pressure equal to 3 cm H_2O, pleural pressure equal to 0, and alveolar pressure equal to 23 (♦), 17 (■), and 7 (●) cm H_2O. From Fung and Sobin (1972a). Reprinted by permission of the authors and the American Heart Association, Inc.

with the effect of a change in the arteriolar pressure of the same magnitude. This situation is aptly described as sluicing or a waterfall phenomenon.

The features of the sluicing flow discussed above had been analyzed earlier by Banister and Torrance (1960), Permutt, Bromberger-Barnea, and Bane (1962) and Permutt et al. (1968) and were attributed to Starling's mechanism and recruitment. In initial assumptions, Fung and Sobin's theory differs from those of Permutt et al. (1968) in two important points: (1) that the alveolar sheet is distensible and that the measured distensibility be used in the calculation, and (2) that according to fluid mechanics, the quasistatic condition prevails in the alveolar sheet. Because of these basic points of departure, the sheet-flow theory provides an explanation of the Starling mechanism and a deduction of sluicing mechanisms without invoking the recruitment hypothesis. Therefore, although the basic hypotheses were different, the predicted pressure–flow relationship is about the same. However, because of the quantitative aspect of Fung and Sobin's theory, they are able to fill in a great many of the details on pulmonary blood flow.

EFFECT OF BIFURCATION ON HEMATOCRIT DISTRIBUTION AND PRESSURE LOSS

In a capillary network, the distribution of flow and hematocrit among the daughter branchings of a bifurcation may fluctuate (Fung, 1973). Because the plasma tends to push the red blood cells in the direction of flow when cell size is comparable to the capillary, the daughter branch with a faster stream gets all the red blood cells from the parent vessel. Some cells may flow into the branch with a slower stream because of the randomness in the red cells' shapes and sizes, nonuniformity in the vessel geometry, and other stochastic factors. Fung's theoretical argument was demonstrated by Svanes and Zweifach (1968), who used a microocclusion technique to slow down the flow in one branch and subsequently to clear that branch of its red cells.

Johnson (1971) measured the average blood opacity, a quantitative index of hematocrit, in individual capillaries of the cat mesentery. For a dichotomous branching, the capillary with higher red cell velocity was found to have a higher opacity, i.e., a higher hematocrit. Bugliarello and Hsiao (1964) had examined the distribution of rigid spheres at a bifurcation. The tube-to-particle-size ratio was approximately 10. Their simplified model study demonstrated that the concentration in the side branch of slower flow is generally lower than in the main branch. Obviously, this uneven distribution of hematocrit at a bifurcation must be considered in evaluating the pressure–flow relationship of a microvascular network.

To determine the additional flow resistance caused by bifurcation, we have recently used the finite-difference technique and the Navier–Stokes equation to compute the flow in a two-dimensional bifurcation (unpublished). In this model, the parent channel is subdivided into two equal channels (see Figure 12). Let u_m be the maximum velocity in the daughter channel of a Poiseuille flow and d be the height of the channel. This bifurcation flow is governed by one dimensionless parameter, the Reynolds number, defined as $\rho u_m d/2\eta$. The conputation technique employed yields a solution for flow with a Reynolds number ranging from 0 to 50.

Let p_{t1} represent the computed total pressure at station 1 far upstream of the bifurcation and p_{t2} that at station 2 far downstream. Then the total energy (or pressure) dissipation from station 1 to 2 is given by

$$\Delta p_t = \frac{W}{Q} \int_{d/2}^{d/2} [p_{t1} u_1(y) - p_{t2} u_2(y)] \, dy \qquad (27)$$

where u_1 and u_2 are the velocities at station 1 and 2, respectively, y is the coordinate perpendicular to the channel wall, and W the width of the channel. If Δp_p represents the sum of the Poiseuille pressure drop over the channel between station 1 and the bifurcation and that between the bifurcation and station 2, we

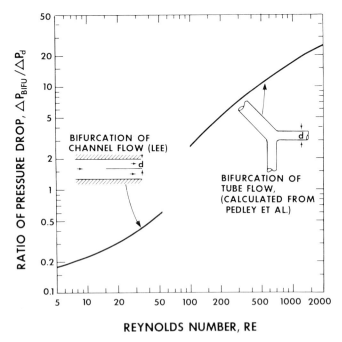

REYNOLDS NUMBER, RE

Figure 12. Additional pressure drop for flow at a bifurcation. The lower curve was computed from a finite-difference technique for a two-dimensional channel. The additional pressure drop at higher Reynolds number was derived from the modeling study of airway dynamics by Pedley et al. (1970). The discrepancy between these two curves is due to the difference in the bifurcation geometry.

define an additional pressure drop due to the bifurcation as

$$\Delta p_{\text{BIFU}} = \Delta p_t - \Delta p_p. \tag{28}$$

With Δp_d as the Poiseuille pressure drop in the downstream channel having a length d, the pressure ratio $\Delta p_{\text{BIFU}}/\Delta p_d$ was computed and plotted in Figure 12 as a function of the Reynolds number. It can be seen that this ratio increases rapidly as the Reynolds number becomes larger.

Because the air flow in a bifurcation is dynamically similar to a fluid flow having the same Reynolds number, we may employ the work of Pedley, Schroter, and Sudlow (1970) on the energy dissipation in human airways to compute the pressure ratio for flows of higher Reynolds number. For the particular bifurcation model used by them, an empirical formula was obtained for Z, the ratio of actual energy dissipation to Poiseuille dissipation. The value of Z is related to the pressure ratio by

$$\Delta p_{\text{BIFU}}/\Delta p_d = (Z - 1)L/D. \tag{29}$$

The Reynolds numbers used in their experiment lay between 180 and 700. The pressure ratio so computed is plotted in Figure 12 against the Reynolds number based on the diameter of the daughter branching.

These experimental results were obtained with relatively short branching network ($L/D = 3.5$). They can be fitted by the following formula:

$$\Delta p_{\text{BIFU}}/\Delta p_d = a + bRe \tag{30}$$

where the two dimensionless constants $a = 0.2$ and $b = 0.025$. Since L/D is large for vascular networks, we employed a bifurcation network composed of standard Nalgene Y-joint (size $\frac{1}{4}$ in.) to measure the effect of bifurcation when L/D is 30. We found the additional pressure drop is well represented by Eq. (30) with $a = 0.2$ and $b = 0.15$ for a Reynolds number ranging from 50 and 3000 (unpublished).

The pressure distribution and the streamline flow in bifurcation with an orthogonal branch was studied by Vawter, Fung, and Zweifach (1974) using a two-dimensional Stokes equation for low-Reynolds-number flows. Although the pressure varies considerably near the bifurcation, it converges rapidly toward a Poiseuillian (linear) distribution within one channel width of the branch. The value of a in Eq. (30) estimated from their computed pressure gradient is similar to our result given in Figure 12.

In the considerations above, the condition of steady state is assumed. Thus inertia is represented by the convective acceleration, with u as the velocity vector. As suggested by Figure 12, the effect of inertia at a bifurcation is small for low-Reynolds-number flow. On the other hand, the interaction between the viscous and inertia force in a bifurcation flow of moderate Reynolds number, say 1,000, may produce a pressure drop equivalent to lengthening the daughter branch by 18 times its diameter. Thus, if there exist a large number of such branchings in a vascular network, the sum of the pressure drops may form a large fraction of the flow resistance of the network.

The discussions above are concerned primarily with branching of one vessel into two vessels of uniform diameter. As found by Zweifach (1975a), the pressure difference between such offshoots is small. For example, the pressure in an arteriolar stem was 61 cm H_2O and the pressure in its two dichotomous branchings was 55 and 56 cm H_2O, respectively. On the other hand, the junctional region of an arteriolar–precapillary side branch is a pinched structure presenting a narrow entry. Its length is about 10–15 μ and its diameter is 3–4 times smaller than the uniform portion of the side branch. The pressure drop across these arteriolar branches ranged from 5 to 30 cm H_2O and associated closely with the ratio of branch diameter to parent diameter. Different branches distributed by a single arteriole have ratios varying from 0.3 to 0.7. Generally, the higher the ratio, the less the pressure drop into the branch.

The large drop across these branches measured by Zweifach (1975a) may be due to the flow resistance of the narrow entry. Based on Figure 7, we take the mean value 0.008 cm H_2O/μ for capillaries as the pressure gradient along the uniform side branch. For a diameter reduction of three, the pressure gradient along the narrow entry is increased to 0.64 cm H_2O/μ (= 0.008 × 3^4). As a result the pressure drop across an entry with a length of 15 μ is 100 cm H_2O (= 0.64 × 15). Vawter et al. (1974) made a more rigorous computation on the pressure gradient along bifurcations with a pinched structure. They showed that the local pressure gradient was increased drastically. Translated in terms of net pressure drop, their result is compatible with the simple estimation made above. This similarity is due to the unique characteristics of low-Reynolds-number flow, which exhibits minimal entrance effect (personal communication with D. Vawter).

On the venous side of the microcirculation, the progressive fall in pressure likewise seems to occur in accord with the branching pattern (Zweifach, 1975a). For example, the pressure in two capillaries was reduced from 36 and 37 cm H_2O, respectively, to 33 cm H_2O in a 26-μ postcapillary venule. The pressure was dropped fruther to 26 cm H_2O in a 32-μ venule and to 19 cm H_2O in the large venule (72 μ) on the perimeter of the repeating module. A comparison of the drop in arteriolar and venular vessels with similar branching ratios showed that the reduction in pressure was consistently greater on the venous side. The reason for this difference is unknown; possibly it was related to the slower flow and an increased frictional resistance in the venules.

PRESSURE–FLOW RELATIONSHIP OF AN ORGAN

To reduce the data on the pressure–flow relationship of an organ, it is conventional to define a peripheral vascular resistance R as

$$R = (P_a - P_v)/Q \tag{31}$$

where P_a is the measured arterial pressure and P_v is the venous one. If the kinetic energy in the artery or the vein is not negligible, e.g., in pulmonary circulation, the term $P_a - P_v$ should be replaced by one similar to that defined in Eq. (27). Because there are many review articles written in this area (see Green, Rapela, and Conrad, 1963, for example), instead of summarizing the results for R, we discuss the difficulties involved in correlating the peripheral vascular resistance with the resistance of single vessels.

In investigating the pressure–flow relation, Benis, Usami, and Chien (1970) employed two Newtonian fluids to perfuse the hind paw of a dog. One was the Albumin-Ringer (AR) solution with a viscosity of 0.97 cp. The other was a high-viscosity (4.5 cp) PAMEG-Ringer (PR) solution. The measured pressure drop across the hind paw for these two perfusates is plotted against the perfusion rate Q in Figure 13. At low pressure, the ratio Q_{PR}/Q_{AR}, which is equal to the resistance ratio R_{AR}/R_{PR}, agrees with the viscosity ratio, indicating purely viscous pressure loss and confirming the absence of vasoactive action by the plasma expander PAMEG. With increasing Δp, Q_{PR}/Q_{AR} decreases progressively and falls below the viscosity ratio, demonstrating the existence of inertial pressure loss. An empirical equation with two parameters A and B,

$$\Delta p = A \eta Q + B Q^2, \tag{32}$$

was found to correlate well with the measurement of pressure and flow. The first term is the pressure drop due to viscous loss and the second due to inertial loss.

For a better understanding of the inertial effect, the Reynolds number, based on the diameter (0.11 cm) of the arterial catheter, was computed and presented in Figure 13 for each data point. For the high-viscosity perfusate, the Reynolds number is relatively small. The nonlinear pressure–flow relationship in Figure 13 reflects mainly the influence of the vascular distensibility on factor A in Eq. (32).

Recently, Benis et al. (1973) reexamined previous experiments done on the hind limb of the dog and showed that at higher perfusion ratio, the ratio of the peripheral vascular resistance falls below the viscosity ratio. In addition, they demonstrated that the ratio of the resistance for two Newtonian perfusates in hind limb fixed in formaldehyde over a period of 1–5 wk is in general agreement with that in freshly isolated hind limbs. From this study, they concluded that the nonlinear pressure loss is not simply due to alteration in vascular geometry related to autoregulation when different perfusates were used.

For the hind limbs of cats, the autoregulation can affect the correct interpretation of the ratio between the peripheral vascular resistance of two Newtonian perfusates (Eliassen, Folkow, and Obug, 1973). They showed that when the hind limb is maximally dilated with papaverine infusion and intermittent exercise, the resistance ratio is essentially constant and coincides with the viscosity ratio. On the other hand, the ratio gradually decreases when no attempts are made to keep the vascular bed maximally dilated.

360   Lee

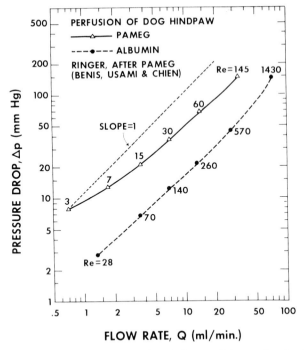

FLOW RATE, Q (ml/min.)

Figure 13. The pressure–flow relationship for hind paw of dog perfused with two New-tonian fluids, PAMEG solution (4.53 cp) and albumin-Ringer (0.97 cp) solution by Benis et al. (1970). The Reynolds number associated with each data point was computed for a diameter of 0.11 cm (that of the arterial catheter). Reference line of slope 1 indicated linear relationship. From S. Chien, 1970, Circulation Research 28:1058. Reprinted by permission of the author and the American Heart Association.

If one idealizes a microvascular network as a sequence of branchings, and considers the flow there fully developed, the linear pressure–flow relation is applicable in Benis's perfusion experiment, since all the Reynolds numbers are smaller then the critical Reynolds number. This idealization leads to a linear relationship between Δp and Q for a rigid network. If the bed is distensible, then the $\Delta p - Q$ curves for perfusates of different viscosity should be parallel to each other. Apparently, this simple model cannot simulate Benis's data.

Let us consider the effect of bifurcation on the pressure–flow relationship of an organ. Based on Eq. (30), the additional pressure drop, Δp_{BIFU} is proportional to the second order of the flow rate. This is in agreement with the second term in Eq. (31). Because $\Delta p_{BIFU} /\Delta p_d = 230$ at the highest Reynolds number (1,450), it is likely that the effect of bifurcation may be sufficient to account for the inertial loss recorded by Benis's experiments.

Another indirect complication from the bifurcation might also have affected the pressure–flow relationship of the paw when it was perfused with AR or PR solution at the same arterial pressure. (The perfusions were done under constant venous pressure.) Since the effect of bifurcation is more pronounced in larger vessels where the Reynolds number is higher, it is possible that more pressure loss occurs over those vessels for the AR perfusion than the PR one. (Note that the former has a higher Reynolds number.) Accordingly, the pressure in the microvessels may be smaller for the former. Because these vessels are distensible, the resistance in the microvessels for the AR perfusion may become much larger than that for the PR perfusion. To illustrate this indirect complication to the pressure–flow relationship, we assume a pressure reduction of 3 cm H_2O in the arterioles. The diameter of the arteriole is reduced by 3–6% (Table 1), which results in a resistance increase in the arteriole of 12–25%. This increase may be significant if there is considerable pressure drop across the arteriole. In summary, even for a simple Newtonian perfusate, the interplay between the pressure drop at bifurcations and the distensibility of the vessels may complicate the separation of viscous and inertial loss. Subsequently, the functional dependence of A and B in Eq. (32) on Δp must be expanded to account for the effect of the pressure redistribution in the microvascular network.

For blood flow in an organ, the following items interact closely with each other:

1. The nonlinear pressure–flow relation of a single vessel (including the Fahraeus–Lindquist effect).
2. The distribution of hematocrit in the microvessels.
3. The pressure loss due to the interaction of the inertial and viscous forces.
4. The mechanical properties of the vessels.
5. The topology of the vascular network.

Because nothing is known about how these quantities are distributed in a vascular bed, quantitative analytic work on the pressure–flow relationship of an organ and its correlation with that of a single vessel cannot yet proceed. It is likely that any suggested discrepancy in the pressure–flow relationship between the in vitro approach using single vessels and in vivo study using whole organs is not due to any intrinsic difference in the biophysical properties of the two systems but due to the use of an oversimplified vascular model that does not account for all five items listed previously and their interaction.

ACKNOWLEDGMENTS

The author wishes to thank Professors Y. C. Fung and G. Cokelet for their helpful comments.

LITERATURE CITED

Adler, M. 1934. Strömung in gekrümmeten Rohren. Ziet. angew. Math. Mech. 14:257–275.

Baez, S., H. Lamport, and A. Baez. 1960. Pressure effects in living microscopic vessels. *In* A. L. Copley and G. Stainsby (eds.), Flow Properties of Blood, pp. 122–136. Pergamon Press, London.

Banister, J., and R. W. Torrance. 1960. Effects of the tracheal pressure upon flow-pressure relations in the vascular bed of isolated lungs. J. Exp. Physiol. 45:352–367.

Barbee, J. M. 1971. The flow of human blood through capillary tubes with inside diameters between 8.7 and 221 microns. Ph.D. Thesis, California Institute of Technology.

Barbee, J. M., and G. R. Cokelet. 1971*a*. The Fahraeus effect. Microvasc. Res. 3:6–16.

Barbee, J. M., and G. R. Cokelet. 1971*b*. Prediction of blood flow in tubes with diameters as small as 29μ. Microvasc. Res. 3:17–21.

Benis, A. M., S. Usami, and S. Chien. 1970. Effect of hematocrit and inertial losses on pressure–flow relations in the isolated hindpaw of the dog. Circ. Res. 28:1047–1068.

Benis, A. M., S. Chien, S. Usami, and K. M. Jan. 1973. Inertial pressure losses in perfused hindlimb: A reinterpretation of the results of Whittaker and Winton. J. Appl. Physiol. 34:383–389.

Blasius, H. 1913. Das Ähnlichkeitsgesetz bei Reibungsvorgängen in Flüssigheiten. Forschg. Arb. Ing.-Wes., No. 131, Berlin.

Bugliarello, G., and C. C. Hsaio. 1964. Phase separation in suspensions flowing through bifurcations: A simplified hemodynamic model. Science 143: 469–471.

Chambers, R., and B. W. Zweifach. 1944. Topography and function of the mesenteric circulation. Am. J. Anat. 75:173–200.

Cokelet, G. R. 1972. The rheology of human blood. *In* Y. C. Fung, N. Perrone, and M. Anliker (eds.), Biomechanics, Its Foundation and Objectives, Chap. 4, pp. 63–103. Prentice-Hall, Englewood Cliffs, N.J.

Dean, W. R. 1927. The streamline motion of a fluid in a curved pipe. Phil. Mag. 4:208–223.

Eliassen, E., B. Folkow, and B. Oberg. 1973. Are there any significant inertial losses in the vascular bed? Acta Physiol. Scand. 87:567–569.

Fahraeus, R. 1929. Suspension stability of blood. Physiol. Rev. 9:241–274.

Fahraeus, R., and T. Lindquist. 1931. The viscosity of the blood in narrow capillary tubes. Am. J. Physiol. 96:562–568.

Frasher, W. G., and H. Wayland. 1972. A repeating modular organization of the microcirculation of cat mesentery. Microvasc. Res. 4:62–76.

Fung, Y. C. 1973. Stochastic flow in capillary blood vessels. Microvasc. Res. 5:34–48.

Fung, Y. C., and S. S. Sobin. 1969. Theory of sheet flow in the lung alveoli. J. Appl. Physiol. 26:472–489.

Fung, Y. C., and S. S. Sobin. 1972*a*. Elasticity of the pulmonary alveolar sheet. Circ. Res. 30:451–469.

Fung, Y. C., and S. S. Sobin. 1972*b*. Pulmonary alveolar blood flow. Circ. Res. 30:470–490.

Gaehtgens, P. A., H. J. Meiselman, and H. Wayland. 1970. Erythrocyte flow velocities in mesenteric microvessels of the cat. Microvasc. Res. 2:151–162.

Glazier, J. B., J. M. B. Hughes, J. E. Maloney, and J. B. West. 1967. Vertical gradient of alveolar size in lungs of dogs frozen intact. J. Appl. Physiol. 23:694–705.

Green, H. D., C. E. Rapela, and M. C. Conrad. 1963. Resistance (conductance) and capacitance phenomena in terminal vascular beds. In W. F. Hamilton and P. Dow (eds.), Handbook of Physiology, Section 2 Circulation, Vol. II, Chap. 28, pp. 935–960. American Physiological Society, Washington, D.C.

Hershey, D., and B. P. Gupta. 1968. The effect of tube diameter on the laminar regime transition for a non-Newtonian suspension (blood). Biorheology 5: 313–321.

Jendrucko, R., and J. S. Lee. 1973. The measurement of hematocrit of blood flowing in glass capillaries by microphotometry. Microvasc. Res. 6:316–331.

Johnson, P. C. 1971. Red cell separation in the mesenteric capillary network. J. Appl. Physiol. 221:99–104.

Lee, J. S., and S. Nellis. 1974. Modelling study on the distribution of flow and volume in the microcirculation of cat mesentery. Ann. Biomed. Eng. 2: 206–216.

Lee, J. S., and M. R. Elsaden. 1969. Slow viscous flow in a lung alveoli model. J. Biomech. 2:187–198.

Lipowsky, H. H., and B. W. Zweifach. 1974. Network analysis of microcirculation of cat mesentery. Microvasc. Res. 7:73–83.

Meiselman, H. J., W. G. Frasher, Jr., and H. Wayland. 1972. In vivo rheology of dog blood after infusions of low-molecular-weight dextran or saline. Microvasc. Res. 4:399–412.

Merrill, E. W., A. M. Benis, E. R. Gilliland, T. K. Sherwood, and E. W. Salzman. 1965. Pressure–flow relations of human blood in hollow fibers at low flow rates. J. Appl. Physiol. 20:954–967.

Merrill, E. W. 1969. Rheology of blood. Physiol. Rev. 49:863–888.

Millsaps, K., and K. Pohlhausen. 1953. Thermal distribution in Jeffery-Hamel flows between nonparallel plane walls. J. Aero. Sci. 20:187–196.

Nellis, S. H., and J. S. Lee. 1974. Dispersion of indicator measured from microvessels of cat mesentery. Circ. Res. 35:580–591.

Pedley, T. J., R. C. Schroter, and M. F. Sudlow. 1970. Energy losses and pressure drop in models of human airways. Respir. Physiol. 9:371–386.

Permutt, S., B. Bromberger-Barnea, and H. N. Bane. 1962. Alveolar pressure, pulmonary venous pressure, and the vascular waterfall. Med. Thorac. 19: 239–260.

Permutt, S., P. Caldini, A. Maseri, W. H. Palmer, T. Sasamori, and K. L. Zierler. 1968. Recruitment versus distensibility in the pulmonary vascular bed. In A. Fishman and H. Hecht (eds.), Pulmonary Circulation and Interstitial Space, pp. 375–387. University of Chicago Press, Chicago.

Renkin, E. M. 1964. Normal regulation of tissue circulation. In H. L. Price and P. J. Cohen (eds.), Effects of Anesthetics on the Circulation, pp. 171–181. Charles C Thomas, Springfield, Ill.

Roos, A., L. J. Thomas, Jr., E. F. Nagel, and D. G. Prommas. 1961. Pulmonary vascular resistance as determined by lung inflation and vascular pressures. J. Appl. Physiol. 16:77–84.

Schlichting, H. 1968. Boundary-Layer Theory. 6th Ed. McGraw-Hill, New York. Chap. 20, 560 p.

Sobin, S. S., Y. C. Fung, H. Tremer, and T. H. Rosenquist. 1972. Elasticity of the pulmonary interalveolar microvascular sheet in the cat. Circ. Res. 30:440–450.

Svanes, S. K., and B. W. Zweifach. 1968. Variations in small blood vessel hematocrits produced in hypothermic rats by micro-occlusion. Microvasc. Res. 1:210–220.

Vawter, D., Y. C. Fung, and B. W. Zweifach. 1974. Distribution of blood flow and pressure from a microvessel into a branch. Microvasc. Res. 8:44–52.

White, C. M. 1929. Streamline flow through curved pipes. Proc. Roy. Soc. London A 123:645–663.

White, C. M. 1932. Fluid friction and its relation to heat transfer. Trans. Inst. Chem. Eng. 10:66–86.

Zweifach, B. W. 1975a. Quantitative studies of microcirculatory structure and function. I. Analysis of pressure distribution in the terminal vascular bed in cat mesentery. Circ. Res. 34:843–857.

Zweifach, B. W., 1975b. Quantitative studies of microcirculatory structure and function. II. Direct measurement of capillary pressure in splanchnic mesenteric vessels. Circ. Res. 34:858–866.

chapter 17

THE SIGNIFICANCE OF PULSATILE MICROHEMODYNAMICS

Joseph F. Gross

BACKGROUND

EXPERIMENTAL TECHNIQUES IN PULSATILE HEMODYNAMICS

MATHEMATICAL THEORY OF PULSATILE FLOW
IN THE MICROCIRCULATION

MASS TRANSFER

NON-NEWTONIAN PULSATILE FLOW

COMMENTS AND FORWARD LOOK

Macroscopic hemodynamics has always been treated as a time-dependent phenomenon because of the easily observable pulsating nature of blood flow in the larger blood vessels. However, the small size of the microvessels and the difficulty in making quantitative observations of the blood flow in them has prevented the formulation of a clear picture of the hemodynamics in the microcirculation. As a result, the assumption has been made that the pulsatility in the macroscopic hemodynamics is damped out—by the compliance of the vasculature and the dissipation in the flow—to produce a steady flow in the microvessels. Through recent advances in instrumentation for quantitative physiologic measurements, however, pulsatility of the blood flow in the microcirculation has been shown to exist. This observation has spurred the development of theoretical models for pulsatile fluid mechanics in the microvessels as well as consideration of the impact of pulsatile hemodynamics in the important mass-transfer processes in the microtissues.

BACKGROUND

The pulsatility of blood flow in the microcirculation was noted at the turn of the century by Krogh (1959), who suggested that the apparent complete damping in

365

the venous circulation was caused by the path differences due to morphology in the microvasculature. This would cause the pulsations to arrive in random phase at the venous end, thus cancelling the pulsation by interference.

Pulsatile flow throughout the microcirculation of the lung was apparent since the first measurement of the pulmonary venous pressure. Until recently, however, there was considerable controversy regarding its cause, i.e., whether it was due to a true pulse transmission of pressure from the pulmonary artery, modified by compliance and resistance properties of the pulmonary vasculature, or whether it was due to the *vis a tergo* action of the heart.

This controversy was resolved by Lee and DuBois (1955), who demonstrated that pulsatility in the absorption of nitrous oxide was directly related to periodic blood flow at the level of the exchange vessels of the lung, and by the direct measurements of Caro and MacDonald (1961), who showed that the pulsation advances in phase through the pulmonary vasculature. Subsequent studies by Rappaport, Bloch, and Irwin (1959) showed that pressures are pulsatile down to 25-μ-diameter pulmonary arterioles. These studies, in conjunction with radiologic studies such as those of Raphael, Steiner, and Greenspan (1969), establish a firm basis for the conjecture that pulsatile pressure is transmitted through the microvasculature of the lung. Although the presence of pulsatile pressure in the lung suggested this phenomenon, pulsatility related to the action of the heart in most other tissues and organs has been assumed to be completely damped in the capillary bed.

Evidence for pulsatile pressure in the microscopic vessels of the mesentery was first provided by Landis (1926, 1927). In his classic work on the direct measurement of capillary pressure, he controlled the motion of the interface between the fluid in a micropipette that punctured the endothelial wall into the capillary lumen and plasma by varying the pressure in the shank of the micropipette. The interface between fluid and plasma was made visible either by adding a concentrated dye or by following the motion of red blood cells at the entrance of the pipette. Intermittant motion, synchronous with the action of the heart, allowed Landis to detect the balance point between the intraluminal hydrostatic microvascular pressure and the pipette pressure and to estimate the magnitude of systolic relative to diastolic excursions. These pulsatile components were observed to persist through the microcirculatory bed to the level of the venous capillaries.

With the development of the pressure servo-nulling technique by Wiederhielm, Woodbury, and Rushmer (1964), the methodology of Landis could be applied to monitor dynamic events. They first utilized this technique in the microcirculation of the frog mesentery and showed that pressures are pulsatile down to 26-μ-diameter arteriolar capillaries.

Pulsatile flow was observed in the mesentery by Bloch (1968), Wayland and Johnson (1967), and Gaehtgens, Meiselman, and Wayland (1970), and in the omentum by Intaglietta, Pawula, and Tompkins (1970), Intaglietta, Tompkins, and Richardson (1970), and Intaglietta, Richardson, and Tompkins (1971). Rosenblum (1969) observed pulsatile flow in arterioles and venules of subarachnoid space. Gaehtgens (1970) measured venous pulsatile pressure in small mesenteric veins. Although these experimental studies provided evidence for significant pulsatile conditions in the microvasculature, most theoretical studies have assumed that flow in the microvessels is steady.

The detailed basis for experimental evidence of pulsatility in microvessels is presented, followed by a discussion of the theoretical models for pulsatile flow in the microcirculation. The concluding section deals with the physiologic implications of pulsatility in the microvessels.

EXPERIMENTAL TECHNIQUES IN PULSATILE HEMODYNAMICS

The earliest observations on the pulsatile nature of flow in the microvessels was made by Krogh (1959), who observed that

> In the capillaries the pulse does not as a rule cause any variation in diameter of the vessels, but the velocity variations can often be very distinctly seen and are practically always present when the flow is too rapid to render them visible . . .

Landis (1926, 1927) used the classical micropipette technique described earlier to measure pressure and noted pulsatility in the measurements through the microcirculation to the level of the venous capillaries.

The capacitance manometer was used by Rappaport et al. (1959) to study pressure in the microvessels (50–250-μ diameters) of the frog mesentery and the rabbit lung. The capacitance manometer consists of a flexible member parallel to a fixed metal plate that together form a variable condenser. The member responds to pressure that changes the capacitance of the condenser. These changes can then be converted into electrical signal charges for making measurements. The transducer was put in a 35-μ-diameter cannula, which was then inserted into the vessel to be measured. The data showed pulsatile pressuregrams in rabbit mesentery and in the pulmonary arterioles of frogs.

The development of the pressure servo-nulling technique by Wiederhielm et al. (1964) extended the Landis technique to include quantitative dynamic measurements of pressure. The principle was to replace the dye by a salt solution that would interface with the plasma in the vessel. The location of the interface was determined by the pressure in the vessel, bringing about an overall change in the resistance of the system as determined by a Bridge circuit. Balancing the Bridge circuit would provide a means of monitoring the interface location and the pressure. The system could also potentially measure pressure in very small capillaries because the micropipette tip diameters were about 1–5μ. Using this technique, they reported pulsatile pressures in the frog mesentery down to 26-μ-diameter capillaries.

Intaglietta, Pawula, and Tompkins (1970), Intaglietta, Tompkins, and Richardson (1970), and Intaglietta et al. (1971) extended and modified the servo-nulling technique through the use of various modifications (see Richardson in Volume III). This made it possible to record dynamic variations in the pressure very accurately down to arterioles of 12-μ diameter.

Using the double-slit techniques, Wayland and Johnson (1967) reported pulsatile velocities in the cat mesentery. The method consists in the on-line measurement of the time delay to maximum cross correlation between the time-varying voltages generated by the images of streaming red blood cells projected onto two adjacent photodetectors aligned in the direction of flow. Intaglietta, Tompkins, and Richardson (1970) extended this approach to real time by the use of electronic cross-correlation techniques. Figure 1 shows an example of the pulsatility in pressure and velocity measurements taken throughout the cat omentum by Intaglietta, Tompkins, and Richardson (1970). Amplitude decay and phase shifts are clearly shown for both velocity and pressure. Recently, Intaglietta and Tompkins (1972) have demonstrated submicron motion of the capillary wall that is synchronous with the systemic pulsatility.

The use of sophisticated electronic techniques and more innovative experimental approaches has revealed convincing evidence for the pulsatility in the microscopic hemodynamics. More important, the measurements are quantitative and provide a quantitative basis for interpretation of the theoretical developments in pulsatile flow in the microcirculation.

MATHEMATICAL THEORY OF PULSATILE FLOW IN THE MICROCIRCULATION

The mathematical analysis of the steady flow of blood in the microcirculation has been treated earlier in this volume, and discussion regarding the interaction of Stokes flow with the non-Newtonian rheology of blood and other mechanical properties of the microvasculature are not repeated here. As pointed out previously, the time-dependent equations of motion of macroscopic hemodynamics have been studied extensively. However, the behavior of the flow system in the microvessels is very different from that in the larger vessels and, as a consequence, the results obtained for arterial flows cannot be used to describe flow in capillaries. In the former case, the pressure forces are balanced by viscous and inertial forces in the fluid. The inertial forces dominate the flow in the larger arteries, but the viscous forces become more important as the characteristic diameter of the vessel decreases. In the microvessels, the Reynolds number is very small, $Re \ll O(1)$, and the inertial forces in the fluid can be neglected [to $O(Re)$] with respect to the viscous forces.

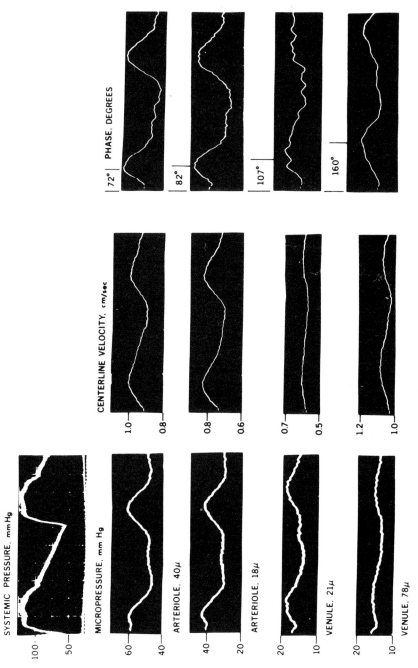

Figure 1. Pulsatile pressure and velocity measurement in cat omentum. Intaglietta et al. (1971); reprinted by permission.

We consider that blood is an incompressible and homogeneous fluid and that the microvessel is a rigid, infinitely long cylinder (see Figure 2). The simplified manometer equation for the flow is given by

$$\rho\frac{\partial \tilde{u}}{\partial \tilde{t}} = -\frac{\partial \tilde{P}}{\partial \tilde{x}}(t) + \frac{1}{\tilde{r}}\frac{\partial^2}{\partial \tilde{r}}\left(\tilde{r}\tilde{\tau}\right).$$ (1)

$$\underbrace{\qquad}_{\text{inertial}}\ \underbrace{\qquad}_{\text{pressure}}\ \underbrace{\qquad}_{\text{viscous}}$$

Equation (1) gives the balance between the inertial, pressure, and viscous forces. It is evident that if the fluid is non-Newtonian, $\tilde{\tau} = \tilde{\tau}(\tilde{u})$, then the system of equations to be solved is nonlinear. If the shear-stress

$$\tilde{\tau} = \mu\frac{\partial \tilde{u}}{\partial \tilde{y}},$$ (2)

where the viscosity equals a constant, then the equation is linear. Both cases are discussed and solutions presented. Following Aroesty and Gross (1972a), non-dimensional variables are introduced:

$$\tilde{\tau} = \frac{P_0 R}{2}\tau,$$

$$\tilde{r} = Rr,$$ (3)

$$\tilde{u} = \frac{P_0 R^2}{2\mu}u,$$

$$\tilde{t} = \frac{t}{\omega},$$

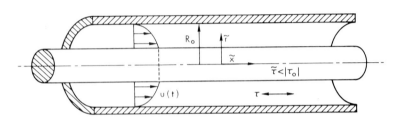

Figure 2. Coordinate system for pulsatile flow in a rigid tube (shown for a Casson fluid).

where P_0 is the absolute magnitude of a typical pressure gradient, R is the tube radius, and μ is the characteristic viscosity at high shear rates. The pressure gradient may then be written

$$-\frac{\partial \tilde{P}}{\partial \tilde{x}} = -P_0 P(t), \quad P_0 = \left| \frac{\partial \tilde{P}}{\partial \tilde{x}} \right|_{\text{average}} \tag{4}$$

The momentum equation may now be written in dimensionless variables:

$$\alpha^2 \frac{\partial u}{\partial t} = -2P(t) + \frac{1}{r} \frac{\partial}{\partial r} (r\tau), \tag{5}$$

where α is the well-known Womersley number,

$$\alpha^2 = \frac{R^2 \omega}{\mu / p}. \tag{6}$$

Clearly, the role of the inertial term in Eq. (5) is determined by the value of α. The characteristic frequency, ω, about 1 sec^{-1}, and the kinematic viscosity (at high shear rates), $\nu = \mu/p \cong 0.03$, will both be independent of vessel diameter. Therefore, $\alpha^2 \cong 30R^2$ when the radius is given in centimeters. For the case of vessels having a diameter of less than 0.2 mm, $\alpha^2 < 0.01$. On the other hand, layer arterial vessels have dimensions of the order of a centimeter and $\alpha^2 \cong O(10)$. This shows that the inertial term can range from a dominating influence in the macrocirculation to a negligible factor in capillaries. In the microcirculation, the range of the Womersley number is from a small value $\sim O(10^{-1})$ to a value of essentially zero. In order to illustrate these differences, a constant viscosity is assumed so that Eq. (5) reduces to

$$\alpha^2 \frac{\partial u}{\partial t} = -2P(t) = \mu \frac{\partial^2 u}{\partial r^2} \quad . \tag{7}$$

The pressure gradient is assumed to be varying sinusoidally, i.e.,

$$P(t) = P_0 e^{i\omega (t-x/c)} e^{-kx}, \tag{8}$$

where c is the phase velocity or displacement speed of wave, x is the physical separation of waves, k is the attenuation constant, and P_0 is the initial amplitude. The wave displacement speed c is related to the phase angle θ by

$$c = \frac{2\pi x \omega}{\theta}. \tag{9}$$

The pressure gradient is reduced as a result of dispersion, viscous damping, and interaction with the vessel wall. Such interaction can be obtained by integrating the continuity equation in the tube, which leads to the following expression:

$$\frac{\partial Q}{\partial x} = -2\pi R v_{\text{fluid}}.$$ (10)

The fluid velocity at the wall can result from the movement of the vessel wall due to ultrafiltration. If only the motion of the wall is considered, then Pollack, Reddy, and Noordergraef (1968) have shown that

$$\frac{\partial Q}{\partial x} = -\frac{3\pi R^2}{E}\frac{(a+1)^2}{(2a+1)}\frac{\partial P}{\partial t},$$ (11)

$$C_m = -\frac{3\pi R^2}{E}\frac{(a+1)^2}{(2a+1)}.$$ (12)

Equation (11) can be written

$$\frac{\partial Q}{\partial x} = C_m \frac{\partial P}{\partial t}.$$ (13)

Where the inertial terms are negligible, the Poiseuille flow in the tube is given by

$$\frac{\partial P}{\partial x} = -\frac{8\mu}{\pi R^4} Q = R_m Q,$$ (14)

and these equations lead to an expression for the behavior of the pressure in the vessel:

$$\frac{\partial^2 P}{\partial x^2} = R_m C_m \frac{\partial P}{\partial t}.$$ (15)

Furthermore, it can be shown that, for $\alpha \ll 1$, the wave speed C is a function of the frequency,

$$C = \sqrt{\frac{R_m C_m}{2\omega}}$$ (16)

and the attenuation constant is given by

$$k = \sqrt{\frac{\omega R_m C_m}{2}}.$$ (17)

Consequently, pulsatile flow in the microvessels is dispersed and highly attenuated. It is important to note that this equation can predict the pressure and flow behavior of the blood in a microvessel if R_m and C_m are known. Both parameters depend only on the morphology and structure of the vessel and, in principle, can be obtained from measurements of microcirculatory beds; see Sobin (1966), Intaglietta and Zweifach (1971), Bloch (1956), Frasher and Wayland (1972), and Fung (1966). This relationship was used in a network model for the microcirculation by Aroesty, Gross, and Gazley (1971) to predict the decay of pressure amplitude and phase-angle shift in a composite bed. They

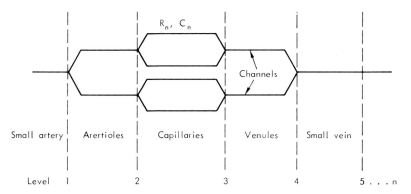

Figure 3. Five-level network model of the microcirculation.

assumed a network model of a microcirculating unit to be given schematically as in Figure 3. The network consists of a sequence of m parallel channels in a series of n levels, each level representing a generation of vessels in the microcirculation. Associated with each level are a resistance R_n and a compliance C_n that contain the viscosity of the blood and the structural properties of the wall. P and Q, the pressure and total flow, are continuous at each juncture between the levels. The time dependence of P and Q are factored out:

$$P = v\, e^{i\omega t},$$
$$Q = f\, e^{i\omega t};$$

(18)

then it can be shown (see Carslaw and Jaeger, 1959) that the flow and pressure at any level can be found from the equation given below:

$$\begin{pmatrix} v_n \\ f_n \end{pmatrix} = \begin{pmatrix} A_n & B_n \\ C_n & D_n \end{pmatrix} \begin{pmatrix} A_{n-1} & B_{n-1} \\ C_{n-1} & D_{n-1} \end{pmatrix} \cdots \begin{pmatrix} A_1 & B_1 \\ C_1 & D_1 \end{pmatrix} \begin{pmatrix} v_1 \\ f_1 \end{pmatrix}$$

(19)

where

$$A_n = \cosh\left[\left(\frac{\omega R_n C_n}{2}\right)^{1/2}(1+i)\right],$$

(20)

$$B_n = -\frac{\sinh\left[\left(\frac{\omega R_n C_n}{2}\right)^{1/2}(1+i)\right]}{\frac{m}{R_n}\left(\frac{\omega R_n C_n}{2}\right)^{1/2}(1+i)}$$

(21)

$$,C_n = -\frac{m}{R_n} \left(\frac{\omega R_n C_n}{2}\right)^{\!\frac{1}{2}} (1+i)\sinh\left[\left(\frac{\omega R_n C_n}{2}\right)^{\!\frac{1}{2}} (1+i)\right] \qquad (22)$$

$$D_n = \cosh\left[\left(\frac{R_n C_n}{2}\right)^{\!\frac{1}{2}} (1+i)\right]. \qquad (23)$$

Calculations were made using the five-level network shown in Figure 3 and composite structural properties and morphologic measurements. A result of this early calculation for the decay of the amplitude of the pressure pulse through the microcirculation is shown in Figure 4. The results for pressure decay and phase-angle shift were in qualitative agreement with the data of Intaglietta et al. (1971) (see Figure 1). Model experiments were made to determine the effect of changing structural properties of vessel dimensions (to test the effect of vasodilation and constriction) in the system. Changing the compliance of the capillaries by an order of magnitude resulted in almost no change in the system behavior. To test for the effects of vasodilation, the vessel diameters were increased by 50%. To test for constriction, they were decreased by 50%. Generally, only the venular portion of the system was affected, and the angles at the exit of the bed showed qualitative agreement with expected behavior: the angle for the case of the vasodilation changed very little, and the angle for the vasoconstriction was about 30% greater than in the normal case.

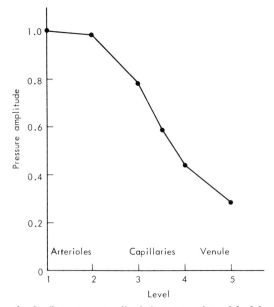

Figure 4. Decay of pulsatile pressure amplitude in a network model of the microcirculation.

A more extensive network model of pulsatile hemodynamics in the microcirculation of the rabbit omentum was studied by Gross, Intaglietta, and
Zweifach (1974). The methodology for the study of the circulation at the
arteriole, capillary, and venule levels in the microcirculation has been described
previously. The results of the measurements are given in Table 1, and the
morphologic data, together with appropriate values for the structural properties
based on Fung (1966), were used in a nine-level model to predict the pulsatile
properties of pressure and flow throughout an omental microcirculating unit.
The results for the attenuation of the pressure amplitude are shown in Figure 5,
which shows the attenuation for different frequencies (4π is the fundamental
one) and for the experimental data. Direct comparison of the data with the
frequency components shows qualitative agreement. It can be seen that the
frequency dependence of the pressure amplitude decay is small. The pressure
plane angle dependence on frequency (or heart rate) shown in Figure 6 is, by
contrast, much greater. The flow phase angle changes only at the arterial and
venous ends of the microcirculation (see Figure 7). There is almost no change in
the capillary section of the bed. The use of vessel size changes (20%) to simulate
the effect of vasoconstrictors and dilators was also studied, and it was again
concluded that pressure phase shift provided a more sensitive parameter than
pressure amplitude. Generally, the changes shown by the model are small as a
result of the diffusion-like behavior of the time-dependent effect in this model.

One of the interesting features of the model is that the morphologic
character of the microcirculatory bed is the major input to the parameters. This
suggests that it will be possible to compare the behavior of pulsatile hemodynamics in different microvascular beds if careful morphologic measurements are
forthcoming. Frasher and Wayland (1972) identified a microcirculatory unit or
module in the cat mesentery. Eriksson and Myrhage (1973) also reported data
on the cat tenuissimus muscle, and similar data are available for the bat wing
(Wiedeman, 1963), and the rat cremaster muscle (Smaje, Zweifach, and Intaglietta, 1970). Since these vascular beds exhibit substantial morphologic differences, it is of interest to compare the distribution of resistance and compliance
in order to establish their influence on the pressure–flow relationship in the
different components of these microvascular networks. Gross and Intaglietta
(1973) compared the resistance and compliance of the microcirculatory units in
cat mesentery, bat wing, rabbit omentum, and cat tenuissimus muscle. The
results for the resistance at each level (see Figure 8) show that the resistance in
the mesentery and omentum remains relatively constant throughout the bed,
while resistance in both bat wing and tenuissimus muscle decreases substantially
from the arterial to the venous end of the bed. Compliance for all the tissues
increases slightly toward the venous end. The decay of pulsatile pressure amplitude shown in Figure 9 indicates that decay takes place primarily on the arterial
side, except for the rabbit omentum, where a substantial amplitude remains after
the mid-capillaries.

Table 1. Pulsatile pressure measurements in the rabbit omentum

Vessel type	Level	No. of measurements[a]	Diameter (μ)		Pressure (cm H$_2$O)		Pressure amplitude (cm H$_2$O)		Pressure phase degrees		RBC velocity (cm/sec)		Velocity amplitude (cm/sec)		Velocity phase (degrees)	
			Ave.	SE	Ave.	SE	Ave.	SE	Ave.	SE	Ave.	SE	Ave.	SE	Ave.	SE
Arteries	1	7P-2V	52	5.8	93	11	14.0	5.4	68	10	3.9	–	0.35	–	65	–
Arteriol	2	5P-2V	20	4.6	44	7.4	8.4	4.0	81	11	0.75	0.15	0.15	–	90	–
Art cap	3	8P-5V	13.6	2.3	38	6.9	3.5	3.0	92	30	0.31	0.06	0.05	0.04	103	23.2
Art cap	4	2P-3V	11.2	–	28	–	1.2	–	90	–	0.28	0.16	0.02	0.005	106	10.2
Mid cap	5	4P-3V	9.5	0.4	25	4.0	1.2	1.0	90	35	0.35	–	0.02	0.005	106	14.0
Ven cap I	6	1V	8.0	–	–	–	1.2	–	–	–	0.40	–	–	–	–	–
Ven cap II	7	4P-5V	11.1	1.1	20	4.0	1.0	1.0	90	35	0.22	0.11	0.02	0.004	112	18.0
Venule	8	1P-7V	25.5	4.2	18	–	2.0	–	100	–	.67	0.28	0.02	0.01	125	17.0
Vein	9	5P-1V	72.0	12.6	16	3.1	0.4	0.5	143	24	3.8	–	0.03	–	140	–

Note: Standard deviation not shown for two measurements.

[a] Designations P and V refer to the number of pressure and velocity measurements performed.

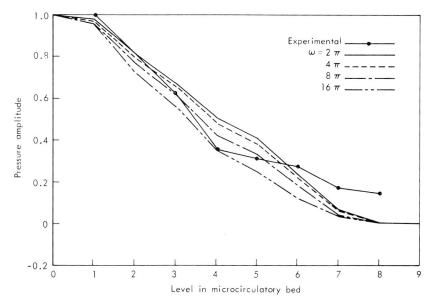

Figure 5. Attenuation of pressure amplitude–frequency dependence and comparison with experiment.

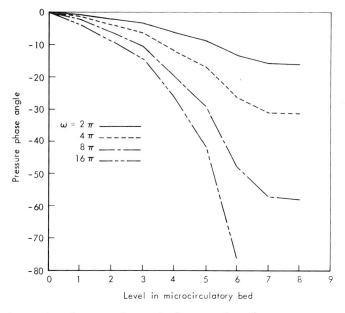

Figure 6. Attenuation of pressure phase-angle–frequency dependence.

378   Gross

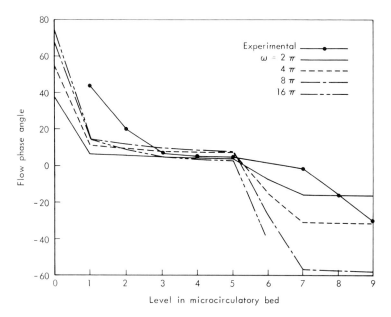

Figure 7. Flow phase-angle shift in the microcirculation with frequency dependence and comparison with data.

The discussion to the present has dealt with the general parameters of pulsatile flow, such as amplitude and phase angle. The detailed shape of the pressure and flow curves can be constructed at different levels in the microcirculatory bed. Gross and Intaglietta (1972) simulated the systemic pressure curve with a sinusoidal series expansion and treated each frequency component to the network analysis. They expressed the intraluminal hydrostatic pressure as follows:

$$P_c(t,b) = P_{co}(b) + \sum^{n} a_n(b) \sin n \left[\omega - \alpha_n(b)\right] t, \qquad (24)$$

where P_c is the intraluminal hydrostatic pressure, P_{co} is the steady component of intraluminal pressure, b is the order of branching, a_n is the frequency component coefficient, α_n is the phase angle, and ω is the frequency.

The components were summed at each level to obtain the pressure trace. These traces were compared with the data of Intaglietta et al. (1971) as shown in Figure 10. The agreement is remarkably good in view of the simplicity of the model and the assumption that blood is a homogeneous Newtonian fluid.

Recently, Ariman, Turk, and Sylvester (1973a, 1973b) and Turk, Sylvester, and Ariman (1973) have studied blood flow using a microcontinuum model. Such a model takes into account the micromotions and deformations in suspensions such as would occur in erythrocytes in plasma. The first two studies

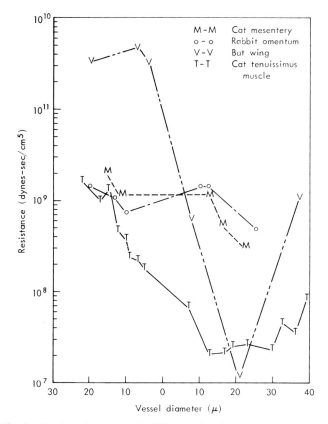

Figure 8. The distribution of resistance in different microtissues.

concern rigid erythrocytes rotating in the plasma. The plasma viscosity, rotational viscosity, and rotational gradient coefficient are determined from the experimental data of Bugliarello and Sevilla (1970) and then used to predict their pulsatile velocity profiles. Excellent agreement is obtained when non-Newtonian effects are absent (see Figure 11). In the case of deformable cells, Ariman et al. (1973a) show that increasing the intensity of red cell deformation leads to an increase of energy dissipation in the flow, and this results in an increase in the degree of blunting of the velocity profile.

MASS TRANSFER

It was pointed out earlier that compliance in the microcirculation might result from fluid movement through the vascular wall. This probability was suggested by Intaglietta et al. (1971) in order to explain the comparatively large phase shifts measured in the cat omentum. The latter implies that a large compliance

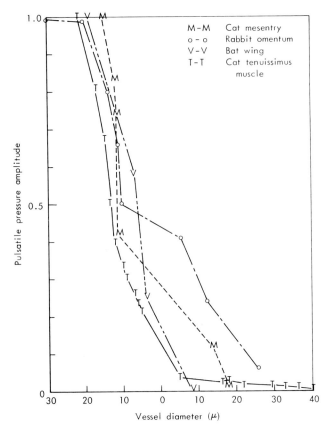

Figure 9. The decay of the pulsatile pressure amplitude in different microtissues.

and visible diameter changes with heart rate should be observed. Intaglietta and Tompkins (1972), using data processing of television microscopy recordings of microvessel diameter, showed diameter changes to be in the submicron range, corresponding to a relatively stiff microvaculature.

The radial velocity component due to ultrafiltration exchange can be expressed as

$$v_f = Kl[P(t) - p], \qquad (25)$$

where K is the Landis–Zweifach capillary filtration coefficient (see Gross and Intaglietta, 1972), and P is a combination of all colloid osmotic and tissue hydrostatic pressures. Equation (25) can be used to compare the "diffusion coefficient" resulting from mechanical compliance effects and ultrafiltration effects. The result is given by

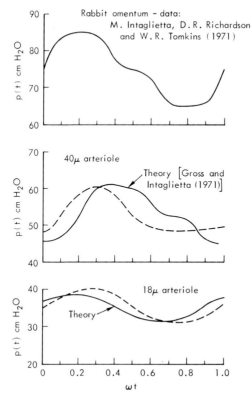

Figure 10. Comparison of measured and calculated velocity profiles in the pulsatile microcirculation.

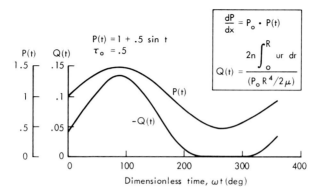

Figure 11. Quasisteady flow rate due to sinusoidal pressure gradient.

$$\frac{D \text{ mech}}{D \text{ exch}} = \frac{3EK}{\omega R}. \tag{26}$$

Estimates of the values of E and K for the capillaries of the rabbit omentum are $E = 3 \times 10^{-6}$ dynes/cm^2 (Fung, 1966) and $K = 10^{-9}$ cm^3/dyne-sec (Zweifach and Intaglietta, 1968). The value of ω is assumed to be 2 sec^{-1}, and $R = 5 \times 10^{-4}$ cm. This value of the ratio in Eq. (26) is of the order of 10 for this system and, therefore, compliance due to ultrafiltration is about 10% of the total compliance.

An extension of this idea was proposed by Aroesty et al. (1971), which included two terms in the expression for the fluid movement across the wall. They assumed that the fluid pressure diffused into the surrounding tissue according to

$$\frac{\partial P}{\partial t} = K_p \, \Delta^2 \, p, \tag{27}$$

where K_p is the diffusion coefficient for fluid pressure. This yields a new equation relating the normal fluid velocity at the wall and the flow:

$$\frac{\partial Q}{\partial x} = 2\pi K R \left[P - \frac{1}{6} \frac{\delta^2}{K_p} \frac{\partial P}{\partial t} \right]. \tag{28}$$

The compliance due to the tissue permeability is then given by

$$C_p = -\frac{\pi \delta^2}{3 \, K_p} \, K. \tag{29}$$

The diffusion time, δ^2/K_p, has not yet been measured, but it could be estimated from transient tissue experiments. Gross and Intaglietta (1972) reported some preliminary results indicating that calculations using the tissue permeability compliance could make a significant difference in the phase angle of the flow compared with the results for mechanical compliance only.

The question of mass transfer intraluminally in the plasma gaps between erythrocyte in bolus flow was studied by Hung, Weissman, and Bugliarello (1971). They used a numerical technique to solve the time-dependent Stokes flow equation in the axial plasma gaps between disk-like erythrocytes that span the entire lumen. They also concluded that the quasisteady solution for the flow would approximate the unsteady secondary flow. They further concluded that the bolus flow is of little importance in the transport of oxygen in the microcirculation.

NON-NEWTONIAN PULSATILE FLOW

The above discussion has focused on a homogeneous model of blood as a fluid having constant viscosity. This is, of course, a serious assumption in the microcirculation, where there is almost no region in which such a condition obtains.

In fact, at this scale of flow, the non-Newtonian, nonhomogeneous aspects of blood flow are likely to be most pronounced. Taylor (1959) and Womersley (1957) analyzed pulsatile flow for large values of the Womersley frequency parameter α. Their results indicated that large changes in the constitutive relations between stress and strain rate did not significantly affect their study.

A comprehensive experimental study in vitro of the pulsatile flow of blood in small rigid tubes has been reported by Bugliarello and Sevilla (1970). They noted that both the flow and the plasma-layer thickness were similar to the steady-state values, i.e., the inertial effects were undetectable.

In the capillaries, a true bolus-type flow usually obtains, and a review of such flows is given by Gross and Aroesty (1972a). When the characteristic diameter of the vessel becomes much larger than the erythrocyte, e.g., about 200 μ, the blood begins to behave as a non-Newtonian fluid. Within certain wall shear stress limits, it has been shown experimentally in vitro by Merrill (1969) that the simple shear behavior of blood may be closely approximated by Casson's equation:

$$\bar{\tau}^{1/2} = \tau_0^{1/2} + \mu \left(\frac{\partial \bar{u}}{\partial \bar{r}} \right)^{1/2}, \tag{30}$$

where τ_0 equals the yield stress. This equation describes the low shear behavior of blood in that a finite stress must be applied to the blood before it will deform and behave as a fluid. The actual value of the yield stress, and, in fact, its very existence, remains a controversial subject. The actual physical process that results in the solid-like behavior is not clearly understood; it is probably related to rouleaux formation in the presence of fibrinogen. Nevertheless, there is ample evidence to demonstrate the yield stress (Cokelet, 1970), and it is included in the analysis.

The existence of a non-Newtonian viscosity introduces a complication into the analysis of the flow. As indicated previously, if the local shear stress in the fluid falls below a certain value τ_0, the velocity gradient in the fluid disappears because the fluid behaves as a solid. Because of the complexity of the shear stress field due to the time-dependent flow, there could be moving solid annuli of blood in the vessel. There is another difficulty that must be treated if the equations are to be solved. Equation (5) can be solved only if the relationship $\tau = \tau(u)$ is known. The Casson equation satisfies that requirement, but in an implicit sense, since the solutions of each of the two equations are independent. Aroesty and Gross (1972b) have solved this system for small values of the Womersley number and demonstrated that the features of the pulsatile system could be very well represented by the quasisteady solution. For the range of vessels where the Casson fluid might be a suitable model for blood flow, the Womersley frequency parameter is quite small. Aroesty and Gross (1972b) show that if the absolute value of the pressure gradient is less than 2 mm H_2O/mm, the quasisteady theory should be appropriate. This theory was used to provide an illustrative example shown in Figure 12. The periodic pressure gradient was given by $P(A) = 1 + 0.5 \sin \omega t$. When the yield stress is large, the flow is strongly non-Newtonian and nonlinear. Figure 12 shows the case when the yield stress is half the average wall stress. Q represents the flow in the vessel, and it is clear that the flow is stopped for almost half of the pressure gradient cycle. Figure 13 shows velocity profiles over a cycle; the dotted lines represent the movement of the yield surface. At a value of $\omega t = 270°$, the solid plug extends to the wall.

The importance and function of the plasma layer in blood flow has received great attention over the years, and it was instructive to see how the thickness of such a layer would influence the results of the calculation. A plasma layer of thickness $Y_1 = 0.01\ R$ and a viscosity equal to 0.25 of the high-shear Casson value was included in the calculation, and the results are shown in Figure 14. The bottom curve for the flow is identical to that in Figure 1. When the plasma layer is included, it is clear that the flow rate is doubled and the plasma acts as a lubricating layer. Results are similar for the case when the yield stress is only 0.10 that of the average wall shear. Note that the flow behavior is not much more sinusoidal. In an effort to compare the determination of non-Newtonian pulsatile flow calculation with an equivalent Newtonian flow, Gross and Aroesty (1971) demonstrated that the use of a Newtonian viscosity based on the average wall shear stress provided the best approximation to the non-Newtonian flow. The high-shear viscosity gave very poor representation (Figure 15). The shape of the flow-rate profile was not well represented by any of the approximations for a high shear stress viscosity.

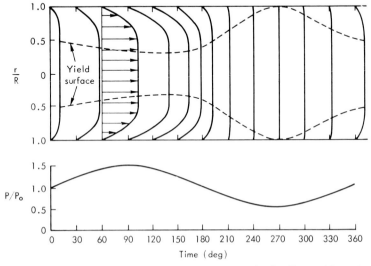

Figure 12. Velocity distribution and yield surface in pulsatile flow with a sinusoidal pressure gradient (no plasma layer).

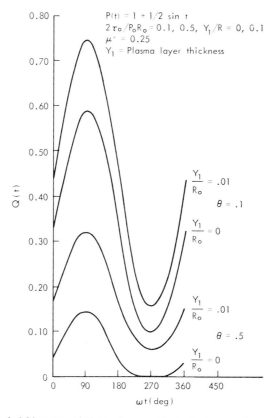

Figure 13. Effect of yield stress and plasma layer on the instantaneous flow rate.

COMMENTS AND FORWARD LOOK

Pulsatile flow in the microcirculation has received great attention, both from theoreticians and experimentalists. The primary thrust of recognition for pulsatility came from the development of quantitative experimental microtechniques for accurate measurement of pressure and flow in the microvessels and the implementation of sophisticated electronic data processing techniques for analysis. The results of these experimental advances made it possible to demonstrate convincingly the pulsatility of pressure and flow in all of the vessels in the microvascular system. Much of this work has been concentrated in the omentum of rabbits and cats and, more recently, in the tenuissimus muscle of the cat. More data need to be taken in other tissues, such as skeletal muscle, mesentery, and adipose tissue, in order to establish chracteristic amplitudes, amplitude decay patterns, and other features of the pulsatile behavior that could provide physiologic insight. The experimental techniques necessary for such investiga-

386   Gross

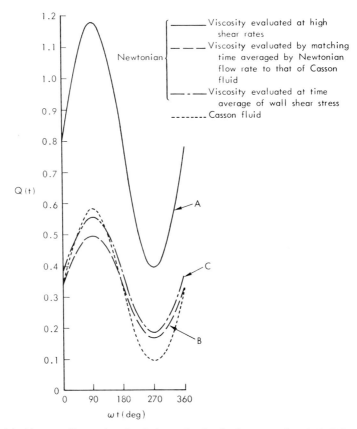

Figure 14. Alternate Newtonian simulations of pulsatile flow rates ($\theta = 0.1$). Taken from a paper presented at the April, 1971, meeting of the Microcirculatory Society in Chicago.

tions are all available. Extensions of the present experimental designs to accommodate special problems of new tissues are still being developed.

The major question to be addressed is the physiologic importance of pulsatility in the microvasculation. Does it really play a critical role in the maintenance of fluid and material balances in the microtissues? This question cannot be answered at the present time either experimentally or theoretically. The pulsatile amplitudes are not large with respect to the pressure levels themselves, but this cannot in itself be construed as a negation of the importance of pulsatility. The values of the hydrostatic and osmotic pressure balances in the microcirculation remain controversial, but it is clear that very small pressure changes (of the order of 1 mm H_2O) are all that are required to bring about substantial shifts in fluid movement. The amount and duration of such shifts could easily depend on the pulsations that have been experimentally observed. An experiment in which steady flow and pulsatile pressure variations are imposed on a tissue could

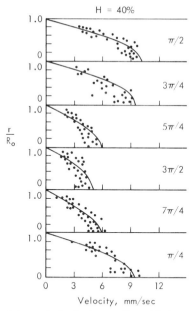

Figure 15. Comparison of theoretical velocity profiles with the experimental pulsatile blood flow data of Bugliarello and Sevilla (1970) at six points in the pressure cycle for a 40 μ tube, hematocrit = 40%. Taken from a paper presented at the 25th Congress of the Physiological Sciences, Munich, July 1976.

provide an interesting qualitative estimate of the effects of pulsatility. It is well known that perfusion for organ preservation must be pulsatile to be successful. Even in experiments employing isogravimetric preparations, steady-state perfusion brings about rapid and substantial edema. This is an important clue to indicate that pulsatility is involved with the homeostatic process. The precise nature of this interaction is just now beginning to receive attention.

The theoretical work outlined above focuses on a very simple model of the pulsatile microcirculation. The contention is that more complexity would involve enormously greater computational effort and probably not provide significantly greater simulation resolution. Such a simple model seems to provide a satisfactory framework for the study of the basic and important features of pulsatile flow, and the agreement with experimental data is encouraging. However, much remains to be done in both fluid mechanics and mass transfer. The latter is most important. The general properties of flow in capillaries and arterioles and in the microvascular beds themselves are known. Studies of the non-Newtonian behavior in the region from 10- to 100-μ vessels have not yet been done, although some work using power-law models to represent the rheologic behavior of blood in this region has been reported (see Gross and Aroesty, 1972b).

The mass-transfer problem for the pulsatile microcirculation is the key to the physiologic importance of pulsatility. A few simple models for pulsatile mass transfer have been presented, but these have not provided theoretical evidence for the postulated fluid movement in the extravascular tissue from the arterial to the venous portion of the microvascular bed. Clearly, there would be no net fluid transfer if some of the fluid that had transferred into the tissue did not remain subsequent to the periodic lowering of the intraluminal pressure. This fluid retention is probably due to molecular drag of the fluid in the tissues, which results in a net fluid transfer to the tissue. Tissue hydrostatic and osmotic pressures could also change as a result of the pressure "diffusion," but no measurements have yet been made. The microcapsule experiments show such changes, but they are all concerned with longer time scales and more intense pressure changes. New theoretical work must include a more realistic model for fluid transfer through tissue and the behavior of pressures in the extravascular tissue.

LITERATURE CITED

Ariman, T., M. A. Turk, and N. D. Sylvester. 1973a. A microcontinuum model of blood with deformable cells. In Y. C. Fung and J. A. Brighton (eds.), ASME Biomechanics Symposium. American Society of Mechanical Engineers, New York.

Ariman, T., M. A. Turk, and N. D. Sylvester. 1973b. A microncontinuum model of blood. In Proceedings of the Fourth Canadian Congress of Applied Mechanics, p. 837.

Aroesty, J., and J. F. Gross. 1972a. The mathematics of pulsatile flow in small vessels. I. Casson theory. Microvasc. Res. 4:1−12.

Aroesty, J., and J. F. Gross. 1972b. Pulsatile flow in small blood vessels. I. Casson theory. Biorheology. 9:33−43.

Aroesty, J., J. F. Gross, and C. Gazley, Jr. 1971. Pulsatile flow in the microvessels. Paper presented at April 1971 Microcirculatory meeting, Chicago. Also, P-4636. The Rand Corporation, Santa Monica, California, 24 p.

Bloch, E. H. 1956. Microscopic observations of the circulating blood in the bulbar conjunction in man in health and disease. Ergeb. Anat. Entwicklungsgeschichte 35:1.

Bloch, E. H. 1968. High speed cinephotography of the microvascular system. In A. L. Copley (ed.), Hemorheology: Proceedings of the First International Conference, pp. 665−667. Pergamon Press, New York.

Bugliarello, G., and J. Sevilla. 1970. Velocity distribution and other characteristics of steady and pulsatile blood flow in fine glass tubes. Biorheology 7:85−107.

Caro, C. G., and D. A. MacDonald. 1961. The relation of pulsatile pressure and flow in the pulmonary vascular bed. J. Physiol. 157:426−453.

Carslaw, H. S., and J. C. Jaeger. 1959. Conduction of heat in solids. Oxford University Press, Cambridge. 510 p.

Cokelet, G. 1972. The rheology of human blood. In Y. C. Fung, N. Perrone, and M. Anliker (eds.), Biomechanics. Its Foundations and Objectives, pp. 63−104 Prentice-Hall, Englewood Cliffs, N.J.

Eriksson, E., and R. Myrhage. 1974. Microvascular dimensions and blood flow in skeletal muscle. Acta Physiol. Scand. 86:211.

Frasher, W. G., and H. Wayland. 1972. A repeating modular organization of the microcirculation of cat mesentery. Microvasc. Res. 4:62–76.

Fung, Y. C. 1966. Microscopic blood vessels in the mesentery. *In* Y. C. Fung (ed.), Biomechanics, pp. 151–166. ASME, New York.

Gaehtgtens, P. A. 1970. Pulsatile pressure and flow in the mesenteric vascular bed of the cat. Pflügers Arch. 316:462–473.

Gaehtgens, P. A., H. J. Meiselman, and H. Wayland. 1970. Erythrocyte flow velocities in mesenteric microvessels of the cat. Microvasc. Res. 2:151–162.

Gross, J. F., and M. Intaglietta. 1973. Effects of morphology and structural properties on microvascular hemodynamics. Bibl. Anat. 11:532–539.

Gross, J. F., and J. Aroesty. 1972*a*. Mathematical models of capillary flow: A critical review. Biorheology 9:225–264.

Gross, J. F., and J. Aroesty. 1972*b*. Power law models in unsteady hemodynamics. Symposium on Biorheology. IV International Biophysics Congress, Moscow.

Gross, J. F., and M. Intaglietta. 1972. Mass transfer in the pulsatile microcirculation. Annual Meeting of the Microcirculatory Society, Chicago, April 1972.

Gross, J. F., and J. Aroesty. 1971. Hemorheology in the pulsatile microcirculation. XXV Congress of the Physiological Sciences, Munich, July 1971. Springer-Verlag, New York. 675 p.

Gross, J. F., M. Intaglietta, and B. W. Zweifach. 1974. Network model of pulsatile hemodynamics in the microcirculation of the rabbit omentum. Am. J. Physiol. 226:1117–1123.

Hung, T. K., M. M. Weissman, and G. Bugliarello. 1971. A numerical model for two-dimensional oscillatory flow and oxygen transfer in the axial plasmatic gaps of capillaries. *In* H. Hartert and A. L. Copley (eds.), Theoretical and Clinical Hemorheology, pp. 60–70. Springer, Heidelberg.

Intaglietta, M. 1971. Pulsatile velocity components in the cat omental microcirculation. Bibl. Anat. 11:74–76. Also, *In* 6th European Conference on Microcirculation, Aalburg. S. Karger, Basel.

Intaglietta, M., and W. R. Tompkins. 1972. On-line measurement of microvascular dimensions by television microscopy. J. Appl. Physiol. 32:546–551.

Intaglietta, M., D. R. Richardson, and W. R. Tompkins. 1971. Blood pressure flow and elastic properties in microvessels of cat omentum. Am. J. Physiol. 221:922–928.

Intaglietta, M., and B. W. Zweifach. 1971. Geometrical model of the microvasculature of the rabbit omentum from in-vivo measurements. Circ. Res. 28: 593–600.

Intaglietta, M., R. F. Pawula, and W. R. Tompkins. 1970. Pressure measurements in the mammalian microvasculature. Microvasc. Res. 2:212–220.

Intaglietta, M., W. R. Tompkins, and D. R. Richardson. 1970. Velocity measurement in the microvasculature of the cat omentum by on-line method. Microvasc. Res. 2:462–473.

Krogh, A. 1959. The anatomy and physiology of capillaries. Hafner, New York. 422 p.

Landis, E. M. 1927. Micro-injection studies of capillary permeability. II. The relation between capillary pressure and the rate at which fluid passes through the walls of single capillaries. Am. J. Physiol. 82:217–238.

Landis, E. M. 1926. The capillary pressure in frog mesentery as determined by micro-injection methods. Am. J. Physiol. 75:548–570.

Lee, G. de J., and A. B. DeBois. 1955. Pulmonary capillary flow in man. J. Clin. Invest. 34:1380–1390.

Lee, G. de J., and A. B. DuBois. 1955. Pulmonary capillary blood flow in man. J. Clin. Invest. 34:1380–1390.

Merrill, E. W. 1969. Rheology of blood. Physiol. Rev. 49:863–888.

Pollack, G. H., R. V. Reddy, and A. Noordergraff. 1968. Input impedence, wave travel and reflections in the human pulmonary arterial tree: Studies using an electrical analog. IEEE Trans. Bio-Med. Eng. 15:151–164.

Raphael, M. J., R. E. Steiner, and R. H. Greenspan. 1969. The origin of the pulmonary densitometric pulse. Br. J. Radiol. 42:824–829.

Rappaport, M. B., E. H. Bloch, and J. W. Irwin. 1959. A manometer for measuring dynamic pressures in the microvascular system. J. Appl. Physiol. 14:651–655.

Rosenblum, W. F. 1969. Erythrocyte velocity and velocity pulse in minute blood vessels on the surface of the mouse brain. Circ. Res. 24:887–892.

Smaje, L., B. W. Zweifach, and M. Intaglietta. 1970. Micropressure and capillary filtration coefficients in single vessels of the cremaster muscle of the rat. Microvasc. Res. 2:96–110.

Sobin, S. S. 1966. The architecture and function of the microvasculature. In Y. C. Fung (ed.), Biomechanics, pp. 132–150. ASME, New York.

Taylor, M. G. 1959. The influence of the anomalous viscosity of blood upon its oscillatory flow. Phys. Med. Biol. 3:273–290.

Turk, M. A., N. D. Sylvester, and T. Ariman. 1973. On pulsatile blood flow. Trans. Soc. Rheol. 17:1–21.

Wayland, H., and P. C. Johnson. 1967. Erythrocyte velocity measurements in microvessels by a two-slit photometric method. J. Appl. Physiol. 22:33–337.

Wiederhielm, C. A., T. W. Woodbury, and R. F. Rushmer. 1964. Pulsatile pressure in the microcirculation of the frog's mesentery. Am. J. Physiol. 207:173–176.

Wiedeman, M. P. 1963. Dimensions of blood vessels from distributing artery to collecting vein. Circ. Res. 12:375–378.

Womersley, J. R. 1957. An elastic tube theory of pulse transmission and oscillatory flow in mammalian arteries. Wright Air Development Center Technical Report, TR-56-514.

Zweifach, B. W., and M. Intaglietta. 1968. Mechanics of fluid movement across single capillaries in the rabbit. Microvasc. Res. 1:83–101.

VASCULARIZATION OF TISSUE

chapter 18

GROWTH AND DIFFERENTIATION OF BLOOD VESSELS

Elof Eriksson and Harvey A. Zarem

The origin of blood vessels has fascinated investigators in embryology, who for many years focused on the formation of the earliest blood vessels in the animal. In 1868 His described the angioblasts as cells of the yolk sack that grew into the embryo and formed all vascular tissues. Subsequent investigators such as Minot (1912), Evans (1912), and Sabin (1917) subscribed to His's angioblast theory. Another theory proposed that all vessels embryologically originated in local intraembryonic mesenchyme; Goethe (1874), Ruckert and Mollier (1906), Maximov (1909), McClure (1921), and Reagen (1917) favored the latter theory, which represents the opinion of the majority of investigators today.

Most information about new vessel formation in the adult has been gathered from studies of the vascularization of regenerating tissues. Essentially the same processes of vessel formation are described under titles such as late inflammation, repair, and wound healing. Several excellent reviews are available, e.g., Clark and Clark (1939), Illig (1961), and Jennings and Florey (1970). Most other reviews, e.g., Zweifach (1973), Grant (1973), Ebert and Grant (1974), and Wilkinson (1974), concentrate on the process of vascularization during the initial inflammatory response to tissue injury.

Advances in electron microscopic techniques have allowed essential contributions during the last two decades; see, e.g., Schoefl (1963), Cliff (1963), Majno (1965), Rhodin (1967, 1968), Palade and Bruns (1968), Karnovsky (1970), Luft (1973), and Casley-Smith (1973). Most recently, new vessel formation in uninjured muscle tissue after chronic stimulation of motor nerves has been studied by Hudlická and Myrhage (1975).

In the following discussion, we use the microvascular morphologic terminology suggested by Wiedeman (1963) and the physiologic terminology used by Folkow and Neil (1971).

MECHANISMS OF NEW VESSEL FORMATION IN THE ADULT

The problems of wound healing and the transplantation of tissue have focused interest on the reestablishment of the vasculature in healing and transplanted tissues. The process of neovascularization has been studied by introducing a transparent chamber into a tissue defect thus permitting in vivo observations of the growth of vessels and tissue cells into a circular space (usually 20–50 μ thick).

According to Sandison's classical method (1924), a transparent chamber is introduced into the rabbit's ear. This method was used extensively by Clark and Clark (1939). Quantitation of the data was performed by Cliff (1965), who combined in vivo microscopic observations with electron microscopy (cf. Jennings and Florey, 1970). Modifications of Sandison's design of the rabbit ear chamber have been used by Barclay, Bruce, and Farid (1959) and Wood et al. (1966), and a further modification of these latter models (Figures 1–3) has been used in our laboratory (Leaf and Zarem 1970a).

Similar techniques have been used for other tissues, such as Algire's (1943) mouse transplant chamber in the skin of the back of the mouse and Branemark's (1959) transparent bone marrow chamber in the tibia of the rabbit. By the use of small titanium chambers (Figures 4 and 5) Brånemark (1971) has been able to study in vivo the regeneration of vessels in humans with little discomfort for the chamber-bearing volunteer.[1] Brånemark elevates a bipedicle skin flap on the inside of the upper arm or forearm. He makes a tube of the bipedicle flap, closes

---

[1] One of the authors (Eriksson) volunteered for this investigation.

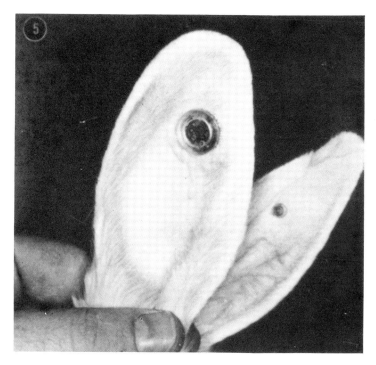

Figure 1. Rabbit with chambers inserted into both ears. *Right background,* the peg protrudes through the dorsal surface of the ear and prevents the dorsal skin from growing across
the optical pathway. Leaf and Zarem (1970a), reprinted by permission.

the skin underneath, and allows time for maturation of the skin tube (Figure 4).
A small transparent chamber with a titanium framing is inserted into the middle
of the skin tube. The ingrowth of vessels into the chamber may be observed
daily with transmitted light (Figure 5) while the volunteer is lying in an
examining chair. After completion of the in vivo observations, the tissue within
the chamber is analyzed in the electron microscope (Brånemark and Ekholm,
1969).

The chamber used in our laboratory (Leaf and Zarem, 1970a) is a modification of Sandison's (1928) design of the rabbit ear chamber, similar to the
chambers used by Barclay et al. (1959) and Wood et al. (1966). This type of
chamber is relatively small; the diameter of the central space is only 10 mm.
Ingrowth and maturation of vessels occurs about twice as fast, and the rate of
infection is low (approximately 25%). Between two parallel transparent surfaces
approximately 20–100 μ apart (the spacers may be varied), vessels grow in from
the surrounding perichondrium and subcutaneous tissues maturing within 3–4
wk (Figures 3 and 6). In the central space of the chamber, which is usually
occupied by a blood clot, budding loops of capillaries progress at a rate of

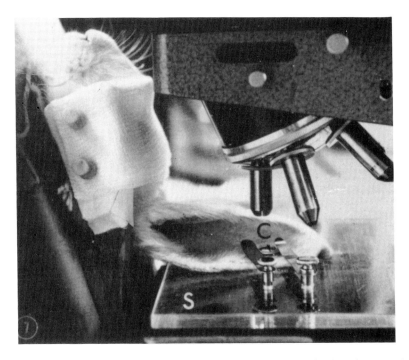

Figure 2. Rabbit ear chamber in the microscope. The chamber (c) is held on the stage with stage clips. The peg fits loosely into a hole in the Lucite stage (s). The rabbit is awake with head and body immobilized. Leaf and Zarem (1970a), reprinted by permission.

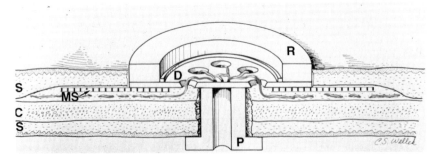

Figure 3. Schematic drawing of a cross section of a rabbit eat with an ear chamber in it. The coverslip of the chamber has been removed in order to show the ingrowing vessels on the top of the perforated Lucite disk (D). S, skin; C, cartilage; MS, mesh skirt anchoring the chamber; R, Lucite ring, P, Lucite peg.

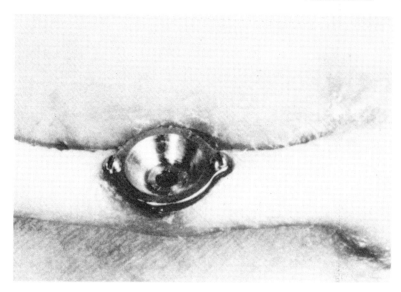

Figure 4. Titanium chamber in a bipedicle skin tube on the inside of the upper arm of a volunteer. Brånemark (1971), reprinted by permission.

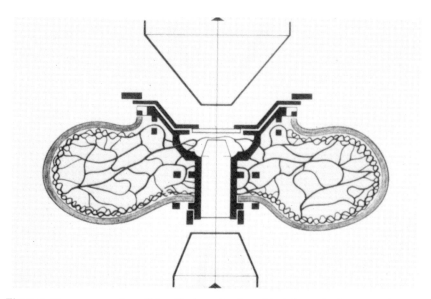

Figure 5. Transverse section of the titanium chamber, skin tube, and microscope elements, as positioned during observation. Brånemark (1971), reprinted by permission.

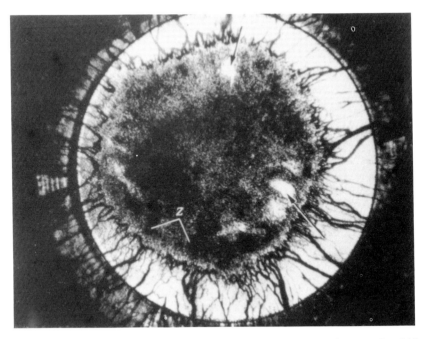

Figure 6. Photomicrography of a recently implanted rabbit ear chamber, showing fairly even invasion by the highly vascular growing fringe. Several clear spaces are visible distal to the growing fringe, two of which are indicated by arrows. These clear spaces are largely within the zone of hemorrhage (Z). × 27. Cliff (1963), reprinted by permission.

approximately 0.4 mm/day (Figure 6). Sandison (1924) and Clark and Clark (1939) and Cliff (1963) found a growth rate of about 0.2 mm/day. The central blood clot seems to stimulate the ingrowth of the vessels (Zarem, 1970*a*; and Clark and Clark, 1939). Brånemark (personal communication) reports that if the central space of the chamber is filled with normal saline only, an exudate of leucocytes and macrophages is followed by fibroblast and endothelial cells that establish a microvasculature. A clear *zone* in front of the ingrowing vessels has been observed. Cliff (1963) observed with light and electron microscopy that fibroblasts migrate in before the endothelial cells.

OBSERVATIONS IN THE LIGHT MICROSCOPE

Formation of a Vessel Plexus

Modern descriptions of the formation of new blood vessels do not differ significantly from that which Thoma (1893) outlined in his study of the vascularization of the tails of tadpoles (Figure 7). Most investigators have favored the basic concept that endothelium begets endothelium.

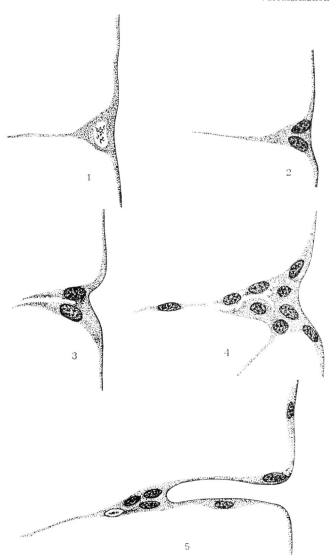

Figure 7. Schematic illustration of capillary sprouting with mitosis of endothelial cells. The mitotic activity takes place mainly at the base of the sprout. The sprout is then canalized and communicates with the lumen of the parent vessel. Thoma's (1893) studies on chick embryo.

The classic work by Clark and Clark (1939) demonstrated that in the tail of a tadpole and in the transparent rabbit ear chamber new capillaries arise from preexisting arterioles, venules, and capillaries by endothelial sprouting (Figures 8 and 9). From the convex side of a curved vessel there is a growth of a solid cord of endothelium. This cord will continue to grow and anastomose with

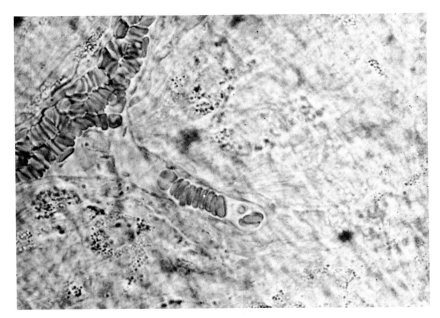

Figure 8. Sprouting vessel as observed in the intravital microscope. × 1100.

another endothelial cord or with a formed vessel. From the beginning, the outgrowing sprouts show small spaces between the endothelial cells, which join to form a lumen. The new capillaries seem to form as solid cords of endothelial cells that become canalized rather than forming directly as hollow tubes. Once the capillaries are perfused, many of them will retract and disappear. Most authors agree that after installation of the chamber, it takes 5–9 days until the first sprouts are seen, and about 3 wk until complete vascularization has occurred.

By using time-lapse cinemicroscopy, Cliff (1965) was able to describe the time sequence of the different steps in the process of neovascularization. The thin open space of the chamber had a diameter of 5–6 mm. It took an average of 9.5 days after insertion for vessels to appear at the border of the chamber. Complete vascularization occurred by 22.7 days. When calculating the rate of growth of sprouts, Cliff found a mean of about 0.12 mm/day, which is lower than the figure from Clark and Clark (1939) of 0.20 mm/day. When connecting with another sprout or vessel, the anastomosis was usually end-to-side or side-to-side. As soon as continuity between the lumen of the new vessel and the rest of the vasculature was established, the vessel filled with red blood cells that pulsated. The new vessels were unusually fragile and permeable (Figure 10). Pressure applied on the coverslip caused many red cells to diapedese through the vessel wall. The room temperature at which the rabbits were kept influenced the rate of vessel growth (Clark, 1918). At a high temperature Clark reported a

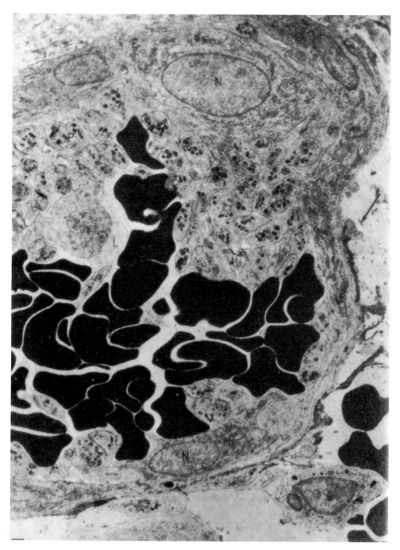

Figure 9. Electron micrograph of a wide vascular sprout growing into a 3-day-old cremaster muscle wound. The luman of this vessel is filled with platelets and red blood cells. Extravasated erythrocytes are shown in the lower right-hand corner. A fine layer of fibrin shreds coats the adventitial aspect of the vessel. Note the cytoplasmic extrusion (large arrow) of the endothelial cell. The small arrow marks a portion of a red blood cell within a cleft in the vascular wall. Stain: Karnovsky. × 3800. Schoefl (1963), reprinted by permission.

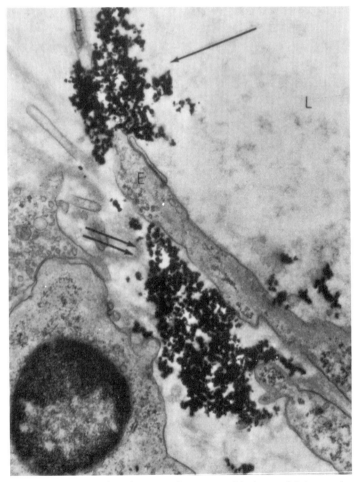

Figure 10. Visualization in the electron microscope of leakage of intravascular carbon particles in a corneal blood vessel. Carbon is escaping through an opening between endothelial cells (large arrows); it has also spilled into the perivascular tissue (double arrow). A structure corresponding to the basement membrane cannot be identified in this picture from a cornea three days after injury. Stain: Karnovsky. × 21,000. Schoefl (1963), reprinted by permission.

growth rate of 0.60 mm/day compared to 0.25 mm/day when the rabbits were kept at 70°F. At 60°F the growth rate was considerably slower. Clark also found the pattern of vasculature very labile. A change in temperature or the application of pressure upon the coverslips would result in the formation of new microvessels and the retraction of others.

When the vascular sprouts have become canalized, they become filled with stagnant red and white cells with occasional slow pulsating movements. Throughout the period of vascularization of the chamber, there is a relative increase in the number of white blood cells present in the newly formed vessels. Most of the white cells are adherent to the vessel wall, and many emigrate through the wall.

Maturation and Differentiation

The newly formed vessels are irregularly dilated and tortuous. Within 48 hr after the appearance of new undifferentiated capillaries, maturation begins (Clark and Clark, 1939). As the slow circulation becomes rapid, the wide, bulging, and tortuous new capillaries become narrow and straight and the endothelial wall visibly thickens (Clark, 1918). The vessels receiving the major blood supply become wide and straight and the new arterioles rapidly develop a thick wall, which Clark and Clark (1943) interpreted as an increase in the number of endothelial cells.

A process of arteriolarization occurred when a vessel with characteristics of a venule connected with an arteriole. The initial event consisted of reversal of flow through the parent venule via the new connection. The flow became rapid and laminar. Subsequently, the walls of the vessel became thick and there appeared to be an accumulation of an additional layer of cells (consistent with pericytes) encircling the orifice of the vessel at its junction with the arteriole.

As the blood vessels progressed centripetally into the center of the chamber (Figure 6), continuous remodeling occurred as a result of sprouting and regression of apparently redundant blood vessels. The remodeling included retraction of some vessels, which began with occlusion or constriction of the lumen and deposition of a refractile material within the lumen. This produced cul-de-sacs with saccular tips. Obliteration of the lumen continued until only a small swelling on the wall of the branching lumen remained. This bulging subsequently disappeared within several days and left no trace of the previously existing vessel.

There is a controversy as to what determines the differentiation of the vessels. Thoma (1893) assumed that up to the point at which the new blood vessels became perfused, genetic factors would decide the growth pattern. After that, further development and differentiation would depend upon the local pressure, flow, and metabolic tissue demands. Clark and Clark (1939), on the other hand, observed that even in the absence of blood flow, there was a differentiation into arterioles, venules, and capillaries. This important issue as well as the question of innervation and pharmacologic reactions of the newly formed vessels, deserve further investigations.

OBSERVATIONS IN THE ELECTRON MICROSCOPE

In 1963, Schoefl and Cliff independently described the ultrastructure of the newly formed vessels. Schoefl (1963) used both light and electron microscopy for the investigation of newly formed vessels in tissue defects produced in the cremaster muscle and in the cornea of rats (Figures 9 and 10). Cliff (1963), using essentially the same methods, studied the vessels formed in a rabbit ear chamber. Studying three different tissues, the investigators arrived at similar conclusions.

Newly formed endothelial cells are described as thinner than normal endothelial cells with greatly varying thicknesses. The cytoplasmic components indicate that the cells are more active and less differentiated than normal. Mitochondria are large and numerous, the endoplasmic reticulum is richly developed, and free ribosomes are sometimes extremely abundant. Pinocytotic vesicles are scanty and irregular in size and shape. The vesicles sometimes are absent over relatively large areas of the endothelial cells (Schoefl, 1963). According to Palade (1961), this is an index of relative undifferentiation. The cytoplasmic membrane appears very plastic with endothelial processes extending both into the lumen and into the surrounding perivascular region (Schoefl, 1963).

The observation of frequent mitotic figures proximal to the tip of the sprout and few in the very tip of the sprout caused both Schoefl (1963) and Cliff (1963) to conclude that the tip of the sprout will advance by migration of endothelial cells produced proximally by mitosis of endothelial cells. This concept seems reasonable since the energy-requiring mitotic process takes place proximally where the blood supply is adequate. Two resting nuclei were never found within one cell, contradicting the suggestion of a syncytial nature of the sprouts.

The changes in capillary permeability of mature capillaries in early tissue injury has recently been reviewed by Crone (1973), Luft (1973), and Catchpole (1973). As evidenced by the injection of different colloidal particles, Schoefl found an increased permeability of the new vessels especially in the areas of junctions and where a basement membrane could not be identified (Figure 10). Early investigation (Sandison, 1924; Clark and Clark, 1939) suggested an increased capillary fragility evidenced by frequent petechiae when slight pressure was exerted on the coverslip. The structural basis for this has been elucidated by observations in the electron microscope. It appeared that the junctions between endothelial cells were loose and there were gaps in the endothelial lining. The basement membrane was thin and occasionally absent. Cliff (1965) found the basement membrane to be formed by fibrillar structures remote from the growing endothelium. Schoefl and Majno (1964) ascribed the loose junctions and gaps to the fact that many endothelial cells of the growing sprout were in a process of migration and, because the zone of increased permeability was very narrow, Schoefl concluded that this was a transient phase.

In his observations of the periendothelial structures, Cliff (1965) described cells that looked like fibroblasts migrating in toward a new vessel, adhering to the wall, encircling it, and forming the periendothelial cell layers. These cells became the muscular and adventitial cell layers. The origin of these cells is not clear, but most investigators assume that they are either fibroblasts or smooth muscle cells that have migrated from muscle-invested vessels in the vicinity. One week after the first fibroblasts have migrated into an area, collagen fibrils appear (Cliff, 1963; Florey, 1970). Most of the fibrils are oriented radially initially, but later they are arranged in a circumferential pattern. Finally, a dense membrane of collagen fibrils is formed.

LYMPHATIC VESSELS

Despite the fact that lymphatics and blood capillaries have similar structure and embryologic origin, lymphatics sprout and anastomose only with lymphatics and blood capillaries only with other blood capillaries (Florey, 1970; Casley-Smith, Chapter 19, this volume). Regenerating lymphatic vessels follow much the same growth pattern as blood vessels, but they start later and grow more slowly than blood capillaries (Clark, 1937; Cliff, 1963).

Cliff (1965) found the growth rate of lymphatic capillaries to be 0.08 mm/day, half the rate of lymphatic capillaries. Clark (1933) questioned the importance of lymphatics in the healing process because he could not see any difference in healing of the chamber tissues whether or not lymphatics were present. Even though our information on the function of the peripheral lymphatics is far from complete, it is reasonable to assume that they have a function in the homeostasis of the healing tissue, especially when one considers the increased capillary permeability. Casley-Smith (1973) and Leak and Burke (1974) have recently reviewed the structure and function of the lymphatic system in early tissue injury.

BLOOD VESSELS IN WOUND HEALING

Vascularization

The formation of blood vessels and granulation tissue in a healing wound follow the same course of events that has been described for granulation tissue in the rabbit ear chamber (Florey, 1970). Even in the surgically clean wound, there is an inflammatory reaction from the mechanical trauma. Even after excellent hemostasis and approximation of the edges of a surgical wound, there is some microscopic bleeding and exudation of plasma, leucocytes, and macrophages into the wound. Fibrin forms a meshwork in the exudate. By 2 or 3 days a rim of new vessels is formed and progresses at a rate of 0.2–0.4 mm/day at the borders of the wound. Fibroblasts with frequent mitoses migrate into the wound. After 4–5 days, reticular fibrils can be discerned and collagen fibrils appear (Florey, 1970), although most of the collagen forms during the second week of healing. If a wound heals secondarily, a large amount of granulation tissue forms in the same way. The granulation tissue is covered with a proteinaceous exudate including fibrin and cells (especially leucocytes and macrophages).

Electron microscopy (Florey, 1970) and scanning electron microscopy (Forrester et al., 1969) in combination with other techniques have recently contributed many important findings. Several recent reviews are available on the subject of wound healing (e.g., Montagna and Billingham, 1964; Newcombe, 1972; Kulonen and Pikkararinen, 1973).

Regulation of the Healing Process

Many factors can interfere with the healing of a wound. Blood supply, infection, size of wound, mechanical tension, metabolic derangements, nutritional deficiencies, and hormonal imbalance have all been implicated in affecting wound healing. Age of the individual seems to be relatively unimportant (Howes and Harvey, 1932). Amino acids, especially the sulfur-containing ones, are necessary for the formation of granulation tissue (Edwards and Dunphy, 1957). Ascorbic acid deficiency decreases the rate of formation of capillary endothelium and collagen fibrils and causes increased capillary fragility (Levenson et al. 1957). Zinc deficiency also interferes with normal wound healing (Newcombe, 1972).

Cortisone and ACTH in large doses retard wound healing. Some studies have been carried out using the cornea of different animals (Alrich, Carter, and Lehman, 1951; Duke-Elder and Ashton, 1951). In the healing process of lesions in the cornea, cortisone or ACTH dramatically decrease the neovascularization as well as the proliferation and migration of fibroblasts. Zarem (1970b) studied the effects of cortisol on the vessels of mouse skin isografts and allografts. It was found that cortisol suppressed the white cell sticking and emigration. Cortisol-treated animals required 9 days to vascularize a skin graft, while in nontreated animals vascularization occurred within 5 days. The general vascular effects of steroids has recently been reviewed by Altura and Altura (1974).

Lindhe and co-workers (Linde, Birch, and Brånemark, 1968; Linde and Brånemark, 1968; Linde, Brånemark, and Birch, 1968) tested the effects of different sex hormones on the process of wound healing in rabbits and in hamsters. In the rabbit ear small wounds were produced and the vascular beds of the wounds were observed in the intravital microscope. They found that vascular proliferation was accelerated by progesterone. As observed in the intravital microscope, estrogen and chorionic gonadotropin caused only minor vascular changes in the healing of a microwound in the hamster cheek pouch. Progesterone treatment seemed to result in a stronger inflammatory reaction than in the healing of the wound in an untreated hamster.

It would be of great interest to isolate and define chemically the factors that regulate the process of wound healing. Many attempts have been made to find a substance that would stimulate wound healing, but so far this has been inconclusive (Florey, 1970).

Stimulation to Vessel Growth—Angiogenesis

Many investigators employing the rabbit ear chamber have commented that blood is a prerequisite for the invasion of vessels into the chamber. Although it has been assumed that there is some factor within tissue or blood that acts as a chemotactic agent to stimulate the new blood vessels, this factor has not been demonstrated. Ryan (1973) has recently discussed the different factors that may influence the growth of vascular endothelium in the skin. Interest in the specific angiogenic factor has also been renewed in the work of tumor angiogenesis, which is discussed later. When studying the microvasculature of the mesentery of the rat in long-term experiments it was found that mechanical trauma, drying, or a subclinical infection would cause a tremendous vascular proliferation (Eriksson et al., 1975).

It has been observed in the mouse transparent chamber studies of Merwin and Algire (1956) and of subsequent investigators using this technique that blood vessels are stimulated to grow if additional tissue is placed in the chamber. There is no new vessel growth (neovascularization) in the areas that are left covered merely by a coverslip. Using this phenomenon of the stimulation of new vessel growth by tissue, O'Donaghue and Zarem (1971) studied the comparative efficacy of fresh and preserved skin grafts in producing neovascularization in the chamber. These authors demonstrated that in the mouse transparent skin chamber vessels grew only in areas where tissue had been placed. The authors concluded that fresh skin isografts, fresh skin allografts, and preserved skin isografts were effective in stimulating neovascularization.

In the same study, purified bovine collagen showed no angiogenic property in the mouse skin chamber. The authors concluded that since the full-thickness skin graft consisted essentially of collagen and blood vessels, the failure of collagen to stimulate new blood vessels suggests that the blood vessels within the skin graft were the key factors in the stimulation of the neovascularization.

Williams (1959) demonstrated that subcutaneous tissue which contained vessels stimulated the growth of blood vessels within a mature rabbit ear chamber so that further vascularization occurred. Using mature chambers, Williams made microscopic incisions in connective tissue without injury to adjacent capillaries or other vessels. These wounds healed with no vascular sprouting, and Williams concluded from these studies that injury to thin connective tissue alone without injury to blood vessels produces no stimulus for endothelial growth or sprouting.

VASCULARIZATION OF AUTOGRAFTS

Whether the revascularization of an autograft takes place by inosculation (anastomoses between the vessels of the recipient bed and the preexisting vessels of the graft) or by ingrowth of a vasculature from the recipient bed into the graft has been a recurring question. The latter alternative was favored by Converse et al. (1957) and Converse and Ballantyne (1962). Birch, Brånemark, and Lundskog (1969) and Lambert (1971) contend that the preexisting vessels of the graft are incorporated into the vasculature at least during the first few weeks. The vascularization of skin grafts has been studied with many different techniques (Malinen et al., 1970). Zarem, Zweifach, and McGehee (1967) and Zarem (1970a) used microscopic observation of the mouse skin transparent chamber. Birch and Branemark (1969) employed a similar technique when they transplanted scrotal skin to rabbit ear chambers where the recipient bed was the outer perichondrium of the ear. Angiography was used by Birch, Branemark, and Lundskog (1969) and Clemmesen (1964). Birch, Branemark, and Nilsson (1969) also used thermography, and Lambert (1971) has employed autoradiography.

   Zarem et al. (1967) examined the mechanism of vascularization of full-thickness skin autografts using the mouse transparent chamber. Vessels observed within the grafted skin have filled primarily with white blood cells. This plexus of immature vessels was seen to progress to a mature complex of arterioles, capillaries, and venules by the eighth day following transplantation. These authors concluded that the primary mechanism of revascularization to a full-thickness skin graft in the mouse was the ingrowth of new vessels. The argument that had been used previously (that the pattern of blood vessels in a grafted skin was similar to the pattern of vessels before grafting) supporting the idea that there was primarily an inosculation between the graft and host vessels was weakened by the observation that the ingrowth of new vessels used the preexisting vessels in some instances as nonviable conduits. With this use of the preexisting vessels to direct the pattern of ingrowth of new vessels, the observation that the vessel patterns were similar before and after grafting does not necessarily demonstrate that the flow through the skin after grafting is through the preexisting vessels per se.

   Lambert (1971) and Folkman et al. (1971) labeled either the vascular endothelium of skin auto- and allografts of the recipient with ^{3}H-thymidine and studied the vascularization of the graft on autoradiographs. They concluded that the graft is vascularized by inosculation and that the graft vascular endothelium survives and constitutes the lining of the graft vascular channels.

   An additional factor that has created some confusion in evaluating the vascularization of transplanted tissues has been the concept that viability of transplanted tissues must be maintained by immediate flow of plasma and/or blood. Today, the term "viable" has become confusing. The criteria for viability may vary from one investigator to another. Enzyme histochemical studies have demonstrated the viability of cells at one level. Tissue cultures have demonstrated the absence or presence of viability by the failure or success of culturing the cells. Clinically, if a large skin graft is placed on the wound and appears to survive for an indefinite period of time, then one would conclude that the skin graft was viable. On the basis of the latter criterion, skin need not be maintained "viable" in any rigid fashion since skin from humans may be removed, stored in a refrigerator for 2 wk, and then replaced successfully. This observation is cited not to indulge in a discussion of viability, but to point out the fallacy of the supposed need to maintain viability of transplanted tissues by immediate re-establishment of vascular flow. The concept of maintaining viability caused earlier investigators to theorize that a *plasmic circulation* served to maintain tissue viability until adequate blood flow was established. Early after grafting, Converse et al. (1957) observed an increased weight of skin grafts, but a "plasmic circulation" could not be confirmed by Birch, Branemark, and Lundskog (1969). Endothelial budding from vessels in the recipient bed and slow irregular circulation from the recipient bed to the graft could be observed within 24–48 hr. The rate of ingrowth of endothelium was 0.5 mm/day. The number of vascular connections and the rate of blood flow within the graft showed an increase during the first week. General vasodilatation disappeared around the tenth day, and pronounced remodeling of the architecture took place. This seemed to be due to the rise in blood flow in the vessels of the recipient bed. Graft vessels that became connected to the large recipient bed vessels became large themselves, while those connected to small recipient bed vessels became small. Odén (1961) found that lymphatic circulation was reestablished in the preexisting graft lymphatics 4–17 days after grafting. During the first week after transplantation, there were white cells sticking to the walls of both graft and recipient bed vessels. Many white and red cells emigrated through the vessel wall.

VASCULARIZATION OF ALLOGRAFTS

The microvasculature in allografts has been examined with a focus on the processes of vascularization and of rejection. A few recent reviews are available (see, e.g., Woodruff, 1960; Malinen et al., 1970; Najarian and Simmonds, 1972).

To further examine these questions, two experimental models were used in our laboratory. In one of them full-thickness skin of one mouse was transferred to a transparent skin chamber of a genetically dissimilar mouse (allograft). The microcirculation of the recipient bed and of the full-thickness skin graft were then observed by in vivo microscopy (Zarem, 1969).

In the mouse transparent chamber active blood flow within the full thickness skin allograft occurred 5 days after transplantation. Early signs of rejection consisted of macrophage infiltrates within the tissues of the grafted skin, endothelial swelling of the graft vessels, and white blood cell sticking, which occurred on the ninth day following transplantation. Rejection of the allografted tissue (cessation of blood flow through the graft) occurred rather abruptly on the thirteenth day following transplantation. Hyperemia in the tissues surrounding the graft was followed by the cessation of flow within the graft and subsequent hemorrhage beneath the graft leading to eschar formation. The majority of the vessels of the allograft appeared as a result of the ingrowth of new vessels, employing the preexisting vessels as nonviable conduits. Cross allograft rejection (eschar formation) occurred several days after microscopic rejection, as judged by the cessation of blood flow within the graft (Zarem, 1969).

The transplanted rabbit ear with a mature transparent chamber served as a model of a whole-organ allograft (Leaf and Zarem, 1970b). In this study it was found that the adherence of many white blood cells to the vascular endothelium preceded the appearance of a perivascular mononuclear infiltrate within the allograft. This phenomenon of white cells sticking to the vascular walls with destruction of the vascular endothelium was so prominent that it was concluded to be the major event in the cessation of blood flow within the allograft microvasculature. It was also found that intravenous administration of cortisol (Zarem, 1970b) and of other immunosuppressive agents (Zarem and Dimitrievich, 1970) delayed the onset of, but did not prevent, the microvascular obstructive changes.

Guttman and Lindquist (1970) found similar events when they investigated rat allograft kidneys in different stages of rejection. From their observations in the electron microscope, they concluded that the primary event was an immunologically specific destruction of renal cells, followed by progressive ischemia causing additional tissue damage. They thought that the microvasculature was altered by nonspecific factors.

Albreksson (1971), in his studies of the vascularization of fresh and preserved bone allografts, studied complete cortical bone segments that were transplanted into diaphyseal defects produced in the rabbit ulna and in the rat tibia. Microangiograms and histochemical and histologic specimens were evaluated with a morphometric technique, and it was found that no rejection occurred and that bone grafts of auto- or allogenous origin were vascularized at the same rate. Freeze-preserved grafts of both types were less readily vascularized.

VASCULARIZATION OF XENOGRAFTS

Different types of xenografts have been used extensively in reconstructive surgery during the last decades. Most of them are nonbiologic in origin, e.g., stainless steel, titanium rubber, and silicone. The nonbiologic xenografts do not become vascularized, and interest is focused upon the interface between graft and recipient. Usually, an inflammatory reaction is seen, depending upon how well the material is tolerated (Zarem, 1968).

There is at least one biologic tissue that is widely used, namely, porcine skin. Pandya and Zarem (1974) transplanted fresh and frozen porcine skin grafts to cover skin defects in the mouse transparent skin chamber. Vascularization of the porcine grafts was compared to that of full-thickness skin autografts as observed by in vivo microscopy. The porcine grafts did not become vascularized in the mouse. The vessels of the recipient bed became dilated and showed evidence of edema. Contrary to this, Toranto, Salyer, and Meyers (1974) showed some ingrowth of vessels into porcine grafts in rabbits at 72 hr before rejection.

GROWTH OF ENDOTHELIUM IN VASCULAR PROSTHESIS

Since 1950 large vessels have been commonly replaced by tubes of different artificial material (Halpert et al., 1960; Florey et al., 1961; Spencer and Imparato, 1974). Early experience indicated that fabric grafts, woven or knitted from artificial fibers, were superior to homografts or impermeable plastic, rubber, glass, or metal tubes (Weslowski, 1962). In homografts, degeneration of the intima and hyalinization and weakening of the media seemed to be the most common reason for failure (Halpert et al., 1960).

Impermeable tubes of glass, plastic, or different metals did show an intimal lining close to the anastomotic sites, but the inside of the remainder of the graft became calcified and progressively stenosed (Weslowski et al., 1961). When woven or knitted porous grafts of Dacron or other synthetic fibers were used, this problem was avoided through the formation of a pseudointimal lining.

The origin of the pseudointimal lining has been investigated. One suggested alternative has been that the endothelium arises by metaplasia from fibroblasts or leucocytes. Florey et al. (1961, 1962) examined the pseudointimal lining of knitted Dacron grafts during the first 12 wk after implantation (Figure 11). As examined under the light and electron microscopes, the inside of the graft was first covered by a thin layer of platelets, leucocytes, and fibrin. The endothelium developed later, growing partly from the endothelium of the aorta at the ends of the graft and partly from small vessels growing in through the pores of the graft (Figure 11). Smooth muscle cells and elastic tissue appear much later.

Regarding Florey's findings in conjunction with the findings of Halpert et al. (1960) and Weslowski et al. (1961), it seems that the establishment of a pseudointimal lining in a prosthetic graft is crucial for the long-term patency of the graft and this requires that the prosthesis have adequate porosity.

VASCULARIZATION OF TUMORS

Many investigators have shown evidence that implanted tumors stimulate neovascularization of both tumor tissue and of the recipient bed (Ide, Baker, and Warren, 1939; Algire and Chalkley, 1945; Cavallo et al., 1972, 1973). It is logical to assume that solid tumors will cease growing when there is no new vascularization. Greene (1941) transplanted various tumors into the anterior chamber of the eye in different animals and showed that in the absence of neovascularization, most tumors will stop growing when they reach a diameter of 2–3 mm and they will then assume a dormant but fully viable state.

Greenblatt and Shubi (1968) implanted melanomas into the hamster cheek pouch stroma. The tumor was separated from the surrounding stroma by a millipore filter. As observed by in vivo microscopy, there was a vasoproliferative response in the surrounding tissues within 3–7 days from implantation of the tumor.

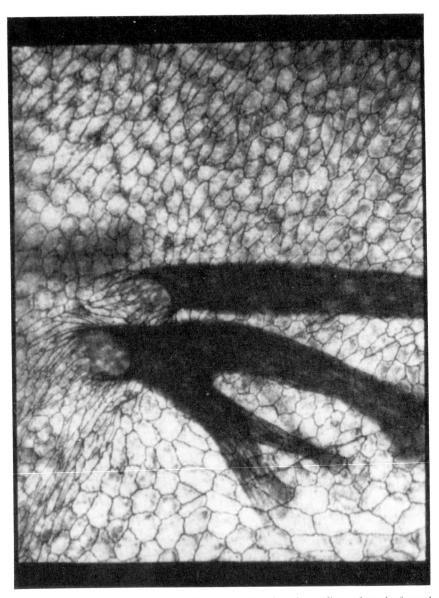

Figure 11. The surface of an aortic fabric graft showing the outlines of newly formed endothelial cells lining the luminal surface. Two small vessels can be seen to branch from the aortic lumen. Stain: Silver nitrate. × 125. Florey, Greer, Poole, and Werthessen (1961), reprinted by permission.

The authors discussed the possibility of an extracellular humoral substance produced by the tumor cells and transmitted through the millipore filter. As an alternative, they considered the possibility of cytoplasmic processes penetrating the filter and thereby establishing a cell-to-cell contact that mediated the vasoproliferative message.

Folkman and collaborators (Folkman, 1971; Folkman et al., 1971; Cavallo et al., 1972, 1973) isolated a "tumor angiogenesis factor" (TAF) (Figure 12). This factor induced mitosis of endothelial cells and formation of new vessels. The concomitant inflammatory reaction was mild. On the other hand, in other experiments where formic acid was injected, a marked inflammatory response was seen but mitotic activity in the endothelium and neovascularization was considerably less than when TAF was injected (Cavallo et al., 1972, 1973). It was also found that pericytes and connective tissue cells were stimulated by TAF to undergo mitosis.

Folkman (1971) states that the tumor is vascularized by sprouting vessels from the recipient bed and not by inosculation. By time-lapse photography, he demonstrated that new capillaries penetrated the tumor implant and within 3 days a blood flow was established in them.

By injection technique and by in vivo observations (Algire and Chalkley, 1945), it has been shown that there is a characteristic vascular architecture for

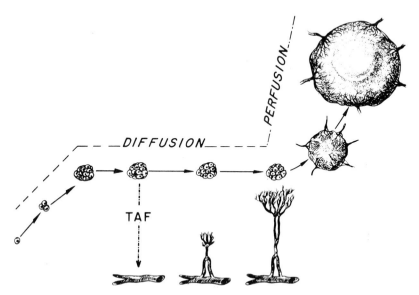

Figure 12. Schematic illustration of tumor angiogenesis. At first the tumor cells are nourished by diffusion. When they reach a certain size, tumor angiogenesis factor (TAF) is secreted and tells the recipient bed to start the formation of a vascular plexus supplying the growing tumor. Folkman (1971), reprinted by permission.

each tumor. Injection techniques have also shown that the topographic site of the tumor determines the structure and branching pattern of its larger vessels.

FUTURE RESEARCH

When reviewing the history of the development of this area of research, it is obvious that most of the valid hypotheses and findings are 100 yr or more old. The major contributions of the present century are based upon a few methodologic innovations and refinements. The transparent chamber technique, electron microscopy, and careful resolution of the time factor and quantitation of data deserve to be mentioned. Using this historical experience as a base for the prediction of the future, one can probably state that the research of the next few decades will not change many of the "old" concepts. With modern techniques employing combinations of subcellular biochemistry, transmission and scanning electron microscopy, autoradiography, ultrastructural tracers, and cell cultures, we will gain more understanding of the process of vascularization of tissues. The main questions are still what controls the speed of the wound-healing process and what determines the final vascular architecture including diffusion distances. These processes might be elucidated from careful studies of the vascularization of the tissues of a growing individual and from studies of the vascularization during activity versus inactivity in the adult. When looking upon the vascular architecture and morphology from the physiologic standpoint, one is often tempted to assume that these parameters are constant. Regarding the changes during the repair of tissue injury, we are probably erroneous in assuming that factors such as capillary diameters and diffusion distances are constant. The potential clinical applications of understanding the process of vascularization of tissues include the stimulation of growth in congenital or traumatic deficiencies, enhancing tissue and organ transplantation capabilities, and the control of neoplasms. These realistic goals continue to stimulate and provoke a growing number of investigators to direct their attention to the microvasculature.

LITERATURE CITED

Albreksson, B. 1971. Repair of diaphyseal defects. Thesis, University of Goteborg. Elanders, Goteborg, pp. 1—95.

Algire, G. H. 1943. Adaptation of transparent-chamber technique to mouse. J. Nat. Cancer Inst. 4:1—11.

Algire, G. H., and H. W. Chalkley. 1945. Vascular reactions of normal and malignant tissues in vivo; vascular reactions of mice to wounds and to normal and neoplastic transplants. J. Natl. Cancer Inst. 6:73—85.

Alrich, E. M., J. P. Carter, and E. P. Lehman. 1951. Effect of ACTH and cortisone on wound healing; Experimental study. Ann. Surg. 133:783—789.

Altura, B. M., and B. T. Altura. 1974. Effects of local anesthetics, antihistamines and glucocorticords on peripheral blood flow and vascular smooth muscle. Anesthesiology 41:197—214.

Barclay, W. R., W. R. Bruce, and Z. Farid. 1959. A simplified rabbit ear chamber. AMA Arch. Pathol. 68:409−412.

Birch, J., and P.-I. Brånemark. 1969. The vascularization of a free full thickness skin graft. I. A vital microscopic study. Scand. J. Plast. Reconstr. Surg. 3:1−10.

Birch, J., P.-I. Brånemark, and J. Lunkskog. 1969. The vascularization of a free full thickness skin graft. II. A microangiographic study. Scand. J. Plast. Reconstr. Surg. 3:11−17.

Birch, J., P.-I. Brånemark, and K. Nilsson. 1969. The vascularization of a free full thickness skin graft. III. An infrared thermographic study. Scand. J. Plast. Reconstr. Surg. 3:18.

Brånemark, P.-I. 1959. Vital microscopy of bone marrow in rabbit. Scand. J. Clin. Lab. Invest., Suppl. II, 38:1−82.

Brånemark, P.-I. 1971. Intravascular Anatomy of Blood Cells in Man, p. 80. S. Karger, Basel.

Brånemark, P.-I., and R. Ekholm. 1969. Pictorial recordings. In W. L. Winters and A. N. Broot (eds.), The Microcirculation, pp. 13−49. Charles C Thomas, Springfield, Ill.

Casley-Smith, J. R. 1973. The lymphatic system in inflammation. In B. W. Zweifach, L. Grant, and R. T. McCluskey (eds.), The Inflammatory Process, Vol. 2, pp. 161−204. Academic Press, New York.

Catchpole, H. R. 1973. Capillary permeability. III. Connective tissue. In B. W. Zweifach, L. Grant, and R. T. McCluskey (eds.), The Inflammatory Process, Vol. 2, pp. 122−148. Academic Press, New York.

Cavallo, T., R. Sade, J. Folkman, and R. S. Cotran. 1972. Tumor angiogenesis. Rapid induction of endothelial mitoses demonstrated by autoradiography. J. Cell. Biol. 54:408−420.

Cavallo, T., R. Sade, J. Folkman, and R. S. Cotran. 1973. Ultrastructural autoradiographic studies of the early vasoproliferative response in tumor angiogenesis. Am. J. Pathol. 70:345−362.

Clark, E. R. 1918. Growth of blood vessels in frog larvae. Am. J. Anat. 23:37−42.

Clark, E. R., and J. C. Sandison. 1931. Observations on circulating blood cells, adventitial (rouget), and muscle cells, endothelium and macrophages in transparent chamber of rabbits ear. Anat. Rec. 50:355−379.

Clark, E. R. 1933. Further observations on living lymphatic vessels in transparent chamber in rabbit ear−Their relation to tissue spaces. Am. J. Anat. 52:273−305.

Clark, E. R. 1937. Observations on living mammalian lymphatic capillaries− Their relation to blood vessels. Am. J. Anat. 60:253−298.

Clark, E. R., and E. L. Clark. 1939. Microscopic observations on growth of blood capillaries in living mammal. Am. J. Anat. 64:251−301.

Clark, E. R., and E. L. Clark. 1943. Caliber changes in minute blood vessels observed in living mammal. Am. J. Anat. 73:215−250.

Clark, E. R., E. L. Clark, and R. O. Rex. 1936. Observations on polymorphonuclear leukocytes in living animal. Am. J. Anat. 59:123−173.

Clemmesen, T. 1964. The early circulation in split-skin grafts. Restoration of blood supply to split-skin autografts. Acta Chir. Scand. 127:1−8.

Cliff, W. J. 1963. Observations on healing tissue: A combined light and electron microscopic investigation. Phil. Trans. 246: (B) 305−323.

Cliff, W. J. 1965. Kinetics of wound healing in rabbit ear chambers: A time lapse cinemicroscopic study. Quart. J. Exp. Physiol. 50:79−89.

Converse, J. M., D. L. Ballantyne, B. O. Rogers, and A. P. Raisbeck. 1957. Plasmatic circulation in the skin. Transplant. Bull. 4:154–156.

Converse, J. M., and D. L. Ballantyne. 1962. Distribution of diphosphopyridine nucleotide diaphorase in rat skin autografts and homografts. Plast. Reconstr. Surg. 30:415–425.

Crone, C. 1973. Capillary permeability. II. Physiological considerations. *In* B. W. Zweifach, L. Grant, and R. T. McCluskey (eds.), The Inflammatory Process, Vol. 2, pp. 95–121. Academic Press, New York.

Duke-Elder, S., and N. Ashton. 1951. Action of cortisone on tissue reaction of inflammation and repair with special reference to eye. Br. J. Opthal. 35:695–707.

Ebert, R. H., and L. Grant. 1974. An experimental approach to the study of inflammation. *In* B. W. Zweifach, L. Grant, and R. T. McCluskey (eds.), The Inflammatory Process, Vol. 1, pp. 4–51. Academic Press, New York.

Edwards, L. C., and J. E. Dunphy. 1957. Methionine in wound healing during protein starvation. *In* M. B. Williamson (ed.), The Healing of Wounds, pp. 47–70. McGraw-Hill, New York.

Eriksson, E., K. Naunheim, B. Geist, and R. L. Replogle. 1975. Unpublished data.

Evans, H. M. 1912. The development of the vascular system. *In* F. Keibel and F. P. Mall (eds.), Manual of Human Embryology, Vol. 2, pp. 507–709. J. B. Lippincott, Philadelphia.

Florey, H. W. 1970. Inflammation: Microscopical observations. *In* H. W. Florey (ed.), General Pathology, pp. 40–123. W. B. Saunders, Philadelphia.

Florey, H. W., S. J. Greer, J. C. F. Poole, and N. T. Werthessen. 1961. The pseudointima lining fabric grafts of the aorta. Br. J. Exp. Pathol. 42:236–246.

Florey, H. W., S. J. Greer, J. Kiser, J. C. F. Poole, R. Telander, and N. T. Werthessen. 1962. The development of the pseudointima lining fabric grafts of the aorta. Br. J. Exp. Pathol. 43:655–660.

Folkman, J., E. Merler, C. Abernathy, and G. Williams. 1971. Isolation of a tumor factor responsible for angiogenesis. J. Exp. Med. 133:275–288.

Folkman, J. 1971. Tumor angiogenesis: Therpeutic implications. New Engl. J. Med. 285, No. 21:1182–1186.

Folkow, B., and E. Neil. 1971. Circulation. Oxford University Press, New York. 593 p.

Forrester, J. C., T. K. Hunt, T. L. Hayes, and R. F. W. Pease. 1969. Scanning electron microscopy of healing wounds. Nature 221:373–374.

Goethe, A. 1874. Ent Wicklungsgeschichte Der Unke Als Grundlage Einer Vergleichenden Morphologic Der Wirbeltiere. Leipzig.

Grant, L. 1973. The sticking and emigration of white blood cells in inflammation. *In* B. W. Zweifach, L. Grant, and R. T. McCluskey (eds.), The Inflammatory Process, Vol. 2, pp. 205–250. Academic Press, New York.

Greenblatt, H., and P. Shubi. 1968. Tumor angiogenesis: Transfilter diffusion studies in the hamster by the transparent chamber technique. J. Natl. Cancer Inst. 41:111–124.

Greene, H. S. N. 1941. Heterologous transplantation of mammalian tumors. I. Transfer of rabbit tumors to alien species. J. Exp. Med. 73:461–474.

Guttman, R. D., and R. R. Lindquist. 1970. The microvasculature during renal allograft rejection. *In* T. I. Malinen and B. S. Linn (eds.), Microcirculation, Perfusion and Transplantation of Organs, pp. 207–218. Academic Press, New York.

Halpert, B., M. E. DeBakey, G. L. Gordon, Jr., and W. S. Henly. 1960. The fate of homografts and prostheses of the human aorta. Surg. Gyn. Obst. 111:659–674.

His, W. 1868. Untersuchungen Über Die Erste Anlage Wirbeltierleibes. F. C. W. Vogel, Leipzig. 237 p.

Howes, E. L., and S. C. Harvey. 1932. Age factor in velocity of growth of fibroblasts in the healing wound. J. Exp. Med. 55:577–590.

Hudlická, O., and R. Myrhage. 1976. Proc. Scand. Physiol. Soc. Kopenhagen (in press).

Ide, A. G., N. H. Baker, and S. L. Warren. 1939. Vascularization of Brown-Pearce rabbit epithelioma transplant as seen in transparent ear chamber. Am. J. Roentgenol. 42:891–899.

Illig, L. 1961. Die Terminale Strombahn, Capillarbett und Mikrozirkulation. Springer, Berlin. 458 p.

Jennings, M. A., and H. W. Florey. 1970. Healing. In H. W. Florey (ed.), General Pathology, pp. 480–548. W. B. Saunders Company, Philadelphia.

Karnovsky, H. J. 1970. Morphology of the capillaries with special reference to muscle capillaries. In C. Crone and N. A. Lassen (eds.), Capillary Permeability, pp. 341–370. Academic Press, New York.

Kulonen, E., and J. Pikkarrainen (eds.). 1973. Biology of the Fibroblast. Academic Press, New York.

Lambert, P. B. 1971. Vascularization of skin grafts. Nature 232:279–280.

Leaf, N., and H. A. Zarem 1970a. Construction and use of a miniaturized rabbit ear chamber. Microvasc. Res. 2, No. 1:77–85.

Leaf, N., and H. A. Zarem. 1970b. Microsurgical transplantation of the rabbit ear with mature transparent chamber. Plast. Reconstr. Surg. 45:332–340.

Leak, L. V., and J. F. Burke. 1974. Early events in tissue injury and the role of the lymphatic system in early inflammation. In B. W. Zweifach, L. Grant, and R. T. McCluskey (eds.), The Inflammatory Process, Vol. 3, pp. 163–236. Academic Press, New York.

Levenson, S. M., H. L. Upjohn, J. A. Preston, and A. Steer. 1957. Effects of thermal burns on wound healing. Ann. Surg. 146:357–368.

Lindhe, J., J. Birch, and P.-I. Brånemark. 1968. Vascular proliferation in pseudopregnant rabbits. J. Periodont. Res. 3:12–20.

Lindhe, J., and P.-I. Branemark. 1968. The effects of sex hormones on vascularization of granulation tissue. J. Periodont. Res. 3:6–11.

Linde, J., P.-I. Brånemark, and J. Birch. 1968. Wounds of oophorectomized hamsters following intramuscular injections of female hormones. J. Periodont. Res. 180–185.

Luft, J. H. 1973. Capillary permeability. I. Structural consideration. In B. W. Zweifach, L. Grant, and R. T. McCluskey (eds.), The Inflammatory Process, Vol. 2, pp. 47–84. Academic Press, New York.

Majno, G. 1975. Ultrastructure of the vascular membrane. In W. F. Hamilton and P. Dow (eds.), Handbook of Physiology, Section 2, Vol. III, pp. 2293–2375. Williams & Wilkins, Baltimore.

Malinen, T. I., B. S. Linn, A. B. Callahan, and W. D. Warren (eds.). 1970. Microcirculation, Perfusion and Transplantation of Organs. Academic Press, New York. 423 p.

Maximov, A. 1909. Untersuchungen, Über Blut und Bindgewebe. Arch. fur Mikr. Anat. BD. 73:444–561.

McClure, C. F. W. 1921. The endothelium problem. Anat. Rec. 22:219–237.

Merwin, R. M., and G. H. Algire. 1956. Role of graft and host vessels in vascularization of grafts of normal and neoplastic tissue. J. Natl. Cancer. Inst. 17:23−33.

Minot, C. S. 1912. The development of the blood, the vascular system and the spleen. I. The origin of the angioblast and the development of the blood. In F. Keibel and F. B. Mall (eds.), Manual of Human Embryology, Vol. 2, pp. 448−534. Lippincott, Philadelphia. pp. 448−534.

Montagna, W., and R. E. Billingham (eds.). 1964. Advances in Biology of Skin, Vol. 5, Wound Healing. MacMillian, New York. 254 p.

Najarian, J. S., and R. L. Simmonds (eds.). 1972. Transplantation. Lea and Febiger, Philadelphia. 797 p.

Newcombe, J. F. 1972. Wound Healing. In W. T. Irvine (ed.), Scientific Basis of Surgery, pp. 433−456. Williams and Wilkins, Baltimore.

Odén, B. 1961. Micro-lymphangiographic studies of experimental skin autografts. Acta Chir. Scand. 121:219−232.

O'Donoghue, M. N., and H. A. Zarem. 1971. Stimulation of neovascularization− Comparative efficacy of fresh and preserved skin grafts. Plast. Reconstr. Surg. 48:474−478.

Palade, G. E. 1961. Blood capillaries of the heart and other organs. Circulation 24:368−388.

Palade, G. E., and R. R. Bruns. 1968. Structural modulations of plasmalemmal vesicles. J. Cell. Biol. 37:633−649.

Pandya, N. J., and H. A. Zarem. 1974. The absence of vascularization in porcine skin grafts. Plast. Reconstr. Surg. 53:211−213.

Reagen, F. P. 1917. Origin of vascular tissues. Am. J. Anat. 21:39−118.

Rhodin, J. A. G. 1967. The ultrastructure of mammalian arterioles and precapillary sphincters. J. Ultrastruc. Res. 18:181−223.

Rhodin, J. A. G. 1968. Ultrastructure of mammalian venous capillaries, venules and small collecting veins. J. Ultrastruc. Res. 25:452−500.

Ruckert, W., and S. Mollier. 1906. Handb. Vergl. Expt. Entwicklungslehre Wirbeltiere. 1:1019−1278.

Ryan, T. J. 1973. The Blood Vessels of the Skin, In A. Jarrett (ed.), Physiology and Pathophysiology of the Skin, Vol. 2, pp. 577−805. Academic Press, New York.

Sabin, F. R. 1917. Origin and development of the primitive vessels of the chick and the pig. Contrits. Embryol. Carnegie Inst. Wash. 6:61−124.

Sandison, J. C. 1924. A new method for the microscopic study of living growing tissues by the introduction of a transparent chamber in the rabbit's ear. Anat. Rec. 28:281−287.

Sandison, J. C. 1928. Observations on growth of blood vessels as seen in transparent chamber introduced into rabbit's ear. Am. J. Anat. 41:475−496.

Schoefl, G. I. 1963. Studies on inflammation. III. Growing capillaries: Their structure and permeability. Virchows Arch. Pathol. Anat. 337:97−141.

Schoefl, G. I., and A. Majno. 1964. Regeneration of blood vessels in wound healing. In W. Montagna and R. E. Billingham (eds.), Advances in Biology of the Skin. Vol. 5, Wound Healing, pp. 173−193. MacMillan, New York.

Spencer, F. C., and A. M. Imparato. 1974. Peripheral arterial disease. In S. I. Schwartz et al. (eds.), Principles of Surgery, pp. 839−912. McGraw-Hill, New York.

Thoma, R. 1893. Untersuchungen Über Die Histogenese Und Histomechanik Des Gefass-systems. Ferdinand Enke, Stuttgart.

Toranto, I. R., K. E. Salyer, and M. B. Meyers. 1974. Vascularization of porcine skin heterografts. Plast. Reconstr. Surg. 54:195–200.
Weslowski, S. A. 1962. Evaluation of Tissue and Prosthetic Vascular Grafts. Charles C Thomas, Springfield, Ill. 167 p.
Weslowski, S. A., C. C. Fries, K. E. Karlson, M. DeBakey, and P. N. Sawyer. 1961. Porosity: Primary determinant of ultimate fate of synthetic vascular grafts. Surgery 50:91–96.
Wiedeman, M. P. 1963. Patterns of the arteriovenous pathways. In W. F. Hamilton and P. Dow (eds.), Handbook of Physiology, Circulation, Section 2, Vol. II. p. 891–933. Williams and Wilkins, Baltimore.
Wilkinson, P. C. 1974. Chemotaxis and Inflammation. Churchill, Livingstone, Edinburgh. 214 p.
Williams, R. G. 1959. Experiments on the growth of blood vessels in thin tissue and in small autografts. Anat. Rec. 133:465–485.
Wood, S. Jr., R. Lewis, Jr., J. H. Mulholland, and J. Knaack. 1966. Assembly, insertion and use of a modified rabbit ear chamber. Bull. Johns Hopkins Hosp. 119:1–5.
Woodruff, M. F. A. (ed.). 1960. The transplantation of tissues and organs. Charles C Thomas, Springfield, Ill. 728 p.
Zarem, H. A. 1968. Silastic implants in plastic surgery. Surg. Clin. North Am. 48:129–142.
Zarem, H. A. 1969. The microcirculatory events within full-thickness skin allografts (homografts) in mice. Surgery 66:392–397.
Zarem, H. A. 1970a. Reestablishment of microvascular flow in transplanted tissues and organs. In T. I. Malinen, B. S. Linn, A. B. Callahan, and W. D. Warren (eds.), Microcirculation, Perfusion and Transplantation of Organs, pp. 201–206. Academic Press, New York.
Zarem, H. A. 1970b. Effects of cortisol on the microvasculature of mouse skin isografts and allografts. Microvasc. Res. 2:86–95.
Zarem, H. A., and G. S. Dimitrievich. 1970. In vivo observations of the effects of imuran on the microvasculature within full thickness mouse skin allografts. Plast. Reconstr. Surg. 45:51–57.
Zarem, H. A., B. W. Zweifach, and J. M. McGehee. 1967. Development of microcirculation in full-thickness autogenous skin grafts in mice. Am. J. Physiol. 212:1081–1085.
Zweifach, B. W. 1973. Microvascular aspects of tissue injury. In B. W. Zweifach, L. Grant, and R. P. McCluskey (eds.), The Inflammatory Process, Vol. 2, pp. 1–46. Academic Press, New York.

LYMPH AND LYMPHATICS

chapter 19

LYMPH AND LYMPHATICS

John R. Casley-Smith

423

There has recently been an increasing awareness of the importance of the roles played by the lymphatic system in the general economy of the body. Earlier it was the most neglected system of all. Recently, fairly comprehensive reviews have been written by Allen (1967), Casley-Smith (1973), Courtice (1971), Földi (1969), Mayerson (1963), Kampmeier (1969), Rusznyák, Földi, and Szabó (1967), and Yoffey and Courtice (1970).

Lymph is the fluid that is contained in lymphatics. It will be seen that its composition and volume depend not only on the composition and volume of the fluid that is present in the tissues, but also on the ways in which the lymphatic system functions. This functioning, in turn, is very dependent on the structure of the lymphatics and its variations from site to site, and from time to time.

In 1963 Mayerson remarked that at that time there were two fundamental problems in lymphology; how material entered the lymphatics, and how it was retained there. It will become apparent that in the subsequent 10 years these questions have largely been answered. The emphasis is now shifting to "why." It is the forces involved in transfers within the blood–tissue–lymph complex, and how circumstances alter these, that are becoming increasingly studied. Interest in function is replacing interest in structure. Nevertheless, structure is extraordinarily important in determining function and it is considered first.

STRUCTURE

General

The gross and light microscopic structure of the lymphatic system are well covered in some of the general reviews mentioned above and are not discussed further. The most peripheral elements of the system are innumerable, small, thin-walled vessels. They often form an approximately two-dimensional plexus (Rodbard, 1969), especially in regions where the connective tissue is lobulated (e.g., glands) or arranged in cylinders (e.g., muscles). They perform the system's primary function of removing material from the tissue. They progressively merge centrally to form the "collecting lymphatics," which perform the system's secondary function of transporting the material to the blood. The peripheral lymphatics are often termed lymphatic capillaries, terminal lymphatics, small lymphatics, lymphatic rootlets, and peripheral lymphatics. All these terms have deficiencies, and I prefer "initial lymphatics," for reasons given elsewhere (Casley-Smith, 1970a). They are usually about 0.5 mm long and of very irregular shape, with "maximal diameters" of some 15–75 μ when completely filled (Casley-Smith, 1975b). They are, however, usually rather flattened, although varying throughout the initial lymphatic cycle.

The initial lymphatics are lined just with endothelium (Figure 1) plus a variable amount of basement membrane. The collecting lymphatics, as soon as they pass centrally, become progressively lined with other elements (Figure 2). These include an internal elastic lamina (which is usually incomplete and

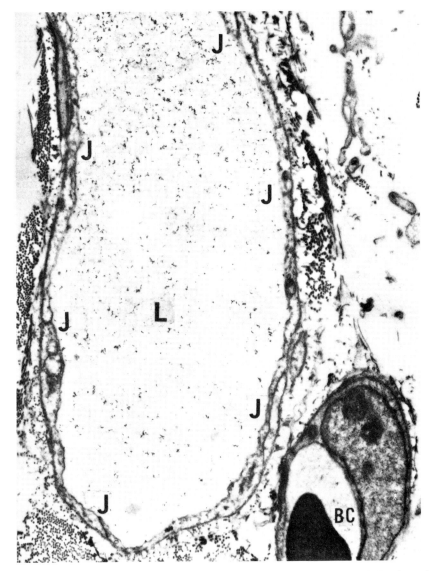

Figure 1. A lymphatic (L) in a normal mouse ear has many closed junctions (J). Its size and other characteristics may be compared with an adjacent blood capillary (BC). 7,000×. (The solid line, in this and all other illustrations represents 1 μ, unless otherwise indicated.)

disappears in the thoracic duct), smooth muscle cells, and connective tissue in general (Casley-Smith, 1969a; Schipp, 1967). There are also many nonmyelinated nerves (Morris, personal communication). The collecting lymphatics have many centrally directed valves; these are very often not of the traditionally described bicuspid form, but are truncated cones (Boussauw and Lauweryns, 1969).

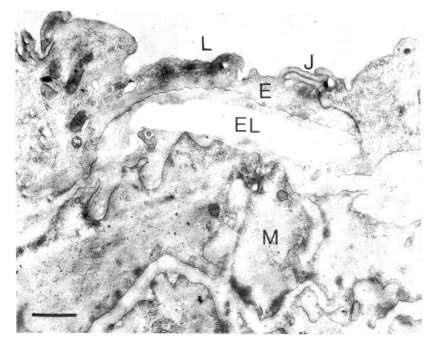

Figure 2. In the rat thoracic duct there is a well-developed internal elastic lamina (EL), but only a very tenuous basement membrane. There are many smooth muscle cells (M), and the endothelium (E) has only closed junctions (J). 12,000×.

The fine structure of the initial lymphatics has been reviewed by Casley-Smith (1967a, 1970a, 1972, 1973), Collin (1969a), Dobbins (1971), Kalima (1971), Lauweryns and Boussauw (1969), Leak (1970), Leak and Burke (1968), Majno (1965), Ottaviani and Azzali (1965), Virágh et al. (1966, 1971), and Yoffey and Courtice (1970). The endothelium is usually a little thicker than blood capillary endothelium, but appears thinner because of the greater diameters of the vessels. It is also rather less electron-opaque (Figure 1) and never has fenestrae (Figures 10, 30, and 31 below). The basement membrane is much less developed in active regions; it is sometimes not visible at all (Figures 3–7). In nondistended vessels, there are frequently lumenal projections of the cells (Figure 3), especially adjacent to junctions. (These may be devices for storing surplus plasma membrane for when the vessels become dilated.) On the ablumenal surfaces of the endothelial cells of the initial lymphatics (but not of the collecting ones) there are processes extending into the connective tissue (Figure 4). Many connective tissue fibrils attach to these and to other regions of the cells, both generally, and at specialized regions which resemble hemidesmosomes. There are two classes of fibrils. Some (~5 nm) are thin, branched, and irregular and may well just be plasma proteins agglutinated here by the fixative.

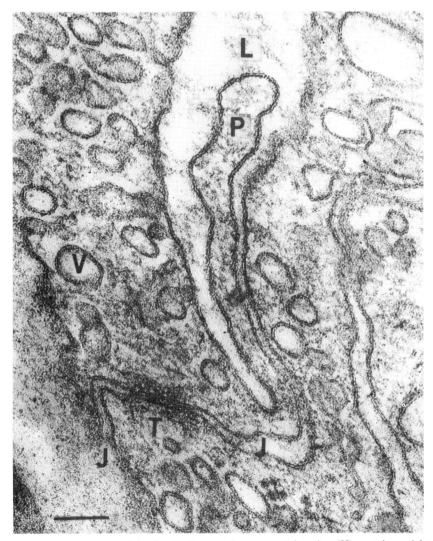

Figure 3. A lymphatic (L) in the diaphragm of a mouse. A junction (JJ) contains a tight portion (T), with its typical fusion of the outer lamellae of the two unit membranes, and intracytoplasmic filaments. There is a lumenal process (P); as is usual, this is adjacent to a junction. There are many small smooth vesicles (V). The basement membrane is almost invisible, 150,000×; the line here is 0.1 μ.

Others (~10 nm) are thicker, straight, long, and probably tubular. These pass into and around the collagen bundles and general ground substance, thus anchoring the cells to these structures. It seems that the anchoring filaments vary in amount with the region; they are infrequent in the intestinal villi (Dobbins, 1971).

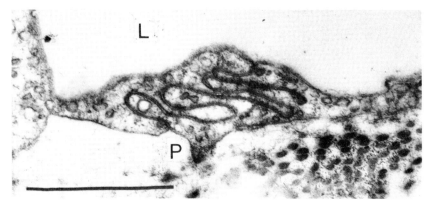

Figure 4. This is a very convoluted junction in a mouse ear lymphatic. An ablumenal projection (P) has some filaments attaching at a hemi-desmosome-like region. 40,000×.

The Endothelial Intercellular Junctions

These are the most important structures in the whole system, for upon them depends both the uptake of material and its retention (Casley-Smith 1970*a*, 1972, 1975*b*). Most of them resemble those in blood capillaries. In cross section, usually near the lumenal side, there is often a region where the two cells come very close together (Figures 1–6). In the zonulae occludentes (Farquhar and Palade, 1963), the outer laminae of their plasma membranes may fuse (tight junction) or be separated by a gap of approximately 6 nm (close junction) (Casley-Smith et al., 1975*b;* Karnovsky, 1968).

Often the cells are parallel for a long distance, separated by about 20 nm (zonula adherens). At times both these specializations are present; at other times there are none. Then the junction is open, with a gap which may be some microns across, but is usually about 0.1 μm (Figures 7–12, and 14 below). (It should be mentioned that the dimensions measured with the electron microscope are probably not exactly those present in vivo but are likely to be fairly close for most objects (Casley-Smith, 1969*b*).) In blood vessels, open junctions are only seen in sinusoids and injured vessels, but in the lymphatic system they occur in all initial lymphatics. In the lymphatics it is the "open" junctions that must be contrasted with the "closed" ones (which is the term I use to include both the "tight" junctions and the "close" junctions). The

Figure 5. A close junction (J) in a mouse diaphragmatic lymphatic (L) has along its length precipitated ferri-ferrocyanide ions. Some vesicles also contain this but, as explained in the text, they are too slow to contribute significantly to the passage of the ions across the endothelial barrier. The technical details are given in Casley-Smith (1967*c*). 80,000×.

Figure 6. Ferritin was injected into the lymphatics (L) of a normal mouse's ear. There is a long, close junction (JJ) that contains little tracer. Some particles are visible in small vesicles (V). 60,000×.

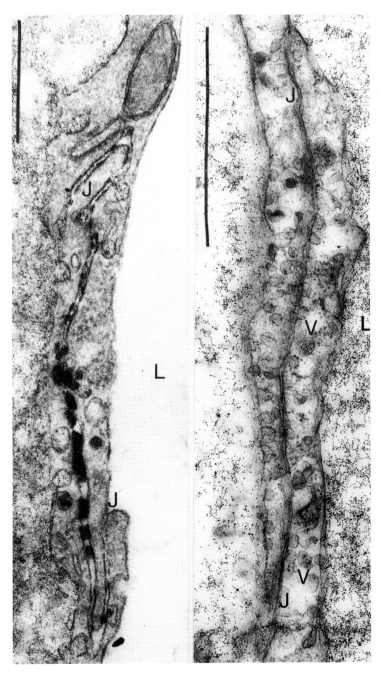

Figure 5   Figure 6

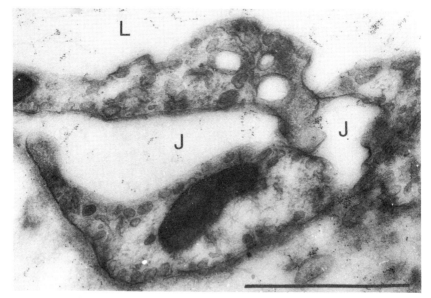

Figure 7. A guinea-pig ear was injured by heat (54°C for 4 min) and ferritin was injected into the lymphatics 5 min before death. There is a complex junction (JJ), open over most of its depth, through which ferritin is passing to the tissues. The pallor of the cytoplasm and the dilated vacuoles are typical of heat injury. 45,000X.

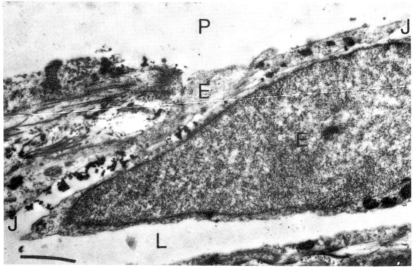

Figure 8. In the diaphragm (of a mouse) the peritoneal cavity (P) and the adjacent lymphatics (L) are frequently united via a junction (JJ) between two endothelial cells (E). This one contains some carbon, which was injected intraperitoneally, but the tissue was fixed during diaphragmatic contraction and it is evident that the junction is not now very permeable to large molecules. 15,000X.

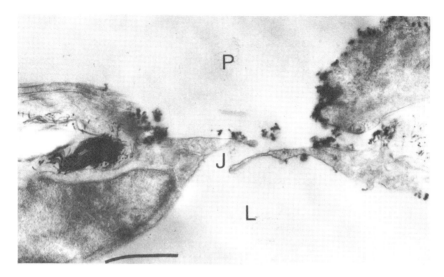

Figure 9. This is also mouse diaphragm but it was fixed in a more relaxed state than the one in Figure 8. The junction is open and permeable to large molecules, etc. The overlapping of the cells indicates how the "inlet-valves" function. 20,000×.

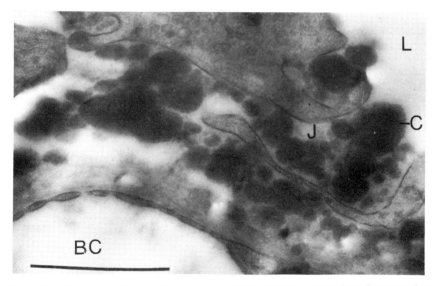

Figure 10. Chylomicra (C), which were produced by feeding a rat maize oil, are passing from the tissue of an intestinal villus into a lymphatic (L) via an open junction (J). Others are entering or leaving the cells via large vesicles. A fenestrated blood capillary (BC) is present; it can be seen that the chylomicra are far too big to pass through the fenestrae. 40,000×.

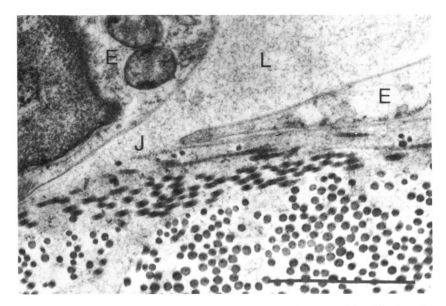

Figure 11. A lymphatic with an open junction, in the ear of a mouse injured by heat (see Figure 7). There is much plasma protein in the lymphatic, but rather less in the surrounding tissue, as was confirmed densitometrically. The dark regions in the tissues are collagen. 40,000×.

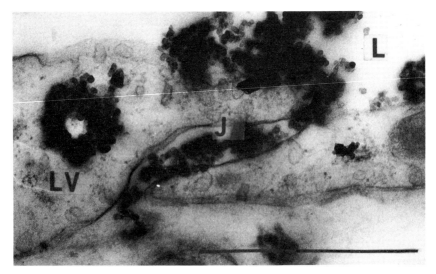

Figure 12. A mouse ear was injured as in Figure 7, and carbon injected into the lymphatics. Some carbon particles may be seen leaving a vessel via an open junction (J). Some are also contained in a large vesicle (LV). 60,000×.

differentiation between close and tight junctions is here not nearly as important as that between open and closed ones.

Electron microscope sections give a false impression of the actual nature of the junctions. It is, of course, evident that they encircle the cells, but it is only through the labor of serial sectioning that an impression is gained of how much individual junctions vary along their lengths (Collan and Kalima, 1974). For most of their lengths around the cells the lymphatic endothelial junctions are much more complex than blood-vascular ones, with many interdigitations probably helping to hold the cells together (Majno, 1965). The interdigitations also occur in the longitudinal direction of the junction (Collan and Kalima, 1974). At places along their lengths, the complex junctions become simpler until they are just two overlapping cells; then the zonulae disappear and this portion of the junction becomes open. The anchoring filaments are here only attached to the more ablumenal of the two cells. After an interval the complexity of the junction reappears and continues until the next open portion. It should be pointed out, however, that these open junctions are not open all the time. As is discussed later, they are closed during tissue compression in the sense of the two cells being forced close together and the gap being impermeable to proteins. They also frequently appear (in the normal random cross sections used in electron microscopy) to be open widely, but only over parts of their depths between the cells (Figure 7). This is likely, because the zonulae only occupy a small portion of the depths of the junctions, usually near the lumen, hence one would expect open channels between the cells along the lengths of the junctions on both sides of an opening.

In quiescent regions, e.g., the pinnae of the mouse ear, there are very few portions of the junctions open (Figure 1); these increase dramatically after injury, especially if edema is present (Figures 7, 11−13, below) (Casley-Smith, 1967a, 1970a, 1972, 1973). They are also much more frequent in active regions, particularly where there is much motion of the tissues (Figures 8−10 and 14) or frequent variations in tissue pressure. In the intestinal villi, Dobbins and Rollins (1970) found that of 254 sections through junctions 6 were open, 10 were close, 89 were tight, and 149 could not be seen clearly enough to be identified. (This means that approximately 2% were open, since if the uncertain ones had been open they would almost certainly have been identified as such.) Other workers using this tissue (Casley-Smith, 1962; Palay and Karlin, 1959; Papp et al., 1962) seem to have found greater numbers of open junctions than this (Figures 10 and 14). Even so, while Dobbins and Rollins (1970) and Ottaviani and Azzali (1965) consider that such numbers are too small for the junctions to contribute significantly to lymphatic filling, it has been shown by calculation that in fact they are more than sufficient (Casley-Smith, 1975b, Elhay and Casley-Smith, 1976). Other compelling evidence indicating the overwhelming importance of the junctions for lymphatic permeability is presented later. As they pass centrally, the junctions in the collecting lymphatics become less frequently open until they are all closed (Figure 2; Casley-Smith, 1969a).

THE EFFECTS OF INFLAMMATION ON LYMPHATIC STRUCTURE

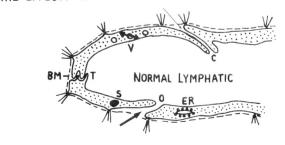

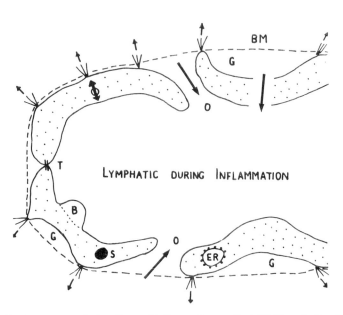

Figure 13. A summary of the effects of inflammation on the initial lymphatics. The vessel is dilated and the cells pulled apart by the filaments attached to the ablumenal surfaces; intervening portions are forced inwards by the raised tissue pressure, leaving gaps (G) between them and the basement membrane (BM). The close junctions (C) become open (O), but the tight ones (T) probably remain closed; however, the convolutions disappear. The very swollen cells stretch and break their plasma membranes, and the vesicle numbers drop, probably as they are incorporated into these membranes. Blebs (B) are seen on the cells and the endoplasmic reticulum (ER) swells to produce vacuoles with and without ribosomes. Fluid and proteins (thick arrows) pass via the indicated paths, in amounts varying with the local circumstances, etc. Symphyosomes (S) are present under both conditions.

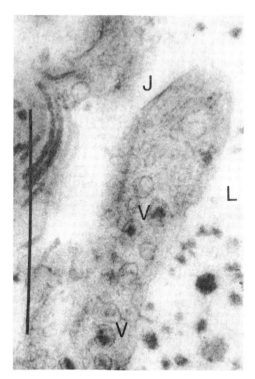

Figure 14. Lipoprotein particles occur in the intestinal tissue of rats fed only glucose for 3 days. They can be seen here in the lumen of a lacteal, which has an open junction, and in small vesicles in the endothelium. 60,000×.

Why do the junctions open? The lack of supporting devices in certain areas is obviously important, as may be the paucity of the basement membranes. The lack of anchoring filaments attached to the inner of the two very flexible cells will allow the junction to be forced out of the way by inflowing fluid; any cells or large particles will act as dilators. The anchoring filaments will pull the cells about during gross movements of the tissues (e.g., adjacent to muscles). but they will have less effect in metabolically active, but relatively motionless regions (e.g., the testis). In edema, however, they are of great importance. Pullinger and Florey (1935) showed that fibers attaching to the lymphatics pulled the vessels open during edema, thus stopping them from being collapsed by the raised tissue pressures. They will also have the effect of moving the cells away from each other, circumferentially, at the open junctions (Figures 11 and 16). The filaments attached to the ablumenal cell of the two will pull this one out into the tissues away from the other. Virágh et al. (1966) queried this action of the fibers, first, because the collagen fibers are not attached directly to the cells. When it was shown that the anchoring filaments perform this function (Casley-

Smith, 1967*b*; Collin, 1969*a*), Virágh, Papp, and Rusznyák (1971) objected that, in the skin, the fibers and filaments do not pass completely from the endothelium to the epithelial layer or the aponeurosis. This objection neglects the considerable viscosity and internal connections of the loose connective tissue, even in edema. The action of the filaments in edema was confirmed by various morphologic pieces of evidence, and also by the action of hyaluronidase, which causes the filaments to slip through the connective tissue and allows the lymphatics to be collapsed by the external pressures (Casley-Smith, 1967*b*). This finding was confirmed by Leak and Burke (personal communication), but not by Virágh et al. (1971). (It is possible that different forms of hyaluronidase were used.) Virágh et al. (1971) at least agree that initially the filaments have this function; it would seem that they will always have this effect, provided that sufficient edema exists in their vicinity. It should be pointed out, however, that collecting lymphatics do not have these filaments; hence they can certainly be collapsed by excessive external pressures, as perhaps the initial lymphatics may be—if the pressures become too high and overcome the effects of edema (Virágh et al., 1971).

When preparing the tissues for electron microscopy it is important that they be treated very gently. Thus, if the pinnae of the ears are depilated (Leak and Burke, 1966), many more open junctions are found than if this is not done (Casley-Smith, 1965). However, certainly not all open junctions are artifacts, as is shown by the frequent finding of tracers, particles, and cells lying in them (Figures 7–12) and by the association of the presence of many open junctions with great increases in lymphatic permeabilities, *vide infra*.

In the case of injury there is another probable cause of the opening of the junctions. It has been shown by Majno, Shea, and Leventhal (1969) that it is very likely that the blood vessel junctions that open during injury do so because of the contraction of their endothelial cells. (However, other factors, e.g., weakening of the intercellular bonds, are certainly not disproved.) Similarly, it has been found that lymphatic endothelial cells (and mesothelial cells) also contract when injured by burning or histamine (Casley-Smith and Bolton, 1973*b*). This contraction occurs maximally in the first few minutes after injury and wears off after 1–2 hr. Intraendothelial fibrils have frequently been observed in the lymphatic endothelium (Casley-Smith and Florey, 1961; Leak, 1970), in blood vessel endothelium (Majno, 1965; Majno et al., 1969), and, significantly, just in the contractile portions of the vasculature of amphioxus (Casley-Smith, 1971*a*). It is probable that these are the contractile elements. Such contractions would be very likely to move one cell over the other at the openable junction sites in lymphatic endothelium, but as mentioned above they would not persist after 1–2 hr.

Vesicles

The small, smooth (~70 nm) vesicles are a prominent feature of endothelium (Figures 3, 5, 6, 14, and 15) but, as is seen later, they are much less important

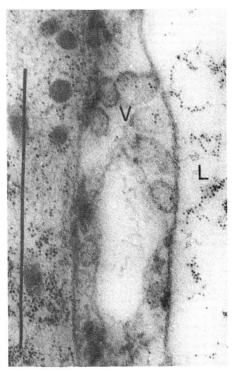

Figure 15. A guinea-pig ear was injured as in Figure 7, and ferritin was injected into the tissues 15 min before death. Ferritin can be seen in the small vesicles of the cell and in the lumen. A portion of the endoplasmic reticulum is dilated. 75,000×.

than the junctions for lymphatic permeability. In the lymphatics they occupy approximately 35% of the non-nuclear cytoplasmic volume, with about half of this being accounted for by their limiting membranes (Casley-Smith, 1969b). About 120 are attached to each square micron of surface area by necks about 10 nm in internal diameter and about 20 nm long. Those free in the cytoplasm number about 300 per μ^2, or about 1000 per μ^3 of cell volume.

Lymphatic endothelium also contains a few smooth and rough elements of the endoplasmic reticulum, and a few ropheosomes ("hairy" or "coated" vesicles ~200 nm) (Figure 16). Phagocytic vesicles (0.1–5 μ) are found if there are particles, etc., to stimulate their formation. Their contents usually stay in them, i.e., in the cells. However, chylomicra seem anomalous in this regard and are transported across the cells, both in the lacteals (Figures 10 and 15) (Casley-Smith, 1962; Dobbins and Rollins, 1970; Palay and Karlin, 1959), and in the lymphatics of the diaphragm (Casley-Smith, 1964). The small vesicles also mutually adhere but then usually separate again. If they contain material that will agglutinate (e.g., carbon particles), this separation does not occur, and the vesicles gradually grow as do their contents (Figure 17). (They stay in cells,

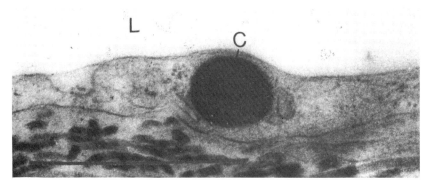

Figure 16. A chylomicron is shown inside a rat lacteal endothelial cell. There is a large indentation to its left, which may be where another left the cell. 60,000X.

which may gradually pass into the tissues and stay there; Casley-Smith, 1964). Such vesicles ("symphyosomes"; Casley-Smith, 1970a) attain the size of 0.1–5 μ and appear very similar to those formed by phagocytosis (Figures 12 and 13 and 18 and 19, below). However, initially, they usually exhibit much more concentrated contents than the phagocytic vesicles. They do not need cellular energy to form, just as the small vesicles do not need it in order to function as transportation mechanisms (Casley-Smith, 1969c; Jennings and Florey, 1967); phagocytic processes, however, need energy. [Probably the small vesicles also need cellular

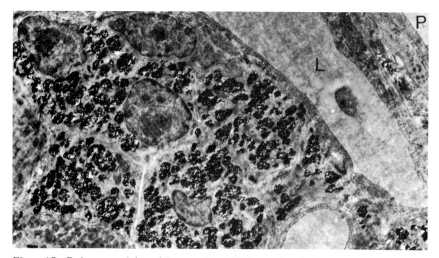

Figure 17. Carbon was injected intraperitoneally into mice 6 wk before death. At first, carbon particles occurred in large vesicles in the lymphatic endothelial cells. These gradually rounded up and left the vessels to lie in the tissues (Casley-Smith, 1964) as shown here. 3,000X.

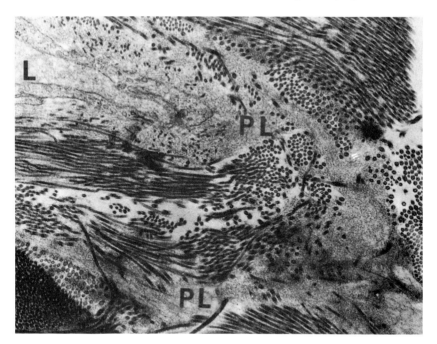

Figure 18. Rat tongues were made lymphedematous by ligating the cervical lymphatics. A lymphatic (L) is shown, as are some prelymphatics (PL) in the connective tissues, between some collagen bundles. 20,000×.

energy to form, but they do not need it to function, joining and leaving the plasma membranes very many times in their (relatively long) lives.]

It has been suggested that the small vesicles move because of Brownian motion (Casley-Smith, 1963; Shea and Karnovsky, 1966). Two models for this process have been proposed (Green and Casley-Smith, 1972; Shea, Karnovsky, and Bossert, 1969), which varied principally in whether it was assumed that vesicles which touched the plasma membranes always fused with them. It was calculated (Green and Casley-Smith, 1972) from the relative numbers of vesicles and the amount they transported that only about 0.004 contacts result in fusion. (This may well be because of the like charges carried by the exterior of the vesicles and the interior of the plasma membranes). The latter model received considerable experimental verification (Casley-Smith and Chin, 1971), and the numerical values were later made somewhat more exact (Casley-Smith and Clarke, 1972; Casley-Smith et al., 1975b). It is considered that about 5.3 vesicles cross vascular endothelial cells (~0.25 μ wide) in each direction, per second, per square micron of capillary surface. Some 50% of those leaving one side eventually return to it, while nearly 50% reach the other side. Their median free lives (between fusions) and mean transit times are 4 sec, and their attachment times are about 6 sec. The cytoplasmic viscosity is about 0.1 poise. (These

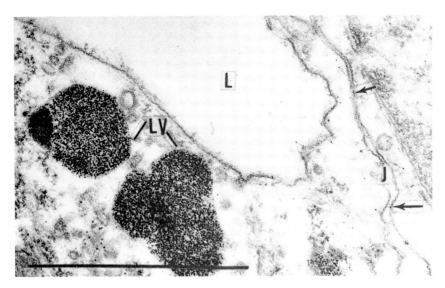

Figure 19. Ferritin was injected into the hind footpad of a mouse, 24 hr before death. In the aortic lymph nodes molecules can be seen in large vesicles (LV) in the lymphatic endothelium and a little in the junctions (arrows). 60,000×.

figures probably apply to the lymphatic endothelium also, but have not been determined here because of technical difficulties in obtaining the flux due to vesicles across the cells). The random movements mean that vesicles slowly carry material, in quanta, in the direction of, and in the amounts proportional to, any concentration gradients existing across the cells.

Recognizing Lymphatics

With the light microscope it is usually fairly simple, on the grounds of size and contents, to distinguish between the initial lymphatics and blood vessels (provided that the lymphatics can be seen at all, e.g., ligating the collecting lymphatics assists in this; Rusznyák et al., 1967). Microinjection also makes the typical lymphatic plexus easily visible, as does the uptake of dyes from deposits, etc. The collecting lymphatics can also be identified in this way. Even easier is to inject lymph nodes with tracers, when the efferent vessels and portions of the afferents are well known. (Traditionally, of course, the "autoinjection" of the mesenteric lymphatics and thoracic duct with lipid after a fatty meal is well known).

Electron microscopy, however, shows a different situation. Sections through initial lymphatics are often no longer than those through blood vessels, the lymphatics may contain red cells, and the vagaries of fixation and the lymphatic cycles can allow some lymphatics to contain more protein than the capillaries and postcapillary venules. Hence individual vessels can be mistaken. Indeed, it is sometimes impossible, on morphologic grounds alone, to identify a particular vessel beyond any doubt. The microinjection, etc., of tracers into the lymphatic system is the only certain way (Casley-Smith, 1965; Casley-Smith and Florey, 1961). The general morphologic features distinguishing lymphatics are: They are usually much bigger than blood capillaries, with very irregular walls, and are often rather collapsed. Their endothelium is usually slightly thicker, but appears thinner because of their larger diameters. They have no fenestrae, are normally paler, and may have open junctions. They are often lumenal projections (but blood vessels may have these, too). The basement membrane is tenuous and may be absent. There are ablumenal projections to which filaments are attached, as they are, irregularly, to the rest of the cell. They normally contain far fewer red cells and less plasma proteins than the blood vessels. Collecting vessels may be distinguished by the relative thinness of their walls in relation to their diameters compared with veins and by their cellular contents; nevertheless, it is much safer to use tracers to tell them apart.

Aside from the absence of fenestrae, none of these criteria are absolute. They are especially fallible in animals more primitive than teleosts, where the blood vessels, particularly the venous capillaries and venules, have many of the characteristics of mammalian lymphatics; *vide infra.*

Prelymphatics

In normal tissues one often sees gaps between the formed elements of the connective tissue, which are easily visible when many tracers or proteins are present. These sometimes end at a lymphatic junction, which is either open or appears openable. These have also been traced by serial sectioning (Collan and Kalima, 1974; Kalima and Collan, 1976). (It is evident that such combinations of paths and open junctions will not normally be seen often, because of the random nature of the sections and the tortuosity of the paths). The paths are particularly prominent in edema when the excess fluid and macromolecules force the cells and fiber bundles further apart (Figure 18). It is obvious that some small regions, at some times, will contain more fluid than others; to many workers this hardly seems sufficient to designate those regions that happen to open at a lymphatic junction with the term prelymphatic.

Some prelymphatics, however, especially in the brain and retina (Casley-Smith, 1976d; Casley-Smith, Földi-Börcsök, and Földi, 1976a; Földi et al., 1968a, 1968b; Ottaviani and Azzali, 1965; Várkonyi et al., 1969, 1970) and perhaps in cortical bone (Deysine, 1976), are particularly large and follow quite definite, well-defined courses in the adventitia of blood vessels. They become dilated and full of protein when the central collecting lymphatics are ligated—just as do the true lymphatics in this artificial lymphedema. If carbon is injected into the cerebral cortex, the prelymphatics carry it into the cervical lymphatics and lymph nodes (Casley-Smith, 1976a). It must therefore be concluded that these nonendothelialized tissue spaces do, in fact, carry protein and fluid from these regions. They act similarly to true lymphatics, and empty into them. Such a system surely deserves a special designation such as prelymphatic pathways, with the more major vessels being prelymphatics. It is then only a matter of degree to apply these names to similar spaces all over the body. After all, it would appear that the fluid-filled spaces, and potential spaces, throughout all the tissues are in continuity. Their effective radii are probably about 60 nm (Casley-Smith et al., 1975a; Chase, 1959, vide infra), but certainly vary greatly with tissue site, activity, injury, etc. It is interesting that in primitive animals, such as amphioxus (Casley-Smith, 1971a; Kampmeier, 1969), all the fluid compartments of the tissues are in continuity; vide infra.

Lymph Nodes

The lymphatic parts of these have morphologies very similar to those of the lymphatics to which they connect. Those in the peripheral nodes have a few open junctions; those in the more central ones do not (Casley-Smith, 1969a). The walls, however, are less thick, especially away from the marginal sinus. The morphology of these and of the other parts of the nodes has been reviewed (Moe, 1963; Pressman, Dunn, and Burtz, 1970; Rusznyák et al., 1967; Yoffey and Courtice, 1970). Intralymphatic tracers are taken up by the endothelial and reticular cells in vesicles and also pass down junctions, probably entering the blood system (Casley-Smith, 1969; Dunn et al., 1970; Pressman et al., 1970).

PERMEABILITY OF THE LYMPHATIC WALL

There are a number of paths through any sheet of cells such as the lymphatic endothelium. These are passages directly through the plasma membranes and cell cytoplasm, via the vesicles, fenestrae (if present), and tight junctions, close junctions, and open junctions. Thus there is really no such thing as "the permeability of endothelium"; rather it is a question of how much of some substance passes along each path, under certain conditions, and at a particular endothelial site (Casley-Smith, 1964).

Initial Lymphatics

The most important path through the initial lymphatic endothelium is the open junctions. A number of workers have observed large amounts of macromolecules, tracers, particles, and cells traversing them (Figures 7–12) (reviewed by Allen, 1967; Casley-Smith, 1970a, 1972, 1973; Leak, 1970; Mayerson, 1963; Yoffey and Courtice, 1970). In particular, it has been shown that lymphatics in sites where they are very permeable have many more open junctions than those in regions where they are less permeable (e.g., the diaphragm and intestinal lymphatics, compared with those in the pinna of the ear). The permeability of the less permeable lymphatics in the quiescent areas such as the ear can be greatly increased by various traumata; such increases are invariably found to be associated with very considerable increases in the numbers of open junctions

(Casley-Smith, 1965). There are also certain regions of the body where the association of open lymphatic junctions with high permeability is especially evident, such as the peritoneal surface of the diaphragm (Figures 8 and 9; Casley-Smith, 1964); the pleural surface does not have these, and the uptake of material into the lymphatics is very much less. It is interesting that von Recklinghausen in 1863 suggested that there might be openings ("stomata") between the peritoneal cavity and the diaphragmatic lymphatics. There was then a century of intense controversy before the electron microscope established that they really exist, at least during expiration. There is very good evidence, then, that the open junctions are particularly important for lymphatic permeability. It has been shown by calculations that even a relatively small percentage of open junctions (1–6%) is quite capable of accounting for great lymphatic permeability (Casley-Smith, 1975b; Elhay and Casley-Smith, 1976).

The close junctions, particularly the close ones, i.e., with about 6-nm gaps, should also be considered. These are certainly almost impermeable (Figures 5 and 6) to all but the smaller macromolecules (~40,000 M.W.; Casley-Smith, 1970a, 1972, 1971, unpublished) but are certainly permeable to fluid and ions as they are in blood vessels (Figure 5; Casley-Smith, 1967c, 1969a, 1972; Casley-Smith et al., 1975b; Karnovsky, 1968; Majno, 1965; Pappenheimer, 1970). Unfortunately, with the electron microscope it is very hard to get accurate quantitative information about the relative importance of these numerous, but narrow junctions, compared with the much fewer, but much wider open, ones. Calculations indicate that the open junctions are much more important, by two to three orders of magnitude (Elhay and Casley-Smith, 1976) during the filling of the lymphatics. During emptying, however, the open junctions become closed and are similar to the close ones. If fluid and ions (but not macromolecules) are forced out of the vessels (vide infra), the two kinds of junctions probably contribute about equally to the increase in permeability. The tight junctions, which may have gaps from about 1 nm, are probably not significant in spite of their relatively greater lengths.

It is possible (Pappenheimer, 1970) that water passes directly through the plasma membranes and the cytoplasm. However, most ions will not do this, but must pass through the junctions. Thus, while direct passage would be of importance when considering the fine details of fluid movements, it is not important in the present context, since the fluid will speedily move back to the increased concentrations of ions. When lymphatic endothelium is badly injured (Figure 13), gaps appear in the plasma membranes and proteins pass directly across the cells (Casley-Smith, 1965); however, this does not normally happen.

The only other path across the lymphatic endothelial barrier is via vesicles (Figures 14 and 15). Evidence from studies on vascular endothelium indicates that the movement of these vesicles is relatively slow and consequently can only transport a very small amount of material compared with the junctions (Carter, Joyner, and Renkin, 1974; Casley-Smith, 1969b, 1970a; Casley-Smith and

Clarke, 1972; Casley-Smith et al., 1975*b*; Garlick and Renkin, 1970; Perry and Garlick, 1975; Renkin, Carter, and Joyner, 1974; Renkin, 1971). Simionescu, Simionescu, and Palade (1975) consider that channels formed of vesicles completely through the endothelium are also responsible for the small pore system; however, these would not give the observed molecular sieving, unlike what can be calculated for the close junctions (Casley-Smith et al., 1975*b*). Thus the small vesicles can account for the slow leakage of proteins from the blood vessels, but not for the more rapid exchange of smaller molecules. It is highly unlikely that this slowness of exchange applies also to the vesicles in the lymphatics. Certainly, experimental results indicate that there is little difference in the relative rates of vesicular transport in the two systems (Casley-Smith, 1964, 1965). The only vesicles that may transport material in significant amounts are the large vesicles that have ingested chylomicra (Figures 10 and 16) (Casley-Smith, 1962; Dobbins and Rollins, 1970; Palay and Karlin, 1959), but even these are relatively infrequent and are probably much less important than the open junctions. In injured blood capillaries (Casley-Smith and Window, 1976) large vacuoles are seen; these probably transport relatively large amounts of macromolecules, but still do not add greatly to the permeability of the endothelium for small molecules.

Selectivity

The open junctions will select against the larger particles and cells because these will be more likely to rebound from the openings and will suffer more friction as they pass along the channels, very much as has been suggested for the small-pore system, i.e., the close junctions (Landis and Pappenheimer, 1963). This will not apply, of course, to the smaller macromolecules, if their diameters are very substantially less than the slit widths. Similar considerations will apply to the much smaller openings into, and out of, the vesicles where the macromolecules will be subjected to molecular sieving. But their smaller diffusion coefficients will allow fluid to enter and leave the newly opened vesicles much more swiftly than the macromolecules themselves. This has been shown experimentally to be the case with ferritin (Casley-Smith and Chin, 1971).

It is interesting that vesicles in the lymphatic endothelium seem to fill with tracers much more readily than those opening at the lumenal surface of blood vessels; the latter fill much more readily if flow is momentarily interrupted (Brandt, personal communication). It may well be that what occurs here is a form of "micro-plasma-skimming." (The flow of blood may keep the larger macromolecules just sufficiently far away from the plasma membranes of the endothelium so that they have far fewer chances of diffusing into the vesicular mouths.)

It would appear almost certain that most (but not all) of the selectivity that causes the differences in concentrations between the substances in the blood and in the lymph occurs at the blood–endothelial barrier (Courtice, 1971; Grotte, 1956; Rusznyák et al., 1967; Yoffey and Courtice, 1970). Further selection may well happen at the blood vessel basement membrane and in the passage through the tissues. There is, however, the strong possibility that the lymph is concentrated by ultrafiltration in the lymphatics (*vide infra*), which is another place where these alterations may occur.

Collecting Lymphatics

Mayerson et al. (1962) and Mayerson (1963) showed that canine leg and mesenteric lymphatics (and the popliteal lymph node) are relatively impermeable to molecules with a molecular weight of more than 6,000, but very permeable to those of less than 2,300. Földi and Zoltán (1965) showed that the thoracic duct is very permeable to ions. Patterson et al. (1958) found that only about 3% of albumin infused into dog leg lymphatics passed to the circulation other than by the thoracic duct, a result similar to those of Garlick and Renkin (1970). Strawitz et al. (1968) also showed that the collecting lymphatics are very permeable to small molecules, but this permeability is rapidly lost as the molecular weight grows greater than 1,000. They recovered 75% of the infused albumin from the lymph and 50% of inulin (M.W. 5,000), but some of that which was lost may have accumulated in the lymphatic endothelium and nodal reticulum (Casley-Smith, 1969*a*) rather than passing directly to the blood. Similarly Rusznyák et al. (1967) have shown that small-molecular-weight fluorescent dyes, unattached to proteins, leave collecting lymphatics very readily, while larger molecular complexes do not.

With the electron microscope the reason for these variations becomes evident. The close junctions, and the tight ones, are readily permeable to ions (Casley-Smith, 1969*d*), while they are relatively impermeable to ferritin, and presumably to other macromolecules (Figure 19) (Casley-Smith, 1969*a*). Some macromolecular tracers are found in the cells in vesicles, and pass through them in this way. As mentioned before, however, this means of passage is very slow; hence the difference in rates of passage of the two classes of molecules can be readily understood. This is similar to the situation in the blood vessels (Carter et al. 1974; Casley-Smith, 1967*c*; Garlick and Renkin, 1970; Grotte, 1956; Karnovsky, 1968; Landis and Pappenheimer, 1963; Renkin, 1971; Renkin et al., 1974). In blood vessels, however, the dividing line between the two classes of molecules is probably rather higher than 1,000 M.W. and approaches 10,000. This difference between the two classes of vessels may possibly be attributable to the relatively much thicker walls of the collecting lymphatics (Figure 2) than those of the blood capillaries and postcapillary venules. Jacobsson and Kjellmer (1964) also demonstrated that the rates of perfusion made great differences in the amounts of small molecules that passed through the walls of these vessels.

FUNCTIONING OF INITIAL LYMPHATICS

It has been shown above that fluid and the macromolecules, particles, etc., pass into the initial lymphatics via the open endothelial intercellular junctions. This occurs during the phase of tissue relaxation, when the lymphatics are not compressed by the surrounding tissues, and are even being pulled open if there is edema (Allen, 1967; Casley-Smith, 1972, 1973, 1975b; Rusznyák et al., 1967; Verzár and McDougal, 1936; Yoffey and Courtice, 1970). The interesting questions here are what forces are involved; how do their magnitudes and directions vary with circumstances; and how do lymphatic volume, lymph protein concentration, and total lymph protein vary both during this period and with different circumstances? Similarly, the lymph is expelled during the compression of the initial lymphatics by the surrounding tissue during muscular contraction, respiration, etc. Attention is now being turned to the forces involved and their possible variations, to differences in the amount and concentration of lymph during this period, and whether some of the fluid components of the lymph are expelled back into the tissues via the temporarily "closed" junctions. Thus it can be seen that our study of the lymphatic system has progressed to the stage where we are concerned with the more intimate details of both the causes and effects of the whole initial lymphatic cycle.

Initial Lymphatic Cycle–The Filling Phase
What forces, then, affect the entry of fluid into the initial lymphatics? It has long been held that there is a slight gradient of hydrostatic pressure from the tissues into the lymphatics (McMaster, 1947; Wiederhielm, 1968). However, the micropipette techniques that yield this measurement have been increasingly criticized (Guyton, 1963, 1969; Guyton, Granger, and Taylor, 1971; Landis and Pappenheimer, 1963; Mayerson, 1963; Rusznyák et al., 1967; Scholander, Hargens, and Miller, 1968). Almost certainly, the "tissue resistance," which is what is measured by micropipettes, really corresponds to the vectorial sum of the true "tissue hydrostatic pressure" and the "solid-tissue pressure" (Guyton, 1969; Guyton et al., 1971). (Solid-tissue pressure is the pressure exerted on relatively large objects, such as the lymphatic walls, by the cells, fiber bundles, and the more solid, continuous, portions of the ground substance.)

Although micropipettes can measure the pressures in lymphatics, reasonably accurately, they can not do so in normal tissues, because here free pools of fluid, of size comparable to the pipette tips, do not exist. They do exist in the wing of the bat (Wiederhielm, 1968), but it is doubtful if these results can be extrapolated to the normal, "dry" tissues of other regions and other animals. [It is probable that bat wings have abnormal tendencies to form edema, as might be expected from their structures; here the "initial" lymphatics are bulbous (Cliff and Nichol, 1970) and contractile in the American species, which is apparently unique.] Of course, in edematous tissue micropipettes are capable of measuring the pressures, and there is quite a large hydrostatic pressure gradient from the tissues of the initial lymphatics. In normal conditions, however, the hydrostatic pressure gradient suggested by Guyton's capsules (1973, 1969) or the wicks of Scholander et al. (1968) is negative, with a magnitude of 5–10 cm of water. The micropipettes only record a positive pressure gradient of about 0.5—1 cm, which as explained above is likely to be fallacious. (The actual pressures found in the initial lymphatics are ±1 cm, which must be carefully distinguished from the much higher pressures found periodically in the collecting lymphatics and which are caused by pressures on, and by, the vessels' walls.) Thus it can be seen that hydrostatic pressure alone is much more likely to impede than to aid the filling of lymphatics in normal tissue.

It has been suggested (Dobbins and Rollins, 1970; Mayerson, 1963; Virágh et al., 1971) that fluid could be actively pumped across the cells in the small cytoplasmic vesicles. This is highly unlikely. The endothelium does not in the least resemble cells where this sort of activity occurs (e.g., gut and renal tubular epithelium). Cyanide does not prevent lymphatic filling (Casley-Smith, 1965; Rusznyák et al., 1967); indeed, by opening more junctions, it assists it. As mentioned earlier, vesicular transport by small vesicles is very slow, occurs in both directions, and is independent of cellular activity. There are far too few phagocytic or ropheocytic vesicles to give active, directed transport. Also, of course, there is considerable evidence that the permeation of the initial lymphatic endothelium is principally via the junctions.

It is conceivable that the first few segments of the collecting vessels could exert a suction force on the initial lymphatics, because the collecting vessels are pulled open, after contraction or compression, by the elasticity of the tissues attached to their walls (Morris, personal communication; Reddy et al., 1975; Taylor et al., 1973). This does not, however, overcome the difficulty that measurements show that the hydrostatic pressures in the initial lymphatics are probably higher than in the tissues (Zweifach, 1973; Zweifach and Intaglietta, 1968). Also, it should be noted that the anchoring filaments are not nearly so frequent on the collecting lymphatics as they are on the initial ones. This would also not explain why so little lymph is produced from paralyzed limbs, although here the collecting lymphatics are presumably still contracting; the absence of variations of the solid-tissue pressure seems to be the reason why there is so little lymph. Although this would not affect any suction by the collecting lymphatics, it would certainly affect the mechanism mentioned below.

One force that is seldom considered is colloidal osmotic pressure (Casley-Smith, 1970b, 1972, 1973, 1975b; Elhay and Casley-Smith, 1976). This neglect has been due to a number of reasons: It has usually (but not invariably, see Rusznyák et al., 1967) been held that the macromolecular concentration of lymph is identical with that of tissue fluids, and it is usually considered that it is impossible to get an osmotic pressure difference across a membrane that has pores many times the diameter of the solute molecules. This last point is undoubtedly true for the smaller molecules (M.W. <5000), but the small diffusion coefficients of molecules of the size of albumin, and above, mean that any small inflow of fluid through a pore will usually prevent the diffusing out, i.e., there is a virtual membrane (Casley-Smith, 1975a). This has been experimentally confirmed in vitro (Figure 20) (Casley-Smith, 1975*a;* Casley-Smith and Bolton, 1973*a*). Effective colloid osmotic pressures, that are 0.7–0.9 of those measured across semi-permeable membranes, were found to exist across pores of 0.1-μ diameter. When the pore diameters were 1 μ, the ratios were 0.5 and 0.9, respectively, for plasma and dilute plasma (one-fourth plasma). It is evident, then, that, contrary to the assumption of Taylor et al. (1973), colloid osmotic pressures will exist across the lymphatic endothelium in spite of the open junctions, provided there is a difference in protein concentration across the membrane. Does one in fact exist?

While this is usually not considered to be the case, it has been found that the mean lymph protein concentration is 3 times that in the connective tissue (Table 1) (Casley-Smith, 1970*b*, 1975*b*, 1976*e;* Casley-Smith and Sims, 1975). Four different methods were used, in lymphatics in both the mouse ear, villus and diaphragm and rat villus, under normal conditions and when gross inflammatory edema was present (Figure 11 and Figures 21–23). (The presence of such edema also avoids the possibility of the "excluded-volume phenomena" of

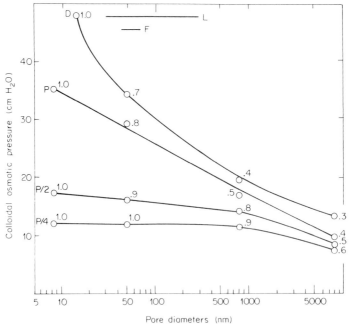

Figure 20. The effective osmotic pressures recorded for various solutes–dextran (D), plasma (P), plasma diluted 1:1 (P/2) and 1:3 (P/4)–plotted against pore diameters (Casley-Smith and Bolton, 1973*a*). The indices at various points show the proportions of osmotic pressure exerted across a semipermeable membrane. The approximate pore diameters of fenestrae (F) and open lymphatic junctions (L) are shown at the top. (The latter are displaced here to the left since they are slits, not cylinders.)

Table 1. Ratios of the mean[a] concentrations of proteins in the lymphatics and in the connective tissues[b]

	Mean	Standard error	Numbers of observations
Densitometry			
Normal ears (initial lymphatics)	2.81	(.049)	50
Lacteals (initial lymphatics)	2.25	(.051)	50
Collecting lymphatics in jejunum	1.17	(.013)	50
Counting lipoproteins			
Lacteals (initial lymphatics)	2.52	(.033)	50
Collecting lymphatics in jejunum[c]	0.96	(.051)	10
Counting ferritin molecules			
Normal ear, initial lymphatics			
0 min after microinjection	1.90	(0.047)	50
20 min after microinjection	3.04	(0.045)	50
2½ hr after microinjection	3.24	(0.081)	50
Heat injured ear,			
2½ hr after microinjection	3.15	(0.044)	50
Combined values			
Mean of all initial lymphatics, except 0 min	2.84	(0.030)	300
Mean of all collecting lymphatics	1.13	(0.017)	60

[a]The values for the initial lymphatics are means, taken randomly over all the initial lymphatic cycles.

[b]The values in parentheses are the Standard Errors of the Means, those in italics are the numbers of observations.

[c]The concentrations here are compared not with those in the adjacent connective tissue, but with those in the tissue adjacent to the initial lymphatics in the mucosa, from which the particles almost certainly originated.

Laurent, 1970.) Arfors (1976) also found a 3 times greater concentration using microchemical methods. Rusznyák et al. (1967) used light microscopy and concluded that the lymph was considerably more concentrated than the tissue fluid, as did Jonsson, Arfors, and Hint (1971), while calculations (Casley-Smith, 1976b) indicate that the concentration of proteins by the initial lymphatics will substantially lower the mean colloidal osmotic pressures and hence the hydrostatic pressures in the tissues. Johnson and Richardson (1974) also found indirect evidence for a concentrating effect. Bruggeman (1976) found that the mean gastric lymph protein concentration obtained adjacent to the stomach is 5.2 g/100 ml, which is higher than earlier determinations of lymph from the gut. Some of these reports were really based on lymph in the smaller collecting ducts. In these, one might well expect a dilution of any concentrated lymph; hence these results indicate that lymph in the initial lymphatics may well be even more concentrated. The direct, electron microscopic results from the initial lymphatics were based on random sections, taken throughout the whole lymphatic cycle. Thus it is highly likely (*vide infra*) that at some parts of the cycle greater

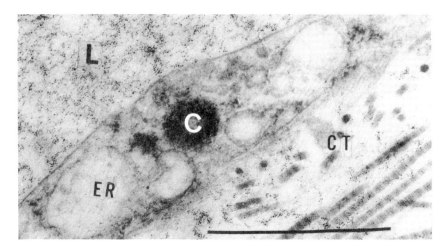

Figure 21. Swollen lymphatic endothelium in a mouse ear injured by heat (as in Figure 7). Ferritin was injected into the connective tissue 2.5 hr before death. There is a much higher concentration of ferritin in the lumen (L) than in the connective tissues (CT), as was confirmed by counting molecules. Also shown is a dilated endoplasmic reticulum (ER) and a centriole (C). 50,000×.

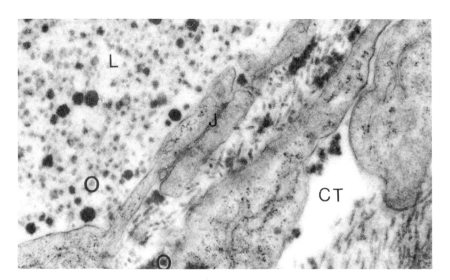

Figure 22. A lacteal (L) contains a much higher concentration of lipoproteins (circled) than does the connective tissue (CT). (This was confirmed by counting molecules.) The lipoproteins were produced as in Figure 14. The paler dots are cross sections of collagen fibers. 30,000×.

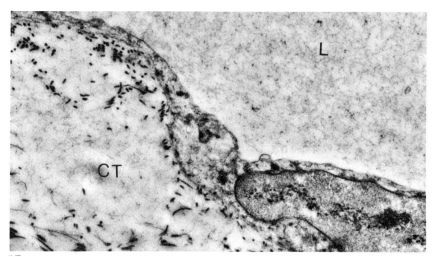

Figure 23. In a lymphatic (L) in a normal mouse's ear there is a much higher concentration of plasma proteins than in the connective tissues (CT), as was confirmed densitometrically. (The thicker, darker fibers are collagen.) 25,000×.

differences exist, as has been shown by direct measurements (Casley-Smith, 1976e). The threefold difference is likely to produce effective osmotic pressure differences (given normal connective tissue protein concentrations) that will easily overcome the outward hydrostatic pressure gradient discussed earlier. (Even if such hydrostatic differences do not exist, e.g., if the tissue hydrostatic pressure is positive—as in edema—or if the negative tissue hydrostatic pressures were shown to be in error, the osmotic differences will still contribute significantly to the lymphatic inflow; Elhay and Casley-Smith, 1976).

Confirmation of the possibility of such effective colloid osmotic pressures across open junctions is provided by the situation in fenestrated blood vessels (Casley-Smith, 1975a, 1975b). These pores (~50 nm in diameter) are quite patent to fluid and proteins. They exist in large numbers in certain regions, e.g., the intestine, endocrines, etc., yet the enormous outpouring of fluid that should occur through such numerous large pores does not happen. Instead, fluid and proteins almost certainly enter the blood capillaries in large amounts through these openings when they occur on the venous limbs of capillaries (vide infra). [Using the data of Casley-Smith et al., 1975a, and a mean capillary hydrostatic pressure of about 10 mm Hg (Johnson and Hanson, 1966) it can be easily calculated that if there were no osmotic pressure across the fenestrae, man would lose approximately 3 liters of fluid each hour into the intestinal tissue alone.] Hence we must conclude that the normal Starling equilibrium exists, with large effective colloidal osmotic pressures across the fenestrae.

While osmotic pressure can account for the inflow of fluid, what happens to proteins? The low diffusion coefficients of proteins, and other macromolecules, particles, and nonmotile cells, will ensure that they are swept along by any bulk flow of fluids (Landis and Pappenheimer, 1963). The transport of proteins by fluid flow through the tissues in accordance with Starling's hypothesis has been experimentally verified in regions with fenestrated capillaries (Casley-Smith, 1970c) and in those with continuous ones (Casley-Smith, in preparation).

If the lymph is much more concentrated than the tissue fluid, proteins will tend to diffuse out of the initial lymphatics via the open junctions, in spite of the inflow of fluid. The extent of this will vary greatly with the circumstances. It has been shown theoretically (Casley-Smith, 1975a; Perry and Garlick, 1975) that, in spite of criticisms (Michel, 1972, 1974), it is indeed very likely that there can be a net uptake of protein due to the solvent drag of the inflowing fluid. A thermodynamic model, and entropy considerations, indicate that the concentration of this fluid is less than the mean of those on the two sides of the membrane; later (Casley-Smith, 1976b), this has been made even more stringent and the inflowing fluid can be shown to be less concentrated than that from which it is flowing. This still, however, allows for the removal of a large amount of protein.

The net transfer of water and of proteins produced by an osmotic pressure gradient, even against a hydrostatic one has been demonstrated in vitro (Figure 24) (Casley-Smith, 1975b). Two stirred compartments were separated by artificial membranes with pores (diameters 50 nm or 0.8 μ). Plasma (7 g/100 ml) was placed in one compartment and plasma diluted 1:3 with Hank's solution in the other. The hydrostatic pressures were varied and the net water and protein transfer were measured. Since the open junctions are slits, they actually correspond to rather smaller circular pores (Pappenheimer, 1970). Thus the 50-nm pores correspond to slits of about 80 nm and the 0.2 μ to slits of 0.3 μ. These span the normal range of open junctions. It can be seen that the preliminary results from this in vitro model indicate that the mechanism proposed for the filling phase (Figure 25) is quite possible from the physical point of view. (Any errors in this system are likely to underestimate the net uptakes.)

Initial Lymphatic Cycle—The Emptying Phase

The emptying phase of the initial lymphatic cycle occurs when the tissues become compressed (Figure 25). This compression will raise the solid tissue pressure to high levels, e.g., about 50 cm H_2O (Elhay and Casley-Smith, 1976; Yoffey and Courtice, 1970) as has been shown by micropipette measurements (accepting that the tissue hydrostatic pressure rises to approximately 0 cm; Guyton, 1969). It is well known that the endothelium is very pliable; hence this greatly increased solid tissue pressure will be transmitted to the lymph, so that the intralymphatic hydrostatic pressure also rises to about 50 cm. If the anchoring filaments are taut and dilating the vessels because of edema, the tissue compression may also have the effect of loosening them and allowing the vessels to collapse, unless overdistension has occurred. This raised pressure in the initial lymphatics will have a number of effects.

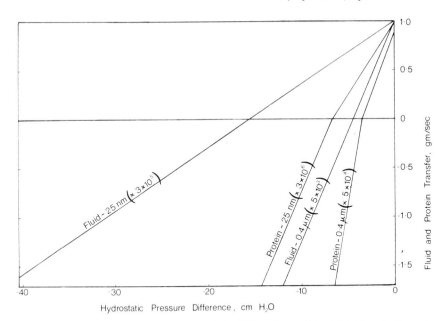

Figure 24. Results of the in vitro model of the filling phase of the initial lymphatic cycle (and of the fenestrated capillary) described in the text. The measured net transfer rates of fluid and of protein are shown for pores of 25 nm and 0.4-μ radii. The rates are plotted in g/sec (per cm² of membrane surface), multiplied by the various indicated factors to bring them to the same scales. Transfer above the 0 line (+) indicates passage from the "tissue" into the "vessel." This relationship exists even in the presence of quite high outward (−) hydrostatic pressure gradients.

Since there is not a large pressure gradient (the net of the hydrostatic and osmotic pressures) directed out of the vessels, lymph will start to flow out. This will result in the very pliable inner leaflets of the open junctions being forced close up against the outer endothelial cells and the surrounding tissues. To this effect will be added the effects of the "telescoping" of the lymphatics during tissue compression (Allen, 1967; Allen and Vogt, 1937). Thus, during the emptying phase, these open junctions come to resemble the close junctions. They are therefore likely to be impermeable to macromolecules, particles, and cells, but still quite permeable to water and small molecules. So these will be forced out of the lymphatics into the tissues, leaving the macromolecules to become more and more concentrated. Thus the initial lymphatics will function as ultrafilters. The amount of this outflow will depend on the net hydrostatic–osmotic pressure difference. The net pressure difference will vary during this phase, becoming less as the lymph becomes more and more concentrated. It has been calculated (Elhay and Casley-Smith, 1976) that the temporally "close" open junctions and the unaltering normally close junctions contribute about equally to this loss of water; the tight junctions probably contribute almost nothing.

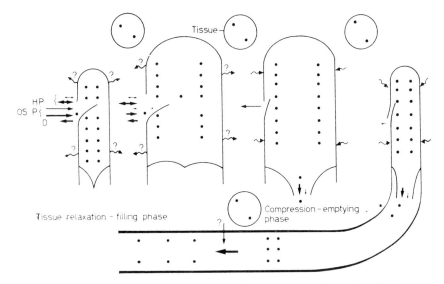

Figure 25. A diagram of the initial lymphatic cycle, passing from left to right. Thick arrows indicate protein movement; thin arrows show movement of water. Their lengths are approximately proportional to the individual forces acting on them at various stages of the cycle. Wavy arrows show the solid-tissue pressures, or pull of the filaments, as occurs during edema. Proteins (dots) are shown in their varying concentrations in the tissues and lymph. The variations in net osmotic pressure (OSP), hydrostatic pressure (HP), and diffusion (D) are indicated, as are the variations in the valves, and the dilution of the concentrated lymph in the collecting lymphatics.

This closure of the open junctions can also be seen to occur when the lymphatics draining a region of fairly nonelastic tissue are ligated (*vide infra*), e.g., the intestinal villi and the parotid gland (Figure 36, below) (Casley-Smith, 1976*a;* Casley-Smith et al., 1974; Dobbins, 1966; Kalima, 1971). Unlike the gross stretching of the tissues and the lymphatics which raised intralymphatic pressure in looser regions (e.g., in the ear, facial skin, and the tongue) (Figure 35, below) (Casley-Smith, 1965, 1973; Casley-Smith et al., 1969, 1974), in nonelastic tissues there is relatively less dilation. Hence instead of the junctions being opened by the cells being forced apart, they are sealed closed by the raised pressure forcing the inner cells against the outer ones. Thus in some regions lymphedema produces open junctions; in others it causes closed ones, which mimic in a more permanent manner the normal temporary closure during the emptying phase.

Another result of the raised intralymphatic hydrostatic pressure is to force some of the lymph onwards into the collecting lymphatics, past the intralymphatic valves. Thus the combination of the open–close junctions acting as inlet valves and the intralymphatic valves cause the initial lymphatics to function as millions of tiny force pumps. It is true, as Drinker (quoted by Mayerson, 1963) remarked, that the pumps are leaky but that nevertheless they still pump.

(In fact, as we are discovering, the leakiness is likely to be essential for their filling and hence for their pumping).

It is important to remember that while, structurally, collecting lymphatics may lie deeply inside a compressed region, the first truly functional collecting lymphatics are those immediately adjacent to the region, but outside it and uncompressed. The compressed collecting lymphatics are still quite permeable to small molecules (*vide supra*) and the hydrostatic pressure along their lengths will be still very high, so they will also leak small molecules. The flow along the collecting lymphatics will be considerably less than might be anticipated, because of the sheer length of the tubes. In the muscles of the larger animals, the lymph may well have to travel 10–20 cm before it reaches an uncompressed collecting lymphatic. By contrast, in the intestinal villi this distance is only 1 mm or less. (This difference is reflected in the relative outflows from the villi as compared with a number of other regions; *vide infra*.) In addition to the effects of the length of the compressed lymphatic system in the compressed regions, there is another important factor. Katz, Chen, and Moreno (1969) have shown that collapsible tubes that are compressed by external pressures slightly greater than those inside the tubes are quite constricted at the ends where the internal pressure is least, i.e., in the direction of flow. (This is to be expected, since the internal pressure gradient must fall slightly along the tube, while the external pressures are constant.) It is uncertain whether this applies to the lymphatic system, but it is likely to do so. If so, it will result in a constricted outlet and even less outflow into the external collecting lymphatics.

The concept of the concentration of lymph in the initial lymphatics and its subsequent redilution in the collecting vessels has recently been criticized (Nicolaysen et al., 1975; Staub, Nicolaysen, and Nicolaysen, 1975; and Vrien, Demling, and Staub, 1975). This group of workers used both conventional fixation and frozen sections for autoradiography of albumin in mouse lungs. They found a dilution along the collecting lymphatics with conventional fixation but not with freezing. One cannot extrapolate from the mouse's lung, with its very short collecting vessels, to collecting vessels in other animals, which are usually very much longer. However, the lung is fairly uniformly compressed, so that true, effective, collecting lymphatics are actually those outside the thoracic cavity (*vide infra*). Some experiments using diaphragmatic lymphatics and ferritin (Casley-Smith, 1976e) support the hypothesis, showing concentration of the lymph during the compression phase and its dilution during filling; they also show that the adjacent collecting lymphatics receive fairly concentrated lymph, which is diluted in the remote collectors, where the solid-tissue pressures are much reduced. This has also been shown using autoradiography of RISA in the jejunum (Casley-Smith and Sims, 1976), where concentration of lymph in the initial lymphatics was noted, as was its dilution in the remote collectors.

The hypothesis about the mode of functioning of the initial lymphatics during the emptying phase implies that quite considerable amounts of water must be forced back into the tissues. As it passes out of the junctions into the tissues it must substantially dilute the proteins in the tissues adjacent to the vessels. (However, about half of these junctions are those that are close even during filling, so only about half of the water dilutes the tissue fluid adjacent to the openable junctions). If this water remained in the vicinity of these junctions, its effect would be to so dilute the proteins that less would be available to be carried into the vessels during the next filling phase to replace those lost in the collecting lymphatics (Taylor et al., 1973, 1976a; Taylor and Gibson, 1975). However, water can easily pass through the tissues by innumerable paths that are unavailable to the proteins (Laurent, 1970), which are confined to the relatively circumscribed prelymphatics. The water expelled from the junctions is at considerable pressure, and will cause a tinly local bleb of edema in the tissues by dilating the prelymphatics. The raised solid-tissue pressure will tend to compress this, thus raising its hydrostatic pressure somewhat above that in the rest of the tissues, but still well below that in the initial lymphatics because of the ease with which water can penetrate the bleb's "wall." Although the water will do this under the influence of the increased pressure, it will have to leave the proteins behind in the prelymphatics. Thus these will be readily available to be swept into the open junctions during the next filling phase. This concept of the water passing into the general ground substance, leaving the proteins in the prelymphatic connective tissue channels as concentrated as before, disposes of Taylor's main objection to this hypothesis. It completely alters his tenet, showing that the concentration of protein in the initial lymphatics will be considerably greater than that in the tissues. There are likely to be two stages of ultrafiltration; one is out of the lymphatics, the second is out of the prelymphatics. (Taylor et al. also did not consider the water leaving the initial lymphatics via the close junctions, which accounts for about half of the ultrafiltration and which is nowhere near the prelymphatics, and hence does not dilute their contents).

This suggested action of the lymphatics during the emptying phase of the cycle implies that relatively little lymph will actually reach the external collecting lymphatics compared with the amount entering the initial lymphatics during filling. While this has not been directly tested, it has been possible to roughly calculate the theoretical maximal outputs of lymphatics from five regions (assuming complete filling and emptying each cycle) and to compare these with the actual outputs (Table 2) (Casley-Smith, 1975b, 1975f). From Table 2 it can be seen that the ratio of actual to theoretical maximal output is 0.1–1% for most regions and 5–30% for the intestinal villi. (As mentioned earlier, this difference is probably accounted for by the great differences in the length of the lymphatic system that is compressed). Of course, the lymphatics are never maximally filled, but even if they were normally only 10% filled, the input is still 10–100 times the output. This is of great importance when Taylor et al.'s (1973) calculations are considered. From these it can be seen that the protein concentrations in the expelled lymph are likely to be many times those in the fluid entering the

Table 2. Actual/theoretical maximal lymph flows

(A) Site	(B) Species	(C) Lymphatic length (cm/cm²)	(D) Maximal diameter (μ)	(E) Area of site (cm²)	(F) Maximal volume (ml)	(G) Cycle length (sec)	(H) Maximal lymph flow (ml/hr)	(I) Actual lymph flow (ml/hr)	Ratio I/H (%)
Jejunum	man	50–70	30	10,000	3	20	500	50	10
	dog			1,000	0.3		50	2.5–15	5–30
	cat			200	0.06		11	2	20
	rat			70	0.02		4	1	30
Diaphragm	rabbit	60–100	75	100	0.4	2.3	600	6	1
	cat	80–130							
Heart	man	50–90	30	1,000	0.4	0.85	2,000	2–3	
	dog	30–70	30	500	0.2	0.6	1,000	1–3	0.2
	pig								
Leg muscle	dog	60	30	2,000	1	1	3,500	2–4	0.1
Lungs	man		33		1	5	700	5–10	1–2
	dog		33		0.2	3.7	200	1–5	
	man		33		10	5	7,000	5–10	0.1–0.2
	dog		33		2	3.7	2,000	1–5	
	man	60	33	34,000	20	5	14,000	5–10	0.05

The details of the estimation of the figures in columns (C) to (I) are given in Casley-Smith (1975b).

vessels. In addition, the outputs were measured well along the collecting lymphatics; here the originally concentrated lymph would be likely to have been diluted again and the ratios should perhaps be further multiplied by a factor of 3. It would appear that the "leaky pump" is very leaky indeed.

Whole Initial Lymphatic Cycle–A Mathematical Model

It was considered necessary to construct a mathematical model of the whole initial lymphatic cycle (Elhay and Casley-Smith, 1976). This used normal physical laws and data we have about dimensions, pressures, etc., to see if the envisaged cycle was compatible with these laws and if it was capable of continuous operation under conditions where no other factors were altered and where the only energy supplied was by adjacent contracting muscles, etc. The dimensions of the junctions, the pressures, etc., are as discussed above. Account is taken of varying lymph protein concentrations that cause the net hydrostatic–osmotic pressures to vary in both filling and emptying, and the amount of back-diffusion of protein to vary during filling.

It has indeed been found, for a wide range of parameters far greater than the likely normal ranges, that the model will act consistently and continuously, thus confirming the hypothesis. One example is shown in Figure 26. Here we assumed a negative tissue hydrostatic pressure of −5 cm, a tissue protein concentration of 2 g/100 ml, a maximum lymph protein concentration of 10 g/100 ml, a compressed vessel length of 10 cm, a maximal diameter of 30 μ, and a change in volume of from 1/10 to 1/3 of maximal. It can be seen that the cycle is continuous, with the total lymph protein varying between 15 and 20×10^{-7} g, i.e., 25% of the protein being pumped along each cycle. From the model it was found that the actual–theoretical-maximal output of water was about 10%, while the actual amount passing to the collecting lymphatics was 30% of that entering, i.e., 70% was ejected back into the tissues. This model also gave a mean ratio of lymph protein–tissue protein concentrations of 3. Thus in several important respects the model gives results similar to those found by observation.

The actual shapes of the various curves are quite interesting and might possibly provide means to test the predictions further. It can be seen how the negative tissue hydrostatic pressure would eventually cause water and protein to leave the vessel if emptying is delayed too long after filling, except that the junctions would close and prevent this. Thus there is an intermediate phase between filling and emptying.

FUNCTIONING OF THE COLLECTING LYMPHATICS

These vessels basically transport macromolecules to the blood. To do this they pump the water in which they are contained. This pumping is achieved with the aid of the intralymphatic valves to prevent back-flow, and the contraction or compression of their walls to provide the motive power (Rusznyák et al., 1967; Yoffey and Courtice, 1970). The contractions are segmental, between the sets

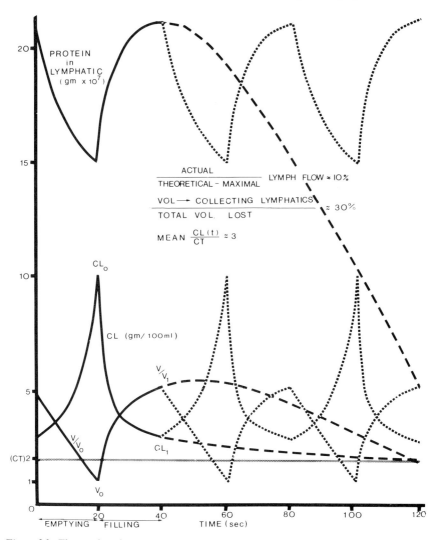

Figure 26. The results of a computer simulation of the initial lymphatic cycle, as described in the text. The total protein in the lymph, its concentration in the lymph (CL) and the tissues (CT), and the volume of lymph (V/VO) are shown. The normal cycle is shown by the continuous and the closely dotted lines. If emptying does not follow maximal filling, the values would follow the dashed line as the assumed net negative hydrostatic pressure overcomes the net positive osmotic pressure, if the junctions did not close and prevent protein from leaving the vessel.

of values. These segments have been termed "lymphangions" (Mislin, 1967). Compression of the collecting lymphatics' walls is often brought about by the contraction of adjacent muscles, respiratory movements, the pulse, etc.

The hydrostatic pressures in the collecting lymphatics, in uncompressed regions, often rise as high as 5–25 cm H_2O (Yoffey and Courtice, 1970). If they are obstructed, the pressures can reach about 150 cm. Using the permeability data of Mayerson et al. (1962), it is easy to see that quite large amounts of water are likely to be forced out of these vessels while these pressures are being applied, only to reenter once they are released and the colloidal osmotic pressure of the newly concentrated lymph exerts itself. When one considers the likely concentration of lymph in the initial lymphatics, its further concentration in the compressed collecting lymphatics, its subsequent dilution in the uncompressed ones, and its continual alterations with the varying pressures, it is evident that it would indeed be remarkable if it bore much resemblance to the tissue fluid from which it originated. One would expect it rather to resemble the fluid in the tissues through which the collecting vessel passed, particularly the fluid in the walls of the lymphatic itself, which may exchange with the vasa lymphorum (Yoffey and Courtice, 1970). [Some workers, however, consider that there is little alteration in the lymph during the passage (Staub et al., 1975; Vriem et al., 1975; Yoffey and Courtice, 1970), but evidence against this view has been presented above.] To these other alterations in the lymph must be added the effects of the addition of lymphocytes at the nodes, plus any addition or removal of macromolecules, etc. (Pressman et al., 1970; Rusznyák et al., 1967).

The lymph is usually discharged into the veins in the neck from the thoracic and right lymph ducts. Other lymphaticovenous communications exist, at least potentially (depending on relative pressures) (Rusznyák et al., 1967; Yoffey and Courtice, 1970). Although these other communications are usually considered only to function if the more central collecting ducts are relatively overloaded, it appears that rather more lymph is produced than can be collected from the thoracic and right lymph ducts, so these other communications may also function normally to some·extent (Yoffey and Courtice, 1970).

CONTROL MECHANISMS OF LYMPHATIC FUNCTION

Initial Lymphatics

The basic reason for the existence of the lymphatic system is to serve the needs of the tissues. As might be expected, therefore, the structure and function of the system have evolved so that the lymphatic output is greatest when the needs of the tissues are greatest.

Tissue metabolism often produces excessive amounts of macromolecules that are too large to pass into the blood vessel system via the junctions and that are too numerous to be carried into them by the vesicles. To these will be added extra plasma proteins escaping from the blood vessels as the metabolically caused vasodilatation increases the surface area of the blood endothelium and makes it thinner—both of which will increase vesicular transport. Because of these extra macromolecules, both from the blood and from metabolism water will also accumulate. Thus the tissues will tend to swell and tissue hydrostatic pressure will rise, becoming less negative. This will increase the flow of water, and macromolecules escaping via the lymphatics. Thus a negative-feedback, homeostatic situation exists. It has been calculated (Elhay and Casley-Smith, 1976) that such a situation even exists intrinsically in the initial lymphatic cycle itself.

In regions with fenestrated capillaries (e.g., the viscera) metabolic products of the tissue will easily enter the blood vessels (*vide infra*), but the dilation of the blood vessels produced by the metabolism will allow more plasma proteins than usual to enter the tissues. As explained later, in spite of the ability of fenestrae to remove large amounts of proteins from the tissues, there will still be a net accumulation, both needing and causing removal by the lymphatics.

To this accumulation are frequently added ingested macromolecules (e.g., in the intestine). The smaller macromolecules will be able to enter the fenestrae, but larger ones (e.g., γ-globulins, lipoproteins and chylomicra) (Figure 10) will not. The larger ones will not add significantly to the colloidal osmotic pressure, and their transport will depend on the flow of fluid produced by that of the smaller ones and any additional plasma proteins. One wonders if this may be the reason for the seemingly unique ability of the chylomicra to be transported across the lymphatic endothelium in large vesicles. If chylomicra are present, but there is little metabolic activity, they may have to rely largely on this mechanism to carry them slowly into the lymphatics.

Muscular activity in itself has a considerable effect on lymphatic functioning. This is not only because of the increased amounts of fluid in the tissues caused by the increased metabolic rate, but because the solid-tissue pressures are greatly increased during muscular contractions. In addition, many muscular activities caused the period of the initial lymphatic cycle to shorten, e.g., in running. There are thus different ways in which the lymphatics, which are so important in muscles, have their output linked to the metabolic state of the muscles, in a homeostatic system.

Metabolically active regions that do not have varying solid-tissue pressures from adjacent muscles are compromised. Some, of course, are greatly affected by respiration, or even by the pulse. It is more difficult to see, however, how organs such as the testes, ovaries, or kidneys achieve the necessary variations in pressure. Periodic transmitted pressures may be an answer; anyone who has watched the gyrations of the scrota of running animals will realize that this is quite likely. But ovaries and kidneys are more puzzling. There is evidence that these tightly encapsulated organs have tissue hydrostatic pressures well above atmospheric. This is perhaps produced by the accumulation of macromolecules, because the lymphatics will not function until this happens. Since the collecting lymphatics external to the organs are able to keep their internal pressures down to about 0, perhaps the initial lymphatics in these organs simply act as ducts, with normally very little pumping activity. Even under these circumstances it can be seen that the removal of macromolecules and fluid will still be homeostatically directed, by flow variations caused by intracapsular hydrostatic pressure variations.

As is well known, the lymphatics are extremely important in inflammation (Casley-Smith, 1973; Rusznyák et al., 1967; Yoffey and Courtice, 1970). The opening of the blood vascular junctions and the destruction of the cells cause many macromolecules and their osmotically associated water to accumulate in the tissues. Here, as has been mentioned, the edema causes the anchoring fibers to become taut, thus dilating the initial lymphatics and opening the junctions. This, together with the positive hydrostatic pressure gradients, will cause rapid lymphatic filling. Again, homeostasis is evident. Any overdistention, however, will prevent the junctions from sealing during the emptying phase, while discontinuities in the vessels' walls (which often are caused by severe injuries) will also tend to vitiate the effects of lymphatic pumping.

Vascular edema, i.e., that produced by raised blood hydrostatic pressures, or lowered blood osmotic ones, is less serious. Here there is no excessive protein to be carried away, so at least in theory all the ultrafiltered small molecules can reenter the blood if conditions are changed. Actually, as the tissue swells, hydrostatic pressures become less negative, and lymph flow increases. When the pressures reach 0 cm, lymph flow is maximal; after this, edema commences, as the lymphatic capacity is exceeded (Guyton, 1969; Guyton et al., 1971; Taylor et al., 1973, 1976b).

Lymphedema is produced by a deficiency in the functioning or capacity of the vessels, which causes the intralymphatic pressures to rise, and the vessels to dilate and their valves to become incompetent. Eventually this extends back to the initial lymphatics. Here there are two possible situations (Casley-Smith, 1973c; Casley-Smith, Földi-Börcsök, and Földi, 1974). If the tissues are loose, these vessels dilate widely and their inlet valves become incompetent (Casley-Smith, Földi, and Zoltán, 1969; Casley-Smith et al., 1974); if the tissues are relatively firm (e.g., the villi) such gross dilation is prevented and the junctions all become closed (Kalima, 1971; Casley-Smith et al., 1974) by the high intralymphatic pressure. A beneficial positive feedback is possible here from any therapy or condition that reduces the extent of the edema and the intralymphatic pressures. The less distended vessels may function better, hence further reducing the edema (Casley-Smith, 1976a).

Collecting Lymphatics

The lymphangions, or segments of the collecting lymphatics, are influenced by a number of factors (Mislin, 1967). When isolated, they have been shown to have varying frequencies that can be influenced by both natural and artificial stimuli. (They normally beat between 8–22 times per minute.) The most important influence is intravascular pressure. When this is raised, and the vessels dilate, the frequency and the strength of the beats increase rapidly. Thus this situation is very similar to Starling's law of the heart, with all its implications of negative feedback and homeostasis. Adrenaline causes an increase in the frequency, which is abolished with ergotamine; the stimulation of the sympathetic system in the intact animal also has this effect. Acetylcholine causes relaxation and inhibits the beat, but it is considered that the adrenergic structures are more important than the cholinergic ones for the regulation of the lymphangions. It is highly likely that the nonmyelinated nerves, frequent in these vessels, serve as afferents from pressure detectors, and as efferents from the sympathetic system to adjust tone and beat. In particular, lymphatic spasm occurs in some conditions, e.g. inflammation, which can be released by chemical or surgical sympathectomy (Rusznyák et al., 1967).

The coordination of the activities of adjacent lymphangions is achieved in different ways. Possibly there is direct passage of the contractile stimulus, but the most important factor is the initiation of contraction in one lymphangion by the dilatation produced by the inflow of lymph from the peripherally adjacent lymphangion, which had contracted slightly earlier.

In a recent, most comprehensive review, Vogel (1972) discusses the pharmacology of the lymph and the lymphatic system. He points out that it is essential to differentiate between drugs (and normal physiologic mechanisms) that affect lymph flow or composition because of their effects on the blood vascular system's components and hemodynamics, those that affect the blood–lymph barrier, and those that affect the lymphatics per se. There are many drugs that affect the lymph by affecting the blood vasculature; in general, it can be said that if the available surface area of the blood vessels in a region or the blood pressure is increased, then lymph flow will rise. In addition, if the permeability of the blood vasculature is increased to macromolecules (i.e., if the blood–lymph barrier is affected), then the amounts of these carried by the lymph will also increase. Their actual concentrations in the lymph will depend on the relative increases in permeability to them, as compared with the amount of increased fluid flow. The results also depend greatly on the region involved. Thus, e.g., Lehmann (1968) found that noradrenaline or angiotensin cause only minimal changes in the lymph flow from the hindleg of a dog, but that there is a great increase in the concentration of dextran (passing from the blood) in the lymph; in the dog liver he found that these substances produced great increases in lymph flow, with a lesser increase in the concentration of dextran. As can be seen, the whole situation regarding drugs affecting either hemodynamics or the blood–lymph barrier is very complex to unravel, not the least because of the possible effects of the connective tissue (Laurent, 1970) on the barrier. Details of the effects of many drugs are given by Vogel (1972).

True lymphotropic drugs are those that act on the tone or on the spontaneous motor activity of lymph vessels. These are also well reviewed by Vogel (1972) and by Mislin (1967, 1972). The importance of these can be seen from the fact that, contrary to earlier opinions, most workers now believe that spontaneous contractions of the lymphangions is almost universal and is of great

464   Casley–Smith

importance for the transport of lymph to the blood. In general, stimuli that directly affect the tone of the blood vasculature, or have neurogenic affects upon it, usually act in a similar fashion on the lymphatics. It is important to remember that anesthetics can greatly depress the activity of the lymphangions— hence some of the earlier confusion about the contractility of lymphatics in various species. It is now known that anesthetics have direct actions on vascular smooth muscle cells (Altura and Altura, 1975; Altura, Edgarian, and Altura, 1976). The effect of certain drugs on lymphangions varies from their effects on blood vessels; some increase both the amplitude and beat frequency of the lymphangions, others decrease both, while yet others increase one and decrease the other. For example (Mislin, 1972), noradrenaline, coumarin, and rutin increase both amplitude (inotropic effect) and frequency (chronotropic effect); papaverin and ergotomine decrease both; histamine and caffeine increase the frequency, but do not alter the amplitude; procaine in low doses increases the frequency, but lowers the amplitude.

A number of drugs, of which coumarin is an example, are known to have the effect of increasing lymph flow (Collard, 1971; Földi-Börcsök, Bedell and Rahlfs, 1971; Mislin, 1971). It seems to act analogously to digitalis on the heart. The efficiency of the contraction of the lymphangions is improved. It should be mentioned that this effect of coumarin is quite distinct from the mode of action of coumarin in causing proteolysis (vide infra). (In many edemas, which coumarin attenuates, the lymphatics are already working at maximal efficiency and coumarin produces no increase in the amount of lymph flow.) It is only in lymphedemas produced by poorly functioning collecting lymphatics or in normal animals that this "digitalis" effect occurs and lymph flow is increased (Földi-Börcsök, 1972).

COMPARATIVE MORPHOLOGY AND FUNCTION OF LYMPHATICS AND BLOOD VESSELS

The gross and light microscopic aspects have been reviewed by Drinker (1942) and more extensively by Kampmeier (1969). The fine structure has been reviewed by Casley-Smith (1971a) and Casley-Smith and Casley-Smith (1975).

In both the vertebrates and the invertebrates one finds that on ascending from the primitive to the more highly developed animals, and in passing from the peripheral vessels to the central ones, the vessels become more complex (Figure 27). In the periphery of primitive animals (e.g., amphioxus, Figure 28) the peripheral vessels have only very scattered endothelial cells with large gaps between them; the vessels simply consist of a basement membrane. At times, even portions of this are absent so that the vessel is partly lined by only the more solid elements of the tissues, much like prelymphatics in mammals. The more central vessels, both arterial and venous, gradually possess more and more continuous endothelium, until all the junctions are closed. Amphiouxus only has

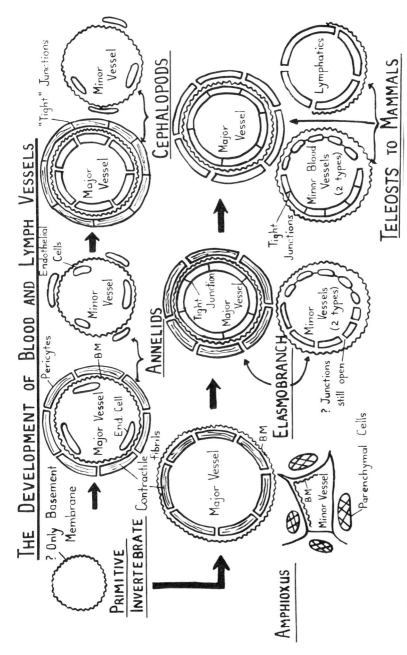

Figure 27. A diagram showing the similar, yet divergent, development of the bascular systems in the vertebrates and invertebrates. The relations of open capillary junctions, fenestrae, and lymphatics are indicated. (The hagfish have been found to occupy a position between amphioxus and elasmobranchs, as might be expected.)

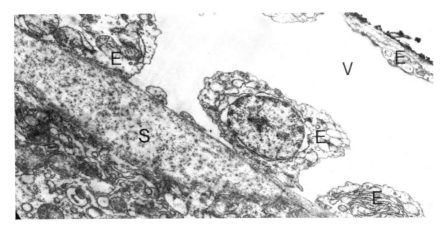

Figure 28. In the gut of amphioxus, the hepatic vein (V) has large openings between its endothelial cells (E). Only a basement membrane lines an adjacent sinusoid (S), which contains lipoproteins. ×5,000.

endothelial cells, which curiously have many contactile fibrils in the dorsal and ventral aortae. Both annelids and hagfish have pericytes, which become continuous in the major vessels and in some regions develop contractile fibrils to propel the blood.

This trend is even more developed in both the higher vertebrates and invertebrates. In the vertebrates it is the junctions of the endothelium that become close and tight, thus keeping most of the blood in the vascular system; in the cephalopods it is apparently the pericyte junctions that develop this capability. In the vertebrates, the elasmobranchs still seem to retain the primitive feature of openable blood vascular junctions in their venous capillaries. These have many features that resemble those of mammalian lymphatics rather than mammalian blood capillaries and venules (Figure 29; Casley-Smith and Mart, 1970). Thus they have many anchoring filaments attached to the exterior of the vessels, a paucity of attachment devices and basement membrane, and occasional open junctions.

It is highly likely that this development in vascular structure is necessitated by the increase in blood vascular hydrostatic pressure which serves the increased metabolisms of the higher animals. In order to maintain Starling's equilibrium, the plasma proteins also increase in parallel with these elevations in hydrostatic pressure. In turn, the development of closed junctions, first in the central vessels where the pressures are high, then throughout the animals, is necessary to withstand these raised pressures and to prevent the excessive leakage of the plasma proteins. Since, however, the vessels contain vesicles, the proteins will continually leak out of the system, as well as pass out of the open junctions on the arterial side of the circulation. The problem then is how to return these proteins to the circulation.

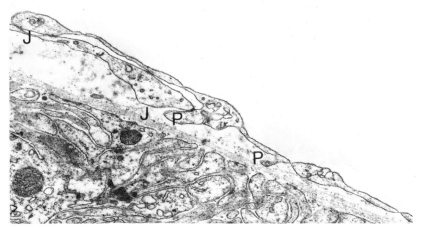

Figure 29. In the kidneys of the elasmobranchs, the venous capillaries have junctions that often appear openable (JJ). There are ablumenal projections (P), to which filaments attach, and poorly developed basement membranes—all features similar to those of mammalian lymphatics. Fenestrae are frequent. ×12,000.

In the primitive animals this is solved very simply by the flow of fluid through the tissues, in accordance with Starling's hypothesis, carrying the excess protein into the blood vessels via the open junctions in the vessels on the venous side of the circulation. Even in the elasmobranch this seems to still be occurring, perhaps aided by the temporary increases in the tissue hydrostatic pressures during swimming motion, etc. In the torpedoes, teleosts, and the higher vertebrates this can no longer happen. The venous junctions are no longer open, perhaps because the blood pressures are increased very sharply in the teleosts as compared to those in the elasmobranchs, especially the pressures in the veins, which pass from negative to positive. A portion of the old blood vascular system, however, was still retained. These evolved initially in the lateral body wall of teleosts and were the first true lymphatics (Kampmeier, 1969; Rusznyák et al., 1967). They later developed in most of the rest of the body. In the regions where they did not form, there were existing prelymphatics, with which they became united. (These occur throughout the body in the most primitive animals; in fact, the development of the vasculature may be looked upon as simply a process whereby certain of these paths became progressively lined.) The lymphatics are able to take up and transmit the proteins because they usually have much lower hydrostatic pressures than the veins, and the periods when these pressures are raised to levels higher than venous pressure occur only intermittently. Thus it is the periodic high-pressure pumping, coupled with much lower pressures during the filling phase, which is so vital for the role of the lymphatic system.

It is of interest, in view of the similarity of some of the roles of lymphatics and fenestrae (*vide infra*), that fenestrae appear to have developed during evolution between the hagfish and elasmobranch stages (Figures 27 and 29). Thus they antedate the true lymphatics.

As is shown later, the fenestrae probably allow considerable local circulation of fluid and macromolecules, from and to the blood vessels, without much passing to the lymphatics. In the more primitive animals the many open junctions probably allow fluid movement, but this ceases when most of the junctions become closed. Perhaps the fenestrae are a device to permit local circulation to continue in the sites, e.g., the viscera, where this may be important. In addition, the fenestrae permit the ready passage of macromolecules into the blood vessels from regions where these appear de novo in the tissues. Thus in the gut of the elasmobranch (Casley-Smith and Mart, 1970) the lipoproteins enter the blood via the fenestrae.

FENESTRATED BLOOD CAPILLARIES

Structure and Permeability

Fenestrated blood capillaries (Figures 10, 30, and 31) are common in many regions of the body, in general, in the viscera. Their occurrence, structure, dimensions, numbers, and permeability are reviewed by Casley-Smith (1971*b*), Casley-Smith et al. (1975*a*), Clementi and Palade (1969), Karnovsky (1968), Majno (1965), Simionescu, Simionescu, and Palade (1972), and Venkatachalam and Karnovsky (1972). They are holes through thin ($\sim$0.1 μ) portions of the endothelium, which are often, but by no means invariably, crossed by a diaphragm (Casley-Smith, 1971; Casley-Smith et al., 1974). The composition of this diaphragm is uncertain, but it is likely to be mucoprotein, probably representing the fused two outer laminae of the two plasma membranes, such as occurs with diaphragms across attached vesicles (Palade and Bruns, 1968). (Since the proportions of diaphragms are about the same in vesicles and in fenestrae, one wonders if the life of a fenestra is similar to the attachment time of a vesicle, $\sim$6 sec; *vide supra*.) Fenestrae are usually about 50 nm in diameter, but sometimes are up to about 200 nm in the renal glomeruli and in the liver (Wisse, 1970).

Their occurrence is very variable. Occasionally, they are found in small numbers in many nonvisceral tissues. In the viscera, however, they are present in almost all regions. They are particularly common in the gut, exocrine and endocrine glands, and the urinary tract. Even in these regions they are variable; this is probably because they predominantly occur on the venous limbs of capillaries (Casley-Smith, 1971*b*). This arteriovenous difference has been found wherever this has been investigated (except in the glomeruli). Thus it has been found to occur in the rete mirabile of the kidney and swim bladder, in the jejunum, the adrenal cortex, the ciliary body, the growing edge of carcinomas

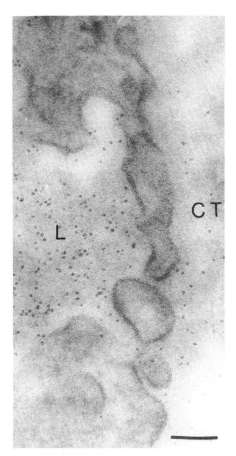

Figure 30. Ferritin was injected into the blood of mice. Here it is seen 4 min later, passing out some fenestrae in an arterial limb of a capillary in the jejunum, from the lumen (L) to the connective tissue (CT). (Details for Figures 30 and 31 are given in Casley-Smith, 1970c.) 125,000×; the line is 0.1 μ.

(Warren, 1970, and personal communication), even among the rare fenestrae in the skin, and the external ocular muscles of rodents (Zed, personal communication). (This latter is unusual since fenestrae are very rare, or absent, in most muscles except the tongue; these are the only muscular areas where they have been found in large numbers; Collin, 1969b).

It was originally thought that the fenestrae were relatively impermeable to macromolecules, but this is now known not to be the case (see reviews above). It has been shown experimentally (Figures 30 and 31) (Casley-Smith, 1970c) that ferritin leaves the vessels mainly via the fenestrae on the arterial limbs and enters them via those on the venous limbs. Since fenestrae in venous limbs are so much more frequent and since the large-molecular-weight tracers, when injected into

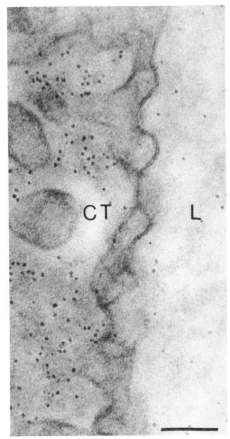

Figure 31. Ferritin was injected into the renal medulla. The ferritin is seen, 8 min after injection, passing from the connective tissues (CT) to the lumen (L). 150,000×; the line is 0.1 μ.

the blood, would almost exclusively enter rather than exit via these fenestrae, it is not surprising that few were seen the leave the vessels. The smaller macromolecules (peroxidase) are able to leave even the venous fenestrae in large amounts, while uptake from the tissues (in the direction of flow) also serves to show their patency (Casley-Smith, 1970c; Hodel, 1970).

Function

A priori, the presence of a few fenestrae on the arterial limbs, and many on the venous limbs, would be ideally suited to allow large amounts of fluid and macromolecules to enter the tissues and to leave them again. The renal glomeruli that are exclusively "arterial" limbs of capillaries are specialized to allow exit; other regions with only venous limb fenestrae, e.g., the retia mirabile, seem specialized for rapid uptake. Possibly the relationship between exit and uptake of fluid needed in a region determines the relative proportions of fenestrae in the two capillary limbs. (Naturally, the "limbs" are only a statistical concept, because of the variable conditions in the capillaries; over a whole region such a generalization is justified). This concept of the functioning of fenestrae fits well with the pattern of fluid flow through the tissues as predicted by Starling's hypothesis, and the carriage of macromolecules by it. The great outward permeability of fenestrated regions is well known (Studer and Potchen, 1971); some direct evidence is becoming available about the role played by fenestrae in the removal of proteins from the tissues. This is discussed later. There are, however, a number of features that need further consideration.

One of these is the osmotic–hydrostatic pressure relationships across the fenestrae. As with the open junctions of lymphatics (*vide supra*), it has been necessary to establish that substantial effective osmotic pressures are possible in the presence of quite large pores. This has been done in vitro (Casley-Smith and Bolton, 1973*a*), where it was shown that effective osmotic pressures (~0.8 of those across the semipermeable membranes) probably occur across fenestrae, as the flow of fluid keeps the proteins in the vessels, establishing a "virtual membrane" across the inner ends of the pores (Casley-Smith, 1975*a*).

Quantitative electron microscopy combined with sterology has allowed us to measure the numbers and dimensions of the fenestrae in the cat intestine (Casley-Smith et al., 1975*a*). Using normal physical laws the capillary filtration and diffusion coefficients could be calculated, and it was found that they were many times greater than those actually observed. Thus it was shown that in this site the fenestrated capillaries are so permeable that the endothelium, while it may influence the passage of macromolecules, has no effect on small molecules; the penetration of these is controlled by the interstitial tissues. Thus these correspond to the tunnel capillaries of Intaglietta and de Plomb (1973), whose calculations and our data allowed us to predict the filtration coefficient that is actually observed. Injured, continuous capillaries (Casley-Smith and Window, 1976) also form temporary tunnel capillaries while their junctions are open. It has been shown (Casley-Smith, 1975*b*) that normally the continuous capillaries of dog skeletal muscle correspond to Intaglietta and de Plomb's tube capillaries, in that measurements of their numbers, junctional dimensions, etc., allow us to predict the capillary filtration coefficient found by experiment, although there is still some interstitial tissue influence on the capillary diffusion coefficient.

The directional permeability of these fenestrae is crucial to this concept and has experimental support (Figures 30 and 31) (Casley-Smith, 1970*c*). At the arterial fenestrae there is no problem; both fluid flow and diffusion of proteins are in the same direction. At the venous fenestrae there is similarly no problem for macromolecules (and indeed small molecules) manufactured at, or ingested into, a region. Here again the local concentrations are such that the direction or diffusion is into the blood, as is the flow of fluid. The only difficulty occurs when one is considering plasma proteins that have passed into the tissues. For these, the flow of fluid is again into the venous fenestrae, but diffusion is directed outward because of the concentration gradients. If the diaphragms of the fenestrae were permanent features, similar to the ground substance, one could see how macromolecules could be forced through them by the flow of fluid, causing them to push a path through the meshwork; by contrast, outward diffusion would be prevented since the flow of fluid would not be available to cause this penetration; in fact, it would oppose it. While it is true that many venous fenestrae have diaphragms, it is probable that this directional permeability can occur in "diaphragmless fenestrae" (Casley-Smith, 1976b). This is because the rapid flow of fluid could still carry more proteins in than could diffuse out. This has been demonstrated both in vitro and in mathematical models (Casley-Smith, 1975a,b, 1976b; Perl, 1975). It should be noted that, if the molecules are substantially smaller than albumin, outward diffusion will often be greater than inward bulk flow; those molecules that are too big will suffer very great molecular sieving and not pass at all.

The in vitro model was the same as that described earlier for the open junction of the lymphatic system (Casley-Smith, 1975b). It could be seen that there is a considerable net inflow of both fluid and proteins in spite of reasonable outwardly directed hydrostatic pressures. A mathematical model (Casley-Smith, 1976b) was constructed by using physical laws for flow through the size of openings for fenestrae and for diffusion. The flow of fluid and the net transfer of proteins were calculated, taking into account the variations in molecular sieving mentioned above, for varying protein concentrations in the connective tissue, and varying net hydrostatic pressure. Some of these results are for "diaphragmless fenestrae" (diameter ~50 nm) shown in Figure 32. If, e.g., −10 cm of water is taken as a reasonable figure for the net hydrostatic pressure difference, on the venous limb it can be seen that the model predicts considerable amounts of inward transfer of both fluids and protein for most reasonable concentrations of protein in the connective tissue. It will be noted that if the hydrostatic pressure difference is made more negative, fluid is still taken up after protein is lost.

It will also be noted that the concentration of the proteins in the fluid leaving the tissues is less than that in the tissues because of molecular sieving and back-diffusion (Casley-Smith, 1976b). Similarly, the fluid passing out of arterial fenestrae will be more concentrated than that in the tissues. Hence the fenestrae alone will not clear the tissues of plasma proteins, although they will maintain a much increased local circulation through them. Thus some other means must be available to remove the surplus proteins, e.g., the lymphatics (Figure 33), as is shown by the fact that there is always a transport of proteins away from fenestrated regions via this system. This concept, that the fenestrae are incapable of removing all the plasma protein from the tissues, is a refinement of the previous hypothesis, which was that they virtually take over the role of the

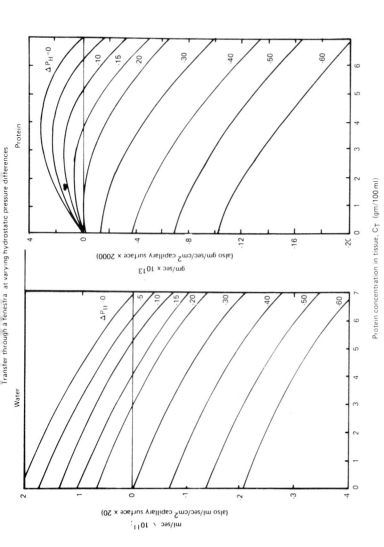

Figure 32. The results of a mathematical simulation of the net water and protein transfer through a diaphragmless 50-nm fenestra, as described in the text. The net transfers vary with the net hydrostatic pressures (P_H, in cm of H_2O) and the concentration of proteins in the tissues (C_T). Transfer above the line implies passage directed out of the capillary. It can be seen that for reasonable estimates of C_T and venous limb P_H (5–15 cm) there will be a net inward transfer of both water and protein. For reasonable arterial limb P_H (20–40 cm) there will be an outward transfer. Simple calculations show that the ratio of protein leaving the tissue, via the fenestrae, to the water doing so, is always less than the concentration of protein in the tissues; hence the latter will tend to become more concentrated through the action of fenestrae alone.

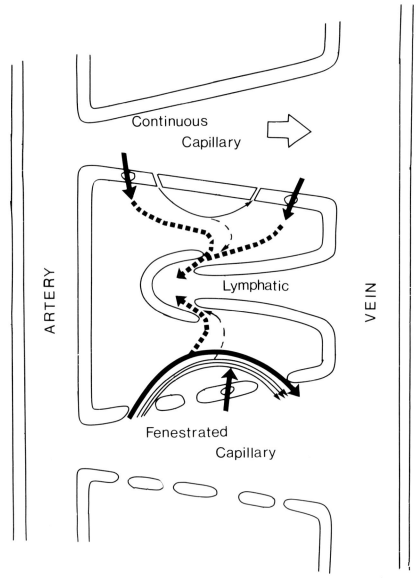

Figure 33. A diagram to show the roles of the blood capillaries and the lymphatics in fenestrated and nonfenestrated regions. The net outward passage of proteins (thick lines) via vesicles and the outward and inward passage of water (thin lines) via close junctions are shown for the continuous capillary. The same occurs for the fenestrated capillary, but the fenestrae also allow an enormous local circulation of water and protein. Some protein, together with its associated water, passes to the lymphatics, from both kinds of capillaries. Protein formed *de novo* in the tissues will pass to both capillaries and to the lymphatics.

lymphatics by removing almost all macromolecules from the tissues (Casley-Smith, 1970c, 1971a,b, 1972). It is still considered that they have this role for proteins ingested, or formed *de novo* in the tissues (*vide infra*). It now seems, however, that in the case of plasma proteins that continually arrive at the tissues, while most return to the blood via the fenestrae, the lymphatics are necessary to carry off the excess. This would also apply if proteins are continually formed *de novo*, or ingested, but not if these only occur periodically, between those times during which they can be cleared from the tissues by the fenestrae.

Recently, Casley-Smith et al. (1975a) quantified the fenestrae in cat jejunum and found that filtration and diffusion were not limited by these structures, but by the interstitial tissue; i.e., the fenestrated capillaries correspond to the "tunnel capillaries" hypothesized by Intaglietta and de Plomb (1973), whose calculations could be combined with the above data on fenestrae to yield a filtration coefficient identical with that observed by physiologic measurements. It was also possible to confirm that much more fluid and protein returns to the venous fenestrae than enters the lymphatics. Fenestrated capillaries could also be shown to permit a nontraumatic approach to the interstitial tissue. It was calculated that the channels through the tissues are about 60 nm in effective radius, at least 40 μ long and are about 60 times more numerous at the blood capillaries than elsewhere in the tissues. This radius corresponds well with Chase's (1959) estimates. This also gives a reasonable agreement with the dimensions of the prelymphatics visible near lymphatics.

Using the data mentioned in the last paragraph it has been possible (Casley-Smith, 1976b) to construct a mathematical model of the changes in protein concentration, osmotic pressure, and resultant hydrostatic pressure in the various regions through which material passes from the arterial-limb fenestrae to those on the venous limbs (Figures 34–36). The calculations concerned with protein concentrations have been confirmed by autoradiographic observations (Casley-Smith and Sims, 1976). It can be shown that the basement membranes here are very important in regulating the passage of macromolecules; this contrasts with their negligible roles in regulating the passage of small molecules (Casley-Smith et al., 1975b). It can also be shown that the concentration of the lymph in the initial lymphatics would increase the "safety margin" against edema by considerably lowering the negative hydrostatic pressure in the tissue channels (Guyton et al., 1971). If the lymphatics do not function at all, this pressure rises, becomes positive, and edema will occur (Figure 36).

ROLE OF THE LYMPHATICS IN EXCHANGE IN NORMAL TISSUE

There are two main classes of substances to consider when discussing the roles of the lymphatics. One of these is the small molecules ($<\sim$2,000 M.W.), including water. In fact, we need really only discuss water since the diffusion of the other small molecules is so rapid that any concentration differences in them will be

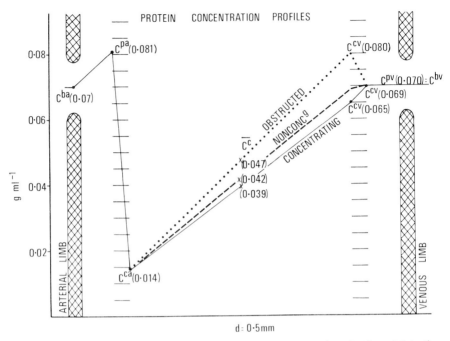

Figure 34. The results of calculations of the protein concentrations in the cat intestine (Casley-Smith, 1975*d*). Values of 26, 6, and 60 nm were assumed for the radii of the fenestrae, at pores through the basement membrane and of the tissue channels. The protein concentrations (in g/ml) are shown at various sites. It can be seen that the arterial-limb membrane causes a backing-up of the protein, which diminishes to a lower concentration just after this effect. The concentration of protein rises as the channel (0.5 mm long) is traversed. Three possible conditions are shown for the lymphatic system (concentrating, nonconcentrating, and obstructed). The effects of these on the mean concentration (C^c) and that near the venous limb (C^{cv}) can be seen; although the lymphatic system does not seem to cause much of a reduction in the protein concentration, the data in Figures 35 and 36 indicate that this is indeed very significant.

equilibrated very rapidly compared with the relatively long time scale of the lymphatic cycle. The second, perhaps even more important, class is that of the macromolecules. In general, these lie between 20,000 and 2,000,000 M.W.; i.e., large enough not to be able to pass through the close junctions of blood capillaries in significant amounts, but small enough so that reasonable concentrations of them can exert significant osmotic pressures. Other classes include the largest macromolecules, ranging in size up to chylomicra, cells, and large cellular fragments.

Small Molecules

There is no question but that the small molecules are predominantly transported by the blood vessels (see reviews by Landis and Pappenheimer, 1963; Renkin,

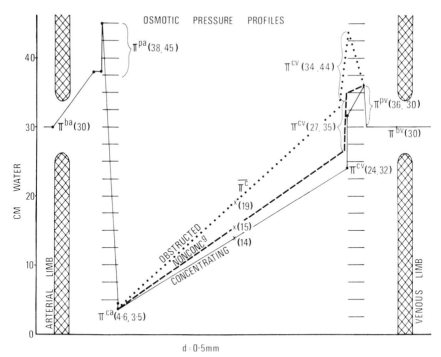

Figure 35. Here are plotted the colloidal osmotic pressures associated with the concentrations shown in Figure 34. The sites pa, ca, cv, and pv all have two pressures shown. This is
because Casley-Smith and Bolton (1973a) found that the radius of the pore influences the
effective osmotic pressure, and this was included in these calculations. (The effect is
different quantitatively from the reflection coefficient normally calculated for smaller
molecules).

1971; Rusznyák et al., 1967; and Yoffey and Courtice, 1970). This is particularly so if the very permeable fenestrae are present (Clementi and Palade, 1969).
It is true that if considerable amounts of water are present in the tissues, lymph
output becomes greatly increased (Taylor et al., 1973). This can be seen in active
muscles (although it is necessary to distinguish carefully between the simple
rapid expulsion of lymph already in the lymphatics, and new lymph formed as a
result of the activity). However, the fact that so many more of the small
molecules pass to the blood than to the lymph indicates that it is the system of
blood vessels which is far more important for their removal. Nevertheless, as
discussed later, the lymphatics exercise a crucial role, qualitatively, although not
quantitatively, in the prevention of vascular edema.

Macromolecules

It is the plasma proteins in the tissues for which the lymphatic system is vital
(Figure 33); they have to carry 50% of the total plasma protein pool back to the

478   Casley–Smith

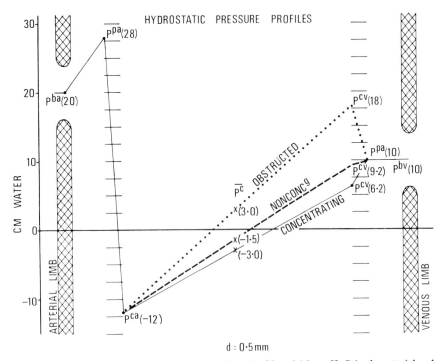

d = 0·5 mm

Figure 36. Hydrostatic pressures were assumed to be 20 and 10 cm H₂O in the arterial and venous limbs. The resulting hydrostatic pressures (using the results of Figure 35) are shown here for the various sites in the tissues. (It was shown that the net pressures across the fenestrae and the membranes are in approximate equilibrium). It can be seen that, if the lymphatics are obstructed, the mean pressure in the tissue channels rises above zero, which will cause edema. In this model, assuming the lymphatics can concentrate proteins, this could result in doubling of the "safety margin" against edema produced by the lymphatic system [cf. the mean pressures (Pᶜ) produced by the concentrating as against the nonconcentrating lymphatics]. This model shows that 80% of the protein entering the tissues passes to the blood via the venous limb fenestrae and only 20% returns via the lymphatic system, yet it can be seen that this latter is essential if edema is to be avoided.

blood every 24 hr (Yoffey and Courtice, 1970). These proteins cannot be removed by the vascular system. They are too big to be carried into the vessels by the flow of fluid entering the close junctions of the venous capillaries and venules. Nevertheless, all along the vessels there is a continual slow net leakage of these proteins via the endothelial vesicles, because of the concentration gradient from the blood to the tissues. In the absence of lymphatics, or of sufficient protein catabolism, the proteins would accumulate in the tissues until their concentrations approximated those in the blood. (Such high rates of catabolism do not normally exist, although they can be produced by the action of coumarin if suitable cells are present in the tissues; *vide infra*.)

In regions with fenestrated capillaries the situation is similar (Figure 33), although somewhat different mechanisms are at work. Here again there is likely to be a net accumulation of proteins in the tissues. This is not only because of the continual leakage of proteins via vesicles all along the vessels, although such vesicles as occur (they are much less frequent here) will undoubtedly add their relatively small contribution to the pool. Instead, there is probably a large, continuous passage of proteins through the tissues; more, however, are added than removed (Casley-Smith, 1975a; Casley-Smith et al., 1975a). The same situation will indeed apply even if there are no arterial-limb fenestrae and only venous-limb ones are present, removing material. This is because even here the fluid removed will contain a smaller concentration of proteins than the tissue fluid (Casley-Smith, 1975a, 1976b). Hence again the lymphatic system is vital for the removal of accumulating plasma proteins in the tissues. (It should perhaps be pointed out that the determinations of blood capillary permeability, which depend on the measurement of the amounts of a tracer in the lymph from a region, will be greatly in error in regions where there are many fenestrae, because of the amounts of material that pass directly back to the blood and do not enter the lymph at all.)

This problem of a net protein outflow from the capillaries does not apply in the cases of proteins that have been ingested or formed *de novo* in a region. Here the concentration gradients will usually be directed from the tissues to the blood. Thus the vesicles will carry the material into the blood, albeit slowly, provided the molecular sizes are such that they can enter these bodies. The fenestrae, if present, will provide a much more permeable path. While the fluid outflow from the arterial-limb fenestrae will interfere with the inward diffusion of the molecules, some uptake is likely even here. On the venous limbs, the fluid flow and the diffusion will be in the same direction and the amount entering the vessels via fenestrae will be quite considerably greater. Thus the lymphatics are likely to be less important for these macromolecules than for the plasma proteins, especially if fenestrae are present. (This will not apply, however, if they are too large to enter fenestrae or vesicles.)

Quantitative Relationships between Lymphatics and Blood Vessels

When considering the question of the relative roles of the lymphatics and blood capillaries, it is evident that quantitative information such as can be supplied by physiologic methods on whole organs is essential. This can provide the numerical evidence necessary to apportion adequately the roles of the two systems in different sites and under different conditions. While there is considerable evidence (Rusznyák et al., 1967; Yoffey and Courtice, 1970) showing that very much larger amounts of the small molecules return to the blood directly rather than via the lymphatics, especially in the organs with fenestrated capillaries, there are very few experiments relating to macromolecules. This is no doubt because experiments involving these are much more difficult to perform—because of the sensitivity of the detection techniques needed, the difficulties caused by possible reentry of the tracer into the region from the blood, the difficulties of introducing the tracer in a physiologic manner, and the length of time necessary. Fortunately, a few experimental results are available, but they need to be supplemented with many more. Unfortunately, however, most give information primarily applicable to ingested and newly formed macromolecules; few give any information about the relative net movements of tissue plasma proteins.

It is certain that particles that are too large to enter vesicles and fenestrae are transported only by the lymph. The most notable member of this class is the chylomicron (Figure 10), but other examples are known, e.g., the γ-globulins ingested *in toto* by neonatal and fetal animals enter the lymph rather than the blood (reviewed by Yoffey and Courtice, 1970) presumably because of extreme molecular sieving. However, quite large macromolecules such as ferritin (Kraehen-buhl et al., 1967) have been observed passing to blood via fenestrae as well as to lymph, as has the smaller peroxidase (Hodel, 1970; Warshaw et al., 1971). In these experiments the tracer entered the connective tissue around the vessels "physiologically" and not by injection. The amounts passing by the two paths are not accurately quantified, and it is evident from the amounts entering the two systems, and the considerably greater blood than lymph flow, that much more probably entered the blood than the lymph.

Using small amounts of injected radio-albumin and other tracers, Jepson, Simeone, and Dobyns (1953) and Szabó, Magyar, and Molnár (1970, 1971, 1973, and personal communication) showed that the amounts of these macro-molecules taken up by the blood and the lymph were approximately equal in regions such as the skin and skeletal muscle where the blood capillaries are nonfenestrated. If the muscle was actively contracting, the relative amounts taken up by the lymph increased some 30 times. [In the heart, however, the clearance via the blood was some 4 times greater than via the lymph; this may be explained by the fact that, unlike the continuous capillaries of skeletal muscle, the capillaries of the subendocardial and intermediate regions of the heart are very permeable to macromolecules (Anversa, Giacomelli, and Weiner, 1973); the "close" junctions are here quite widely open and presumably function similarly to fenestrae.] By contrast, in regions where there are many fenestrated capil-laries (renal cortex, medulla, and liver) the uptake by the vascular system was very much more than via the lymphatics. [The liver has now been shown to possess large fenestrae rather than open junctions (Wisse, 1970).] In the pan-creas and the intestine, however, the transport by blood and lymph appeared about equal. It should be realized that such experiments using the injection of tracer (as against microinjection with vital microscopic control) can never be free from the possibility that material was just injected into injured blood vessels;

still, this possibility applies equally in both the fenestrated and nonfenestrated regions.

It is fortunate, therefore, that some other kinds of experiments have given very similar results. These (Courtice, Adams, and Shannon, 1976; Szabó, 1976a,b; Szabó et al., 1972, 1973, and personal communication) were done by using increased metabolism and injurious stimuli to induce the release of enzymes (20,000–100,000 M.W.) from various regions. Again it was found that substantial amounts of these passed into the blood as well as into the lymph. In nonfenestrated regions the amounts were roughly comparable, although rather greater for the blood (taking into account the much greater blood flow). In fenestrated regions, e.g., the intestine and liver, the amounts passing to the blood were very much greater than those passing to the lymph. It should be pointed out that such experiments as these apply only to the uptake of proteins appearing in the tissues *de novo* and not to the net passage of plasma proteins.

A different approach was used by Swann (1960) and Swann et al. (1961), investigating the permeability of the various compartments detectable by tracer analysis, in the kidney and the intestine. These results indicate that 11 mg of albumin/sec/100 g tissue can leave the very fenestrated blood vessels of the kidney while 3.7 mg albumin/sec/100 g tissue escape in the intestine (again presumably mainly via the fenestrae). Calculated lymphatic transport of albumin from these two regions is 0.04 and 0.02 mg/sec/100 g tissue, respectively. This indicates that the amount leaving, and presumably mostly reentering, the blood is 200–300 times that passing to the lymphatics. Additional proof of this blood–lymph transport difference was furnished by the fact that the (apparently) extravascular compartment could be filled with radio-albumin in 10 min, and could be washed out again in 10 min. During this time lymph flow would have been negligible.

The calculations of Casley-Smith et al. (1975a) indicate that 8 mg of albumin/min/100 g of jejunum tissue return to the blood, via the fenestrae, while only about 1 mg passes to the lymphatics. This agrees with the observation of Studer and Potchen (1971) on the rate of passage of albumin out of the vessels, which certainly does not leave via the lymphatics. This is 25 times less than the estimate of Swann et al. For reasons given in Casley-Smith et al. (1974a), it is considered that Swann et al. most certainly overestimated the amount returning to the blood. Even so, it can be seen that at least 90% of the albumin in the tissues seems to pass to the fenestrated capillaries in this region and only 10% to the lymph. While this proportion no doubt varies considerably with the region, it is likely to be considerably greater in, e.g., the kidneys. In the model (Casley-Smith, 1976b; Figure 34) it was found that about 20% of the protein entering the tissues was removed via the lymphatics, while about 80% went via the venous fenestrae. This quantitatively small amount could be shown to be qualitatively vital; it is essential for lowering the mean protein concentration in the tissues (and the resultant osmotic pressure and hydrostatic pressures) sufficiently to yield a negative tissue pressure rather than a positive one. Hence edema would be avoided (Guyton et al., 1971). It does appear, therefore, from a number of approaches, that the bulk of the tissue protein passes to the fenestrated capillaries (if these are present) while the lymphatics perform the essential task of removing the excess that would otherwise accumulate in the tissues.

ROLE OF THE LYMPHATICS IN EXCHANGE IN EDEMATOUS TISSUES

As Földi (1969) has remarked, any edema is a sign that the lymphatic system has failed. This is because no matter what conditions cause the fluid to accumulate in the tissues, the lymphatic system will remove it. In the case of low-protein (0.1–0.5 g/100 ml) edemas this will be simply by carrying large amounts of low-protein lymph; for edemas with high protein concentrations (1–5 g/100 ml), it is the protein that must be removed. It is very necessary to distinguish, however, between the relative significance of the roles of the lymphatics in the main classes of edema. (It is also important to realize that the various kinds of edema sometimes occur together; e.g., mechanical insufficiency can add its effects in inflammation).

Low-Protein Edemas

These are caused by the disturbances in the Starling equilibrium (Földi, 1969, Rusznyák et al., 1967; Yoffey and Courtice, 1970). Thus increased hydrostatic pressure, or reduced colloid osmotic pressure, cause excess water outflow compared with inflow. Because the permeability of the blood vascular walls is essentially unaltered, the fluid that passes to the tissues will have a very low protein content. (If, however, the hydrostatic pressure increases too much, the junctions will be opened and extra protein will escape, too). As the fluid accumulates in the tissues, the tissue hydrostatic pressure rises and causes lymph flow to increase (Taylor et al., 1973, 1976b). When the limit of the lymphatic capacity is reached, the tissue hydrostatic pressure becomes positive, and the further fluid accumulation causes edema to commence. From this it can be seen that here the lymphatics are acting as "safety valves" (Földi, 1969) or "spill-ways" (Drinker, 1942), tending to protect the tissue from "overflowing" with fluid and keeping the tissue hydrostatic pressures below zero. When the spillways become full, they can no longer keep the pressure down; once these become equal to atmospheric, the tissues swell rapidly and edema is visible.

This mere description of the mechanisms involved does not really allow us to judge the relative importance of the increased lymph flow in this situation. Certainly it provides a measure of defense against edema, but then so does the reduction of the tissue osmotic pressure and the increase in its hydrostatic pressure. It seems (Taylor et al., 1973, 1976b) that these amounts are about 7.4, 4, and 6.5 mm Hg, respectively, in the dog subcutaneous tissue, yielding the total 18 mm Hg increase in capillary pressure necessary to cause edema. Thus the lymphatic system here contributes about 40% of the "safety factor" against edema.

In the light of the earlier discussion about the relative lack of importance of the lymphatic system for the removal of small molecules from the tissues, it is interesting to consider what is happening in low-protein edema. Undoubtedly many more small molecules are passing to the blood vessels than to the lymphatics. This is because all that happens is that the alteration in the hydrostatic—osmotic pressure relationships simply moves the balance point between inflow and outflow so far along the blood vascular system toward the venous end that there is a *net* outflow. Thus there will still be a very great inflow of the small molecules into the blood vessels—much more than into the lymphatics. All the lymphatics really do in preventing edema is to remove the small extra amount that is necessary to restore the net balance. Thus the contribution of the lymphatic system here is quantitatively negligible, but qualitatively vital.

High-Protein, High-Flow Edemas

These occur when there is a considerable leakage of high-protein fluid from the blood vessels (Casley-Smith, 1973a; Földi, 1969; Rusznyák et al., 1967; Yoffey and Courtice, 1970). This usually follows injuries that open many blood vascular intercellular junctions (Majno, 1965). (One wonders, however, if they could be produced in regions with many fenestrated capillaries by simply raising the venous pressure enough to reverse the flow through a sufficient proportion of the fenestrae; although at least in the intestine this is less likely because of "autoregulation.") This situation is more complicated than the low-protein edemas. Again the lymphatics will be tending to provide the additional amount of fluid removal necessary to restore the balance between fluid outflow and inflow in the tissues. However, while most of the small molecules will still be able to reenter the blood vessels, with only a relatively small number having to pass to the lymphatics, the situation is very different for the protein.

While increased tissue protein concentrations will cause increases in both fenestral and vascular uptake, there is no mechanism by which increased blood vascular uptake could reduce the net outflow. Hence it must be removed by the lymphatics or by protein catabolism. Although undoubtedly a certain amount of such catabolism occurs (*vide infra*), a considerable amount of the proteins must normally have to be removed by the lymphatic system If this does not occur sufficiently, the accumulated protein will retain fluid by virtue of its osmotic action (Figures 11 and 37). Thus the edema will remain as long as the excess protein does. Hence in high-protein edemas we have two causes: excess fluid leakage, and protein accumulation causing even more excess fluid. In the first case the lymphatics function as they do in low-protein edemas, tending to maintain the balance between fluid outflow and inflow. In the second, they are very important for the removal of the proteins, which otherwise will retain fluid.

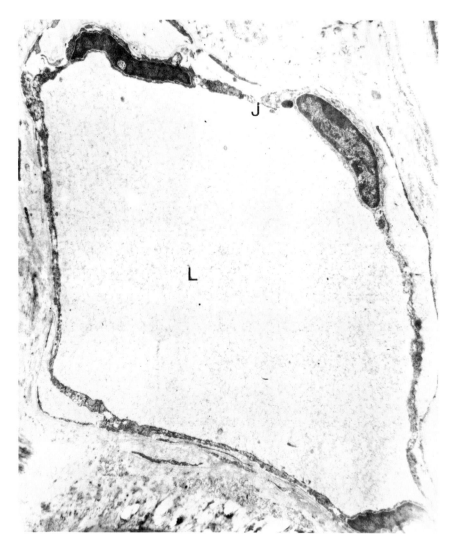

Figure 37. In a mouse ear, injured by heat as in Figure 7, a very dilated lymphatic (L) contains a high concentration of protein, as does the connective tissue. An open junction (J) is present. The endothelium is dense and shrunken, with some vacuoles. 3,000×.

Unfortunately, there have been relatively few experiments designed to determine the importance of the functioning of the lymphatics in this form of edema (and even fewer for low-protein edemas). It has, however, been shown (Table 3; Casley-Smith and Piller, 1974) that after a standardized mild burn (54°C, 60 sec) the edema produced in rats' legs is much greater if the lymphatics are occluded. Hence the lymphatic system must be of considerable importance in limiting the

Table 3. Mean leg weights of rats under various conditions

Treatment	Number	Mean	Standard error	Significance
Normal	24	11.5 g	0.139	N.S.
Normal + coumarin	22	11.5	0.095	
Burned	25	15.1	0.360	$p<0.0001$
Burned + coumarin	22	13.1	0.115	
Lymphedema	22	14.6	0.253	$p<0.0001$
Lymphedema + coumarin	22	12.2	0.311	
Lymphedema/burned	22	19.4	0.272	$p<0.0001$
Lymphedema/burned + coumarin	23	14.0	0.371	

In each group, except the normal, the amount of edema was significantly reduced by the action of coumarin. The difference between the lymphedema/burned and lymphedema group was also very significant ($p<0.0001$), as was that between the lymphedema/burned and burned groups.

amount of edema for this sort of inflammation. Many more such experiments are needed to determine the general importance of the lymphatic system in preventing edema under varying conditions.

High-Protein, Low-Flow Edemas

These lymphedemas occur when the lymphatic system fails because it is incapable of removing the normal amounts of protein from the tissues. This may be caused by the congenital lack of lymphatics, their blockage, or malfunction of their pumping mechanisms in either the collecting or the initial vessels (Casley-Smith, 1973a,c; Földi, 1969, Rusznyák et al., 1967; Yoffey and Courtice, 1970). The principal difference between this form of edema and the preceding one is that here there is no increased leakage from the blood vessels, but the normal net protein outflow is not removed by the lymphatics, and accumulates. This, osmotically, causes water to accumulate in the tissues as well. After a period the accumulated fluid stretches the tissue, making it more difficult to cure the condition, and the proteins seem to cause increased fibrosis in the tissues, possibly because altered protein induces a chronic inflammatory response. This fibrosis can be very massive and produces many of the typical changes in elephantiasis, although infection is needed to cause the complete syndrome.

If the lymphedema is caused by blockage of the lymphatics, i.e., if the pumping is normal, the pressures in the peripheral collecting lymphatics rise very greatly (to ~150 cm; Yoffey and Courtice, 1970) as the lymphangions react to distension. This, together with the distension of the vessels, causes the adjacent valves to become incompetent and so the distension and incompetency extend peripherally by a chain reaction. As mentioned earlier, even many of the inlet valves of the initial lymphatics will become incompetent (Figure 38) if the

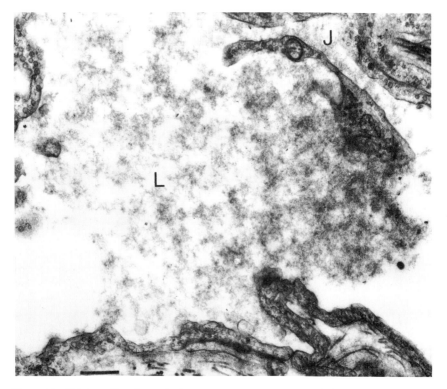

Figure 38. This is a dilated lymphatic in a rat tongue that was made lymphedematous as in Figure 18. There is considerable protein in the lumen, and an open junction (J). 10,000×.

tissues are loose enough to permit it; or all become sealed closed, if the tissues do not permit the vessels to dilate too much (Figure 39; Casley-Smith, 1976a; Casley-Smith et al., 1974). In either case the tissues and the nonfunctional lymphatics become filled with a stagnant, high-protein fluid (Figures 18, 38, and 39). Of course, there will still be an overall exchange of both proteins and fluid between the tissues and the blood, by diffusion via the vesicles, junctions and the fenestrae if they are present. However, this will only be molecular interchange; there will be no net removal. When considering lymphedema the problem appears to be not so much why edema occurs, but why it stops or what the factors are that cause equilibrium to occur in severe lymphedema.

One can understand the mechanism causing the net outflow of fluid to stop, namely, raised tissue hydrostatic pressure. What is hard to comprehend is why the normal outward diffusion of plasma proteins from the blood vessels does not continue until the tissue fluids contain the same concentration of proteins as the blood does. (Although the concentration of proteins can become high, approximately 5 g/100 ml, it does not equal that of blood.) This may possibly be due to the osmotic pressures exerted by the ground-substance mucopolysaccharides

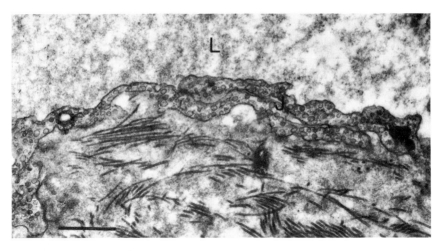

Figure 39. In the parotid glands of rats, with lymphedema as in Figures 18 and 38, the junctions (J) are not forced open by the raised intralymphatic pressures. On the contrary, the firmer surrounding connective tissue does not allow the vessels to dilate so much; hence the pressure seals all the junctions, instead of opening many of them. The high protein concentrations in the lymph and the tissue can be seen. 15,000×.

(Laurent, 1970), or the effects of their exclusion volume, which may produce a concentration of proteins in the tissue fluids, which artifactually disappears when just the fluid is sampled. A further possibility is that the many macrophages, etc. that come to lie in the lymphedematous region (Kalima, 1971), may cause proteolysis. The amount of this may well vary with the protein concentration, and hence produce an equilibrium situation at fairly high protein concentrations. Such a mechanism probably does occur normally (*vide infra*), but its quantitative importance as compared with the other two factors just mentioned is at present unknown.

Therapy of Edema—General

There are certain general forms of therapy for all edemas that are designed to improve lymph flow: gentle massage, elevation of the part, etc. (Casley-Smith, 1976*a;* Földi, 1969, 1976). To these can be added pressure bandages to decrease fluid outflow from blood vessels, and to increase lymphatic drainage, cold to cause constriction of blood vessels, or heat to cause extra fluid to leave the blood and wash accumulated proteins into the lymphatics. (Naturally, clinical skill is necessary do determine which of these to apply, and when.) The use of diuretics is valuable in low-protein edemas. They are useless, however, for the removal of protein; thus they are valueless in the low-flow, high-protein edemas and probably also in the high-flow, high-protein ones. All they will do in this instance is to cause a temporary dehydration, which will disappear very rapidly.

There are a number of surgical techniques by which absent or relatively nonfunctioning lymphatics can be supplemented by lymphatics from another region. These have been reviewed in a recent book (Clodius, 1976). There is also a recently investigated group of drugs that have great promise in the treatment of all forms of high-protein edemas. These are the benzopyrones and related compounds such as rutin, pyridoxine, and pantothenic acid. Coumarin actually has at least two roles. One is to have a "digitalis" type of action on the lymphangions of the collecting lymphatics; thus it can make the beat stronger and more effective in the cases where this is the cause of lymphedema. It also, however, has a most surprisingly marked, and presumably unrelated, effect on the proteins in the tissue themselves.

Effect of Benzo-pyrones on Protein in the Tissues

This has been reviewed by Casley-Smith (1976c), Casley-Smith and Piller (1974), and Casley-Smith et al., (1974). It has been shown by a number of workers that coumarin (~25 mg/kg) and rutin (~450 mg/kg), either separately or together greatly reduce the amount of edema after thermal or dextran injury, and other lymphatic ligation (Figures 40 and 41; Table 3; Casley-Smith and Piller, 1974). They are likely to be effective, then, in all high-protein edemas. (This is not so

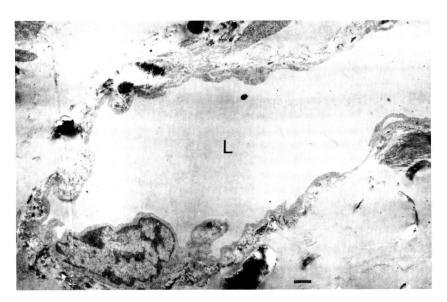

Figure 40. Rat legs were burned, much like the mouse ear in Figure 37, with very similar findings. Some animals were treated with a mixture of coumarin and troxerutin (Venalot, Schaper and Brümmer, West Germany). A typical lymphatic from one of these is seen here and may be compared with Figures 11 and 37. The dilation is less and there is much less protein in the lymph and the tissues. 5,000×.

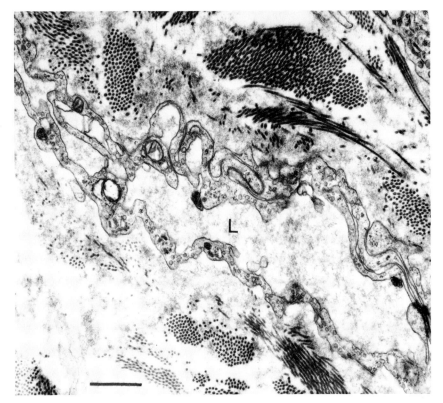

Figure 41. In the lymphedematous rat tongue, compounds with effects similar to coumarin (pantothenic acid and pyridoxine) also greatly reduce the amounts of protein in the lymph and tissues (cf. Figures 18, 38, and 39) and somewhat reduce the dilation of the lymphatics and the numbers of open junctions (Figure 38). 15,000×.

significant in inflammation where there are other therapies, but is very important in lymphedema where the only alternatives are prolonged, relatively ineffective physical methods, or complex surgery).

While coumarin does increase lymph flow in normal tissues, in thermal edemas where the lymphatics are functioning maximally there is no significant increase in lymph flow (Földi-Börcsök, 1972). Since the drugs are also effective where the lymphatics are ligated (Figure 41; Casley-Smith et al., 1969; Tables 3 and 4, Casley-Smith and Piller, 1974), this indicates that the mode of action of coumarin is not just to increase lymph flow.

Experiments with a variety of injurious stimuli under normal conditions on rabbit skin (Casley-Smith, 1976c; Piller, 1976b) indicate that, far from reducing the vascular outflow of protein, coumarin and rutin both injure the vessels more. Thus they slightly increase the amount of protein reaching the tissues, however, they remove proteins so effectively that this extra amount is also removed. It

Table 4. The clearances $(K)^a$ of protein, PVP, and the ratio protein/PVP in rat legs

Treatment	N	$K_{prot.}$ (mean ± S.E.)	K_{PVP} (mean ± S.E.)	K_{ratio} (mean ± S.E.)
Normal	11	−0.0677 ± 0.0046	−0.0596 ± 0.0033	−0.0080 ± 0.0071
Normal + C[b]	10	−0.0811 ± 0.0088[c]**	−0.0404 ± 0.0030***	−0.0307 ± 0.0088***
Burned	12	−0.0680 ± 0.0079	−0.0500 ± 0.0024	−0.0127 ± 0.0080
Burned + C	9	−0.0750 ± 0.0058*	−0.0388 ± 0.0079***	−0.0354 ± 0.0053***
Lymphedema	9	−0.0378 ± 0.0034	−0.0326 ± 0.0039	−0.0052 ± 0.0040
Lymphedema + C	10	−0.0620 ± 0.0032***	−0.0423 ± 0.0194	−0.0197 ± 0.0056***
Lymphedema/burned	8	−0.0269 ± 0.0075	−0.0203 ± 0.0180	−0.0067 ± 0.0230
Lymphedema/burned + C	11	−0.0350 ± 0.0031**	−0.0324 ± 0.0048*	−0.0048 ± 0.0050

^{a}K signifies the normal clearance constant; when K is more negative the rate of clearance is greater. $K_{ratio} = K_{prot} - K_{PVP}$ for each animal, and shown as the mean ± S.E. for the group. The time intervals are days.

^{b}C shows that the group was given 25 mg/kg of coumarin per day.

^{c}NS = $p > 0.05$; * = $0.05 > p > 0.01$; ** = $0.01 > p > 0.001$; *** = $0.001 > p$.

It can be seen that the coumarin invariably increased the clearance of protein. In the normal and burned groups it decreased that of PVP, while slightly increasing it in the two lymphedematous groups. In the first three groups the K_{ratio} was significantly increased, indicating that the protein clearance was increased considerably more than was that of the similar sized PVP. In the lymphedema/burned group the relative clearance was not significantly increased. This was probably because the edema was so greatly reduced by the coumarin (Table 3) that the lessened intercapillary distance caused both substances to clear much more rapidly than before.

should be noted that rutin reduces the amount of leakage from the capillaries in scurvy and dextran injury (Casley-Smith, 1976c,d; Hammersen, 1972) but evidently it still slightly injures normal vessels. It is thus apparent that coumarin and rutin do not remove protein by reducing vascular leakage.

By exclusion, the only mode of action that these drugs can have is to increase the amount of proteolysis. (This has also been suggested as the mode of action of cortisol, Houck and Sharma, 1969). That this is in fact what happens has been shown by a number of experiments (Casley-Smith, 1976c; Piller and Casley-Smith, 1975). Using radio-albumin it was shown that the label does in fact disappear from normal lymphedematous and thermally injured areas much faster if coumarin is administered. (This, incidently, shows that the removal of protein is not just due to endocytosis by the cells, although this might be the initial step in proteolysis. If so, it must be followed by the release of the fragments and their escape from the tissues). If radio-polyvinylpyrrolidone (PVP) is injected simultaneously, it can be shown that the clearance of this similar-sized, nonmetabolizable molecule is relatively unaffected by coumarin, indicating that the proteins may be undergoing lysis (Table 4). This is confirmed by finding significantly more labeled protein fragments in animals treated with coumarin (Table 5). The electron microscope also indicates that these drugs are similarly acting ones, and remove protein from the tissues (Figures 40 and 41; Casley-Smith, 1976a,c; Casley-Smith et al., 1969, 1974b).

How is this lysis effective in removing edema? A priori, one would expect it to produce more edema, by producing many smaller molecules that would add

Table 5. Ratio of ^{51}Cr-labeled protein fragments (M.W. $<$ 1,000) to the amount of total label (proteins + fragments)

Treatment	N	Mean ratio ± S.E.
Normal	12	0.384 ± 0.0164
Normal + coumarin	10	0.425 ± 0.0194[a]
Burned	11	0.320 ± 0.020
Burned + coumarin	9	0.394 ± 0.012[a]

Coumarin (25 mg/kg) was injected into rats 50.5 hr before death; one hind leg of one of the groups was burned at 50 hr before death. ^{51}Cr-plasma protein was injected into the leg 47 hr before death. The rat was frozen and homogenized. Total ^{51}Cr was estimated, as was that fraction precipitated by trichloroacetic acid (TCA), which was associated with polypeptides. $<$~1,000 M.W. (Completely free label was excluded by dialysis.) It can be seen that under both conditions coumarin increased the amount of proteolysis.
[a]$p < 0.001$

to the osmotic pressure of the tissues. The protein fragments, however, are small enough to be able readily to enter the blood vessels via their close junctions and they will suffer less molecular sieving in the tissues, their diffusion coefficients are high, and consequently their concentration gradients will be directed into the vessels. Hence the fragments will be rapidly removed from the tissues, and thus the lysis of proteins will result in the reduction of osmotic pressure and the reduction in the edema.

It is unknown where the lysis occurs. Cortisol seems to produce both intra- and extracellular proteolysis (Houck and Sharma, 1969). Whether this is the case here is uncertain. Incubation experiments have shown that these drugs are incapable of causing the lysis themselves and so must stimulate the production of lytic enzymes in some cells, most likely the macrophages that are present in large numbers in both inflammatory foci and lymphedemas. It has been shown (Bolton and Casley-Smith, 1975) that coumarin increases the normal lysis of proteins by macrophages approximately 2.5 times. In addition, poisoning the macrophages with silica (Piller, 1976) makes the drugs no longer effective in high-protein edemas.

These drugs are cheap, can be taken orally or by injection, and have remarkably little toxicity. (Although coumarin is the parent molecule of dicoumarol, it has no anticoagulant action, nor has dicoumarol any proteolytic action). They should prove to be of very great value in all forms of high-protein edema, particularly in lymphedema, which is otherwise very difficult to treat. Not only do they stimulate the cells that normally lyse protein (and which accumulate in high numbers just where there are excess proteins), but the drugs are absorbed onto the plasma proteins and so are concentrated at the sites containing excess protein (Casley-Smith, 1976c). It should be noted, however, that the lymphedema has to be relatively recent, e.g., less than a year to respond to drug treatment at once, and before extensive fibrosis has occurred. However, even with fibrosis, symptomatic relief of the feeling of tension is reported (Földi, 1976; Casley-Smith, 1976c), and the reduction in the amount of protein present seems to allow the natural turnover of connective tissue to result in its gradual removal so that even here there is a reduction of the limb volume (Piller and Clodius, 1976). These drugs have not only revealed more of the details of the blood–tissue–lymph interactions, but look extremely promising therapeutically.

This therapeutic action may be very valuable not only in the diseases mentioned so far, but in many others. It is becoming increasingly apparent that many diseases have a previously unsuspected lymphatic component. This sometimes may be crucial; at other times it may simply add to the general disorder of the body (Dumont and Witte, 1969; Földi, 1969; Rusznyák et al., 1967; Yoffey and Courtice, 1970). Such diseases include those that affect the heart, lungs, kidney, intestine, liver, brain, and pancreas; it even appears from esophageal varices are dilated lymphatic–venous anastomoses. One might expect that benzo-pyrones, etc., will find a role in the treatment of all these syndromes.

LITERATURE CITED

Allen, L. 1967. Lymphatics and lymphoid tissues. Ann. Rev. Physiol. 29:197–224.

Allen, L., and E. Vogt. 1937. Mechanism of lymphatic absorption from serous cavities. Am. J. Physiol. 119:776–782.

Altura, B. M., H. Edgarian, and B. T. Altura. 1976. Differential effects of ethanol and mannitol on contraction of arterial smooth muscle. J. Pharmacol. Exp. Ther. 197:352–361.

Altura, B. T., and B. M. Altura. 1975. Barbiturates and aortic and venous smooth muscle function. Anesthesiology 43:432–444.

Anversa, P., F. Giacomelli, and J. Wiener. 1973. Regional variations in capillary permeability of ventricular myocardium. Microvasc. Res. 6:273–285.

Arfors, K. 1976. In M. Witte and C. Witte (eds.), Proceedings of the Fourth International Congress on Lymphology, Tucson. University of Arizona Press, Tucson.

Bolton, T., and J. R. Casley-Smith. 1975. The in vitro demonstration of proteolysis by macrophages and its increase with coumarin. Experientia 31:271–273.

Boussauw, L., and J. M. Lauweryns. 1969. Reconstructions graphiques des valvules lymphatiques pulmonaries. C. R. Ass. Anat. (54e Reunion, Sofia) 145:104.

Bruggeman, T. M. 1976. Protein content of gastric lymph. In M. Witte and C. Witte (eds.), Proceedings of the Fourth International Congress on Lymphology, Tucson. University of Arizona Press, Tucson.

Carter, R. D., W. L. Joyner, and E. M. Renkin. 1974. Effects of histamine and some other substances on molecular selectivity of the capillary wall to plasma proteins and dextran. Microvasc. Res. 7:31–48.

Casley-Smith, J. R. 1962. The identification of chylomicra and lipoproteins in tissue sections and their passage into jejunal lacteals. J. Cell. Biol. 15:259–277.

Casley-Smith, J. R. 1963. Pinocytic vesicles: An explanation of some of the problems associated with the passage of particles into and through cells via these bodies. Proc. Austral. Soc. Med. Res. 1:58 (Abst.).

Casley-Smith, J. R. 1964. Endothelial permeability—The passage of particles into and out of diaphragmatic lymphatics. Quart. J. Exp. Physiol. 49:365–383.

Casley-Smith, J. R. 1965. Endothelial permeability. II. The passage of particles through the lymphatic endothelium of normal and injured ears. Br. J. Exp. Pathol. 46:35–49.

Casley-Smith, J. R. 1967a. The fine structures, properties and permeabilities of the endothelium. And: The fine structures and permeabilities of lymphatics under some pathological conditions. In J. M. Collette, G. Jantet, and E. Schoffeniels (eds.), New Trends in Basic Lymphology, pp. 19–39 and 124–137. S. Karger, Basil.

Casley-Smith, J. R. 1967b. Electron microscopical observation on the dilated lymphatics in oedematous regions and their collapse following hyaluronidase administration. Br. J. Exp. Pathol. 48:680–686.

Casley-Smith, J. R. 1967c. An electron microscopical study of the passage of ions through the endothelium of lymphatic and blood capillaries, and through the mesothelium. Quart. J. Exp. Physiol. 52:105–113.

Casley-Smith, J. R. 1969a. The structure of normal large lymphatics: How this determines their permeabilities and their ability to transport lymph. Lymphology 2:15–25.

Casley-Smith, J. R. 1969*b*. The dimensions and numbers of small vesicles and the significance of these for endothelial permeability. J. Microsc. 90:251–268.

Casley-Smith, J. R. 1969*c*. Endocytosis: The different energy requirements for the uptake of particles by small and large vesicles into peritoneal macrophages. J. Microsc. 90:15–30.

Casley-Smith, J. R. 1969*d*. The permeability of the large lymphatics to ions, studied with the electron microscope. Experientia 25:374–375.

Casley-Smith, J. R. 1970*a*. How the lymphatic system overcomes the inadequacies of the blood system. And: The dilation of lymphatics by oedema and their collapse following hyaluronidase. And: The transportation of large molecules, by small vesicles, through the endothelium. *In* M. Viamonte et al. (eds.), Progress in Lymphology II, pp. 51–54, 122–124, 255–260. Thieme, Stuttgart.

Casley-Smith, J. R. 1970*b*. Osmotic pressure: A probably important force for the entrance of material into lymphatics. *In* J. Gruwez (ed.), Proceedings of the Third International Congress on Lymphology, Brussels, p. 148 (Abstr.).

Casley-Smith, J. R. 1970*c*. The functioning of endothelial fenestrae on the arterial and venous limbs of capillaries, as indicated by the differing directions of passage of proteins. Experientia 26:852–853.

Casley-Smith, J. R. 1971*a*. The fine structures of the vascular system of amphiouxus: implications in the development of lymphatics and fenestrated blood vessels. Lymphology 4:79–94.

Casley-Smith, J. R. 1971*b*. Endothelial fenestrae in intestinal villi: Differences in their numbers, etc., between the arterial and venous ends of capillaries. Microvasc. Res. 3:49–68.

Casley-Smith, J. R. 1972. The role of the endothelial intercellular junctions in the functioning of the initial lymphatics. Angiologica 9:106–131.

Casley-Smith, J. R. 1973. The lymphatic system in inflammation. *In* B. W. Zweifach, L. Grant, and R. C. McCluskey, (eds.), The Inflammatory Process. 2nd Ed. Vol. 2, pp. 161–204. Academic Press, New York.

Casley-Smith, J. R. 1975*a*. A theoretical support for the transport of macromolecules by osmotic flow across a leaky membrane against a concentration gradient. Microvasc. Res. 9:43–48.

Casley-Smith, J. R. 1975*b*. The entrance of material into initial lymphatics and their relationship with fenestrated blood capillaries. *In* M. Witte and C. Witte (eds.), Proceedings of the Fourth International Congress on Lymphology, Tucson, University of Arizona Press, Tucson, and submitted to Microvasc. Res.

Casley-Smith, J. R. 1976*a*. The structural basis for the conservative therapy of lymphoedema. *In* L. Clodius (ed.), The Pathophysiology and Treatment of Lymphoedema. Thieme, Stuttgart.

Casley-Smith, J. R. 1976*b*. Calculations relating to the passage of fluid and protein out of arterial-limb fenestrae, through basement membranes and connective tissue channels, and into venous-limb fenestrae and lymphatics. Microvasc. Res. 12:13–34.

Casley-Smith, J. R. 1976*c*. The actions of the benzo-pyrones on the blood–tissue–lymph system. Folia Angiol. 24:7–15.

Casley-Smith, J. R. 1976*d*. The prelymphatic pathways of the brain; lymphostasis, and the benzo-pyrones. *In* M. Földi (ed.), III Ringelheim Symposium. Springer, Berlin.

Casley-Smith, J. R. 1976*e*. The concentrating of proteins in the initial lymphatics and their rediluting in the collecting lymphatics. Folia Angiol. In press.

Casley-Smith, J. R. 1976*f*. The efficiencies of the initial lymphatics. Microvasc. Res. In press.

Casley-Smith, J. R., and T. Bolton. 1973*a*. The presence of large effective colloidal osmotic pressures across large pores. Microvasc. Res. 5:213−216.

Casley-Smith, J. R., and T. Bolton. 1973*b*. Electron microscopy of the effects of histamine and thermal injury on the blood and lymphatic endothelium, and the mesothelium of the mouse's diaphragm, together with the influence of coumarin and rutin. Experientia 29:1386−1388.

Casley-Smith, J. R., and J. R. Casley-Smith. 1975. The fine structures of endocrine capillaries in the hagfish: Implications for the phylogeny of lymphatics and fenestrated capillaries. Rev. Suisse. Zool. 82:35−40.

Casley-Smith, J. R., and J. C. Chin. 1971. An experimental determination of some of the parameters involved in the uptake and transport of material by small vesicles. J. Microsc. 93:167−689.

Casley-Smith, J. R., and H. I. Clarke. 1972. The numbers and dimensions of vesicles in the capillaries of the hind legs of dogs, and their relation to vascular permeability. J. Microsc. 96:263−267.

Casley-Smith, J. R., and H. W. Florey. 1961. The structure of normal small lymphatics. Quart. J. Exp. Physiol. 46:101−106.

Casley-Smith, J. R., M. Földi, and Ö. T. Zoltán. 1969. The treatment of acute lymphoedema with pantothenic acid and pyridoxin. Lymphology 2:63−71.

Casley-Smith, J. R., E. Földi-Börcsök, and M. Földi. 1974. Fine structural aspects of lymphoedema in various tissues, and the effects of treatment with coumarin and troxerutin. Br. J. Exp. Pathol. 55:88−93.

Casley-Smith, J. R., E. Földi-Börcsök, and M. Földi. 1976*a*. The prelymphatic pathways of the brain as revealed by cervical lymphatic obstruction and the passage of particles. Br. J. Exp. Pathol. 57:179−188.

Casley-Smith, J. R., E. Földi-Börcsök, and M. Földi. 1976*b*. Fine structural aspects of the influence of lymphatic blockage on cold injury to the brain and skin, and the effects of benzo-pyrones. Arnz.-Forsch. (Drug Res.). In press.

Casley-Smith, J. R., H. S. Green, J. L. Harris, and P. J. Wadey. 1975*b*. The quantitative morphology of skeletal muscle capillaries in relation to permeability. Microvasc. Res. 10:43−64.

Casley-Smith, J. R., and P. Mart. 1970. The relative antiquity of fenestrated blood capillaries and lymphatics, and their significance for the uptake of large molecules. Experientia 26:508−510.

Casley-Smith, J. R., P. J. O'Donoghue, and K. W. J. Crocker. 1975*a*. The quantitative relationships between fenestrae in jejunal capillaries and connective tissue channels; proof of "tunnel-capillaries." Microvasc. Res. 9:78−100.

Casley-Smith, J. R., and N. B. Piller. 1974. The mode of action of coumarin and related compounds in lymphoedema. *In* L. Clodius (ed.), The Pathophysiology and Treatment of Lymphoedema, Thieme, Stuttgart; Folia Angiol. Suppl. 3:33−60.

Casley-Smith, J. R., and M. A. Sims. 1976. Protein concentrations in regions with fenestrated and continuous blood capillaries, and in initial and collecting lymphatics. Microvasc. Res. (submitted for publication).

Casley-Smith, J. R., and J. Window. 1976. Quantitative morphological correlations of alterations in capillary permeability, following histamine and moderate burning in the mouse diaphragm; and effects of benzopyrones. Microvasc. Res. 11:279−305.

Chase, W. H. 1959. Extracellular distribution of ferrocyanide in muscle. A.M.A. Arch. Pathol. 67:525–532.

Clementi, F., and G. E. Palade. 1969. Intestinal capillaries. I. Permeability to peroxidase and ferritin. J. Cell Biol. 41:33–58.

Cliff, W. J., and P. A. Nicol. 1970. Structure and function of lymphatic vessels of the bat's wing. Quart. J. Exp. Physiol. 55:112–121.

Clodius, L. (ed.). 1976. The Pathophysiology and Treatment of Lymphoedema. Thieme, Stuttgart.

Collan, Y., and T. V. Kalima. 1974. Topographical relations of lymphatic endothelial cells in the initial lymphatics of the intestine. Lymphology 7: 175–184.

Collard, M. 1971. Radiologische Studie über die Wirkung von Pharmaka auf die Lymphgefässe der unteren Extremitaten. Fortschr. Röntgenstr. 115:643–649.

Collin, H. B. 1969a. The ultra-structure of conjunctival lymphatic anchoring filaments. Exp. Eye Res. 8:102–105.

Collin, H. B. 1969b. The ultra-structure of fenestrated blood capillaries in extraocular muscles. Exp. Eye Res. 8:16–20.

Courtice, F. C. 1971. Lymph and plasma-proteins: Barriers to their movement throughout the extra-cellular fluid. Lymphology 4:9–17.

Courtice, F. C., E. P. Adams, and A. D. Shannon. 1976. Lysosomal enzymes in lymph and plasma in shock and limb ischemia. In M. Witte and C. Witte (eds.), Proceedings of the Fourth International Congress on Lymphology, University of Arizona Press, Tucson.

Deysine, M. 1976. Lymphatic space in cortical bone, anatomy and physiology. In M. Witte and C. Witte (eds), Proceedings of the Fourth International Congress on Lymphology, University of Arizona Press, Tucson.

Dobbins, W. O. 1966. Electron microscopic study of the intestinal mucosa in intestinal lymphangelectasia. Gastroenterology 51:1004–1017.

Dobbins, W. O. 1971. Intestinal mucosal lacteal in transport of macromolecules and chylomicrons. Am. J. Clin. Nutrition 24:77–90.

Dobbins, W. O., and E. L. Rollins. 1970. Intestinal mucosal lymphatic permeability: an electron microscopic study of endothelial vesicles and cell junctions. J. Ultrastruct. Res. 33:29–59.

Drinker, C. K. 1942. Lane Medical Lectures: The Lymphatic System Stanford University Press, Palo Alto.

Dumont, A. E., and M. H. Witte. 1969. Clinical usefulness and thoracic duct cannulation. Advan. Intern. Med. 15:51–71.

Dunn, R. F., M. W. Burtz, and P. W. Ward. 1970. Ultrastructural evidence for the lymph node-venous transport of carbon particles. J. Ultrastruct. Res. 30:249 (Abstr.).

Elhay, S., and J. R. Casley-Smith. 1976. Mathematical model of the initial lymphatic. Microvasc. Res. In press.

Farquhar, M. G., and G. E. Palade. 1963. Junctional complexes in various epithelia. J. Cell Biol. 17:375–412.

Földi, M. 1969. Diseases of Lymphatics and Lymph Circulation. Charles C Thomas, Springfield, Ill.

Földi, M. 1976. On the conservative treatment of lymphoedema (mechanical methods). In L. Clodius (ed.), The Pathophysiology and Treatment of Lymphoedema. Thieme, Stuttgart.

Földi, M. B. Csillik, and Ö. T. Zoltán. 1968a. Lymphatic drainage of the brain. Experientia 24:1283–1287.

Földi, M., B. Csillik, T. Várkonyi, and Ö. T. Zoltán. 1968b. Lymphostatic cerebral hemangiopathy. Ultrastructural alterations in blood capillaries of the brain after blockage of cervical lymph drainage. Vox. Sang. 2:214−222.

Földi, M. and Ö. T. Zoltán. 1965. Permeability of the thoracic duct. Lancet 1:914.

Földi-Börcsök, E. 1972. Effect of external lymph drainage and coumarin treatment on thermal injury in the rat hind leg. Br. J. Pharmacol. 46:254−259.

Földi-Börcsök, E., F. K. Bedell, and V. W. Rahlfs. 1971. Die antiphlogistische und ödemhemende Wirkung von Cumarin aus Melelotus officinalis. Arzneimittel. Forsch. (Drug Res.) 21:2025−2029.

Garlick, D. G., and E. M. Renkin. 1970. Transport of large molecules from plasma to interstitial fluid and lymph in dogs. Am. J. Physiol. 219:1595−1605.

Green, H. S., and J. R. Casley-Smith. 1972. Calculations on the passage of small vesicles across endothelial cells by Browian motion. J. Theoret. Biol. 35: 103−111.

Grotte, G. 1956. Passage of dextran molecules across the blood-lymph barrier. Acta Chir. Scand. III, Suppl. 211:419−420.

Guyton, A. C. 1963. A concept of negative interstitial pressure based on pressures in implanted perforated capsules. Circ. Res. 12:399−414.

Guyton, A. C. 1969. Interstitial fluid pressure-volume relationships and their regulation. In J. Wolstenholme (ed.), Circulatory and Respiratory Mass Transport, Ciba Foundation Symposium pp. 4−20. J. Churchill, London.

Guyton, A. C., H. J. Granger, and A. E. Taylor. 1971. Interstitial fluid pressure. Physiol. Rev. 51:527−563.

Hammersen, F. 1972. The fine structure of different types of experimental edemas for testing the effect of vasoactive drugs demonstrated with a flavonoid. Angiologica 9:326−354.

Hodel, Ch. 1970. Ultrastructural studies on the absorption of protein markers by the greater omentum. Eur. Surg. Res. 2:435−449.

Houck, J., and V. Sharma. 1969. Enzyme induction in skin and fibroblasts by antiinflammatory drugs. In A. Bertelli and J. Houck (eds.), Inflammation Biochemistry and Drug Interaction, pp. 85−96. Excerpta Medica Foundation, Amsterdam.

Intaglietta, M., and E. P. de Plomb. 1973. Fluid exchange in tunnel and tube capillaries. Microvasc. Res. 6:153−168.

Jacobsson, S., and I. Kjellmer. 1964. Flow and protein content of lymph in resting and exercising skeletal muscle. Acta. Physiol. Scand. 60:278−285.

Jennings, M. A., and H. W. Florey. 1967. An investigation of some properties of endothelium related to capillary permeability. Proc. Roy. Soc. London Ser. B 167:39−63.

Jepson, R., F. Simeone, and B. Dobyns. 1953. Removal from skin of plasma protein labeled with radioactive iodine. Am. J. Physiol. 175:443−448.

Johnson, P. C., and J. M. Hanson. 1966. Capillary filtration in the small intestine of the dog. Circ. Res. 19:766−733.

Johnson, P. C., and D. R. Richardson. 1974. The influence of venous pressure on filtration forces in the intestine. Microvasc. Res. 7:296−306.

Jonsson, J., K. E. Arfors, and H. C. Hint. 1971. Studies on relationships between the blood and lymphatic systems within the microcirculation. In Fourth European Conference on Microcirculation, Aalborg, pp. 214−218. S. Karger, Basel.

Kalima, T. V. 1971. The structure and function of intestinal lymphatics and the influence of impaired lymph flow on the ileum of rats. Scand. J. Gastroent. 6, Supp. 10.

Kalima, T. V., and Y. Collan. 1976. A serial section study of lymphatic "inlet-valves" in intestinal villi. *In* M. Witte and C. Witte (eds.), Proceedings of the Fourth International Congress on Lymphology, Tucson. University of Arizona Press, Tucson.

Kampmeier, O. F. 1969. Evolution and Comparative Morphology of the Lymphatic System. Charles C Thomas, Springfield, Ill.

Karnovsky, M. J. 1968. The ultrastructural basis of transcapillary exchanges. J. Gen. Physiol. 52:64s—95s.

Katz, A. I., Yu Chen, and A. H. Moreno. 1969. Flow through a collapsible tube. Biophys. J. 9:1261—1279.

Kraehenbuhl, J. P., E. Gloor, and B. Blanc. 1967. Résorption intestinale de la ferritine chez deux espéces animales aux possibilités d'absorption protéique néonatale différentes. Z. Zellforsch. 76:170—186.

Landis, E. M., and J. R. Pappenheimer. 1963. Exchange of substances through the capillary walls. *In* W. F. Hamilton and P. Dow (eds.), Handbook of Physiology, Section 2, Circulation II, pp. 961—1034. Waverly Press, Baltimore.

Laurent, T. C. 1970. The structure and function of the intercellular polysaccharides in connective tissues. *In* C. Crone and N. A. Lassen (eds.), Capillary Permeability, pp. 261—277. Academic Press, New York.

Lauweryns, J. M., and L. Boussauw. 1969. The ultrastructure of pulmonary lymphatic capillaries of newborn rabbits and of human infants. Lymphology 2:108—129.

Leak, L. V. 1970. Electron microscopic observations of lymphatic capillaries and the structural components of the connective tissue-lymph interface. Microvasc. Res. 2:361—391.

Leak, L. V., and J. F. Burke. 1966. Fine structure of the lymphatic capillary and the adjoining connective tissue area. Am. J. Anat. 118:785—809.

Leak, L. V., and J. F. Burke. 1968. Ultrastructural studies on the lymphatic anchoring filaments. J. Cell Biol. 36:129—149.

Lehmann, H. D. 1968. Über Lymph-Fluss und Lymph-Zusammensetzung der Leber des Hundes in Abhängigkeit von der Hämodynamik. Naunyn-Schmiedebergs Arch. Pharmak. Exp. Pathol. 260:168—169, and unpublished work quoted by Vogel (1972).

Majno, G. 1965. Ultrastructure of the vascular membrane. *In* W. F. Hamilton and P. Dow (eds.), Handbook of Physiology, Section 2, Circulation 3, pp. 2293—2375. Waverly Press, Baltimore.

Majno, G., S. M. Shea, and M. Leventhal. 1969. Endothelial contraction induced by histamine-type mediators. J. Cell Biol. 41:647—672.

Mayerson, H. S. 1963. The physiologic importance of lymph. *In* W. F. Hamilton and P. Dow (eds.), Handbook of Physiology, Section 2, Circulation 2, pp. 1035—1073. Waverly Press, Baltimore.

Mayerson, H. S., R. M. Patterson, A. McKee, S. J. LeBrie, and P. Mayerson. 1962. Permeability of lymphatic vessels. Am. J. Physiol. 203:98—106.

McMaster, P. D. 1947. The relative pressures within cutaneous lymphatic capillaries and the tissues. J. Exp. Med. 86:293—308.

Michel, C. C. 1972. Flow across the capillary wall. *In* D. H. Bergel (ed.), Cardiovascular Fluid Dynamics, Vol. 2, pp. 241—298. Academic Press, New York.

Michel, C. C. 1974. The transport of solute by osmotic flow across a leaky membrane. Microvasc. Res. 8:122—125.

Mislin, H. 1967. Structural and functional relationships of the mesenteric lymph vessels. In J. M. Collette, G. Jantet, and E. Schoffeniels (eds.), New Trends in Basic Lymphology, pp. 87—96. Birkhäusern, Stuttgart.

Mislin, H. 1971. Die Wirkung von Cumarin aus Melilotus officinalis auf die Funktion des Lymphangions. Arzneitmittel. Forsch. (Drug Res.) 21:852—853.

Mislin, M. 1972. Die motorik der Lymphgefässe und die Regulation der Lymphherzen. In H. Meesen (ed.), Lymph Vessel System (Lymphgefässe System), In Handbuch der Allgemeinen Pathologie. 3rd Ed., 6th Part, pp. 219—238. Springer-Verlag, Berlin.

Moe, R. E. 1963. Fine structure of the reticulum and sinuses of lymph nodes. Am. J. Anat. 112:311—318.

Nicolaysen, G., A. Nicolaysen, and N. C. Staub. 1975. A quantitative radioautographic comparison of albumin concentration in different sized lymph vessels in normal mouse lungs. Microvasc. Res. 10:138—152.

Ottaviani, G., and G. Azzali. 1965. Ultrastructure des capillaires lymphatiques. In International Symposium Morphologie Histochimie Paroi Vasculaire, Fribourg, Vol. 2, p. 325.

Palade, G. E., and R. R. Bruns. 1968. Structural modulations of plasmalemmal vesicles. J. Cell Biol. 37:633—649.

Palay, S. L., and L. J. Karlin. 1959. An electron microscopic study of the intestinal villus I and II. J. Biophys. Biochem. Cytol. 5:363—371, 373—383.

Papp, M. E., P. Rohlich, I Rusznyák, and I. Törö. 1962. An electron microscopic study of the central lacteal in the intestinal villus of the cat. Z. Zellforsch. Mikrosk. Anat. 57:475—486.

Pappenheimer, J. R. 1970. Osmotic reflection coefficients in capillary membranes. In C. Crone and N. A. Larsen (eds.), Capillary Permeability, pp. 278—290. Academic Press, New York.

Patterson, R. M., C. L. Ballard, K. Wasserman, and H. S. Mayerson. 1958. Lymphatic permeability to albumin. Am. J. Physiol. 194:120—124.

Perl, W. 1975. Convection and permeation of albumin between plasma and interstitium. Microvasc. Res. 10:83—94.

Perry, M., and D. Garlick. 1975. Transcapillary efflux of gamma globulin in rabbit skeletal muscle. Microvasc. Res. 9:119—126.

Piller, N. B. 1976a. The ineffectiveness of coumarin treatment on thermal oedema of macrophage-free rats. Br. J. Exp. Pathol. 57:170—178.

Piller, N. B. 1976b. Benzopyrones: Their selective injury to rabbit vascular endothelium. Clin. Exp. Pharmacol. Physiol. 3:127—143.

Piller, N. B., and J. R. Casley-Smith. 1975. The effects of coumarin on protein and PVP clearance from rat legs with various high protein oedemas. Br. J. Exp. Pathol. 56:439—443.

Piller, N. B., and L. Clodius. 1976. The use of the tissue tonometer as a diagnostic aid in lymphoedema. Eur. J. Clin. Invest. In press.

Pressman, J. J., R. F. Dunn, and M. V. Burtz. 1970. Direct communication between lymph nodes and veins. In M. Viamonte et al. (eds.), Progress in Lymphology II, pp. 77—78. Thieme, Stuttgart.

Pullinger, B. D., and H. W. Florey. 1935. Some observations on the structure and functions of lymphatics; their behavior in local oedema. Br. J. Exp. Pathol. 16:49—61.

Recklinghausen, F. von. 1863. Zur Fettresorption. Virchow's Arch. 26:172–208.

Reddy, N. P., T. A. Krouskop, and P. H. Newell. 1975. A note on the mechanisms of lymph flow through the terminal lymphatics. Microvasc. Res. 10:214–216.

Renkin, E. M. 1971. Diffusional components of trans-capillary exchange. *In* Proceedings of the 25th International Congress of the Physiological Society Vol. 8, p. 263. (Abstr.).

Renkin, E. M., R. D. Carter, and W. L. Joyner. 1974. Mechanisms of the sustained action of histamine and bradykinin on transport of large molecules across capillary walls in the dog paw. Microvasc. Res. 7:49–60.

Rodbard, S. 1969. The capsular barrier between the interstitial fluid and the source of the lymph. Curr. Mod. Biol. 3:27–34.

Rusznyák, I., M. Földi, and G. Szabó. 1967. Lymphatics and Lymph Circulation. 2nd Ed. Pergamon Press, London.

Schipp, R. 1967. Structure and ultrastructure of mesenteric lymphatic vessels. *In* J. M. Collette, G. Jantel, and E. Schoffeniels (eds.), New Trends in Basic Lymphology, pp. 50–55. Birkhauser, Stuttgart.

Scholander, P. F., A. R. Hargens, and S. L. Miller. 1968. Negative pressure of the interstitial fluid of animals. Science 161:321–328.

Shea, S. M., and M. J. Karnovsky. 1966. Brownian motion: A theoretical explanation for the movement of vesicles across the endothelium. Nature 212:353–355.

Shea, S. M., M. J. Karnovsky, and W. H. Bossert. 1969. Vesicular transport across endothelium: Simulation of a diffusion model. J. Theoret. Biol. 24:30–42.

Simionescu, N., M. Simionescu, and G. E. Palade. 1972. Permeability of intestinal capillaries. J. Cell Biol. 53:365–392.

Simionescu, N., M. Simionescu, and G. E. Palade. 1975. Permeability of muscle capillaries to small heme-peptides. Evidence for the existence of patent trans-endothelial channels. J. Cell Biol. 64:586–607.

Staub, N. C., G. Nicolaysen, and A. Nicolaysen. 1975. Constant albumin concentration along lung lymphatics in normal mice. *In* Proceedings of the Fifth International Congress on Lymphology, p. 49 (Abstr.).

Strawitz, J. G., K. Eto, H. Mitsuoka, C. Olney, F. W. Pairent, and J. M. Howard. 1968. Molecular weight dependence of lymphatic permeability. Microvasc. Res. 1:58–67.

Studer, R., and J. Potchen. 1971. The radioisotopic assessment of regional microvascular permeability to macromolecules. Microvasc. Res. 3:35–46.

Swann, H. G. 1960. The functional distension of the kidney. Texas Rep. Biol. Med. 18:566–595.

Swann, H. G., H. F. Stegal, W. D. Collings, and N. A. Miles. 1961. Red cell and albumin circulation in the ileum. Am. J. Physiol. 201:943–950.

Szabó, G. 1976a. Lymphatic and venous transport of intracellular enzymes. *In* M. Witte and C. Witte, Proceedings of the Fourth International Congress on Lymphology, Tucson. University of Arizona Press, Tucson.

Szabó, G. 1976b. The passage of proteins to blood and lymph. *In* M. Földi (ed.), III Ringelheim Symposium. Springer, Berlin.

Szabó, G., E. Anda, and E. Vándor. 1972. The effect of muscle activity on the lymphatic and venous transport of lactic dehydrogenase. Lymphology 5:111–114.

Szabó, G., Z. Magyar, and G. Molnár. 1970. The importance of lymphatic and venous pathways in the transport of large molecules. And: The transport of macromolecules from the intestinal wall. *In* Proceedings of the Third International Congress on Lymphology, Brussels, pp. 51 and 137 (Abstr.).

Szabó, G., Z. Magyar, and G. Molnár. 1971. Transport of macromolecules from the tissues. *In* Proceedings of the 25th International Congress on the Physiological Sciences, Vol. 9, p. 549 (Abstr.).

Szabó, G., Z. Magyar, and G. Molnár. 1973. Lymphatic and venous transport of colloids from the tissues. Lymphology 6:69—79.

Taylor, A. E., W. H. Gibson, H. J. Granger, and A. C. Guyton. 1973. The interaction between intracapillary and tissue forces in the overall regulation of interstitial fluid volume. Lymphology 6:192—208.

Taylor, A. E., and W. H. Gibson. 1975. Concentrating ability of lymphatic vessels. Lymphology 8:43—48.

Taylor, A. E., W. H. Gibson, and A. C. Guyton. 1976a. Model of the concentrating ability of lymphatics. In M. Witte and C. Witte (eds.), Proceedings of the Fourth International Congress on Lymphology, Tucson. University of Arizona Press, Tucson.

Taylor, A. E., W. H. Gibson, and A. C. Guyton. 1976b. Subcutaneous tissue safety factors in edema formation. *In* M. Witte and C. Witte (eds.), Proceedings of the Fourth International Congress on Lymphology, Tucson. University of Arizona Press, Tucson.

Várkonyi, T., B. Csillik, Ö. T. Zoltán, and M. Földi. 1969. Über de feinstrukturellen die feinstrukturellen Veranderungen im Grosshirn bei der lymphogenen Enzapholopathie der Ratte. Beitr. Pathol. Anat. 139:344—361.

Várkonyi, T., J. Polgár, Ö. T. Zoltán, B. Csillik, and M. Földi. 1970. Lymphostatic retinal haemangiopathy. Experientia 26:67—68.

Venkatachalam, M. A., and M. J. Karnovsky. 1972. Extravascular protein in the kidney. Lab. Invest. 27:435—444.

Verzár, F., and E. J. McDougall. 1936. Absorption from the Intestine. Longmanns, London.

Virágh, Sz., M. Papp, E. Törö, and I. Rusznyák. 1966. Cutaneous lymphatic capillaries in dextran-induced oedema of the rat. Br. J. Exp. Pathol. 47:563—567.

Virágh, Sz., M. Papp, and I. Rusznyák. 1971. The lymphatics in oedematous skin. Acta Morph. Hung. 19:203—212.

Vogel, G. 1972. The pharmacology of the lymph and the lymphatic system. *In* H. Meessen (ed.), Lymphgefäss-System (Lymph-Vessel System), 6th part of Handbuch der Allgemeinen Pathologie. 3rd Ed. pp. 363—404. Springer, Berlin.

Vreim, C. E., R. H. Demling, and N. C. Staub. 1975. Protein composition of lung fluids during edema. *In* Proceedings of the Fifth International Congress on Lymphology, p. 47 (Abstr.).

Warren, B. A. 1970. The ultrastructure of the microcirculation of the advancing edge of Walker 256 carcinoma. Microvasc. Res. 2:443—453.

Warshaw, A. L., W. A. Walker, R. Cornell, and K. J. Isselbacher. 1971. Small intestinal permeability to macromolecules. Lab. Invest. 25:675—684.

Wiederhielm, C. A. 1968. Dynamics of trans-capillary fluid exchange. J. Gen. Physiol. 52:29s—63s.

Wisse, E. 1970. An electron microscopic study of the fenestrated endothelial lining of rat liver sinusoids. J. Ultrastruct. Res. 31:125—150.

Yoffey, J. M., and F. C. Courtice. 1970. Lymphatics, Lymph and Lympho-myeloid Complex. Academic Press, New York.

Zweifach, B. W. 1973. Microcirculation. Ann. Rev. Physiol. 35:117–150.

Zweifach, B. W., and M. Intaglietta. 1968. Mechanics of fluid movement across single capillaries in the rabbit. Microvasc. Res. 1:83–88.

AUTHOR INDEX

Page numbers in italics indicate text pages; page numbers in roman indicate reference pages.

SUBJECT INDEX